HIGH-RISK
PREGNANCY

EDITOR
JOHN T. QUEENAN, MD

EDITORIAL COMMITTEE
NANCY C. CHESCHEIR, MD
GARY D.V. HANKINS, MD
BRIAN M. MERCER, MD

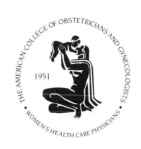

THE AMERICAN COLLEGE OF
OBSTETRICIANS
AND GYNECOLOGISTS
WOMEN'S HEALTH CARE PHYSICIANS

CONTINUING MEDICAL EDUCATION

ACCME Accreditation

The American College of Obstetricians and Gynecologists (ACOG) is accredited by the Accreditation Council for Continuing Medical Education (ACCME) to provide continuing medical education for physicians.

AMA PRA Category 1 Credit™ and ACOG Cognate Credit

The American College of Obstetricians and Gynecologists (ACOG) designates this educational activity for a maximum of 25 AMA PRA Category 1 Credit(s)™ or up to a maximum of 25 Category 1 ACOG cognate credit(s). Physicians should only claim credit commensurate with the extent of their participation in the activity.

High-Risk Pregnancy was planned and produced in accordance with the Standards for Enduring Materials of the Accreditation Council for Continuing Medical Education. Any discussion of unapproved use of products is clearly cited in the appropriate critique.

Current guidelines state that continuing medical education (CME) providers must ensure that CME activities are free from the control of any commercial interest. The editor and contributing authors declare that neither they nor any business associate nor any member of their immediate families has material interest, financial interest, or other relationships with any company manufacturing commercial products relative to the topics included in this publication or with any provider of commercial services discussed in this publication except for Zane A. Brown, MD, who is a speaker for GlaxoSmithKline, Inc.; Carolyn Gardella, MD, MPH, who is on the speakers' bureau for GlaxoSmithKline, Inc.; Kennneth J. Moise, Jr, MD, who is a consultant for Sequenom, Inc., assisting in the development of a free fetal DNA assay for determining the fetal RhD status; Rhoda Ashley Morrow, PhD, who is a consultant for Biokit USA; and Anna Wald, MD, MPH, who has received grants from GlaxoSmithKline, Inc., Antigenics, Roche, and Vical and is a consultant for Novartis, Powdermed, and Medigene and a speaker for Merck Vaccines. All potential conflicts have been resolved.

Library of Congress Cataloging-in-Publication Data

High-risk pregnancy / edited by John T. Queenan.
     p. ; cm.
 Includes bibliographical references.
 ISBN 978-1-932328-27-1
 1. Pregnancy--Complications. I. Queenan, John T. II. American College of Obstetricians and Gynecologists.
 [DNLM: 1. Pregnancy, High-Risk. 2. Pregnancy Complications. WQ 240 H63745 2007]

 RG571.H442 2007
 618.2--dc22

                                    2006037353

ISBN: 978-1-932328-27-1

12345/10987

CONTENTS

[†]Deceased February 5, 2004

ACKNOWLEDGMENTS

The chapters in this book were originally published in the following issues of *Obstetrics & Gynecology*

Malone FD, D'Alton ME. First-trimester sonographic screening for Down syndrome. (2003;102:1066–79)*

Casey BM, Leveno KJ. Thyroid disease in pregnancy. (2006;108:1283–92)

Ramin SM, Vidaeff AC, Yeomans ER, Gilstrap LC III. Chronic renal disease in pregnancy. (2006;108:1531–9)

Dombrowski MP. Asthma and pregnancy. (2006;108:667–81)

Sibai BM. Chronic hypertension in pregnancy. (2002;100:369–77)

Branch DW, Khamashta MA. Antiphospholipid syndrome: obstetric diagnosis, management, and controversies. (2003;101:1333–44)

Lockwood CJ. Inherited thrombophilias in pregnant patients: detection and treatment paradigm. (2002;99:333–41)

Catalano PM. Management of obesity in pregnancy. (2007;109:419–33)

Gabbe SG, Graves CR. Management of diabetes mellitus complicating pregnancy. (2003;102:857–68)

Resnik R. Intrauterine growth restriction. (2002;99:490–6)

Silver RM. Fetal death. (2007;109:153–67)

Sibai BM. Diagnosis and management of gestational hypertension and preeclampsia. (2003;102:181–92)

Sibai BM. Diagnosis, controversies, and management of the syndrome of hemolysis, elevated liver enzymes, and low platelet count. (2004;103:981–91)

Iams JD. Prediction and early detection of preterm labor. (2003;101:402–12)

Harger JH. Cerclage and cervical insufficiency: an evidence-based analysis. (2002;100:1313–27)

Mercer BM. Preterm premature rupture of the membranes. (2003;101:178–93)

Goldenberg RL. The management of preterm labor. (2002;100:1020–37)

Meis PJ. 17 hydroxyprogesterone for the prevention of preterm delivery. (2005;105:1128–35)*

Moise KJ Jr. Management of rhesus alloimmunization in pregnancy. (2002;100:600–11)

Oyelese Y, Smulian JC. Placenta previa, placenta accreta, and vasa previa. (2006;107:927–41)

Oyelese Y, Ananth CV. Placental abruption. (2006;108:1005–16)

Krivak TC, Zorn KK. Deep vein thrombosis and pulmonary embolism in obstetrics and gynecology. (2007;109:761–77)

Sheffield JS, Cunningham FG. Urinary tract infection in women. (2005;106:1085–92)

Gibbs RS, Schrag S, Schuchat A. Perinatal infections due to group B streptococci. (2004;104:1062–76)

Brown ZA, Gardella C, Wald A, Morrow RA, Corey L. Genital herpes complicating pregnancy. (2005;106:845–56)

Minkoff H. Human immunodeficiency virus infection in pregnancy. (2003;101:797–810)

Freeman RK. Problems with intrapartum fetal heart rate monitoring interpretation and patient management. (2002;100:813–26)

Hankins GDV, Speer M. Defining the pathogenesis and pathophysiology of neonatal encephalopathy and cerebral palsy. (2003;102:628–36)

Moise KJ Jr. Umbilical cord stem cells. (2005;106:1393–1407)

*For the Society of Maternal–Fetal Medicine

PREFACE

During the past 50 years, unsurpassed advances in the management of high-risk pregnancies have been witnessed. Perhaps the most dramatic example of this progress is the conquest of the Rh problem.

At one time, Rh-erythroblastosis fetalis resulted in fatality of the babies in 50% of pregnancies of immunized, Rh-negative women: one half died in utero and one half in the newborn nursery. With William Liley's ingenious work in the 1960s, at last we had tools to treat this disease. The first tool was amniotic fluid analysis of bilirubin levels, indicating the degree of fetal disease. The next tool was fetal transfusion to combat potentially fatal fetal anemia. Sensitized Rh-negative mothers were referred to Rh clinics where they could be evaluated and treated systematically. With this breakthrough, the concept of high-risk pregnancy management was born. In this process, obstetricians made impressive advances in improving fetal evaluation and therapy. Enormous strides also were made by neonatologists in managing newborn anemia, hyperbilirubinemia, and prematurity. The final triumph in the conquest was the development of Rh-immune prophylaxis.

The concept of high-risk pregnancy management was applicable to many other problems, and clinics specializing in diabetes, hypertension, and preterm labor began to appear in larger medical centers. The evaluation and treatment of diabetes has improved so much that having a baby today has become a safe reality for most women with diabetes. Successes in preventing preterm birth and preeclampsia have been incremental and ongoing, but much work is still needed.

Today the major challenges in the field of high-risk pregnancy remain preterm birth and preeclampsia. Our many tools include assays, ultrasonography, Doppler ultrasonography, neonatal ventilatory support, steroids to prevent respiratory distress syndrome, and surfactant to treat the condition. Let me suggest that our biggest challenge is knowing how and when to use these tools to manage these clinical problems optimally. To answer some of these questions, the Maternal–Fetal Medicine Unit Network of the National Institute of Child Health and Human Development has systematically evaluated key clinical questions and provided invaluable answers. Other investigators from the United States and countries around the world have conducted important research studies that have shaped our understanding of pregnancy and the treatment of its complications. Nonetheless, evidence-based information is available for only 30–40% of conditions encountered in clinical practice. Accordingly, we have to rely on the expertise and wisdom of authorities.

Five years ago, the editors of *Obstetrics & Gynecology* decided to develop a source of clinical information and guidance by launching the Clinical Expert Series. Important clinical subjects in obstetrics and gynecology were identified. Then, after much consultation with clinical leaders in the United States and abroad, we selected outstanding experts to present the various subjects. Their assignment was to perform a thorough review, eliciting evidence-based information. The authors supplemented the evidence by drawing on their considerable clinical expertise to describe how they would manage a situation. The articles were extensively peer reviewed and then published in *Obstetrics & Gynecology*. The Clinical Expert Series, according to surveys, is widely read and one of the most popular features in the journal. Therefore, the editors decided to make these articles available to all practitioners involved in the care of patients with high-risk pregnancies.

In creating this book, we invited authors of high-risk pregnancy articles in the Clinical Expert Series to update their original work. Each of the articles has been extensively revised and updated. The list of authors represents a "Who's Who" of experts in high-risk pregnancy management, and their collective expertise is reflected in the contents. An editorial committee of experts was assembled to guide this project. Doctors Nancy C. Chescheir, Gary D. V. Hankins, and Brian M. Mercer have critiqued each article and edited and offered advice on the development of this book. Dr. Roger P. Smith contributed his expertise, writing the continuing medical education test questions for this book. I stand in awe of their breadth and depth of medical knowledge. In this undertaking, we were guided by the skill and wisdom of the Director of Publications of the American College of Obstetricians and Gynecologists (ACOG), Rebecca D. Rinehart, and her talented staff, and assisted by the diligent efforts of Heidi Logothetti, editorial assistant in the journal office.

The ACOG Committee Opinions and Practice Bulletins provide clinical practice guidelines. These guidelines are developed by committees and present recommendations that are generally relevant to and attainable by all practitioners in the United States. However, they should not be construed as dictating an exclusive course of treatment or procedure to be followed. They serve as a foundation on which clinical judgment is based. As such, the recommendations made by an expert in one setting, such as those conveyed in this book, may differ from those in practice guidelines.

This book is meant to be an authoritative guide for the management of high-risk pregnancies. New knowledge is developing continually, so this book should be used in conjunction with current information from journals and other sources. The authors have provided recommendations and approaches to treatment for clinical settings they have experienced. The most important factor for a sucessful outcome to a high-risk pregnancy is you, the physician, and the decisions you make. I hope this book helps you in this endeavor.

—John T. Queenan, MD
Deputy Editor, *Obstetrics & Gynecology*

CONTRIBUTORS

CANDE V. ANANTH, PhD, MPH
University of Medicine and Dentistry of New Jersey
Robert Wood Johnson Medical School
New Brunswick, New Jersey

D. WARE BRANCH, MD
University of Utah School of Medicine
Salt Lake City, Utah

ZANE A. BROWN, MD
University of Washington School of Medicine
Seattle, Washington

BRIAN M. CASEY, MD
University of Texas Southwestern Medical School
Dallas, Texas

PATRICK M. CATALANO, MD
Case Western Reserve University
School of Medicine
Cleveland, Ohio

NANCY C. CHESCHEIR, MD
Vanderbilt University School of Medicine
Nashville, Tennessee

LAWRENCE COREY, MD
University of Washington School of Medicine
Seattle, Washington

F. GARY CUNNINGHAM, MD
University of Texas Southwestern Medical School
Dallas, Texas

MARY E. D'ALTON, MD
Columbia University College of Physicians
and Surgeons
New York, New York

MITCHELL P. DOMBROWSKI, MD
St. John Hospital
Detroit, Michigan

ROGER K. FREEMAN, MD
Long Beach Memorial Medical Center
Long Beach, California

STEVEN G. GABBE, MD
Vanderbilt University School of Medicine
Nashville, Tennessee

CAROLYN GARDELLA, MD, MPH
University of Washington School of Medicine
Seattle, Washington

RONALD S. GIBBS, MD
University of Colorado School of Medicine
Denver, Colorado

LARRY C. GILSTRAP III, MD
University of Texas Medical School
Houston, Texas

ROBERT L. GOLDENBERG, MD
University of Alabama School of Medicine
Birmingham, Alabama

CORNELIA R. GRAVES, MD
Vanderbilt University School of Medicine
Nashville, Tennessee

GARY D. V. HANKINS, MD
University of Texas Medical Branch
Galveston, Texas

JAMES H. HARGER, MD[†]
University of Pittsburgh School of Medicine
Pittsburgh, Pennsylvania

JAY D. IAMS, MD
Ohio State University College of Medicine
Columbus, Ohio

†Deceased February 5, 2004

MUNTHER A. KHAMASHTA, MD, PhD
King's College London School of Medicine
London, United Kingdom

THOMAS C. KRIVAK, MD
University of Pittsburgh School of Medicine
Pittsburgh, Pennsylvania

KENNETH J. LEVENO, MD
University of Texas Southwestern Medical School
Dallas, Texas

CHARLES J. LOCKWOOD, MD
Yale University School of Medicine
New Haven, Connecticut

FERGAL D. MALONE, MD
Rotunda Hospital
Dublin, Ireland

PAUL J. MEIS, MD
Wake Forest University School of Medicine
Winston-Salem, North Carolina

BRIAN M. MERCER, MD
Case Western Reserve University School of Medicine
Cleveland, Ohio

HOWARD MINKOFF, MD
State University of New York
Downstate Medical Center
Brooklyn, New York

KENNETH J. MOISE JR, MD
Baylor College of Medicine
Houston, Texas

RHODA ASHLEY MORROW, PhD
University of Washington School of Medicine
Seattle, Washington

JOHN OWEN, MD
University of Alabama School of Medicine
Birmingham, Alabama

YINKA OYELESE, MD
University of Medicine and Dentistry of New Jersey
Robert Wood Johnson Medical School
New Brunswick, New Jersey

SUSAN M. RAMIN, MD
University of Texas Medical School
Houston, Texas

ROBERT RESNIK, MD
University of California, San Diego
School of Medicine
La Jolla, California

STEPHANIE SCHRAG, PhD
Centers for Disease Control and Prevention
Atlanta, Georgia

ANNE SCHUCHAT, MD
Centers for Disease Control and Prevention
Atlanta, Georgia

JEANNE S. SHEFFIELD, MD
University of Texas Southwestern Medical School
Dallas, Texas

BAHA M. SIBAI, MD
University of Cincinnati College of Medicine
Cincinnati, Ohio

ROBERT M. SILVER, MD
University of Utah School of Medicine
Salt Lake City, Utah

ROGER P. SMITH, MD
University of Missouri
Kansas City School of Medicine
Kansas City, Missouri

JOHN C. SMULIAN, MD, MPH
University of Medicine and Dentistry of New Jersey
Robert Wood Johnson Medical School
New Brunswick, New Jersey

MICHAEL SPEER, MD
Baylor College of Medicine
Houston, Texas

ALEX C. VIDAEFF, MD
University of Texas Medical School
Houston, Texas

ANNA WALD, MD, MPH
University of Washington School of Medicine
Seattle, Washington

EDWARD R. YEOMANS, MD
University of Texas Medical School
Houston, Texas

KRISTIN K. ZORN, MD
University of Pittsburgh School of Medicine
Pittsburgh, Pennsylvania

PART I

GENETICS

CHAPTER 1

First-Trimester Screening for Down Syndrome

FERGAL D. MALONE AND MARY E. D'ALTON

Significant advances have been made in antenatal screening for Down syndrome over the past few decades. Initially, invasive prenatal diagnosis for Down syndrome with amniocentesis or chorionic villus sampling (CVS) was offered only to women of advanced maternal age (older than 35 years at delivery) or those who previously had an affected child. Subsequently, invasive diagnosis was offered to women younger than 35 years who had abnormal second-trimester multiple-marker serum screening results and also to those with abnormal second-trimester ultrasound signs—so-called "soft-markers"—of Down syndrome. The most efficient multiple-marker screening test in the second trimester is the "quad" screen, comprising alpha-fetoprotein (AFP), human chorionic gonadotropin (hCG), unconjugated estriol (E_3), and Inhibin-A. This approach yields sensitivity for Down syndrome of up to 81%, when ultrasonographic dating is used, for a 5% false-positive rate (1, 2).

Interest has been directed toward first-trimester screening with the use of ultrasound and serum screening markers. In a survey of perinatologists in the United States, 46% used nuchal translucency ultrasonography and 27% used the serum markers pregnancy-associated plasma protein A and hCG during the first trimester to screen for Down syndrome (3).

The purpose of this review is to summarize the current data that have resulted in a shift toward first-trimester screening and to articulate the implementation issues that need to be addressed before the use of nuchal translucency-based screening programs becomes more widespread.

Fetal Nuchal Translucency

Nuchal translucency refers to the normal subcutaneous fluid-filled space between the back of the fetal neck and the overlying skin (Fig. 1-1). By adhering to a standard ultrasound technique, it is possible to obtain accurate measurements of this area in most fetuses between 10 weeks and 14 weeks of gestation. The components of one commonly accepted nuchal translucency ultrasound technique are summarized in Box 1-1. These criteria were used successfully in the recently completed First and Second Trimester Evaluation of Risk (FASTER) trial in the United States (1). There is a direct correlation between an increased nuchal translucency measurement and risk for Down syndrome, other aneuploidies, major structural malformations, and adverse pregnancy outcome (1, 2, 4, 5). Figure 1-2 demonstrates an increased nuchal translucency observed in a fetus subsequently shown to have Down syndrome. There are several hypotheses regarding the pathophysiology of large nuchal translucency measurements, and it is unlikely that a single common etiology for this ultrasound sign

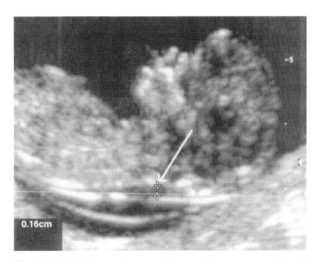

Fig. 1-1. Nuchal translucency ultrasound measurement at 13 weeks of gestation in a chromosomally normal fetus, measuring 1.6 mm. Various features of good nuchal translucency ultrasound technique are evident in this image: adequate image magnification, midsagittal plane, neutral neck position, inner-to-inner caliper placement perpendicular to the fetal body axis (as indicated by white arrow), and separate visualization of the overlying fetal skin and amnion. (Malone FD, D'Alton ME. First-trimester sonographic screening for Down syndrome. Obstet Gynecol 2003;102:1066–79.)

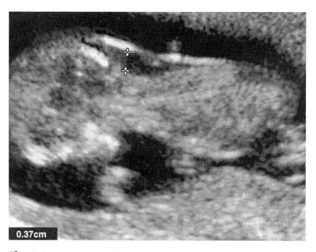

Fig. 1-2. Increased nuchal translucency measurement of 3.7 mm at 12 weeks of gestation in a fetus with Down syndrome. (Malone FD, D'Alton ME. First-trimester sonographic screening for Down syndrome. Obstet Gynecol 2003;102:1066–79.)

underlies all associated abnormalities. Possible etiologies include cardiac failure secondary to structural malformation, abnormalities in the extracellular matrix, and abnormal or delayed development of the lymphatic system (5,6).

Nuchal Translucency Screening for Down Syndrome

Most early studies of nuchal translucency-based screening were performed on patients at high risk for fetal aneuploidy, with sensitivities for Down syndrome ranging from 46% to 62% (4). These studies were useful in establishing that an association exists between increased nuchal translucency measurements and Down syndrome. However, because they were mostly small, retrospective studies of patients drawn from select high-risk populations, they could not address the role of nuchal translucency measurement in general population screening. Extrapolation of results from select high-risk popu-

lations to general population screening will overestimate the true performance of a screening test.

A recent meta-analysis of 30 studies on the performance of nuchal translucency-based screening focused only on an unselected general population (7). The studies composing this meta-analysis are summarized in Table 1-1 (8–36). In combination, these studies described 316,311 patients who were screened with nuchal translucency ultrasonography during the first trimester. A total of 1,177 fetuses with Down syndrome were ascertained in this population, for a prevalence of 3.7 per 1,000 pregnancies. However, many of these studies had a Down syndrome prevalence of 5 per 1,000 or greater, suggesting that these were unlikely to be representative of the general patient population. Such studies likely overstate the true performance of nuchal translucency-based screening in the unselected general population.

The largest of these studies was conducted by the Fetal Medicine Foundation in London, in which 96,127 unselected patients at 22 centers had nuchal translucency ultrasonography performed between 10 weeks and 14 weeks of gestation (13). That series reported sensitivity for Down syndrome of 82% with a false-positive rate of 8%, which is equivalent to 77% sensitivity for a 5% false-positive rate.

However, the calculation of the Down syndrome detection rate in that study has been called into question. In this study, it was calculated that, in the absence of any form of screening in the population of 96,127 patients, there would have been 266 live births of infants at term with Down syndrome (13). This calculation was based on the maternal age and gestational age distribution of the enrolled participants. However, it is known that as many as 40% of fetuses alive at 10–14 weeks of gestation with

Down syndrome will not survive to term but instead will result in a spontaneous intrauterine demise (37). Therefore, if 266 infants with Down syndrome were present in a population at term, that would imply that at least 443 fetuses with Down syndrome must have been alive at 10–14 weeks of gestation, which is the time the screening test was performed (443 times 0.40 = 177 and 443 minus 177 = 266 term live births). Therefore, the quoted Down syndrome detection rate of 268 of 326 (82%) should have been more correctly stated as 268 of 443, or 60% (38).

Table 1-1. Studies of Nuchal Translucency Screening in Unselected Patient Populations

Authors	Number of fetuses	Prevalence	Trisomy 21 Sensitivity n (%)	False-Positive Rate (%)	Positive Predictive Value (%)	LR(+)	LR(-)
Kornman et al (8)	537	13	2/7 (29)	6.4	5.6	5	0.8
Taipale et al (9)	6,939	9	4/6 (67)	0.8	6.7	83	0.3
Hafner et al (10)	4,233	1.7	3/7 (43)	1.7	4.1	25	0.6
Economides et al (11)	2,256	3.5	5/8 (63)	1	17.9	63	0.4
Theodoropoulos et al (12)	3,550	3.1	10/11 (91)	2.6	9.9	35	0.1
Snijders et al (13)	96,127	3.4	268/326 (82)	8	3.4	10	0.2
Pajkrt et al (14)	1,473	6.1	6/9 (67)	1.8	18.2	37	0.3
DeBiasio et al (15)	1,467	8.9	8/13 (62)	6.7	7.5	9	0.4
Quispe et al (16)	424	16.5	7/7 (100)	1.7	50	59	
Whitlow et al (17)	6,443	3.6	13/23 (57)	0.3	37.1	188	0.4
Schwarzler et al (18)	4,523	2.7	10/12 (83)	4.9	4.3	17	0.2
Thilaganathan et al (19)	9,802	2.1	16/21 (76)	4.7	3.3	16	0.3
Krantz et al (20)	5,809	5.7	24/33 (73)	5	7.6	15	0.3
O'Callaghan et al (21)	1,000	8	6/8 (75)	6.2	8.8	12	0.3
Niemimaa et al (22)	1,602	3.1	3/5 (60)	11.6	1.6	5	0.5
Schuchter et al (23)	9,342	2	11/19 (58)	2.3	5	25	0.4
Audibert et al (24)	4,130	2.9	9/12 (75)	4.9	4.3	15	0.3
Michailidis et al (25)	7,447	3.1	19/23 (83)	4.5	5.4	18	0.2
Gasiorek-Wiens et al (26)	21,959	9.6	174/210 (83)	8.9	8.2	9	0.2
Zoppi et al (27)	10,157	6.3	58/64 (91)	9.6	5.7	9	0.1
Brizot et al (28)	2,557	3.9	7/10 (70)	6.5	4	11	0.3
Wayda et al (29)	6,841	2.5	17/17 (100)	4.3	5.5	23	
Schuchter et al (30)	4,939	2.8	8/14 (57)	4.9	3.2	12	0.5
Murta and Franca (31)	1,152	12.2	9/14 (64)	4.2	15.8	15	0.4
Rozenberg et al (32)	6,234	3.4	13/21 (62)	2.8	7	22	0.4
Crossley et al (33)	17,229	2.6	20/37 (54)	5	2.3	11	0.5
Lam et al (34)	16,237	2.2	24/35 (69)	5	2.9	14	0.3
Bindra et al (35)	14,383	5.7	64/82 (79)	5	8.3	16	0.2
Comas et al (36)	7,536	5	38/38 (100)	5	9.4	20	
Morris et al (37)	39,983	2.1	54/85 (63)	5	2.6	13	0.4
Total	316,311	3.7	910/1,177(77.3)	5.9	4.7	13.1	0.24
(Pooled 95% confidence interval)			(75, 80)	(5.8, 6)	(4.5, 4.8)	(12.7, 13.5)	(0.22, 0.27)

Abbreviations: LR(+), likelihood ratio for trisomy 21 given positive result; LR(-), likelihood ratio for trisomy 21 given negative result.
Malone FD, D'Alton ME. First-trimester sonographic screening for Down syndrome. Obstet Gynecol 2003;102:1066–79.

When data from all studies from the meta-analysis in Table 1-1 were pooled, the overall sensitivity for Down syndrome was 77%, with a false positive rate of 6%. The overall odds of carrying a fetus with Down syndrome, given a positive nuchal translucency screening result, were approximately 1 in 20 (positive predictive value 4.7%, 95% confidence interval [CI], 4.5–4.8) (7). There is considerable variability in these studies, however, with sensitivities varying from 29% to 100%, false-positive rates varying from 0.3% to 11.6%, and positive predictive values ranging from 1.6% to 50%.

The performance characteristics of this meta-analysis have recently been validated by the FASTER trial, a multicenter prospective study from 15 centers in the United States in which 38,167 patients had first trimester combined serum and ultrasound screening for Down syndrome completed (1). The detection rate for nuchal translucency with maternal age decreased from 70% at 11 weeks of gestation to 64% at 13 weeks of gestation, respectively, for a 5% false-positive rate (1). Another NIH-funded multicenter prospective study of 8,216 patients from the United States showed similar results, with a Down syndrome detection rate of 69%, for a 5% false-positive rate, for nuchal translucency at 10 weeks to 14 weeks of gestation, with maternal age (39).

Interpreting Literature on Nuchal Translucency-Based Screening

Underascertainment of Cases of Down Syndrome

All interventional studies of Down syndrome screening in which there is anything less than 100% karyotype information on all enrolled patients will be subject to underascertainment bias. This is because cases of Down syndrome are more likely to result in demise in utero, and, therefore, early pregnancy losses and stillborn fetuses are likely to represent significant numbers of cases of Down syndrome. In a review of this topic, in which studies were grouped as being either "subject to ascertainment bias" or "not subject to ascertainment bias," the mean sensitivity for Down syndrome was 77% in the former but only 55% in the latter (40).

Almost all of the studies listed in Table 1-1 are subject to significant underascertainment bias. The more recent NIH-funded prospective studies from the United States likely yield more reliable results regarding the true performance of nuchal translucency-based screening because significant attempts were made to obtain pregnancy outcome or karyotype information on cases of stillborn fetuses or early pregnancy loss, which are groups likely to represent cases of Down syndrome (1, 39).

Success Rate of Obtaining Adequate Nuchal Translucency Measurement

Many studies do not provide any information on the success rate of obtaining a nuchal translucency measurement. Some studies suggest a 100% success rate of obtaining a nuchal translucency measurement (40), but none provides information on the adequacy of these images once obtained. Given that nuchal translucency ultrasonography, which requires considerable training and experience to master, is very operator-dependent, attention needs to be paid not only to obtaining a measurement but also to obtaining a satisfactory measurement.

Although some investigators from the Fetal Medicine Foundation suggest that a 100% success rate of obtaining nuchal translucency ultrasonography is possible (35), this might not be attainable. In the multicenter Scottish Trial of first-trimester screening, in which nuchal translucency training and quality control was provided by the Fetal Medicine Foundation, one acceptable measurement was obtained in only 73% of cases, and three acceptable measurements were obtained in only 52% (41). It is inappropriate to quote Down syndrome detection rates based only on the subgroup of patients in which nuchal translucency ultrasonography was successful. Such calculations should be based on all patients who presented for screening. For example, in the Scottish Trial, the sensitivity for Down syndrome was 54% (5% false-positive rate) for patients in whom nuchal translucency was successful but was only 44% when all patients who desired screening were included (41).

In the recently published FASTER trial, the success rate at obtaining nuchal translucency measurements was 95% (1). It should be noted that this high degree of technical success occurred in the very regulated setting of a prospective research trial, with highly experienced trained ultrasonographers. It is unclear if this success rate can be achieved on a routine basis in regular clinical practice in the general obstetric community.

Controlled Comparisons Between Alternative Screening Programs

The current standard for Down syndrome screening in the United States relies on second-trimester multiple-marker serum screening and maternal age. Before this standard can be replaced by a new screening paradigm, novel approaches to screening should be compared with current methods. It is inappropriate to compare first-trimester screening performance derived from one study with second-trimester screening performance derived from another study because the prevalence of Down syndrome will necessarily be different between both populations. Until recently, most comparisons for screening performances at different gestational ages were derived from the use of mathematical models and data from multiple studies. Recently completed trials in the United States (FASTER) and the United Kingdom (SURUSS [Serum, Urine and Ultrasound Screening Study]) have for the first time provided such comparative data on which the range of screening tests currently available can be directly compared (1, 2). Figure 1-3 summarizes the comparative performance of the various screening options from the FASTER trial and demonstrates that first-trimester combined screening has very similar performance to second-trimester quad marker serum screening (1). Only when performed at 11 weeks of gestation does first-trimester combined screening have a significantly better performance than second-trimester quad marker serum screening. It also is important to realize that only the combination of first-trimester nuchal translucency ultrasonography with first-trimester serum markers comes close to the performance of second-trimester quad marker serum screening. Nuchal translucency alone, without being combined with serum markers, has significantly inferior performance characteristics (1).

Nuchal Translucency Screening Techniques

Combined Testing With First-Trimester Serum Markers

Research in first-trimester maternal serum screening has consistently shown that pregnancies with fetal Down syndrome are associated with higher levels of total hCG and of the free β subunit of hCG (with a median multiple of the median [MoM] of 1.83 in affected cases) and lower levels of pregnancy-associated plasma protein A (with a median MoM of 0.38 in affected cases) (42). Studies of the combination of free β subunit of hCG, pregnancy-associated plasma protein A, and maternal age uniformly demonstrate a sensitivity for Down syndrome of approximately 60%, with a 5% false-positive rate (42). This uniformity is in contrast to studies of nuchal translucency in Table 1-1, which demonstrate significant variability in quoted detection rates.

These first-trimester serum markers are largely independent of nuchal translucency, which would imply that both serum and ultrasound approaches can be combined into a single protocol more effective for screening than either used alone. Two large prospective studies have now been published from the United States, validating the performance of such combined first-trimester screening. The Biochemistry, Ultrasound, Nuchal translucency (BUN) study evaluated 8,514 patients and demonstrated a Down syndrome detection rate of 79%, at a 5% false-positive rate, or 64% at a 1% false-positive rate (39). The FASTER trial evaluated 38,033 patients and demonstrated even better Down syndrome detection rates and showed that performance varied significantly by gestational age (1). For a 5% false-positive rate, the Down syndrome detection rates were 87%, 85%, and 82% at 11, 12, and 13 weeks of gestation, respectively. For a 1% false-positive rate, the Down syndrome detection rates were 73%, 72%, and 67% at 11, 12, and 13 weeks of gestation, respectively (1).

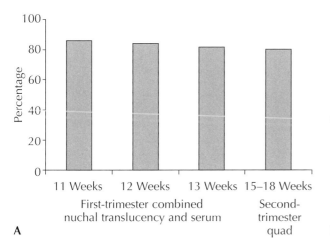
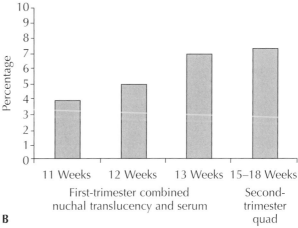

Fig. 1-3. Comparison of first- and second-trimester screening for Down syndrome. **A.** Detection rates of combined first-trimester screening at 11, 12, and 13 weeks of gestation compared with second trimester quad marker serum screening performed at 15–18 weeks of gestation (each at a 5% false-positive rate). **B.** False-positive rates of combined first-trimester screening at 11, 12, and 13 weeks of gestation compared with second-trimester quad marker serum screening performed at 15–18 weeks of gestation (each for 85% detection rate). (Data from Malone FD, Canick JA, Ball RH, Nyberg DA, Comstock CH, Bukowski R, et al. First-trimester or second-trimester screening, or both, for Down's syndrome. N Engl J Med 2005;353:2001–11.)

Combined Testing With First- and Second-Trimester Serum Markers

Incorporating nuchal translucency and maternal serum markers obtained in the first trimester with maternal serum analytes from the second trimester to provide patients with a single risk assessment has been proposed as an alternative to quoting separate Down syndrome risks in each trimester. Four different methods have been described that allow combinations of screening tests in both trimesters: 1) independent sequential, 2) stepwise sequential, 3) integrated screening, and 4) contingent screening.

Independent sequential screening is not recommended because it is associated with an unacceptably high false-positive rate and provides inaccurate risk calculations. This form of screening involves immediately providing first-trimester results to patients, with high-risk patients having definitive diagnosis by means of CVS and with low-risk patients returning at 15 weeks of gestation for further screening. This further screening is provided by means of the second-trimester quad serum marker test, and its risks are calculated independently of the previously performed first-trimester screening. Because each screening test using this approach has its own false-positive rate, it is not surprising that the overall population screen-positive rate would be quite high. Additionally, at least 80% of cases of Down syndrome will have been picked up by the first-trimester component of screening, thereby greatly reducing the prevalence of Down syndrome in the second trimester. The positive predictive value of the second-trimester component of screening will be greatly reduced, and the risks quoted for an individual patient will be less accurate.

Stepwise sequential screening is performed in much the same way as independent sequential screening. In the former, however, the earlier first-trimester marker results also are incorporated into the final second-trimester risk calculation algorithm. This effectively controls the overall false-positive rate and maximizes the accuracy of risks quoted to patients. In the FASTER Trial, independent sequential screening provided a 94% Down syndrome detection rate but at an 11% false-positive rate, whereas stepwise sequential screening performed significantly better, with a 95% detection rate at only a 5% false-positive rate (1).

Another option for combining screening tests in both trimesters is integrated screening. This approach involves measuring nuchal translucency and pregnancy-associated plasma protein A in the first trimester, but no results are provided at that time to the patient. All patients return at 15 weeks of gestation, at which time serum AFP, hCG, unconjugated E_3, and Inhibin-A are measured and are combined with the earlier first trimester markers. A single Down syndrome risk result is then provided based on all markers. The advantage of this approach is its simplicity because patients will not receive potentially conflicting first- and second-trimester results and its safety because it will have the lowest possible false-positive rate (43). The FASTER Trial demonstrated very similar performance between integrated and stepwise sequential screening, with both providing 95% detection rates at 4% and 5% false-positive rates, respectively (1). Although integrated testing has been introduced at a few centers, it remains controversial, with concerns about withholding a potentially significant first-trimester finding until after the second-trimester testing has been completed (44). Although many patients might prefer the speed of having a first-trimester screening test, others might prefer the efficiency and safety of a single screening result that maximizes the detection rate while minimizing the false-positive rate.

The most recently suggested option for combining screening tests in both trimesters is known as contingent screening. This involves triage of patients after first-trimester screening, depending on the risk results obtained. For patients with extremely high-risk results, such as 1 in 30 or greater, immediate diagnostic testing with CVS is provided. For patients with extremely low-risk results, such as 1 in 1,500 or lower, no further screening tests are performed because it is highly unlikely that they would change the initial first-trimester result to high risk. Only those patients with intermediate risk results, such as risks between 1 in 30 and 1 in 1,500, are offered second-trimester screening. Once these second-trimester markers are obtained, a final risk is calculated based on all available marker results, and amniocentesis is available if the final risk is elevated. Although prospective studies of this form of screening are not yet available, modeling would suggest that it will have a Down syndrome detection rate and false-positive rate very similar to stepwise sequential and integrated screening but with only a fraction of patients needing to return in the second trimester for additional testing (45). If confirmed by prospective implementation studies, this form of screening may be attractive from a cost-effectiveness perspective.

Cystic Hygroma

It has been recently noted that a subset of fetuses with very large nuchal translucency measurements that have an extremely high risk of fetal aneuploidy or other adverse pregnancy outcomes can be effectively identified in the first trimester. This finding has been described as septated cystic hygroma, and is present when the nuchal translucency space is enlarged, extending along the entire length of the fetus, and in which septations are clearly visible (Fig. 1-4) (46). Septated cystic hygroma is seen in more than 1 in 300 first-trimester pregnancies. In a recent prospective study of routine first-trimester ultrasound screening, septated cystic hygroma was shown to have a 50% chance of being associated with fetal aneuploidy, with most cases being Down syndrome, as well as cases of Turner syndrome and trisomy 18 (46). Additionally, among cystic hygroma cases confirmed as being euploid, approximately 50% had a major structural fetal malformation, with most being cardiac malformations, as well as other malformations such as skeletal dysplasias. When compared with simple increased nuchal translucency, septated cystic hygroma cases were 5 times more likely to be aneuploid, 12 times more likely to have cardiac malformations, and 6 times more likely to result in fetal or neonatal demise (46).

The practical benefit of being able to counsel patients in the first trimester following the identification of septated cystic hygroma is that there is no need to delay decision making while awaiting serum marker results or using computerized risk calculation algorithms. When faced with a 50% chance of fetal aneuploidy, it is reasonable to offer such patients the immediate option of CVS. If fetal aneuploidy has been excluded, a detailed fetal anatomical evaluation, including fetal echocardiography, should be performed at 18–20 weeks of gestation (46).

Nasal Bone in the First Trimester

An association between absence of the fetal nose bones on first-trimester ultrasound screening and Down syndrome has been described (47). For this study, 701 fetuses with increased nuchal translucency were evaluated for the presence or absence of the nose bones during first-trimester ultrasonography. The fetal nasal bones could not be visualized in 73% of Down syndrome fetuses (43 of 59) and in only 0.5% of unaffected fetuses (3 of 603). The authors also felt that the absence of the fetal nose bone was not related to nuchal translucency thickness and, therefore, could be combined into a single ultrasound screening modality, with a predicted sensitivity of 85% for a 1% false-positive rate (47). This study was challenged by a subsequent report of five consecutive Down syndrome cases, each of which reportedly had a visible nasal bone (48). However, the five images presented in this latter report do not represent optimal views to evaluate the fetal nose bone.

Adequate imaging of the fetal nasal bone can be technically challenging in the first trimester and, therefore, careful attention should be paid to correct technique to ensure consistency. The nasal bone should be visualized on ultrasonography along the midsagittal plane with a perfect fetal profile. The fetal spine should be down, with slight neck flexion. Two echogenic lines at the fetal nose profile should be visualized; the superficial echogenic line is the nasal skin, and the deeper echogenic line represents the nasal bone. This deeper echogenic line representing the nasal bone should be more echolucent at its distal end (Fig. 1-5). Care should be taken not to perform this evaluation with the ultrasound beam parallel to the plane of the nose bone because this might erroneously lead to a conclusion of absent nasal bones.

Several other studies evaluating the role of first-trimester nasal bone ultrasonography as a screening test for fetal Down syndrome also have been published; however, all were limited by being derived from high-risk

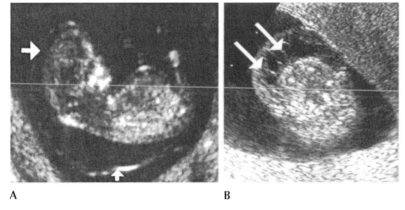

A   **B**

Fig. 1-4. Septated cystic hygroma at 12 weeks of gestation. **A**. Midsagittal ultrasound view of a fetus with septated cystic hygroma, demonstrating increased nuchal translucency space extending along the entire length of the fetus. **B**. Transverse view through the fetal neck of the same fetus demonstrating obvious septations (arrows). (Malone FD, Canick JA, Ball RH, Nyberg DA, Comstock CH, Bukowski R, et al. First-trimester or second-trimester screening, or both, for Down syndrome. Obstet Gynecol 2005;106:288–94.)

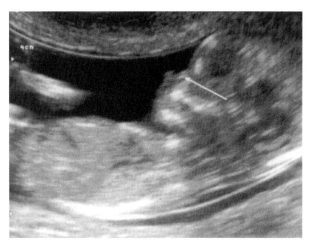

Fig. 1-5. Nasal bone image of a euploid fetus at 13 weeks of gestation. Various features of good nasal bone technique are evident in this image: a good midsagittal plane, clear fetal profile, downward-facing spine, slight neck flexion, and two echogenic lines, representing the overlying fetal skin and the nasal bone. The white arrow represents the fetal nose bone, which loses its echogenicity distally. (Malone FD, D'Alton ME. First-trimester sonographic screening for Down syndrome. Obstet Gynecol 2003;102:1066–79.)

patient populations or lacking adequate pregnancy outcome ascertainment (49). The largest study of first-trimester fetal nasal bone ultrasonography published to date, and in which an unselected general patient population has been evaluated, did not confirm a useful role for this form of screening (49). In a prospective study of 6,324 patients having nasal bone ultrasonography by trained and experienced ultrasonographers, adequate views of the fetal profile were obtained in only 76% of cases, and none of the 11 cases of fetal Down syndrome were found to have absent nasal bones (49).

Although it is possible that there may be a role for first-trimester fetal nasal bone ultrasonography in the hands of select experts as a second-line screening tool in high-risk patients, there are currently insufficient data to recommend the use of this form of ultrasonography as a general population screening tool.

Multiple Gestations

Prenatal risk assessment for Down syndrome in multiple gestation pregnancies has been quite limited before the advent of nuchal translucency-based screening. Maternal serum screening has not been widely used in the setting of multiple gestations because of the potential for discordancy between twins and the impact of different placentas on the various analytes. It seems that the nuchal translucency distribution does not differ significantly in singleton compared with twin pregnancies, which implies that the Down syndrome detection rates should be similar. The false-positive rate of nuchal translucency

screening might be higher in monochorionic twins because some complications unique to monochorionic gestations, such as twin-to-twin transfusion syndrome, might present with increased nuchal translucency measurement (50). Although additional research on the efficacy of this screening method in multiple gestations is still needed, nuchal translucency measurement should at least represent an improvement over serum screening in multiple gestations. Currently, some centers are already using nuchal translucency ultrasonography to assist in selecting fetuses for reduction in higher-order multiple gestations.

Implementing Nuchal Translucency Into Clinical Practice

Nuchal translucency ultrasonography has pushed prenatal screening for Down syndrome into the first trimester and might lead to major advances in prenatal care. However, there are several practical issues that must be resolved before all obstetric providers should consider implementing this form of screening into routine obstetric practice.

Quality Control

The extent of quality-control measures among earlier studies of nuchal translucency screening likely accounts for the large inconsistencies in quoted Down syndrome detection rates. Nuchal translucency ultrasonography is extremely operator dependent and will be a poor technique for general population screening if strict guidelines and ongoing quality-control systems are not maintained (51). In one multicenter study in which adequate training and quality control was not addressed, the overall sensitivity for Down syndrome was only 31% (51). Appropriate training, adherence to a standard technique, and experience are key to its success as a reliable screening tool. Criteria that might help maintain stable and high-quality nuchal translucency ultrasound technique are summarized in Box 1-1.

Initial training in nuchal translucency ultrasonography, however, is only one element of the quality control needed to optimize this technique. Systems must also be put in place at each local ultrasound practice to ensure that ongoing quality assurance is maintained. How such ongoing quality control is maintained optimally is unclear. Options include regular review of a sampling of nuchal translucency ultrasound images by an independent evaluator, although this might be quite impractical on a national basis. Another alternative might be to track individual ultrasonographers' median nuchal translucency measurements and standard deviations over time. This quality assurance technique has the advantage of being easier to standardize and automate, thereby being more practical for national screening.

Another practical problem with nuchal translucency quality control is what to do when an individual ultrasonographer's median measurements drift or image quality deteriorates. How should retraining or correction of errors in technique be applied? Who would be responsible for carrying this out? Should a certification or credentialing system be put in place to ensure that only those with adequate training perform this type of screening? Who should administer such a system? What should be done if an individual ultrasonographer's images do not improve despite retraining? Leadership at a national basis is clearly needed to adequately address each of these implementation issues. Currently in the United States, the Society for Maternal–Fetal Medicine provides a voluntary system for the training of ultrasonographers and physicians in the nuchal translucency technique and also provides a mechanism to validate the quality of imaging.

Interpretation of Results

Mean nuchal translucency measurements increase by approximately 17% each week from 10 weeks to 14 weeks of gestation (52). Therefore, it is inappropriate to use a single millimeter cutoff to interpret nuchal translucency measurements for routine pregnancy screening. More appropriate options include using the 95th percentile for a particular gestational age or MoMs. Unfortunately, such cutoff values are not easily available in the published literature, and all require a software program to adequately integrate other background data, such as maternal age and maternal serum marker results, into the risk assessment.

The validation of such commercially available software programs in specific populations also is uncertain at this time. For example, it is unclear whether it is valid to use generic population medians to interpret nuchal translucency measurements or whether such medians for risk calculations should be center specific or ultrasonographer specific. In one study that addressed the importance of differences in center-specific medians, a Scottish trial of 15 centers evaluating 17,229 patients had individual center nuchal translucency median MoMs ranging from 0.7 MoMs to 1.4 MoMs (41). Ideally the median MoM should be 1. The consequences of such large variability in MoMs between centers could be dramatic. The Down syndrome risk quoted to a 37-year-old patient with a nuchal translucency measurement of 1 mm might vary up to fivefold by having nuchal translucency MoMs that range from 0.7 to 1.4, with quoted risks ranging from 1:1,400 to 1:285. Further studies are needed to evaluate the role and feasibility of center-specific or ultrasonographer-specific medians in a national Down syn-

drome screening program. In the recently completed SURUSS trial from the United Kingdom, the use of ultrasonographer-specific medians resulted in an improvement of 5% in overall Down syndrome detection rates, compared with use of center-specific medians (2).

Implications for Second-Trimester Serum Screening

Implementing a national nuchal translucency screening program in isolation will likely have a negative impact on current second-trimester serum screening programs because the positive predictive value of second-trimester screening might be reduced as much as sixfold after first-trimester screening (53). The number of fetuses with Down syndrome still alive during the second trimester will be significantly reduced because many such fetuses will have already been diagnosed in the first trimester. Sequential screening without appropriate modifications of second-trimester serum marker cutoffs will increase the overall false-positive rate, resulting in an increased number of amniocenteses and procedure-related pregnancy losses (1, 54, 55). Furthermore, sequential screening introduces two independent risk results, which might create unnecessary confusion and anxiety for the patient (56). The only way to adequately ensure against such inefficiency is to either provide a single integrated risk result from both trimesters or to modify the second-trimester risk cutoffs to allow for prior first-trimester screening. It is unclear how such risk modification arrangements can be accomplished if first-trimester screening is implemented in an uncoordinated manner.

Another approach to avoid confusion between uncoordinated first- and second-trimester screening programs would be to drop second-trimester serum screening entirely. However, if Down syndrome screening is limited to the first trimester only, there will likely be a negative impact on neural tube defect detection, which relies on second-trimester maternal serum AFP evaluation. Maternal serum AFP assessment is of no value in the first trimester. Therefore, to drop it completely from antenatal care programs might lead to more cases of spina bifida being missed prenatally. Furthermore, a large proportion of prenatal patients do not present for prenatal care early enough in pregnancy to avail of first-trimester screening. Therefore, second-trimester maternal serum screening will likely remain useful.

Currently, second-trimester multiple-marker serum screening is supported by a well-established and successful quality assurance program. It is unclear how effective a national first-trimester ultrasound screening quality assurance program would be, although the Society for Maternal–Fetal Medicine has developed a system to accomplish this goal. This uncertainty will add to the difficulty in simply dropping second-trimester serum screening.

Implications for Second-Trimester Ultrasonography

Nuchal translucency screening will not obviate the need for second-trimester ultrasonography for the detection of structural fetal abnormalities. The "genetic ultrasonogram," which evaluates structural malformations and a range of second-trimester soft markers for aneuploidy, such as short femurs, echogenic bowel, echogenic intracardiac foci, and nuchal fold, has gained widespread acceptability. A national policy of first-trimester screening will likely have a negative impact on the performance of the genetic ultrasonogram. The positive predictive value of these ultrasound soft markers for aneuploidy will decrease because the number of aneuploid fetuses entering the second trimester will be reduced. It is currently not known what the relevance of these soft markers will be in a population of fetuses that has already undergone nuchal translucency-based screening. If the genetic ultrasonogram continues without allowance for the lower prevalence of second-trimester aneuploid fetuses, it is likely that more unnecessary amniocenteses will be performed without significant improvement in detection rates. The best way to incorporate the genetic ultrasonogram into a practice in which first trimester screening has already been performed is to rely on likelihood ratios. If a soft marker for Down syndrome is seen at a second-trimester ultrasound examination, the appropriate likelihood ratio for that marker should be multiplied by the final Down syndrome risk quoted from first-trimester screening, rather than multiplying by the maternal age-related risk.

Availability of Early Prenatal Diagnosis

One of the most compelling arguments in favor of nuchal translucency-based screening for Down syndrome is the shift to earlier diagnosis through CVS at 10–13 weeks of gestation. Chorionic villus sampling is not as widely available as amniocentesis on a national basis (3). Early amniocentesis in the first trimester is no longer considered an acceptable alternative to CVS because of its higher association with fetal loss, fetal clubfoot, and procedure failure (57). If first-trimester screen-positive patients do not have ready access to CVS, they might experience increased anxiety, waiting 3–4 weeks for an opportunity to undergo amniocentesis at 15 weeks of gestation. Therefore, a policy of first-trimester screening for aneuploidy should not be implemented unless first-trimester diagnosis with CVS is locally available. If a patient desires the benefit of first-trimester screening, but CVS is not easily available, then the optimal approach might be to provide the first-trimester result at 16 weeks of gestation as part of a single integrated screening result in combination with second-trimester serum markers.

Choosing the Correct Combination of Screening Tests

With the increasing range of Down syndrome screening tests available to obstetric providers today, there is a need for accurate comparative data to evaluate the best combination of tests to implement into practice. The comparative performance of each type of Down syndrome screening recently has been described from the FASTER trial (1). These results have shown that the most inefficient test, associated with the highest screen-positive rate, is nuchal translucency ultrasonography performed on its own. First-trimester screening seems to derive much of its efficiency by combining nuchal translucency with pregnancy-associated plasma protein A and free β subunit of hCG evaluation. An integrated screen, incorporating nuchal translucency and pregnancy-associated plasma protein A in the first trimester, together with AFP, hCG, unconjugated E_3, and Inhibin-A assessments in the second trimester, seems to be the single most efficient test. In a center without easy access to high-quality nuchal translucency ultrasonography, another reasonable alternative might be a serum-only test, incorporating pregnancy-associated plasma protein A assessments in the first trimester with those of AFP, hCG, unconjugated E_3, and Inhibin-A in the second trimester, with a single risk being quoted.

It is unlikely that a single screening test will be suitable for all practitioners and their patients. The decision as to which screening test to incorporate into local clinical practice will be based on factors such as gestational age at presentation, availability of high-quality nuchal translucency ultrasonography, and availability of first trimester invasive testing with CVS. Some patients might be most interested in the earliest possible screening result; for such patients, combined first trimester nuchal translucency and serum screening might be desired. Other patients might be more interested in the most efficient test, maximizing their detection rate and minimizing the need for amniocentesis; for such patients, a single integrated screen result combining first- and second-trimester approaches might be desired. Still other patients might not present for care sufficiently early to take advantage of first-trimester screening; for these patients, there should be the option of second-trimester serum screening and genetic ultrasonography.

Informed consent regarding the variety of prenatal screening tests for aneuploidy should be an integral part of the screening process itself. Because of the complexity of choices regarding the different screening options and because of the range of abnormal outcomes associated with increased nuchal translucency, it will be vital to provide all patients with pretest genetic counseling before embarking on these newer forms of screening.

Current and Future Status of Nuchal Translucency Screening in the United States

From a review of the current literature, it is clear that nuchal translucency ultrasonography is the single most powerful prenatal screening marker for fetal Down syndrome. The comprehensive comparative data now available confirm that if first-trimester screening is implemented, the only test that should be recommended at this time is nuchal translucency combined with first-trimester serum. Nuchal translucency screening alone should not be performed in singleton pregnancies because it is inferior to both first-trimester combined screening or second-trimester quad marker screening. Nuchal translucency should be expressed as an MoM, and median nuchal translucency values should be maintained and monitored carefully, just like any other laboratory analyte. However, before such first-trimester screening can be endorsed for use in routine clinical practice, a range of implementation issues needs to be addressed. It is precisely because nuchal translucency has such great potential that it must be implemented in a coherent and organized manner. If these implementation issues can be resolved on a national basis, first-trimester screening will likely become a fundamental part of 21st century antenatal care.

References

1. Malone FD, Canick JA, Ball RH, Nyberg DA, Comstock CH, Bukowski R, et al. A comparison of first trimester screening, second trimester screening, and the combination of both for evaluation of risk for Down syndrome. N Engl J Med 2005;353:2001–11.

2. Wald NJ, Rodeck C, Hackshaw AK, Walters J, Chitty L, Mackinson AM. First and second trimester antenatal screening for Down's syndrome: The results of the Serum, Urine and Ultrasound Screening Study (SURUSS). J Med Screen 2003;10:56–104.

3. Egan JF, Kaminsky LM, DeRoche ME, Barsoom MJ, Borgida AF, Benn PA. Antenatal Down syndrome screening in the United States in 2001: A survey of maternal-fetal medicine specialists. Am J Obstet Gynecol 2002;187:1230–4.

4. Malone FD, Berkowitz RL, Canick JA, D'Alton ME. First trimester screening for aneuploidy: Research or standard of care? Am J Obstet Gynecol 2000;182:490–6.

5. Nicolaides KH, Heath V, Cicero S. Increased fetal nuchal translucency at 11-14 weeks. Prenat Diagn 2002;22:308–15.

6. Moscoso G. Fetal nuchal translucency: A need to understand the physiological basis. Ultrasound Obstet Gynecol 1995;5:6–8.

7. Malone FD, D'Alton ME, for the Society for Maternal Fetal Medicine. First trimester sonographic screening for Down syndrome. Obstet Gynecol 2003;102:1066–79.

8. Kornman LH, Morssink LP, Beekhuis JR, De Wolf BT, Heringa MP, Mantingh A. Nuchal translucency cannot be used as a screening test for chromosomal abnormalities in the first trimester of pregnancy in a routine ultrasound practice. Prenat Diagn 1996;16:797–805.

9. Taipale P, Hiilesmaa V, Salonen R, Ylostalo P. Increased nuchal translucency as a marker for fetal chromosomal defects. N Engl J Med 1997;337:1654–8.

10. Hafner E, Schuchter K, Liebhart E, Philipp K. Results of routine fetal nuchal translucency measurement at weeks 10-13 in 4233 unselected pregnant women. Prenat Diagn 1998;18:29–34.

11. Economides DL, Whitlow BJ, Kadir R, Lazanakis M, Verdin SM. First trimester sonographic detection of chromosomal abnormalities in an unselected population. Br J Obstet Gynaecol 1998;105:58–62.

12. Theodoropoulos P, Lolis D, Papageorgiou C, Papaioannou S, Plachouras N, Makrydimas G. Evaluation of first trimester screening by fetal nuchal translucency and maternal age. Prenat Diagn 1998;18:133–7.

13. Snijders RJ, Noble P, Sebire N, Souka A, Nicolaides KH. UK multicenter project on assessment of risk of trisomy 21 by maternal age and fetal nuchal-translucency thickness at 10-14 weeks of gestation. Lancet 1998;351:343–6.

14. Pajkrt E, van Lith JM, Mol BW, Bilardo CM. Screening for Down's syndrome by fetal nuchal translucency measurement in a general obstetric population. Ultrasound Obstet Gynecol 1998;12:163–9.

15. De Biasio P, Siccardi M, Volpe G, Famularo L, Santi F, Canini S. First-trimester screening for Down syndrome using nuchal translucency measurement with free β-hCG and PAPP-A between 10 and 13 weeks of pregnancy—the combined test. Prenat Diagn 1999;19:360–3.

16. Quispe J, Almandoz A, de Quiroga M, Isabel M. Traslucencia nucal fetal, un marcador de alteraciones cromosomicas en el primer trimestre. Ginecol Obstet 1999;45:183–6.

17. Whitlow BJ, Chatzipapas IK, Lazanakis ML, Kadir RA, Economides DL. The value of sonography in early pregnancy for the detection of fetal abnormalities in an unselected population. Br J Obstet Gynaecol 1999;106:929–36.

18. Schwarzler P, Carvalho JS, Senat MV, Masroor T, Campbell S, Ville Y. Screening for fetal aneuploidies and fetal cardiac abnormalities by nuchal translucency thickness measurement at 10-14 weeks of gestation as part of routine antenatal care in an unselected population. Br J Obstet Gynaecol 1999;106:1029–34.

19. Thilaganathan B, Sairam S, Michailidis G, Wathen NC. First trimester nuchal translucency: Effective routine screening for Down's syndrome. Br J Radiol 1999;72:946–8.

20. Krantz DA, Hallahan TW, Orlandi F, Buchanan P, Larsen JW, Macro JN. First-trimester Down syndrome screening using dried blood biochemistry and nuchal translucency. Obstet Gynecol 2000;96:207–13.

21. O'Callaghan SP, Giles WB, Raymond SP, McDougall V, Morris K, Boyd J. First trimester ultrasound with nuchal translucency measurement for Down syndrome risk estimation using software developed by the Fetal Medicine Foundation, United Kingdom—the first 2000 examinations in Newcastle, New South Wales, Australia. Aust N Z J Obstet Gynaecol 2000;40:292–5.

22. Niemimaa M, Suonpaa M, Perheentupa A, Seppala M, Heinonen S, Laitinen P, et al. Evaluation of first trimester maternal serum and ultrasound screening for Down's syndrome in Eastern and Northern Finland. Eur J Hum Genet 2001;9:404–8.

23. Schuchter K, Hafner E, Stangl G, Ogris E, Philipp K. Sequential screening for trisomy 21 by nuchal translucency measurement in the first trimester and serum biochemistry in the second trimester in a low-risk population. Ultrasound Obstet Gynecol 2001;18:23–5.

24. Audibert F, Dommergues M, Bennattar C, Taieb J, Thalabard JC, Frydman R. Screening for Down syndrome using first-trimester ultrasound and second-trimester maternal serum markers in a low-risk population: A prospective longitudinal study. Ultrasound Obstet Gynecol 2001;18:26–31.

25. Michailidis GF, Spencer K, Economides DL. The use of nuchal translucency measurement and second trimester biochemical markers in screening for Down's syndrome. Br J Obstet Gynaecol 2001;108:1047–52.

26. Gasiorek-Wiens A, Tercanli S, Kozlowski P, Kossakiewicz A, Minderer S, Meyberg H, et al. Screening for trisomy 21 by fetal nuchal translucency and maternal age: A multicenter project in Germany, Austria and Switzerland. Ultrasound Obstet Gynecol 2001;18:645–8.

27. Zoppi MA, Ibba RM, Floris M, Monni G. Fetal nuchal translucency screening in 12,496 pregnancies in Sardinia. Ultrasound Obstet Gynecol 2001;18:649–51.

28. Brizot ML, Carvalho MH, Liao AW, Reis NS, Armbruster-Moraes E, Zugaib M. First-trimester screening for chromosomal abnormalities by fetal nuchal translucency in a Brazilian population. Ultrasound Obstet Gynecol 2001;18:652–5.

29. Wayda K, Kereszturi A, Orvos H, Horvath E, Pal A, Kovacs L, et al. Four years experience of first-trimester nuchal translucency screening for fetal aneuploidies with increasing regional availability. Acta Obstet Gynecol Scand 2001;80:1104–9.

30. Schuchter K, Hafner E, Stangl G, Metzenbauer M, Hofinger D, Philipp K. The first trimester 'combined test' for the detection of Down syndrome pregnancies in 4939 unselected pregnancies. Prenat Diagn 2002;22:211–5.

31. Murta CG, Franca LC. Medida da translucencia nucal no rastreamento de anomalies cromossomicas. Rev Bras Ginecol Obstet 2002;24:167–73.

32. Rozenberg P, Malagrida L, Cuckle H, Durand-Zaleski I, Nisand I, Audibert F, et al. Down's syndrome screening with nuchal translucency at 12+0-14+0 weeks and maternal serum markers at 14+1 – 17+0 weeks: A prospective study. Hum Reprod 2002;17:1093–8.

33. Crossley JA, Aitken DA, Cameron AD, McBride E, Connor JM. Combined ultrasound and biochemical screening for Down's syndrome in the first trimester: A Scottish multicenter study. Br J Obstet Gynaecol 2002;109:667–76.

34. Lam YH, Lee CP, Sin SY, Tang R, Wong HS, Wong SF, et al. Comparison and integration of first trimester nuchal translucency and second trimester maternal serum screening for fetal Down syndrome. Prenat Diagn 2002;22:730–5.

35. Bindra R, Heath V, Liao A, Spencer K, Nicolaides KH. One-stop clinic for assessment of risk for trisomy 21 at 11-14 weeks: A prospective study of 15,030 pregnancies. Ultrasound Obstet Gynecol 2002;20:219–25.

36. Comas C, Torrents M, Munoz A, Antolin E, Figueras F, Echevarria M. Measurement of nuchal translucency as a single strategy in trisomy 21 screening: Should we use any other marker? Obstet Gynecol 2002;100:648–54.

37. Morris JK, Wald NJ, Watt HC. Fetal loss in Down syndrome pregnancies. Prenat Diagn 1999;19:142–5.

38. Haddow JE. Antenatal screening for Down's syndrome: Where are we and where next? Lancet 1998;352:336–7.

39. Wapner R, Thom E, Simpson JL, Pergament E, Silver R, Filkins K, et al. First trimester screening for trisomies 21 and 18. N Engl J Med 2003;349:1405–13.

40. Mol BW, Lijmer JG, van der Meulen J, Pajkrt E, Billardo CM, Bossuyt PM. Effect of study design on the association between nuchal translucency measurement and Down syndrome. Obstet Gynecol 1999;94:864–9.

41. Crossley JA, Aitken DA, Cameron AD, McBride E, Connor JM. Combined ultrasound and biochemical screening for Down's syndrome in the first trimester: A Scottish multicenter study. Br J Obstet Gynaecol 2002;109:667–76.

42. Canick JA, Kellner LH. First trimester serum screening for aneuploidy: Serum biochemical markers. Semin Perinatol 1999;23:359–68.

43. Wald NJ, Watt HC, Hackshaw AK. Integrated screening for Down's syndrome based on tests performed during the first and second trimesters. N Engl J Med 1999;341:461–7.

44. Cuckle H. Time for a total shift to first-trimester screening for Down's syndrome. Lancet 2001;358:1658–9.

45. Cuckle H, Benn P, Wright D. Down syndrome screening in the first and/or second trimester: Model predicted performance using meta-analysis parameters. Semin Perinat 2005;29:252–7.

46. Malone FD, Ball RH, Nyberg DA, Comstock CH, Saade GR, Berkowitz RL, et al. First-trimester septated cystic hygroma: Prevalence, Natural history, and pediatric outcome. Obstet Gynecol 2005;106:288–94.

47. Cicero S, Curcio P, Papageorghiou A, Sonek J, Nicolaides KH. Absence of nasal bone in fetuses with trisomy 21 at 11-14 weeks of gestation: An observational study. Lancet 2001;358:1665–7.

48. De Biasio PD, Venturini PL. Absence of nasal bone and detection of trisomy 21. Lancet 2002;359:1344–5.

49. Malone FD, Ball RH, Nyberg DA, Comstock CH, Saade G, Berkowitz RL, et al. First-trimester nasal bone evaluation for aneuploidy in the general population. Obstet Gynecol 2004;104:1222–8.

50. Sebire NJ, Souka A, Skentou H, Geerts L, Nicolaides KH. Early prediction of severe twin-to-twin transfusion syndrome. Hum Reprod 2000;15:2008–10.

51. Haddow JE, Palomaki GE, Knight GJ, Williams J, Miller WA, Johnson A. Screening of maternal serum for fetal

Down's syndrome in the first trimester. N Engl J Med 1998;338:955–61.

52. Scott F, Boogert A, Sinosich M, Anderson J. Establishment and application of a normal range for nuchal translucency across the first trimester. Prenat Diagn 1996;16:629–34.

53. Kadir RA, Economides DL. The effect of nuchal translucency measurement on second-trimester biochemical screening for Down's syndrome. Ultrasound Obstet Gynecol 1997;9:244–7.

54. Hackshaw AK, Wald NJ. Inaccurate estimation of risk in second trimester serum screening for Down syndrome among women who have already had first trimester screening. Prenat Diagn 2001;21:741–6.

55. Platt LD, Greene N, Johnson A, Zachary J, Thom E, Krantz D, et al. Sequential pathways of testing after first-trimester screening for trisomy 21. Obstet Gynecol 2004;104:661–6.

56. Hackshaw AK, Wald NJ. Assessment of the value of reporting partial screening results in prenatal screening for Down syndrome. Prenat Diagn 2001;21:737–40.

57. Canadian Early and Mid-Trimester Amniocentesis Trial (CEMAT). Randomized trial to assess safety and fetal outcome of early and midtrimester amniocentesis. Lancet 1998;351:242–7.

PART II

MEDICAL COMPLICATIONS

CHAPTER 2

Thyroid Disease in Pregnancy

BRIAN M. CASEY AND KENNETH J. LEVENO

*I*nterest in thyroid dysfunction complicating pregnancy has increased greatly during the past decade. This increased interest has been largely fueled by two reports in 1999 that suggested offspring of women with variously defined hypothyroidism identified during pregnancy, to include overt and subclinical disease, are at increased risk of impaired neurodevelopment (1, 2). There also have been reports linking subclinical hypothyroidism with an increased risk for preterm birth (3, 4). As a result, several national endocrine authorities have recommended routine screening for hypothyroidism during pregnancy (5). The rationale for routine screening of pregnant women hinges on the reported prevalence of subclinical hypothyroidism and the potential benefits of treatment during pregnancy. Importantly, if universal screening during pregnancy was adopted in the United States, most women who would be identified would have subclinical hypothyroidism (3). However, one of the most important U.S. Preventive Services Task Force criteria for recommending screening of asymptomatic individuals is a demonstrated improvement in important health outcomes of those individuals identified through screening (6, 7). The position of the American College of Obstetricians and Gynecologists has been that it is premature to recommend routine screening for subclinical hypothyroidism because there is no good evidence that identification and treatment improves maternal or infant outcomes (8).

Pregnancy is associated with significant, but reversible, changes in maternal thyroid physiology that can lead to confusion in the diagnosis of thyroid abnormalities. There is moderate thyroid enlargement as a result of pregnancy hormone-induced glandular hyperplasia and increased vascularity. Ultrasound evaluation of the thyroid gland during pregnancy shows an increase in volume, whereas its echo structure remains unchanged (9). This enlargement, although not pathologic, may prompt biochemical evaluation of thyroid status during pregnancy. As shown in Figure 2-1, there are well described changes in thyroid function tests during pregnancy that are related to 1) an estrogen-mediated

increase in circulating levels of thyroid-binding globulin, which is the major transport protein for thyroid hormone; 2) thyroid stimulation because of a "spillover" effect, especially in the first trimester, by human chorionic gonadotropin (hCG), which shares some structural homology with thyrotropin (thyroid-stimulating hormone [TSH]); and 3) a relative decrease in availability of iodide related to increased renal clearance and overall losses to the fetus and placenta (10). Further complicating the diagnosis of thyroid dysfunction during pregnancy are the effects that several abnormal pregnancy conditions, such as gestational trophoblastic disease and hyperemesis gravidarum, have on thyroid function studies.

Especially relevant is the intimate relationship between maternal and fetal thyroid function, particu-

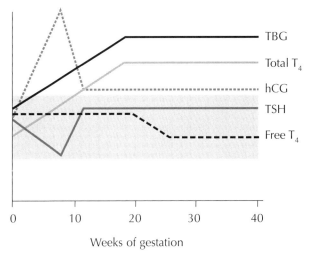

Fig. 2-1. The pattern of changes in serum concentrations of thyroid function studies and human chorionic gonadotropin according to gestational age. The shaded area represents the normal range of thyroid-binding globulin, total thyroxine, thyroid-stimulating hormone or free T_4 in the nonpregnant woman. Abbreviations: hCG, human chorionic gonadotropin; T_4, thyroxine; TBG, thyroid-binding globulin; TSH, thyroid-stimulating hormone. (Modified from Brent GA. Maternal thyroid function: interpretation of thyroid function tests in pregnancy. Clin Obstet Gynecol 1997;40:3–15.)

larly during the first half of pregnancy. The fetal thyroid gland begins concentrating iodine and synthesizing thyroid hormone after 12 weeks of gestation. Any requirement for thyroid hormones before this time is supplied by the mother, and it is during this time that thyroid hormones are most important to fetal brain development (11). However, significant fetal brain development continues considerably beyond the first trimester, making thyroid hormone also important later in gestation. Importantly, although overt maternal thyroid failure during the first half of pregnancy has been associated with several pregnancy complications and intellectual impairment in offspring (12–15), it is currently less clear whether milder forms of thyroid dysfunction have similar effects on pregnancy and infant outcomes (7).

Overt Hypothyroidism

Overt hypothyroidism complicates 1–3 of 1,000 pregnancies and is characterized by vague, nonspecific signs or symptoms that are often insidious in onset and easily confused with symptoms attributable to pregnancy. Initial symptoms include fatigue, constipation, cold intolerance, and muscle cramps. These may progress to insomnia, weight gain, carpal tunnel syndrome, hair loss, voice changes, and intellectual slowness. Women who report that such symptoms have worsened over the previous year are more likely to have overt thyroid disease (16).

The most common cause of primary hypothyroidism in pregnancy is chronic autoimmune thyroiditis (Hashimoto's thyroiditis). It is a painless inflammation with progressive enlargement of the thyroid gland characterized by diffuse lymphocytic infiltration, fibrosis, parenchymal atrophy, and eosinophilic change. Other important causes of primary hypothyroidism include endemic iodine deficiency and a history of either ablative radioiodine therapy or thyroidectomy. Secondary hypothyroidism is pituitary in origin. For example, Sheehan's syndrome from a history of obstetric hemorrhage is characterized by pituitary ischemia and necrosis with subsequent deficiencies in some or all pituitary hormones. Other causes of secondary hypothyroidism include lymphocytic hypophysitis and a history of a hypophysectomy. Tertiary or hypothalamic hypothyroidism is very rare. Central hypothyroidism refers to inadequate stimulation of the thyroid gland because of a defect at the level of the pituitary or hypothalamus.

Women with overt hypothyroidism are at an increased risk for pregnancy complications such as early pregnancy failure, preeclampsia, placental abruption, low birth weight, and stillbirth (Table 2-1) (12, 13, 17). Treatment of women with overt hypothyroidism has been associated with improved pregnancy outcomes.

Table 2-1. Pregnancy Complications in 96 Women With Overt or Subclinical Hypothyroidism as Reported by Davis, Leung, and Their Colleagues (12, 13, 17)

	Hypothyroidism	
Complications	Overt n = 39	Subclinical n = 57
Preeclampsia	12 (31%)	9 (16%)
Abruptio placentae	3 (8%)	0
Postpartum hemorrhage	4 (10%)	1 (2%)
Cardiac dysfunction	1 (3%)	1 (2%)
Birth weight less than 2,000 g	10 (26%)	6 (11%)
Stillbirths	3 (8%)	1*

*Caused by syphilis.
Casey BM, Leveno KJ. Thyroid disease in pregnancy. Obstet Gynecol 2006;108:1283–92.

Diagnostic Approach

The presence or absence of a pathologically enlarged thyroid gland (ie, goiter) depends on the cause of hypothyroidism. Women in areas of endemic iodine deficiency or those with Hashimoto's thyroiditis are much more likely to have a goiter. Other signs of hypothyroidism include periorbital edema, dry skin, and prolonged relaxation phase of deep tendon reflexes. The diagnosis of clinical hypothyroidism during pregnancy is particularly difficult because many of the aforementioned signs or symptoms also are common to pregnancy. Thyroid testing should be performed on symptomatic women or those with a history of thyroid disease (8).

The mainstay for the diagnosis of thyroid disease is the measurement of serum TSH. Serum TSH is more sensitive than free thyroxine (T_4) for detecting hypothyroidism and hyperthyroidism. If the TSH level is abnormal, then evaluation of free T_4 is recommended. A disadvantage of this TSH first-testing strategy is that unusual thyroid conditions characterized by discordant TSH and free T_4 test results may go undetected. The diagnosis of overt hypothyroidism is generally established by an elevated serum TSH concentration and a low serum free T_4 concentration. The reference range for serum TSH concentrations in nonpregnant individuals is 0.45–4.5 mU/L. However, recent data indicate that more than 95% of normal individuals have a TSH level below 2.5 mU/L and that those with a TSH level between 2.5 and 4.5 mU/L have an increased risk of progression to overt disease (18). This finding has led some researchers to recommend a decrease in the upper limit of the TSH reference range to 2.5 mIU/L (19), whereas other researchers suggest that this change would only increase the diagnosis of subclinical hypothyroidism without clear evidence of a benefit from treatment (20). We are, therefore, of the view that a reduction in the upper limit of normal for TSH levels is currently unwarranted.

During early pregnancy, there is a decrease in serum TSH levels and a modest increase in free thyroxine levels because of the structurally related thyroid-stimulating activity of hCG (10) (Fig. 2-1). These physiologic changes confound the diagnosis of hypothyroidism during pregnancy and highlight the need for gestational age-specific TSH level thresholds. Such thresholds have been reported and are based on a large population-based study of pregnant women (21). As shown in Figure 2-2, the upper limit of the statistically defined normal range for TSH levels (97.5th percentile) in the first half of pregnancy was 3 mU/L (21). Moreover, if population-specific medians for TSH levels are determined for each trimester at a particular laboratory, these data indicate that the upper limit of TSH levels during the first trimester should be 4 multiples of the median and 2.5 multiples of the median for the second and third trimester in singleton gestations. The upper limit for twin gestations should be 3.5 multiples of the median in the first trimester and 2.5 multiples of the median in the second and third trimesters (21).

The effects of changes in free T_4 levels during normal pregnancy have been the subject of much controversy, particularly with the advent of automated free hormone immunoassays. The diagnostic accuracy of these free T_4 tests is dependent on protein binding, especially given the physiologic changes in thyroid-binding globulin and other proteins during pregnancy (22). (Fig. 2-1) Although there is a significant decrease in free T_4 levels in

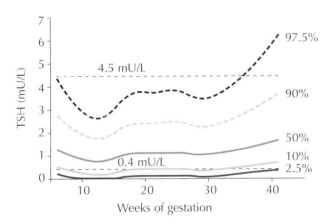

Fig. 2-2. Gestational age-specific thyroid-stimulating hormone nomogram derived from 13,599 singleton and 132 twin pregnancies as reported by Dashe and colleagues (21). Abbreviation: TSH, thyroid-stimulating hormone. (Modified from Dashe JS, Casey BM, Wells CE, McIntire DD, Byrd EW, Leveno KJ, Cunningham FG. Thyroid-stimulating hormone in singleton and twin pregnancy: importance of gestational age-specific reference ranges. Obstet Gynecol 2005;106:753–7.)

late gestation when compared with nonpregnant women or those in the first trimester, overall, free T_4 concentrations remain within the reference range (0.7–1.8 ng/dL) throughout pregnancy (10). Therefore, we recommend using nonpregnant free T_4 level thresholds for diagnosis of hypothyroidism until pregnancy-specific free T_4 level thresholds are available.

It may be helpful to confirm the presence of antimicrosomal antibodies in pregnant women with hypothyroidism. Specifically, the presence of antithyroid antibodies may identify a population of women at a particular risk for pregnancy complications, postpartum thyroid dysfunction, and progression to symptomatic disease (23, 24). One recent study revealed that 50% of women identified with thyroid peroxidase antibodies at 16 weeks of gestation developed postpartum thyroid dysfunction, and one in four of these women went on to develop permanent overt hypothyroidism within the year (25).

Therapeutic Approach

The goal of treatment in pregnant women with overt hypothyroidism is clinical and biochemical euthyroidism. Levothyroxine sodium is the treatment of choice for routine management of hypothyroidism. The starting dose usually is 1–2 mcg/kg/d or approximately 100 mcg/d. Thyroid-stimulating hormone is then measured at 6–8 week intervals, and the levothyroxine dose is adjusted in 25–50-mcg increments. The therapeutic goal is a TSH level between 0.5 mU/L and 2.5 mU/L (26) (Fig. 2-3). As shown in Figure 2-4, serum TSH values can be misleading during early therapy for hypothyroidism because it takes 6 weeks or more for pituitary TSH secretion to reequilibrate to the new thyroid hormone status. Assessment of free T_4 levels may be helpful when monitoring response to treatment.

Women with a history of hypothyroidism before conception should have a serum TSH level evaluation at their first prenatal visit. Approximately one half of these women will require an increase in thyroid replacement therapy during pregnancy. Because of the increased likelihood of biochemical hypothyroidism during early pregnancy, some authors have recommended that the levothyroxine dose be increased routinely by 30% in pregnant women at the time that pregnancy is confirmed (27). However, this practice has not been shown to be beneficial and, because there is a significant potential for overtreatment in such women, we believe that thyroid treatment should be guided by thyroid function studies performed at initiation of prenatal care (16). In women with well-controlled thyroid disease, it is recommended that thyroid function studies be repeated during each trimester. Notably, several drugs can interfere with

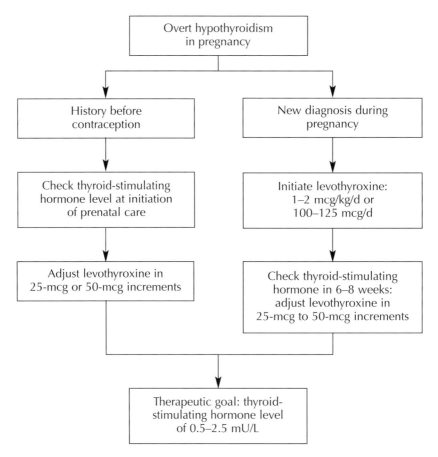

Fig. 2-3. Management algorithm for pregnant women with a history of hypothyroidism or those newly diagnosed during pregnancy. (Casey BM, Leveno KJ. Thyroid disease in pregnancy. Obstet Gynecol 2006;108:1283–92.)

levothyroxine absorption (eg, cholestyramine, ferrous sulfate, aluminum hydroxide antacids) or its metabolism (eg, phenytoin, carbamazepine, and rifampin).

Follow-up

After delivery, levothyroxine therapy should be returned to the prepregnancy dose and the TSH level checked 6–8 weeks postpartum. Breastfeeding is not contraindicated in women treated for hypothyroidism. Levothyroxine is excreted into breast milk but levels are too low to alter thyroid function in the infant or to interfere with neonatal thyroid screening programs (28). Periodic monitoring with an annual assessment of serum TSH concentration generally is recommended given that changing weight and age may modify thyroid function.

Subclinical Hypothyroidism

Reports suggesting increased fetal wastage or subsequent neurodevelopmental complications in the offspring of women with mild hypothyroidism have prompted recommendations that levothyroxine be prescribed to restore the TSH level to the reference range (5). However, there are no published intervention trials specifically assessing the efficacy of such treatment to improve neuropsychologic performance in offspring of women with subclinical hypothyroidism (ie, elevated TSH and normal free T_4 levels). As a result, routine screening and treatment of subclinical hypothyroidism during pregnancy is not recommended by the American College of Obstetricians and Gynecologists. It is acknowledged, however, that obstetricians are under increasing pressure to screen and treat for maternal subclinical hypothyroidism despite uncertainty whether such therapy would be beneficial. Indeed, national endocrinology organizations have emphasized the need for large clinical trials to address this issue. Until such studies are complete, we continue to recommend against routine screening for and treatment of subclinical hypothyroidism during pregnancy.

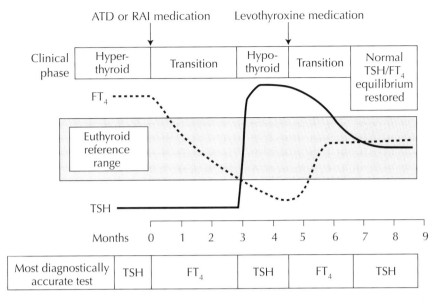

Fig. 2-4. Thyroid-stimulating hormone and free thyroxine values during transition periods after treatment for hyperthyroidism or hypothyroidism. Abbreviations: ATD, antithyroid drugs; FT_4, free thyroxine; RAI, radioactive iodine; TSH, thyroid-stimulating hormone. (Reproduced with permission of the National Academy of Clinical Biochemistry, Washington, DC. Laboratory medicine practice guidelines: laboratory support for the diagnosis of thyroid disease. Larchmont (NY): Mary Ann Liebert; 2003.)

Isolated Hypothyroxinemia

Maternal isolated hypothyroxinemia, defined as a normal range TSH level with a low free T_4 level, recently has been linked to impaired fetal neurodevelopment (2, 11). Specifically, offspring of Dutch women from an iodine-sufficient area and with isolated hypothyroxinemia, defined by a free T_4 level below the 10th percentile at 12 weeks of gestation, were reported to have significant developmental delay as measured by Bayley Scales of Infant Development (2, 29). Low serum free T_4 levels with paradoxically normal or even slightly decreased serum TSH levels are classically suggestive of central hypothyroidism, which is a rare condition. Central hypothyroidism is usually caused by pituitary macroadenomas, pituitary surgery, or irradiation. Isolated hypothyroxinemia also has been associated with iodine insufficiency because of an autoregulatory response by the thyroid gland that leads to an isolated low free T_4 level (30). Finally, laboratory inaccuracy from technical interference also should be considered when discordant thyroid test results are encountered (22).

When considering the impact of pregnancy on thyroid hormone status (Fig. 2-1) and the increased pressure on obstetricians to screen for thyroid dysfunction during pregnancy, there will likely be an increase in the number of pregnant women identified with low free T_4 but normal TSH levels. Similar to subclinical hypothyroidism, however, there are no reports indicating that

treatment of such isolated hypothyroxinemia is beneficial for either mother or her offspring. Therefore, we believe that treatment of such women, in the absence of central hypothyroidism, is unwarranted and should be considered experimental.

Overt Hyperthyroidism

Overt hyperthyroidism complicates approximately 2 of 1,000 pregnancies. Pregnant women with hyperthyroidism are at increased risk for spontaneous pregnancy loss, congestive heart failure, thyroid storm, preterm birth, preeclampsia, fetal growth restriction, and associated increased perinatal morbidity and mortality (31, 32). The most common cause of overt hyperthyroidism is Graves' disease, an organ-specific autoimmune process whereby thyroid-stimulating autoantibodies attach to and activate TSH receptors. In pregnant women with a history of Graves' disease, however, thyroid-stimulating antibody activity may actually decrease, leading to chemical remission during pregnancy (33). Other causes of overt hyperthyroidism include functioning adenoma or toxic nodular goiter, thyroiditis, and excessive thyroid hormone intake.

Gestational transient thyrotoxicosis is a unique form of hyperthyroidism associated with pregnancy. It is typically associated with hyperemesis gravidarum, and can be caused by high levels of hCG resulting from molar pregnancy. These high hCG levels lead to TSH-receptor stimulation and temporary hyperthyroidism. Women with gestational transient thyrotoxicosis are rarely symptomatic, and treatment with antithyroxine drugs has not been shown to be beneficial. With expectant management of hyperemesis gravidarum, serum free T_4 levels usually normalize in parallel with the decrease in hCG concentrations as pregnancy progresses beyond the first trimester. Notably, TSH levels may remain partially depressed several weeks after free T_4 levels have returned to the normal range. Gestational transient thyrotoxicosis has not been associated with poor pregnancy outcomes (Table 2-2).

Diagnostic Approach

As with hypothyroidism, clinical features of hyperthyroidism can easily be confused with those typical of pregnancy. Symptoms may include nervousness, heat intolerance, palpitations, thyromegaly or goiter, failure to gain weight or weight loss, and exophthalmos. Although nausea is common in early pregnancy, the occurrence of hyperemesis gravidarum in conjunction with weight loss can signify overt hyperthyroidism. Thyroid testing may be beneficial in these circumstances. Otherwise, routine testing in women with hyperemesis gravidarum is not recommended.

The diagnosis of overt hyperthyroidism can reliably be confirmed by evaluating serum TSH and free T_4 levels. In women with a depressed serum TSH level (less than 0.45 mIU/L), clinical hyperthyroidism is confirmed by an elevation of free T_4 (more than 1.8 ng/dL) concentration. However, as is true when diagnosing hypothyroidism during pregnancy, one must consider the impact of gestational age on measurement of TSH levels. For example, the 2.5th percentile for TSH levels during the first half of pregnancy in one study decreased to less than 0.1 mU/L (21). Despite the effect of pregnancy on maternal thyroxine levels, use of nonpregnant free T_4 level thresholds is recommended (0.7–1.8 ng/dL). Rarely, symptomatic hyperthyroidism is caused by an abnormally high serum T_3 level in women with normal free T_4 levels (T_3 thyrotoxicosis). In women with depressed TSH levels but with normal free T_4 levels, evaluation of free T_3 levels or the T_3 index may explain the presence of hypermetabolic symptoms. Evaluation of TSH receptor antibodies also has been shown to be helpful in assessing women with Graves' disease and may be associated with neonatal hypothyroidism (35, 36).

Therapeutic Approach

Treatment to achieve adequate metabolic control in women with hyperthyroid disease has been associated with improved pregnancy outcome (31, 32, 34) (Fig. 2-5). Thyrotoxicosis during pregnancy can nearly always be controlled by use of thioamide drugs. Some clinicians prefer propylthiouracil because it partially inhibits the conversion of T_4 to T_3 and crosses the placenta less readily than methimazole. Although not proved, methimazole use in early pregnancy has been associated with esophageal and choanal atresia as well as aplasia cutis in the fetus (37–39). Transient leukopenia occurs in approximately 10% of pregnant women treated with thioamides but usually does not necessitate cessation of therapy. In approximately 0.2% of women, agranulocytosis develops suddenly and mandates discontinuation of the drug. Agranulocytosis is not dose related, and because of its acute onset, serial leukocyte counts during therapy have not been helpful in prevention. Therefore, women given thioamide drugs should discontinue medication immediately if they develop a fever or sore throat until complete evaluation for agranulocytosis can be performed.

The dose of thioamide is empirical. In nonpregnant women, the American Thyroid Association recommends an initial daily dose of 100–600 mg for propylthiouracil or 10–40 mg for methimazole (40). It has been our experience that women with overt hypothyroidism diagnosed during pregnancy require a higher average daily propylthiouracil dose, and we recommend a starting dosage of at least 300 mg/d. The goal of treatment during pregnancy is to maintain free T_4 levels in the upper normal range using the lowest possible dose of thioamide (41). Improvement in free T_4 levels is generally seen in 4 weeks, and the median time to normalization of the TSH concentration is 6–8 weeks (42, 43). Importantly, caution against overtreatment is recommended because it may result in maternal or fetal hypothyroidism. Serial ultra-

Table 2-2. Pregnancy Outcomes in 239 Women With Overt Hyperthyroidism as Reported by Davis, Kriplani, Millar, and Their Colleagues (12, 31, 34)

Factor	Treated and Euthyroid n = 149	Uncontrolled Thyrotoxicosis n = 90
Maternal Outcome		
Preeclampsia	17 (11%)	15 (17%)
Heart failure	1	7 (8%)
Death	0	1
Perinatal Outcome		
Preterm delivery	12 (8%)	29 (32%)
Growth restriction	11 (7%)	15 (17%)
Stillborn	0/59	6/33 (18%)
Thyrotoxicosis	1	2
Hypothyroid	4	0
Goiter	2	0

Casey BM, Leveno KJ. Thyroid disease in pregnancy. Obstet Gynecol 2006;108:1283–92.

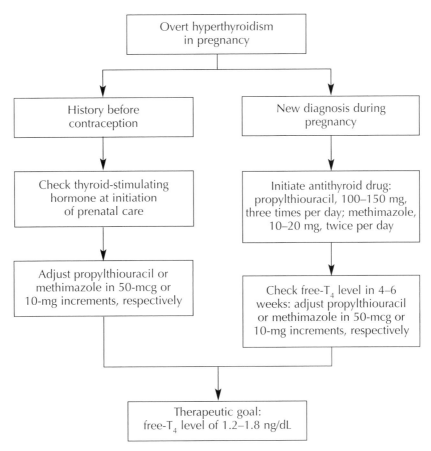

Fig. 2-5. Management algorithm for pregnant women with a history of hyperthyroidism or those newly diagnosed during pregnancy. (Casey BM, Leveno KJ. Thyroid disease in pregnancy. Obstet Gynecol 2006;108:1283–92.)

sound assessment of fetal thyroid size to assist in management of pregnant women taking thioamide drugs has been reported (35, 43). However, routine ultrasound evaluation of the fetal thyroid is currently not recommended.

There are alternatives for treatment of overt hyperthyroidism that are rarely undertaken during pregnancy. For example, thyroidectomy typically is reserved for treatment outside of pregnancy. Occasionally, however, women who cannot adhere to medical therapy or in whom therapy is toxic may benefit from surgical management (44). Ablative radioactive iodine is contraindicated in pregnancy because it can destroy the fetal thyroid. It has been recommended that women avoid pregnancy for 6 months after radio-ablative therapy (45).

Thyroid Storm or Heart Failure

Thyroid storm is an acute, life-threatening exacerbation of thyrotoxicosis. The classic findings are fever, tachycardia, tremor, nausea, vomiting, diarrhea, dehydration, and delirium or coma. Thyroid storm is rare in pregnancy

and its diagnosis is based entirely on clinical grounds in women with laboratory test results consistent with overt hyperthyroidism. Heart failure because of cardiomyopathy from excessive thyroxine in women with uncontrolled hyperthyroidism is more common in pregnant women (46).

Treatment of thyroid storm or thyrotoxic heart failure is similar. They both should be treated as medical emergencies in an intensive care setting (47). Specific treatment consists of 1g of propylthiouracil, given orally or crushed and placed through a nasogastric tube. This drug is continued in 200-mg doses every 6 hours. One hour after administration of the initial propylthiouracil dose, iodide is given to inhibit thyroid release of T_3 and T_4. It is given every 8 hours as 500–1,000 mg of intravenous sodium iodide, or it can be given orally as 5 drops of supersaturated solution of potassium iodide or as 10 drops of oral Lugol's solution every 8 hours. If there is a history of iodine-induced anaphylaxis, lithium carbonate, 300 mg every 6 hours, is given instead (48). Most authorities also recommend dexamethasone be given intravenously as 2 mg every 6 hours for 4 doses to further block peripheral conversion of T_4 to T_3. Treatment with a β-blocker to control tachycardia usually is reserved for heart rates of 120 beats per minute or higher. Propranolol, labetalol, and esmolol have all been used successfully in pregnancy (49).

Follow-up

Women with Graves' disease should be monitored closely after delivery because recurrence or aggravation of symptoms is not uncommon in the first few months postpartum. In asymptomatic women, TSH and free T_4 level evaluation should be performed approximately 6 weeks postpartum. Both propylthiouracil and methimazole are excreted in breast milk, but propylthiouracil is largely protein bound and does not seem to pose a significant risk to breastfed infants. Methimazole has been found in breastfed infants of treated women in amounts sufficient to cause thyroid dysfunction; however, at low doses (10–20 mg/d) it does not seem to pose a major risk to nursing infants (50). The American Academy of Pediatricians considers both compatible with breastfeeding (51).

Subclinical Hyperthyroidism

Subclinical hyperthyroidism is defined as a serum TSH concentration below the statistically defined lower limit of the reference range when serum free T_4 and free T_3 concentrations are within their reference range (7). Subclinical hyperthyroidism affects 1.7% of pregnant women and is more frequently diagnosed with the use of extremely sensitive, third-generation serum TSH assays (52). Its prevalence is higher in iodine-insufficient areas and increases with age. Subclinical hyperthyroidism has been reported to have long-term adverse sequelae that include osteoporosis, cardiovascular morbidity, and progression to overt thyrotoxicosis or thyroid failure. During pregnancy, however, the diagnosis of subclinical hyperthyroidism has not been found to be associated with adverse outcomes (52). In fact, subclinical hyperthyroidism may even have a protective effect against the development of hypertension during pregnancy (52).

At present, there is no convincing evidence that subclinical hyperthyroidism should be treated in nonpregnant individuals. Therefore, treatment during pregnancy seems especially unwarranted because maternal antithyroid drugs cross the placenta. Further studies are necessary to ascertain whether there are any adverse long-term fetal effects of maternal subclinical hyperthyroidism. The potential for long-term adverse sequelae in the mother suggests that women identified with subclinical hyperthyroidism may benefit from periodic surveillance later in life.

Postpartum Thyroiditis

Transient autoimmune thyroiditis has been identified in up to 10% of women during the first year after childbirth (53, 54). Histologically, a destructive lymphocytic thyroiditis is identified. The likelihood of developing postpartum thyroiditis antedates pregnancy and is related to increasing serum levels of thyroid autoantibodies. Women with high antibody titers in early pregnancy are most commonly affected (55). In clinical practice, however, thyroiditis is infrequently diagnosed because it typically develops months after delivery and has vague and nonspecific symptoms. These include depression, carelessness, and memory impairment (56). Risk factors other than antithyroid antibodies include previous thyroid dysfunction or a family history of thyroid or other autoimmune disease. For example, as many as 25% of women with insulin-dependent diabetes mellitus develop postpartum thyroid dysfunction (57).

There are two recognized clinical phases of postpartum thyroiditis. In the first phase, between 1 month and 4 months after delivery, approximately 4% of all women develop transient thyrotoxicosis from excessive release of thyroid hormone from glandular disruption (58). The onset is abrupt, and a small, painless goiter often is found. Fatigue and palpitations are the most common symptoms in women with early postpartum thyroiditis. Antithyroid medications such as thioamides are typically ineffective, and approximately two thirds of these women return to a euthyroid state. If symptoms are severe, however, a β-blocker may be given. In the second phase, between 4 months and 8 months postpartum, 2–5% of women develop hypothyroidism (53, 59). Importantly, hypothyroidism can even develop within 1 month of the onset of thyroiditis. Thyromegaly and other symptoms are common and more prominent than during the thyrotoxic phase. Thyroxine replacement is recommended for at least 6–12 months. Most women identified with postpartum thyroiditis will return to the euthyroid state within 12 months of delivery. Women who experience either type of postpartum thyroiditis have approximately a 30% risk of developing permanent hypothyroidism (60, 25).

References

1. Haddow JE, Palomaki GE, Allan WC, Williams JR, Knight GJ, Gagnon J, et al. Maternal thyroid deficiency during pregnancy and subsequent neuropsychological development of the child. N Engl J Med 1999;341:549–55.

2. Pop VJ, Kuijpens JL, van Baar AL, Verkerk G, van Son MM, de Vijlder JJ, et al. Low maternal free thyroxine concentrations during early pregnancy are associated with impaired psychomotor development in infancy. Clin Endocrinol (Oxf) 1999;50:149–55.

3. Casey BM, Dashe JS, Wells CE, McIntire DD, Byrd W, Leveno KJ, et al. Subclinical hypothyroidism and pregnancy outcomes. Obstet Gynecol 2005;105:239–45.

4. Stagnaro-Green A, Chen X, Bogden JD, Davies TF, Scholl TO. The thyroid and pregnancy: a novel risk factor for very preterm delivery. Thyroid 2005;15:351–57.

5. Gharib H, Tuttle RM, Baskin HJ, Fish LH, Singer PA, McDermott MT, et al. Consensus Statement #1. Subclinical Thyroid Dysfunction: a joint statement on management form the American Association of clinical Endocrinologists, the American Thyroid Association, and The Endocrine Society. Thyroid 2005;15:24–8.

6. U.S. Preventative Services Task Force, Agency for Healthcare Research and Quality. Available at: www.ahrq.gov/clinic/ 3rduspstf/thyrrs.htm. Retrieved August 16, 2006.

7. Surks MI, Ortiz E, Daniels GH. Sawin CT, Col NF, Cobin RH, et al. Subclinical thyroid disease: scientific review and guidelines for diagnosis and management. JAMA 2004;291:228–38.

8. Clinical management guidelines for obstetrician–gynecologists. ACOG Practice Bulletin No. 37. American College of Obstetricians and Gynecologists. Obstet Gynecol 2002;100:387–96.

9. Rasmussen NG, Hornnes PJ, Hegedus L. Ultrasonography determined thyroid size in pregnancy and postpartum: the goitrogenic effect of pregnancy. Am J Obstet Gynecol 1989;160:1216–20.

10. Glinoer D, de Nayer P, Bourdoux P, Lemone M, Robyn C, van Steirteghem A, et al. Regulation of maternal thyroid during pregnancy. J Clin Endocrinol Metab 1990;71: 276–87.

11. Morreale de Escobar G, Obregon MJ, Escobar del Rey F. Is neuropsychological development related to maternal hypothyroidism or to maternal hypothyroxinemia? J Clin Endocrinol Metab 2000;85:3975–87.

12. Davis LE, Leveno KJ, Cunningham FG. Hypothyroidism complicating pregnancy. Obstet Gynecol 1988;72:108–12.

13. Leung AS, Millar LK, Koonings PP, Montoro M, Mestman JH. Perinatal outcome in hypothyroid pregnancies. Obstet Gynecol 1993;81:349–53.

14. Cao XY, Jiang XM, Dou ZH, Rakeman MA, Zhang ML, O'Donnell K, et al. Timing of vulnerability of the brain to iodine deficiency in endemic cretinism. N Engl J Med 1994;331:1739–44.

15. Delange F, de Benoist B, Pretell E, Dunn JT. Iodine deficiency in the world: where do we stand at the turn of the century. Thyroid 2001;11:437–47.

16. Canaris GJ, Manowitz NR, Mayor G, Ridgway EC. The Colorado thyroid disease prevalence study. Arch Intern Med 2000;160:526–34.

17. Abalovich M, Gutierrez S, Alcaraz G, Maccallini G, Garcia A, Levalle O. Overt and subclinical hypothyroidism complicating pregnancy. Thyroid 2002;12:63–8.

18. Vanderpump MP, Tunbridge WM, French JM, Appleton D, Bates D, Clark F, et al. The incidence of thyroid-disorders in the community: a twenty-year follow-up of the Whickham Survey. Clin Endocrinol (Oxf) 1995;43:55–68.

19. Wartofsky L, Dickey RA. The evidence for a narrower thyrotropin reference range is compelling. J Clin Endocrinol Metab 2005;90:5483–8.

20. Surks MI, Goswami G, Daniels GH. The thyrotropin reference range should remain unchanged. J Clin Endocrinol Metab 2005;90:5489–96.

21. Dashe JS, Casey BM, Wells CE, McIntire DD, Byrd EW, Leveno KJ, et al. Thyroid-stimulating hormone in singleton and twin pregnancy: importance of gestational age-specific reference ranges. Obstet Gynecol 2005;106:753–7.

22. Mandel SJ, Spencer CA, Hollowell JG. Are detection and treatment of thyroid insufficiency in pregnancy feasible? Thyroid 2005;15:44–53.

23. Stagnaro-Green A, Roman SH, Cobin RH, el Harazy E, Alvarez-Marfany M, Davies TF. Detection of at-risk pregnancy by means of highly sensitive assays for thyroid autoantibodies. JAMA 1990;264:1422–5.

24. Glinoer D, Soto MF, Bourdoux P, Lejeune B, Delange F, Lemone M, et al. Pregnancy in patients with mild thyroid abnormalities: maternal and neonatal repercussions. J Clin Endocrinol Metab 1991;73:421–7.

25. Premawardhana LD, Parkes AB, Ammari F, John R, Darke C, Adams H, Lazarus JH. Postpartum thyroiditis and long-term thyroid status: prognostic influence of thyroid peroxidase antibodies and ultrasound echogenicity. J Clin Endocrinol Metab 2000;85:71–5.

26. Dickey RA, Wartofsky L, Feld S. Optimal thyrotropin level: normal ranges and reference intervals are not equivalent. Thyroid 2005;15:1035–9.

27. Alexander EK, Marqusee E, Lawrence J, Jarolim P, Fischer GA, Larsen PR. Timing and magnitude of increases in levothyroxine requirements during pregnancy in women with hypothyroidism. N Engl J Med 2004;351:241–9.

28. Franklin R, O'Grady C, Carpenter L. Neonatal thyroid function: comparison between breast-fed and bottle-fed infants. J Pediatr 1985;106:124–6.

29. Pop VJ, Brouwers EP, Vader HL, Vulsma T, van Baar AL, de Vijlder JJ. Maternal hypothyroxinaemia during early pregnancy and subsequent child development: a 3-year follow-up study. Clin Endocrinol (Oxf) 2003;59:282–8.

30. Pedraza PE, Obregon MJ, Escobar-Morreale HF, del Rey FE, de Escobar GM. Mechanisms of adaptation to iodine deficiency in rats: thyroid status is tissue specific. Its relevance for man. Endocrinology 2006;147:2098–108.

31. Davis LE, Lucas MJ, Hankins GD, Roark ML, Cunningham FG. Thyrotoxicosis complicating pregnancy. Am J Obstet Gynecol 1989;160:63–70.

32. Millar LK, Wing DA, Leung AS, Koonings PP, Montoro MN, Mestman JH. Low birth weight and preeclampsia in pregnancies complicated by hyperthyroidism. Obstet Gynecol 1994;84:946–9.

33. Kung AW, Jones BM. A change from stimulatory to blocking antibody activity in Graves' disease during pregnancy. J Clin Endocrinol Metab 1998;83:514–8.

34. Kriplani A, Buckshee K, Bhargava VL, Takkar D, Ammini AC. Maternal and perinatal outcome in thyrotoxicosis complicating pregnancy. Eur J Obstet Gynecol Reprod Biol 1994;54:159–63.

35. Luton D, Le Gac I, Vuillard E, Castanet M, Guibourdenche J, Noel M, et al. Management of Graves' disease during pregnancy: the key role of fetal thyroid gland monitoring. J Clin Endocrinol Metab 2005;90:6093–8.

36. Weetman AP. Graves' disease. N Engl J Med 2000;343: 1236–48.

37. Milham S Jr. Scalp defects in infants of mothers treated for hyperthyroidism with methimazole or carbimazole during pregnancy. Teratology 1985;32:321.

38. Mandel SJ, Cooper DS. The use of antithyroid drugs in pregnancy and lactation. J Clin Endocrinol Metab 2001;86:2354–9.

39. Karlsson FA, Axelsson O, Melhus H. Severe embryopathy and exposure to methimazole in early pregnancy. J Clin Endocrinol Metab 2002;87:947–9.

40. Singer PA, Cooper DS, Levy EG, Ladenson PW, Braverman LE, Daniels G, et al. Treatment guidelines for patients with hyperthyroidism and hypothyroidism. Standards of Care Committee, American Thyroid Association. JAMA 1995;273:808–12.

41. Ecker JL, Musci TJ. Treatment of thyroid disease in pregnancy. Obstet Gynecol Clin North Am 1997;24:575–89.

42. Ecker JL, Musci TJ. Thyroid function and disease in pregnancy. Curr Probl Obstet Gynecol Fertil 2000;23:109–22.

43. Cohen O, Pinhas-Hamiel O, Sivan E, Dolitski M, Lipitz S, Achiron R. Serial in utero ultrasonographic measurements of the fetal thyroid: a new complementary tool in the management of maternal hyperthyroidism in pregnancy. Prenat Diagn 2003;23:740–2.

44. Davison S, Lennard TW, Davison J, Kendall-Taylor P, Perros P. Management of a pregnant patient with Graves' disease complicated by thionamide-induced neutropenia in the first trimester. Clin Endocrinol (Oxf) 2001;54:559–61.

45. International Commission on Radiological Protection. Release of patients after therapy with unsealed radionuclides [published erratum appears in Ann ICRP. 2004;34:281]. Ann ICRP 2004;34:1–79.

46. Sheffield JS, Cunningham FG. Thyrotoxicosis and heart failure that complicate pregnancy. Am J Obstet Gynecol 2004;190: 211–7.

47. Zeeman GG, Wendel GD Jr, Cunningham FG. A blueprint for obstetric critical care. Am J Obstet Gynecol 2003;188:532–6.

48. Burch HB, Wartofsky L. Life-threatening thyrotoxicosis. Thyroid storm. Endocrinol Metab Clin North Am 1993;22:263–77.

49. Bowman ML, Bergmann M, Smith JF. Intrapartum labetalol for the treatment of maternal and fetal thyrotoxicosis. Thyroid 1998;8:795–6.

50. Cooper DS. Antithyroid drugs: to breast-feed or not to breast-feed. Am J Obstet Gynecol 1987;157:234–5.

51. American Academy of Pediatricians, Committee on Drugs. American Academy of Pediatricians 2001;108:776–89.

52. Casey BM, Dashe JS, Wells CE, McIntire DD, Leveno KJ, Cunningham FG. Subclinical hyperthyroidism and pregnancy outcomes. Obstet Gynecol 2006;107:337–41.

53. Amino N, Tada H, Hidaka Y, Izumi Y, et al. Postpartum autoimmune thyroid syndrome. Endocr J 2000;47:645–55.

54. Dayan CM, Daniels GH. Chronic autoimmune thyroiditis. N Engl J Med 1996;335:99–107.

55. Pearce EN, Farwell AP, Braverman LE. Thyroiditis [published erratum appears in N Engl J Med 2003;349:620]. N Engl J Med 2003;348:2646–55.

56. Hayslip CC, Fein HG, O'Donnell VM, Friedman DS, Klein TA, Smallridge RC. The value of serum antimicrosomal antibody testing in screening for symptomatic postpartum thyroid dysfunction. Am J Obstet Gynecol 1988;159:203–9.

57. Alvarez-Marfany M, Roman SH, Drexler AJ, Robertson C, Stagnaro-Green A. Long-term prospective study of postpartum thyroid dysfunction in women with insulin dependent diabetes mellitus. J Clin Endocrinol Metab 1994;79:10–6.

58. Lucas A, Pizarro E, Granada ML, Salinas I, Foz M, Sanmarti A. Postpartum thyroiditis: epidemiology and clinical evolution in a nonselected population. Thyroid 2000;10:71–7.

59. Jansson R, Dahlberg PA, Karlsson FA. Postpartum thyroiditis. Baillieres Clin Endocrinol Metab 1988;2:619–35.

60. Muller AF, Drexhage HA, Berghout A. Postpartum thyroiditis and autoimmune thyroiditis in women of childbearing age: recent insights and consequences for antenatal and postnatal care. Endocr Rev 2001;22:605–30.

CHAPTER 3

Chronic Renal Disease in Pregnancy

SUSAN M. RAMIN, ALEX C. VIDAEFF, EDWARD R. YEOMANS, AND LARRY C. GILSTRAP III

$\mathcal{R}$enal disease during pregnancy is relatively uncommon. In a population-based study of pregnant women with kidney disease, the diagnosis of renal disease before pregnancy was only 0.03% (1). There is, however, a paucity of scientific data regarding the general topic of renal disease in pregnancy on which to base clinical management and counseling recommendations.

The present review focuses on the impact of chronic renal disease on pregnancy outcome. Our primary goal was to examine pregnancy outcome in women with chronic renal disease, especially with regard to the degree of renal insufficiency. A secondary objective was to examine the effect of pregnancy on the progression of renal disease. As very aptly pointed out in one study, "the potential impact of pregnancy is best considered by categories of functional renal status before conception" (2).

A PubMed, MEDLINE, and Ovid search of the literature from January 1990 through December 2005 was accomplished. Studies were limited to the English language and those including human subjects. The keywords used were "chronic renal disease or insufficiency in pregnancy" or "pregnancy outcome," "incidence and epidemiology of renal disease in pregnancy" and "pregnancy outcome in women with mild, moderate, moderate-to-severe, and severe renal insufficiency." We also looked at keyword combinations such as "adverse fetal and maternal outcomes," "natural history of women with chronic renal disease or insufficiency," or "impaired renal function and kidney disease in pregnancy." Studies of pregnant women with preexisting renal disease were included if both outcome data and degree of renal insufficiency were reported.

Of the articles we reviewed, 23 met our inclusion criteria. Our search of the literature did not reveal any randomized clinical trials or meta-analyses. The available information is derived from opinion, reviews, retrospective series, and limited prospective observational series. Large observational studies included in major texts during this time period were also reviewed if they included maternal or perinatal outcome data and the degree of renal insufficiency.

Mild renal insufficiency was defined as a serum creatinine level of 0.9–1.4 mg/dL (3, 4). Moderate renal insufficiency was defined as a serum creatinine level of 1.5–2.5 mg/dL (5). Severe renal insufficiency was defined as a serum creatinine level greater than 2.5 mg/dL (2, 5, 6). Some investigators use 1.5–2.9 mg/dL to define moderate renal insufficiency and 3 mg/dL or greater to define severe renal insufficiency.

Incidence

We could not ascertain the exact incidence of chronic renal disease in pregnancy from the available literature. Because pregnant women are not routinely screened for renal dysfunction, the condition often is unrecognized (especially in those with mild dysfunction). However, it does seem reasonable to conclude that chronic renal disease in pregnancy is uncommon. For example, in an 18-year review from Parkland Memorial Hospital, there were only 37 women whose pregnancies were complicated by moderate-to-severe renal insufficiency for an approximate incidence of 2 per 10,000 women (5). In a more recent review in 2004 (7), the prevalence of moderate chronic renal insufficiency was 6 per 10,000 births in women in their hospital from 1989 to 1999. A review of Colorado birth and death certificates from 1989 to 2001 found 911 births from women with a diagnosis of kidney disease out of 747,368 births for a frequency of 0.12% (12 per 10,000) (8).

There are several possible reasons why chronic renal insufficiency is uncommonly associated with pregnancy. First and foremost is the fact that many women with significant renal insufficiency or renal failure are either beyond childbearing age or infertile (9). Another important reason may be incomplete reporting or data collection. For example, in a review of preexisting maternal medical conditions, the use of the combination of birth certificates and hospital discharge data was superior to that of birth certificate data alone for confirming renal disease in pregnancy (10). Additionally, the incidence of mild renal disease is often not included in many of the reported series.

Physiology and Pathophysiology

It is important for the practicing clinician to be cognizant of the various physiologic and anatomic changes involving the urinary system that are induced by pregnancy. Probably the most significant of these is the increase in glomerular filtration rate and renal plasma flow, which starts very early in pregnancy and exceeds nonpregnant levels by 50%. This, in turn, results in a significantly higher endogenous creatinine clearance (110–150 mL/min) and lower serum creatinine (0.5–0.8 mg/dL) and serum urea nitrogen (9–12 mg/dL) levels. Anatomically, there is a slight increase in kidney size and marked dilation of the renal pelves, calyces, and ureters (Figs. 3-1, 3-2). To compensate for a 10-mm reduction in P_{CO_2} (averages 28–30 mm Hg), the kidneys excrete more

bicarbonate in pregnancy, which results in a 4–5 mEq/L decrease in serum bicarbonate (averages 20–22 mEq/L). Serum osmolality also decreases by approximately 10 mOsm/L (serum sodium 5 mEq/L).

There are many different causes of chronic renal disease or end-stage renal disease in pregnancy, each with its own intrinsic pathophysiologic mechanism of disease. Some of the more common causes include type 1 diabetes, glomerulonephritis, hypertension, lupus nephritis, immunoglobulin A (IgA) nephropathy, and polycystic kidney disease. It is beyond the scope of this review to discuss the pathophysiology of each disease entity separately. However, summarized in Table 3-1 are specific renal diseases associated with pregnancy and outcomes (2). The natural history of renal disease during and after pregnancy most often relates to prepregnant renal function and the presence or absence of hypertension. There also is no consensus about whether pregnancy may adversely affect specific renal diseases.

Overview of Chronic Renal Disease and Pregnancy

Although pregnant women with chronic renal disease are at an increased risk for both maternal and perinatal morbidity, many such pregnancies can be expected to result

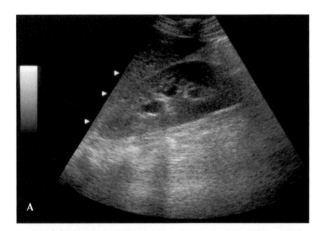

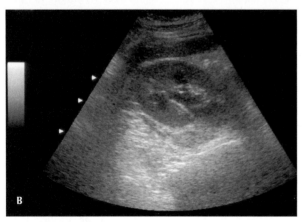

Fig. 3-1. Ultrasound images in the longitudinal (**A**) and transverse (**B**) planes of the right kidney demonstrate moderate dilation of the collecting system consistent with hydronephrosis in a woman whose pregnancy is at 24 weeks of gestation. (Courtesy of Dr. Diane Twickler, University of Texas Southwestern Medical School, Dallas, TX.)

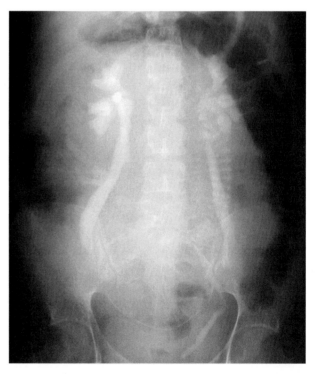

Fig. 3-2. One-shot intravenous pyelogram at 30 minutes of a woman in the late third trimester of pregnancy with moderate hydronephrosis and contrast in the renal collecting system. (Courtesy of Dr. Diane Twickler, University of Texas Southwestern Medical School, Dallas, TX.)

Table 3-1. Chronic Renal Disease and Pregnancy

Renal Disease	Effects
Chronic glomerulonephritis and focal glomerular sclerosis	Increased incidence of high blood pressure late in gestation but usually no adverse effect if renal function is preserved and hypertension is absent before gestation. Some disagree, believing coagulation changes in pregnancy exacerbate disease, especially immunoglobulin A nephropathy, membranoproliferative glomerulonephritis, and focal glomerular sclerosis.
Immunoglobulin A nephropathy	Some cite risks of sudden escalating or uncontrolled hypertension and renal deterioration. Most note good outcome when renal function is preserved.
Chronic pyelonephritis (infectious tubulointerstitial disease)	Bacteriuria in pregnancy and may lead to exacerbation.
Reflux nephropathy	In the past, some emphasized risks of sudden escalating hypertension and worsening of renal function. Consensus now is that results are satisfactory when preconception function is only mildly affected and hypertension is absent. Vigilant screening for urinary tract infections is necessary.
Urolithiasis	Ureteral dilatation and stasis do not seem to affect natural history, but infections can be more frequent. Stents have been successfully placed, and sonographically controlled ureterostomy has been performed during gestation.
Polycystic kidney disease	Functional impairment and hypertension are usually minimal in childbearing years.
Diabetic nephropathy	No adverse effect on the renal lesion. Increased frequency of infections, edema, or preeclampsia.
Systemic lupus erythematosus	Prognosis is most favorable if disease is in remission 6 or more months before conception. Some authorities increase steroid dosage in immediate postpartum period.
Periarteritis nodosa	Fetal prognosis is poor. It is associated with maternal death. Therapeutic abortion should be considered.
Scleroderma	If onset occurs during pregnancy, there can be rapid overall deterioration. Reactivation of quiescent scleroderma can occur during pregnancy and postpartum.
Previous urologic surgery	Depending on original reason for surgery, there may be other malformations of the urogenital tract. Urinary tract infection is common during pregnancy, and renal function may undergo reversible decrease. There is no significant obstructive problem, but cesarean delivery might be necessary for abnormal presentation or to avoid disruption of the continence mechanism if artificial sphincters or neourethras are present.
After nephrectomy, solitary and pelvic kidneys	Pregnancy is well tolerated. It might be associated with other malformations of the urogenital tract. Dystocia rarely occurs with a pelvic kidney.

Davison JM, Lindheimer MD. Renal Disorders. In: Creasy RK, Resnik R, Iams JD, editors. Maternal–fetal medicine: principles and practice. 5th ed. Philadelphia (PA): Saunders; p. 901–23. Copyright © 2004, with permission from Elsevier.

in a successful outcome. Maternal morbidity associated with chronic renal disease includes the development of preeclampsia, deterioration of renal function and end-stage renal disease, preterm delivery, anemia, chronic hypertension, and cesarean delivery (1, 3, 5, 11–14). One report noted that 40% of pregnant women with chronic renal insufficiency had preeclampsia, 48% anemia, and 56% chronic hypertension (7). In addition, the pre-

maturity rate was 60%, and the cesarean delivery rate was 52%.

In a review of 46 pregnancies in 38 women with chronic renal insufficiency, 22% had preeclampsia, 22% preterm delivery, and 13% growth restriction (4). The cesarean delivery rate was 24%. The low incidence of complications in this review can be traced to the fact that nearly 90% of the women had only mild renal insufficiency.

Only two (4.4%) of the newborns required admission to the neonatal intensive care unit (NICU).

A study of 82 pregnancies in 67 women with moderate-to-severe renal insufficiency showed a prematurity rate of 59%, fetal growth restriction rate of 37%, cesarean delivery rate of 59%, and an infant survival rate of 93% (3). A review of 43 pregnancies in 40 women reported an overall pregnancy loss rate of 32.6% (14). A study of 43 pregnancies in 30 women showed a "success rate" for live births of 82% after excluding first-trimester abortions (15). The reason for the variances in outcome in the literature is becase of the different degrees of renal insufficiency and various types of primary renal disease in the pregnant women studied.

Hypertension is an indicator for poor pregnancy outcome. It is fair to conclude that pregnant women with minimal renal dysfunction and normal blood pressures have more than a 90% chance of a successful outcome (16). Moreover, it is unlikely that pregnancy in this group will affect the progression of renal disease (16). Summarized in Table 3-2 is the effect of blood pressure and renal deterioration on pregnancy outcome (2). The effects of pregnancy on other renal disease entities such as diabetic nephropathy, lupus nephropathy, membranoproliferative glomerulonephritis, scleroderma, and periarteritis nodosa are summarized in Table 3-1 (2).

Pregnancy Outcome According to the Degree of Renal Insufficiency

The degree of impairment of renal function appears to be the major determinant for pregnancy outcome. Most outcome studies lack an appropriate control group, and the estimates of comparative risk are generally flawed. In addition to the severity of renal disease (Table 3-3), the presence or absence of hypertension with or without superimposed preeclampsia (Table 3-2) also appears to

be a significant prognostic feature influencing outcome (2, 14). In a unique approach, a regression model was used in one study for the prediction of successful pregnancy outcome (4); the only clinical predictor was preexisting hypertension ($P = .01$). Interestingly, these authors found that other often-cited prognostic factors, such as the type of renal disease and the serum creatinine (prepregnancy and second-trimester), did not correlate with successful pregnancy outcome ($P > .1$) (4). Despite these findings, most evidence supports the premise that the degree of renal functional impairment does predict the outcome of pregnancy.

Mild Renal Insufficiency

Women with mild renal disease (ie, serum creatinine 0.9–1.4 mg/dL) have a lower risk of adverse pregnancy outcomes than those with more advanced renal disease. The aforementioned series (4) included 89% with mild renal disease. There were no stillbirths and the complication rate was very low (4.4–22%). In another report by this group on some of the same patients, the authors reported that the outcome was good even when taking into account the type or etiology of renal disease (21). For example, the live birth rate was 98% in the women with primary renal disease, 96% in the women with diabetic nephropathy, and 89% in the women with a renal allograft. Although an assessment of renal function at 2 years postpartum revealed that 5% of the women with renal insufficiency (mostly mild) had an increase in serum creatinine defined as more than 1 mg/dL above baseline, none of the women progressed to end-stage renal disease (4). Thus, based on our review of the available data, it would appear that the perinatal outcome for pregnant women with mild renal insufficiency is only slightly affected, and irreversible deterioration of maternal renal function is uncommon.

Table 3-2. Effect of Blood Pressure and Renal Deterioration (Alone or Together) on Nonsuccessful Obstetric Outcome

	Hypertension (%)	Renal Deterioration (%)	Both (%)
Absent throughout pregnancy	6	7	7
Present at some time during pregnancy	12	12	19
Present and managed from first trimester	10	—	13
Present from first trimester and not managed	50	40	55
Present only during third trimester	8	9	10

Estimated from Cunningham et al, 1990 (5); Abe, 1996 (17); Jones and Hayslett, 1996 (3); Jungers et al, 1996 (18); Jungers et al, 1997 (15); Jungers and Chauveau (19).

Davison JM, Lindheimer MD. Renal disorders. In: Creasy RK, Resnik R, Iams JD, editors. Maternal–fetal medicine: principles and practice. 5th ed. Philadelphia (PA): Saunders; p. 901–23. Copyright © 2004, with permission from Elsevier.

Table 3-3. Pregnancy Prospects for Women With Moderate and Severe Chronic Renal Disease

Problems in Pregnancy (%)	Successful Obstetric Outcome (%)	Long-Term Problems (%)	End-Stage Renal Failure Within 1 Year (%)
90 (81–97)	84 (65–93)	50 (30–57)	15 (10–23)

Values are means, with ranges in parentheses. Data are from 107 women in 125 pregnancies from Jones and Hayslett, 1996 (3); Jungers and Chauveau, 1997 (20).

Davison JM, Lindheimer MD. Renal Disorders. In: Creasy RK, Resnik R, and Iams JD, editors. Maternal–fetal medicine principles and practice. 5th ed. Philadelphia (PA): Saunders, p. 901–23.2. Copyright © 2004, with permission from Elsevier.

Moderate-to-Severe Renal Insufficiency

The rate of complications is clearly higher in pregnant women with moderate-to-severe renal insufficiency than in women with mild renal disease. Chronic hypertension, preeclampsia, anemia, fetal growth restriction, and prematurity are common complications in pregnant women with moderate-to-severe renal insufficiency. In one observational study, there were 37 pregnancies complicated by chronic renal disease that was moderate (serum creatinine level 1.4–2.5 mg/dL) to severe (serum creatinine level greater than 2.5 mg/dL) (5). In the 26 women with moderate renal disease, 62% had chronic hypertension, 58% had preeclampsia, and 73% had anemia. Of the women with moderate renal disease, 80% of those with hypertension versus 30% without hypertension developed superimposed preeclampsia. These 26 women had a live-birth rate of 88% (23 of 26 women, excluding two spontaneous abortions and one stillbirth), a fetal growth restriction rate of 35%, and preterm birth rate of 30%. In the 11 women with severe renal insufficiency, 82% had chronic hypertension, 64% had preeclampsia, and 100% had anemia (5). The fetal outcomes in these women with severe renal disease include a live-birth rate of 64% (7 of 11 women, excluding the two elective abortions and two spontaneous abortions), fetal growth restriction rate of 43%, and preterm birth rate of 86%. There were no stillbirths in the 11 women with severe insufficiency. In this series, five women with moderate renal insufficiency and one with severe disease had worsening of renal function (50% or greater increase in serum creatinine during gestation).

Our review of the literature indicates that, unlike pregnant women with mild renal insufficiency, women with moderate-to-severe renal disease are at risk for worsening of renal function during pregnancy or postpartum. Almost 50% of the pregnant women with a serum creatinine of 1.4 mg/dL or greater had an increase in serum creatinine during pregnancy to a mean of 2.5 mg/dL in the third trimester (3). The risk of accelerated progression to end-stage renal disease is highest when the serum creatinine level is above 2 mg/dL at the beginning of pregnancy (3). Within 6 months after delivery, 23% of such women had progression to end-stage renal disease.

The degree of renal function impairment is not the only prognosticator. Renal disease associated with hypertension increases the risk of maternal and neonatal adverse outcomes to an even greater extent. An increase in fetal loss by a factor of 10 has been reported when hypertension was present at conception at comparable serum creatinine levels (15).

Proteinuria

Proteinuria may also be an indicator for chronic renal disease. For example, in a review of 65 pregnancies in 53 asymptomatic women with significant proteinuria (greater than 500 mg/d) and no known preexisting renal disease or diabetes, renal insufficiency coexisted in 62%, and 40% had chronic hypertension (22). Although 93% of 53 pregnancies resulted in live newborns (excluding abortions), almost one half were delivered prematurely and almost one quarter had growth restriction. Importantly, 20% of the 53 women with follow-up had progressed to end-stage renal disease at a median of 5 years. These authors concluded that asymptomatic proteinuria was associated with both adverse pregnancy outcome and long-term progression of renal disease (22). Unfortunately, neither the frequency of "significant" proteinuria on dipstick nor the proportion of women screened with a 24-hour urine collection who had more than 500 mg/24 h can be determined from their study (22).

In pregnant women with asymptomatic proteinuria, we recommend the following during routine prenatal care. First, identify the pregnant woman who has persistent 2-plus protein or more on dipstick. Second, obtain a 24-hour urine collection for protein and creatinine clearance or at least a spot urine collection for a protein/creatinine ratio (23). Additionally, pregnant women with proteinuria plus renal insufficiency are candidates after delivery for short- and long-term follow-up of renal function and should be referred to a nephrologist.

Management

Prepregnancy or Early Prenatal Counseling

We counsel women that fertility is somewhat dependent upon the degree of renal insufficiency, as is pregnancy outcome (24). We also counsel women that renal disease may progress during pregnancy, especially in those with moderate-to-severe disease (24, 25). Most pregnancies with moderate-to-severe renal insufficiency will result in a premature birth (25). Moreover, women with serum creatinine levels greater than 2 mg/dL should be counseled that they have a one-in-three chance of progressing to end-stage renal disease within 1 year postpartum (6, 26). Pregnant women requiring dialysis are at an even higher risk for complications and adverse pregnancy outcomes.

Pregnancy outcome is also related to the degree of hypertension, the effectiveness of antihypertensive therapy, and the presence or absence of superimposed preeclampsia (6, 16). It is important to counsel pregnant women about the increased risk of adverse outcomes and the need for blood pressure control and to explain to them that the antihypertensive medications belonging to the angiotensin-converting enzyme inhibitor group (ie, ACE inhibitors) and angiotensin-receptor blockers are contraindicated during pregnancy because these drugs have the potential for causing teratogenic effects (hypocalvaria) and damage to fetal kidneys (renal failure, oliguria, and demise) (24). Angiotensin-converting enzyme inhibitors and angiotensin-receptor blockers should be discontinued before attempting pregnancy or as soon as possible in the first trimester after pregnancy is diagnosed. There are some women with severe hypertension and chronic renal disease in whom discontinuation of these agents may not be clinically feasible. It also is important to control blood pressure in these women and to assess renal function. One of the reasons to prescribe antihypertensive medication in pregnant women with mild chronic hypertension is the presence of underlying renal disease, and we use these agents to maintain diastolic blood pressure at 90 mm Hg or less.

During Pregnancy

Management guidelines for pregnant women with chronic renal disease are based solely on retrospective and observational series and opinions. We believe that the care of pregnant women with underlying renal disease should entail a multidisciplinary approach at a tertiary center and include a maternal–fetal medicine specialist and a nephrologist. Pregnant women with chronic renal disease often require more frequent prenatal visits for maternal and fetal monitoring depending on the severity of their renal insufficiency. We prefer to monitor these women every 2 weeks until 30–32 weeks of gestation and then weekly for the remainder of the pregnancy.

In addition to the routine prenatal laboratory tests, baseline renal function should be assessed and then repeated at least every 4–6 weeks throughout pregnancy. This evaluation should include but is not limited to a serum creatinine, serum urea nitrogen, electrolytes, albumin, cholesterol, hemoglobin, hematocrit, platelet count, urinalysis, and urine culture. In addition, a 24-hour urine collection for volume, creatinine clearance, and protein to monitor for worsening of renal function or the development of preeclampsia is also recommended. Indications for renal biopsy during pregnancy are controversial. At present there are no scientific data on which to base specific clinical recommendations regarding renal biopsy during pregnancy. Moreover, specialists prefer to defer the procedure to the postpartum period because of the associated complications, which include gross hematuria, perirenal hematoma, and severe flank pain.

Maternal anemia that occurs in pregnant women with chronic renal disease is caused by decreased erythropoietin production and shortened red cell survival. This anemia can be managed with oral iron therapy, recombinant erythropoietin, intravenous iron, or blood transfusions. We consider recombinant erythropoietin when the hematocrit falls below 19%. The clinician should be cognizant of the fact that erythropoietin may cause or aggravate preexisting hypertension.

We usually institute fetal surveillance such as the biophysical profile at 30–32 weeks of gestation. However, it may sometimes be necessary to begin at 28 weeks of gestation or earlier, depending on the degree of renal insufficiency, hypertension, fetal growth restriction, and past obstetric outcome (ie, prior stillbirth). A baseline ultrasonography is performed for dating, and fetal growth is monitored every 4–6 weeks by ultrasonography in pregnant women with chronic renal insufficiency. In the absence of maternal or fetal deterioration, consideration should be given to delivery at or near term.

Dialysis During Pregnancy

The indications for acute dialysis during pregnancy are similar to those in nonpregnant individuals. The indications include severe refractory metabolic acidosis, retention of toxins, electrolyte imbalance, especially severe refractory hyperkalemia, and volume overload leading to congestive heart failure or pulmonary edema unresponsive to diuretics. Dialysis may be initiated earlier in pregnancy during the course of acute renal failure when the serum urea nitrogen levels reach 60–80 mg/dL or greater or the serum creatinine exceeds 5–7 mg/dL (9, 27) because of the increased risk of fetal demise.

There are little scientific data regarding chronic dialysis in pregnancy. However, the data from a large registry of pregnancy in dialysis patients have been analyzed (28). In a survey of 2,299 dialysis units involving more than 6,000 women aged 14–44 years (1,699 peritoneal dialysis and 4,531 hemodialysis), 184 pregnancies occurred in women who were on dialysis before conception and 57 in women who were initially dialyzed during pregnancy (28). Not surprisingly, the infant survival was better in those women who began dialysis during pregnancy (73.6%) than in those who conceived after dialysis was initiated (40.2%) (28). The overall infant survival rate was not significantly different between the peritoneal dialysis group (37%) and the hemodialysis group (39.5%). There were two maternal deaths in this series, and five women were admitted to the intensive care unit for hypertensive crisis (79% of the women had some degree of hypertension). Anemia was common, with 26% requiring erythropoietin and 77% requiring blood transfusions (28). Newborn complications also were common. For example, 84% of those born to mothers who conceived after starting dialysis were premature. Eleven newborns had congenital anomalies.

In a review of six studies from 1992 through 2002 of dialysis patients and pregnancy, a pregnancy rate of 1–7% and an infant survival rate of 30–50% were reported (29). The spontaneous abortion rate from three of the studies ranged from 12% to 46%. Four studies provided information on complications. The incidence of hydramnios ranged from 42% to 79% (three studies), the cesarean delivery rate from 46% to 53% (two studies), and the incidence of hypertension from 42% to 79% (three studies) (29). The etiology of the development of hydramnios in pregnant women on dialysis is unknown. It has been hypothesized that the hydramnios develops secondary to the elevated placental blood urea nitrogen levels resulting in fetal solute diuresis and increased amniotic fluid volume (29). The mean pregnancy duration was approximately 32 weeks, and the mean birth weight ranged from 1,164 g to 1,542 g.

Increased dialysis time (more than 20 h/wk) may improve outcome (28). In a review of dialysis in pregnant women with chronic renal disease, more intensive, frequent dialysis or prolonged dialysis to increase the chance of successful pregnancy outcome is recommended (9). A definitive statement on the true advantages or disadvantages of more intensive, frequent, or prolonged dialysis in pregnant women cannot be ascertained because of the lack of scientific data on the effect of dialysis on maternal or fetal outcomes. However, the literature does contain case reports, small observational studies, and retrospective studies that seem to support the premise that more intensive, frequent, or prolonged

dialysis may be associated with improved pregnancy outcomes (ie, live births) if predialysis serum urea nitrogen levels are maintained between 30 mg/dL and 50 mg/dL (9). It has been hypothesized that, by increasing the frequency of dialysis in pregnant women, their serum urea nitrogen levels between dialysis treatments will be decreased as will their risk for developing hydramnios, preterm labor, and preterm delivery (29). Excessive volume reduction with dialysis may affect fetal well-being. Recommendations for the management of dialysis in the pregnant woman are as follows (29): 1) Maternal volume depletion and hypotension should be avoided during dialysis. The maternal diastolic blood pressure should be maintained at 80–90 mm Hg. 2) A nonreusable, biocompatible, smaller surface area dialyzer can reduce ultrafiltration rate during treatments. 3) The amount of bicarbonate and potassium in the dialysate should be adjusted based on serum chemistries to avoid electrolyte imbalances that may result from increased frequency of dialysis. 4) Protein intake should be 1.8 g/kg/d, and one can expect a 1 lb weight gain per week. 5) Water-soluble vitamin supplements including folate, 1 mg/d, should be taken. 6) Erythropoietin also can be administered at the time of dialysis treatment to maintain a target hemoglobin level of 10–11 g/dL. A 50% higher erythropoietin dose is usually required in pregnancy, and intravenous supplemental iron will likely be necessary to maintain iron saturation at 30% or greater. 7) Frequent dialysis should be performed (4–6 times per week after the first trimester) (29).

Summary

Even mild chronic renal disease occurs uncommonly during pregnancy. It seems reasonable to conclude that the incidence of moderate-to-severe chronic renal disease is less than 1 in 1,000 pregnancies.

Although pregnant women with chronic renal disease are at an increased risk of both maternal and perinatal morbidity, many such pregnancies can be expected to result in a successful pregnancy outcome. Adverse pregnancy outcome is related to the presence of hypertension and the degree of renal insufficiency. Maternal complications include preeclampsia, worsening chronic hypertension, deterioration of renal function and end-stage renal disease, increased risk of cesarean delivery, increased preterm delivery, and anemia. Screening and prenatal care can be provided by the obstetrician, who should be aware of the effect of pregnancy on disease as well as the effect of the disease on pregnancy. Counseling and management of selected complications and issues regarding timing and mode of delivery can be addressed by a specialist in maternal–fetal medicine. Consultation with a nephrologist for consideration or initiation of dialysis in both acute and chronic cases is essential. Fetal and new-born complications include growth restriction, prematurity, and increased perinatal morbidity and mortality. Pregnant women with chronic renal disease should have a tailored management plan based on the underlying specific renal disease entity and the degree of renal insufficiency.

Longitudinal studies of women who have varying degrees of renal insufficiency are needed to provide better data with which to counsel such women about the associated risks. Postpartum women with renal disease also should be referred to a nephrologist for both short- and long-term follow-up.

References

1. Fink JC, Schwartz SM, Benedetti TJ, Stehman-Breen CO. Increased risk of adverse maternal and infant outcomes among women with renal disease. Paediatr Perinat Epidemiol 1998;12:277–87.

2. Davison JM, Lindheimer MD. Renal disorders. In: Creasy RK, Resnik R, Iams JD, editors. Maternal–fetal medicine principles and practice. 5th ed. Philadelphia (PA): Saunders; 2004. p. 901–23.

3. Jones DC, Hayslett JP. Outcome of pregnancy in women with moderate or severe renal insufficiency [published erratum appears in N Engl J Med 1997;336:739]. N Engl J Med 1996;335:226–32.

4. Bar J, Orvieto R, Shalev Y, Peled Y, Pardo Y, Gafter U, et al. Pregnancy outcome in women with primary renal disease. Isr Med Assoc J 2000;2:178–81.

5. Cunningham FG, Cox SM, Harstad TW, Mason RA, Pritchard JA. Chronic renal disease and pregnancy outcome. Am J Obstet Gynecol 1990;163:453–9.

6. Davison JM. Renal disorders in pregnancy. Curr Opin Obstet Gynecol 2001;13:109–14.

7. Trevisan G, Ramos JG, Martins-Costa S, Barros EJ. Pregnancy in patients with chronic renal insufficiency at Hospital de Clinicas of Porto Alegre, Brazil. Ren Fail 2004; 26:29–34.

8. Fischer MJ, Lehnerz SD, Hebert JR, Parikh CR. Kidney disease is an independent risk factor for adverse fetal and maternal outcomes in pregnancy. Am J Kidney Dis 2004; 43:415–23.

9. Shemin D. Dialysis in pregnant women with chronic kidney disease. Semin Dial 2003;16:379–83.

10. Lydon-Rochelle MT, Holt VL, Cardenas V, Nelson JC, Easterling TR, Gardella C, et al. The reporting of pre-existing maternal medical conditions and complications of pregnancy on birth certificates and in hospital discharge data. Am J Obstet Gynecol 2005;193:125–34.

11. Jungers P, Houillier P, Forget D, Henry-Amar M. Specific controversies concerning the natural history of renal disease in pregnancy. Am J Kidney Dis 1991;17:116–22.

12. Abe S. An overview of pregnancy in women with underlying renal disease. Am J Kidney Dis 1991;17:112–5.

13. Purdy LP, Hantsch CE, Molitch ME, Metzger BE, Phelps RL, Dooley SL, et al. Effect of pregnancy on renal function in patients with moderate-to-severe diabetic renal insufficiency. Diabetes Care 1996;19:1067–74.

14. Holley JL, Bernardini J, Quadri KH, Greenberg A, Laifer SA. Pregnancy outcomes in a prospective matched control study of pregnancy and renal disease. Clin Nephrol 1996; 45:77–82.

15. Jungers P, Chauveau D, Choukroun G, Moynot A, Skhiri H, Houillier P, et al. Pregnancy in women with impaired renal function. Clin Nephrol 1997;47:281–8.

16. Lindheimer MD, Katz AI. Gestation in women with kidney disease: prognosis and management. Baillieres Clin Obstet Gynaecol 1994;8:387–404.

17. Abe S. Pregnancy in glomerulonephritic patients with decreased renal function. Hypertens Pregn 1996;15: 305–11.

18. Jungers P, Houillier P, Chauveau D, Choukroun G, Moynot A, Skhiri H, et al. Pregnancy in women with reflux neph-ropathy. Kidney Int 1996;50:593–9.

19. Jungers P, Chauveau D, Choukroun G, Moynot A, Skhiri H, Houillier P. Pegnancy in women with impaired renal function. Clin Nephrol 1997;47:281–8.

20. Jungers P, Chauveau D Pregnancy in renal disease. Kidney Int 1997;52:871–85.

21. Bar J, Ben-Rafael Z, Padoa A, Orvieto R, Boner G, Hod M. Prediction of pregnancy outcome in subgroups of women with renal disease. Clin Nephrol 2000;53:437–44.

22. Stettler RW, Cunningham FG. Natural history of chronic proteinuria complicating pregnancy. Am J Obstet Gynecol 1992;167:1219–24.

23. Rodriguez-Thompson D, Lieberman ES. Use of a random urinary protein-to-creatinine ratio for the diagnosis of significant proteinuria during pregnancy. Am J Obstet Gynecol 2001;185:808–11.

24. Hou S. Pregnancy in chronic renal insufficiency and end-stage renal disease. Am J Kidney Dis 1999;33:235–52.

25. Epstein FH Pregnancy and renal disease [published erratum appears in N Engl J Med 1996;335:759]. N Engl J Med 1996;335:277–8.

26. Baylis C. Impact of pregnancy on underlying renal disease. Adv Ren Replace Ther 2003; 10:31–9.

27. Lindheimer MD, Grunfeld JP, Davison JM Renal disorders. In: Baron WM, Lindheimer MD, editors. Medical disorders during pregnancy. 3rd ed. St. Louis (MO): Mosby Inc; 2000. p. 39–70.

28. Okundaye I, Abrinko P, Hou S. Registry of pregnancy in dialysis patients. Am J Kidney Dis 1998;31:766–73.

29. Holley JL, Reddy SS. Pregnancy in dialysis patients: a review of outcomes, complications, and management. Semin Dial 2003;16:384–7.

CHAPTER 4

Asthma and Pregnancy

Mitchell P. Dombrowski

Asthma may be the most common potentially serious medical condition to complicate pregnancy (1). Asthma is characterized by chronic airway inflammation with increased airway responsiveness to a variety of stimuli and airway obstruction that is partially or completely reversible (1). Insight into the pathogenesis of asthma has changed with the recognition that airway inflammation is present in nearly all cases. Current medical management for asthma emphasizes treatment of airway inflammation to decrease airway responsiveness and prevent asthma symptoms. Approximately 4–8% of pregnancies are complicated by asthma (2, 3). In general, the prevalence, morbidity, and mortality from asthma are increasing.

Diagnosis

The enlarging uterus elevates the diaphragm about 4 cm, with a reduction of the functional residual capacity (Fig. 4-1). However, there are no significant alterations in

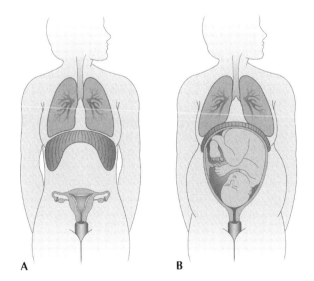

Fig. 4-1. Effect of enlarging pregnancy on the chest and pulmonary anatomy. **A**. Nonpregnant woman. **B**. Woman in the third trimester of pregnancy. Illustration: John Yanson. (Dombrowski MP. Asthma and pregnancy. Obstet Gynecol 2006;108:667–81.)

forced vital capacity, peak expiratory flow rate (PEFR) or forced expiratory volume in 1 second (FEV_1) in normal pregnancy. Shortness of breath at rest or with mild exertion is common and is often referred to as physiologic dyspnea of pregnancy. Asthma is characterized by paroxysmal or persistent symptoms including breathlessness, chest tightness, cough, and sputum production. The diagnosis of asthma is based on a history of symptoms and spirometry. Patients with asthma will have an improvement in FEV_1 after administration of a short-acting inhaled β_2-agonist. They also will have increased sensitivity to inhaled methacholine, although this is not usually administered during pregnancy.

In 2004, the National Asthma Education and Prevention Program Working Group on Asthma and Pregnancy defined mild intermittent, mild persistent, moderate persistent, and severe persistent asthma according to symptomatic exacerbations (wheezing, cough, dyspnea or all three) and objective tests of pulmonary function (Box 4-1). The most commonly used measures are the PEFR and FEV_1. The National Asthma Education and Prevention Program guidelines did not list the need for regular medication to be a factor for classifying asthma severity during pregnancy. However, patients with mild asthma by National Asthma Education and Prevention Program criteria, but who required regular medications to control their asthma, were similar to those with moderate asthma with respect to asthma exacerbations (4). Pregnant patients requiring regular systemic corticosteroids to control asthma symptoms were similar to severe asthmatics with respect to exacerbations.

The Effects of Asthma on Pregnancy

Asthma has been associated with considerable maternal morbidity. In a large prospective study, patients with mild asthma had an exacerbation rate of 12.6% and hospitalization rate of 2.3%; those with moderate asthma had an exacerbation rate of 25.7% and hospitalization rate of 6.8%; and severe asthmatics had an exacerbation

---

BOX 4-1

ASTHMA SEVERITY CLASSIFICATION

Mild intermittent asthma*
- Symptoms twice per week or less
- Nocturnal symptoms twice per month or less
- PEFR or FEV_1 80% predicted or more, variability less than 20%

Mild persistent asthma
- Symptoms more than twice per week but not daily
- Nocturnal symptoms more than twice per month
- PEFR or FEV_1 80% predicted or more, variability 20–30%

Moderate persistent asthma
- Daily symptoms
- Nocturnal symptoms more than once per week
- PEFR or FEV_1 more than 60% to less than 80% predicted, variability more than 30%
- Regular medications necessary to control symptoms

Severe asthma
- Continuous symptoms and frequent exacerbations
- Frequent nocturnal symptoms
- PEFR or FEV_1 60% predicted or less, variability more than 30%
- Regular oral corticosteroids necessary to control symptoms

*Data from National Institutes of Health, National Heart, Lung, and Blood Institute. National Asthma Education Program. Report of the Working Group on Asthma and Pregnancy: management of asthma during pregnancy. 1993 Available at: http://www.nhlbi.nih.gov/health/prof/lung/asthma/astpreg.txt. Retrieved June 28, 2006.

Abbreviations: FEV_1, forced expiratory volume in 1 second; PEFR, peak expiratory flow rate.

Dombrowski MP. Asthma and pregnancy. Obstet Gynecol 2006;108:667–81.

---

rate of 51.9% and a hospitalization rate 26.9% (4). The effects of pregnancy on asthma are variable, and in a large prospective study, 23% improved and 30% become worse during pregnancy (4). One of the most important conclusions to be made from this study is that pregnant asthmatic patients, even with mild or well-controlled disease, need to be monitored by PEFR and FEV_1 testing during pregnancy.

The Effects of Pregnancy on Asthma

Existing studies on the effects of asthma on pregnancy outcomes have had inconsistent results with regard to maternal and perinatal outcomes. For example, asthma has been reported to be associated with increased perinatal mortality (5), hyperemesis gravidarum (6), hemorrhage (2, 6, 7), hypertension or preeclampsia (6–13), preterm birth (6, 10, 11, 14–16), hypoxia at birth (6), low birth weight (6, 17), increased cesarean delivery (7, 9, 10, 17, 14) small for gestational age or intrauterine growth restriction (10, 11, 18), gestational diabetes (7, 14), and malformations (10). In contrast, asthma also has been reported not to be associated with preterm birth (2, 5, 17–20), birth injury (6), reduced gestational age (8, 9, 21–23), reduced mean birth weight (8, 9, 17, 22–24), increased perinatal mortality (6, 7, 9, 19, 23, 25), low Apgar score (9), neonatal respiratory difficulty (9), malformations (2, 6, 9, 11, 19), antepartum or postpartum hemorrhage or both (11, 17, 21), perinatal complications (12, 17), gestational hypertension or preeclampsia (14, 18, 19, 26) intrauterine growth restriction (14, 19) increased cesarean delivery (2, 20, 25), low birth weight (2, 19–21, 25) gestational diabetes (2, 12), or respiratory distress syndrome (2).

Many of the older studies have a number of methodologic inadequacies, including low power; different inclusion criteria; lacking or inadequate control for confounders; little or no information regarding asthma severity, management, or control; and time frames that do not reflect current management. Until recently, there have been few large prospective studies of asthma during pregnancy.

There have been two recent, large, multicenter, prospective cohort studies evaluating the effects of maternal asthma perinatal outcomes that contained information regarding asthma severity and management (27, 28). In a 2003 study, preterm delivery was not associated with asthma diagnosis or severity (27). However, the need for treatment with oral corticosteroids or theophylline was significantly associated with a decrease in gestational age at delivery. Small for gestational age was significantly increased among those with daily symptoms or moderate persistent severity. No specific medication type was observed to lead to an increased risk of fetal growth restriction. Preeclampsia was significantly increased among the cohort who had daily asthma symptoms and among those who required theophylline (29). These data suggest that poor asthma control, by causing acute or chronic maternal hypoxia, may be the most remedial responsible factor and support the important generalization that adequate asthma control during pregnancy is important in improving maternal and fetal outcome.

The National Institute of Child Health and Human Development and National Heart, Lung, and Blood Institute (NHLBI) conducted a multicenter, prospective, observational cohort study involving 16 centers with preterm delivery less than 32 weeks of gestation as the primary outcome (28). In the study were enrolled 873 subjects with mild asthma, 814 with moderate asthma, 52 with severe asthma, and 881 nonasthmatic controls. There were no significant differences in the rates of preterm delivery less than 32 weeks or less than 37 weeks gestation. Of all outcomes explored (including preterm delivery, gestational diabetes, preeclampsia, preterm labor, chorioamnionitis, oligohydramnios, cesarean delivery, low birth weight, small for gestational age, and congenital malformations), only the cesarean delivery rate was significantly increased in the group of patients with moderate to severe asthma. Among the cohort with severe asthma, there was a significantly increased incidence of gestational diabetes and delivery at less than 37 weeks of gestation compared with controls by logistic regression adjusted for confounding variables. Oral corticosteroid use was significantly associated with both preterm delivery at less than 37 weeks of gestation and birth weight less than 2,500 g (30). There were no significant differences for neonatal outcomes except for discharge diagnosis of neonatal sepsis among the group with mild asthma, a finding that may be related to type 1 error.

Participants in the National Institute of Child Health and Human Development and NHLBI study had excellent maternal and perinatal outcomes despite a high frequency of asthma exacerbations. These findings do not contradict the possibility that suboptimal control of asthma during pregnancy is associated with increased risk to the mother or baby. In fact, this study did find a relationship between lower FEV_1 during pregnancy and an increased risk of low birth weight and prematurity (31). Both studies indicate that classification of asthma severity with therapy tailored according to asthma severity can result in excellent perinatal and maternal outcomes. This generally confirms the findings of two earlier and smaller prospective cohort studies (19, 21) in which asthma was managed by asthma specialists.

Putting the Literature Into Perspective

There is considerable consistency among prospective studies of the effects of asthma on maternal and perinatal outcomes. The results of eight prospective studies reporting maternal and neonatal outcomes of at least 100 participants in locations at or near sea level, have been published in the English-language literature, (Table 4-1). One can conclude from these studies that cohorts with mild or moderate asthma during pregnancy can have excellent maternal and perinatal outcomes. The two largest studies (28, 29), reported an increase of preterm delivery at less than 37 weeks of gestation among subjects who had severe asthma, required oral corticosteroids, or

both. In addition, in two studies an increase in preeclampsia was reported (9, 27), although one of these only found this in patients with daily symptoms (27). In three studies, increased cesarean delivery was reported (9, 21, 28), although one of these was only in patients with moderate to severe asthma (28). In one study, an increased incidence of gestational diabetes with severe asthma was reported, (28) and in one, an increased risk of small for gestational age in infants of mothers with daily asthma symptoms was found (27).

In contrast, there is much less consensus among retrospective studies of asthma in pregnancy. Nearly every possible pregnancy complication has been associated with asthma by at least one retrospective publication. In 1993, the National Asthma Education and Prevention Program of the NHLBI recommended antiinflammatory treatment for pregnant women with moderate or severe asthma. Studies that enrolled patients after the 1993 National Asthma Education and Prevention Program recommendations tended to have fewer adverse pregnancy outcomes associated with asthma. This again supports the concept that optimal asthma management can mitigate adverse pregnancy outcomes. Patients with poorly controlled asthma complicated by severe exacerbations are at significant risk for maternal and fetal morbidity and mortality.

A potential explanation for the inconsistencies among many studies with regard to the effect of asthma on obstetric and neonatal outcomes may include the fact that most studies of asthma during pregnancy did not attempt to classify asthma severity. Classification of asthma severity has important clinical implications with regard to asthma morbidity and tailoring optimal treatment regimens (32, 33). Failure to classify severity may result in suboptimal asthma control, thereby increasing risks for adverse maternal or neonatal outcomes. Oral corticosteroid treatment per se may confound maternal and neonatal outcomes. Some positive findings may be attributed to chance or caused by confounders such as ethnicity, smoking status, socioeconomic status, hypertension, and others. Asthma medications and poor asthma control leading to hypoxia have been hypothesized to explain some of these observations (34). There are some data to support a correlation with poor asthma control indicated by increased hospitalization for exacerbations and decreased FEV_1 values with low birth weight and ponderal index (25, 34, 35). Studies have shown that patients with more severe asthma may have the greatest risk for complications during pregnancy (10, 14, 15, 36), whereas better-controlled asthma is associated with decreased risks (19, 27, 28). Prospective studies have tended to find fewer significant adverse associations, possibly because of better asthma surveillance and treatment.

Table 4-1. Prospective Cohort Studies Reporting Obstetric and Neonatal Outcomes

Outcome	Dombrowski et al 2004 (28) (N = 1,739)	Bracken et al 2003 (27) (N = 872)	Stenius 1996 (21) (N = 504)	Schatz 1995 (19) (N = 486)	Mihrshahi 2003 (12) (N = 340)	Jana 1995 (25) (N = 182)	Stenius 1988 (9) (N = 181)	Minerbi-Codish 1998 (20) (N = 101)
Preterm less than 32 weeks of gestation	No	NR	NR	NR	NR	NR	NR	NR
Preterm less than 37 weeks of gestation	No (yes, if severe)	No (yes, if oral steroids)	No	No	No	No	NR	No
Preeclampsia	No	No (yes, if daily symptoms	No	No	No	NR	Yes	No
Cesarean delivery	Yes, (if moderate or severe)	NR	Yes, (if elective)	NR	No	No	Yes	No
Gestational diabetes	No (yes, if severe)	NR	No	No	NR	NR	No	No
Small for gestational age	No	No (yes, if daily symptoms)	NR	No	NR	NR	NR	No
Malformation	No	NR	No	No	NR	No	NR	No
Antenatal hemorrhage	NR	NR	No	NR	NR	No	No	NR
Postnatal hemorrhage	No	NR	NR	NR	NR	NR	NR	NR
RDS or HMD	No	NR	NR	No	NR	NR	No	NR
NEC	No	NR	NR	No	NR	NR	NR	NR
Perinatal death	No	NR	No	No	NR	No	No	NR
NICU admission	No	NR	No	NR	No	NR	No	NR

Yes = significantly increased, No = no significant association, NR = not reported.

Abbreviations: HMD, hyaline membrane disease; NEC, necrotizing enterocolotis; NICU, neonatal intensive care unit; RDS, respiratory distress syndrome.

Reprinted from Dombrowski MP. Outcomes of pregnancy in asthmatic women. Immunol Allergy Clin North Am 2006;26:81–92. Copyright © 2006, with permission from Elsevier.

There are important caveats when interpreting this literature. The excellent maternal and perinatal outcomes were achieved at centers that tended to manage asthma actively in pregnancy. In addition, women who enroll in research studies tend to be more compliant and better motivated than the general public. The lack of finding more adverse outcomes among pregnant women with severe asthma also may be a function of the relatively small numbers of this cohort and the resulting lack of power to find adverse outcomes that were statistically significant. Nonetheless, these prospective studies are reassuring in their consensus of good pregnancy outcomes among women with asthma. Asthma should not be considered to be a benign condition, however, because active asthma management was a part of these studies and may have affected outcomes.

Asthma Management

The ultimate goal of asthma therapy during pregnancy is to maintain adequate oxygenation of the fetus by prevention of hypoxic episodes in the mother. Other goals include achievement of minimal or no maternal symptoms day or night, minimal or no exacerbations, no limitations of activities, maintenance of normal or near-normal pulmonary function, minimal use of short-acting β_2-agonists, and minimal or no adverse effects from medications. Consultation or comanagement with an asthma specialist is appropriate, as indicated, for evaluation of the role of allergy and irritants, evaluation of complete pulmonary function study results, or evaluation of the medication plan if there are complications in achieving the goals of therapy or the patient has severe asthma.

A team approach is helpful if more than one clinician is managing the asthma and the pregnancy. The effective management of asthma during pregnancy relies on four integral components: 1) objective measures for assessment and monitoring, 2) avoidance or control of asthma triggers, 3) patient education, and 4) pharmacologic therapy.

Objective Measures for Assessment and Monitoring

Subjective measures of lung function by either the patient or physician provide an insensitive and inaccurate assessment of airway hyperresponsiveness, airway inflammation, and asthma severity. The FEV_1 after a maximal inspiration is the single best measure of pulmonary function. When adjusted for confounders, a mean FEV_1 less than 80% predicted has been found to be significantly associated with increased preterm delivery at less than 32 weeks of gestation, preterm delivery at less than 37 weeks of gestation, and birth weight less than 2,500 g (31). However, measurement of FEV_1 requires a spirometer. The PEFR correlates well with the FEV_1 and has the advantage that it can be measured reliably with inexpensive, disposable, portable peak flow meters (Fig. 4-2).

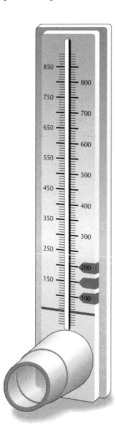

Fig. 4-2. Typical peak flow meter. Illustration: John Yanson. (Dombrowski MP. Asthma and pregnancy. Obstet Gynecol 2006;108:667–81.)

Patient self-monitoring of PEFR provides valuable insight into the course of asthma throughout the day, assesses circadian variation in pulmonary function, and helps detect early signs of deterioration so that timely therapy can be instituted. Patients with persistent asthma should be evaluated at least monthly and those with moderate to severe asthma should have daily PEFR monitoring (37). The typical PEFR in pregnancy should be 380–550 L/min. Each patient should establish her "personal best" PEFR, then calculate her individualized PEFR zones: green zone, more than 80% of personal best; yellow zone, 50–80% of personal best; and red zone, less than 50% of personal best PEFR.

Avoidance or Control of Asthma Triggers

Limiting adverse environmental exposures during pregnancy is important for controlling asthma. Irritants and allergens that provoke acute symptoms also increase airway inflammation and hyperresponsiveness. Avoiding or controlling such triggers can lessen asthma symptoms, airway hyperresponsiveness, and the need for medical therapy. Association of asthma with allergies is common; 75–85% of patients with asthma have skin test results that are positive for common allergens, including animal dander, house dust mites, cockroach antigens, pollens, and molds. Other common nonimmunologic triggers include tobacco smoke, strong odors, air pollutants, food additives such as sulfites, and certain drugs, including aspirin and β-blockers. Another trigger can be strenuous physical activity. For some patients, exercise-induced asthma can be avoided with inhalation of albuterol 5–60 minutes before exercise.

Specific measures for avoiding asthma triggers include using allergen-impermeable mattress and pillow covers, removing carpeting, weekly washing of bedding in hot water, avoiding tobacco smoke, inhibiting mite and mold growth by reducing humidity, and leaving the house when it is vacuumed. Animal dander control includes weekly bathing of the pet, keeping furry pets out of the bedroom, or removing the pet from the home. Cockroaches can be controlled by poison or bait traps and eliminating exposed food or garbage.

Patient Education

Patients should be made aware that controlling asthma during pregnancy is especially important for the well-being of the fetus. The patient should understand that she could reduce symptoms by limiting asthma triggers. The patient should have a basic understanding of the medical management during pregnancy, including self-monitoring of PEFRs and the correct use of inhalers. Patients should be instructed on proper PEFR technique. They should make the measurement while standing, take a maximum inspiration, and note the reading on the peak flow meter.

Pharmacologic Therapy

The goals of asthma therapy include relieving bronchospasm, protecting the airways from irritant stimuli, mitigating pulmonary and inflammatory response to an allergen exposure, and resolving the inflammatory process in the airways leading to improved pulmonary function with reduced airway hyperresponsiveness. A step-care therapeutic approach uses the least amount of drug intervention necessary to control the severity of asthma.

Asthma Pharmacotherapy

It is safer for pregnant women with asthma to be treated with asthma medications than it is for them to have asthma symptoms and exacerbations (37). Current pharmacologic therapy emphasizes treatment of airway inflammation to decrease airway hyperresponsiveness and prevent asthma symptoms. Typical dosages of commonly used asthma medications are listed in Table 4-2. Low, medium, and high doses of inhaled corticosteroids are presented in Table 4-3. Although it is assumed that asthma medications are equally effective during pregnancy, differences in maternal physiology and pharmacokinetics may affect the absorption, distribution,

Table 4-2. Typical Dosages of Asthma Medications

Medicine	Dosage
Albuterol MDI	2–8 puffs as needed
Salmeterol MDI	2 puffs, twice daily
Fluticasone and salmeterol DPI	1 inhalation, twice daily (dose depends on severity of asthma)
Montelukast	10-mg tablet at night
Zafirlukast	20 mg, twice daily
Prednisone	20–60 mg/d for active symptoms
Theophylline	Start 10 mg/kg, target serum levels of 5–12 mcg/mL (decrease dosage by half if treated with erythromycin or cimetidine)
Ipratropium	
MDI	4–8 puffs as needed
Nebulizer	3 mL (0.5 mg), every 30 minutes for 3 doses, then every 2–4 hours as needed
Cromolyn MDI	2–4 puffs, 3 or 4 times daily

Abbreviations: DPI, dry powder inhaler; MDI, metered-dose inhaler
Dombrowski MP. Asthma and pregnancy. Obstet Gynecol 2006;108:667–81.

metabolism, and clearance of medications during pregnancy. Endocrinologic and immunologic changes during pregnancy include elevations in free plasma cortisol, possible tissue refractoriness to cortisol (38), and changes in cellular immunity (39).

Step Therapy

The step-care therapeutic approach increases the number and frequency of medications with increasing asthma severity (Table 4-4). Based on the severity of asthma, medications are considered to be "preferred" or "alternative." Patients not optimally responding to treatment should be "stepped up" to more intensive medical therapy. Once control is achieved and sustained for several months, a step-down approach can be considered but should be undertaken cautiously and gradually to avoid compromising the stability of the asthma control. For some patients, it may be prudent to postpone until after birth attempts to reduce therapy that is effectively controlling the patient's asthma (37). In the case of a patient who has a favorable response to an alternative drug before becoming pregnant, it would be preferable to maintain the therapy that successfully controls the patient's asthma before pregnancy. However, when initiating new treatment for asthma during pregnancy, preferred medications should be considered rather than alternative treatment options (37).

A burst of oral corticosteroids is indicated for exacerbations not responding to initial β_2-agonist therapy, regardless of asthma severity. Additionally, patients who require increasing amounts of inhaled albuterol therapy to control their symptoms may benefit from oral corticosteroids. In such cases, a short course of oral prednisone, 40–60 mg/d for one week, followed by 7–14 days of tapering, may be effective.

Inhaled Corticosteroids

Inhaled corticosteroids are the preferred treatment for the management of all levels of persistent asthma during pregnancy (37). Airway inflammation is present in nearly all cases; therefore, inhaled corticosteroids have been advocated as first-line therapy for patients with mild asthma (40). The use of inhaled corticosteroids among nonpregnant asthmatics has been associated with a marked reduction in fatal and near-fatal asthma (41). Inhaled corticosteroids produce clinically important improvements in bronchial hyperresponsiveness that appear dose related (42) and include prevention of increased bronchial hyperresponsiveness after seasonal exposure to allergen (43, 44). Continued administration also is effective in reducing the immediate pulmonary response to an allergen challenge. In a prospective observational study of 504 pregnant subjects with asthma, 177

Table 4-3. Comparative Daily Doses for Inhaled Corticosteroids

		Dosage Level		
		Low Dose	Medium Dose	High Dose
Beclomethasone MDI	42 mcg per puff	4–12 puffs	12–20 puffs	More than 20 puffs
	84 mcg per puff	2–6 puffs	6–10 puffs	More than 10 puffs
Triamcinolone MDI	100 mcg per puff	4–10 puffs	10–20 puffs	More than 20 puffs
Budesonide DPI	200 mcg per puff	1–2 puffs	2–3 puffs	More than 3 puffs
Fluticasone MDI	44 mcg per puff	2–6 puffs		
	110 mcg per puff	2 puffs	2–6 puffs	More than 6 puffs
	220 mcg per puff		1–3 puffs	More than 3 puffs
Flunisolide MDI	250 mcg per puff	2–4 puffs	4–8 puffs	More than 8 puffs

Total daily puffs are usually divided as twice per day or three times per day.
Abbreviations: DPI, dry powder inhaler; MDI, metered-dose inhaler
Dombrowski MP. Asthma and pregnancy. Obstet Gynecol 2006;108:667–81.

Table 4-4. Medical Management of Asthma

	Management	
Type	Preferred	Alternative
Mild intermittent asthma	No daily medications, albuterol* as needed	
Mild persistent asthma	Low-dose inhaled corticosteroid	Cromolyn, leukotriene receptor antagonist, or theophylline (serum level 5–12 mcg/mL)
Moderate persistent asthma	Low-dose inhaled corticosteroid and salmeterol or medium-dose inhaled corticosteroid or (if needed) medium-dose inhaled corticosteroid and salmeterol	Low-dose or (if needed) medium-dose inhaled corticosteroid and leukotriene receptor antagonist or theophylline (serum level 5–12 mcg/mL)
Severe persistent asthma	High-dose inhaled corticosteroid and salmeterol and (if needed) oral corticosteroid	High-dose inhaled corticosteroid and theophylline (serum level 5–12 mcg/mL) and oral corticosteroid if needed

*Albuterol, 2–4 puffs as needed for peak expiratory flow rate or forced expiratory volume in 1 second less than 80%, asthma exacerbations, or exposure to exercise or allergens; oral corticosteroid burst if inadequate response to albuterol, regardless of asthma severity.
Data from National Institutes of Health, National Heart, Lung, and Blood Institute. National Asthma Education Program. Report of the Working Group on Asthma and Pregnancy: management of asthma during pregnancy. 1993 Available at: http://www.nhlbi.nih.gov/health/prof/lung/asthma/astpreg.txt. Retrieved June 28, 2006.

patients were not initially treated with either inhaled budesonide or inhaled beclomethasone (21). This cohort had a 17% acute exacerbation rate compared with only a 4% rate among those treated with inhaled corticosteroids from the start of pregnancy.

The National Asthma Education and Prevention Program Working Group reviewed 10 studies, including 6,113 patients who took inhaled corticosteroids during pregnancy for asthma (37). There is no evidence linking inhaled corticosteroid use and increases in congenital malformations or adverse perinatal outcomes. Included among these studies was the Swedish Medical Birth Registry that had 2,014 infants whose mothers had used inhaled budesonide in early pregnancy (45). Because there are more data on using budesonide during pregnancy than on using other inhaled corticosteroids, the National Asthma Education and Prevention Program considered budesonide to be a preferred medication. However, if a woman's asthma is well controlled by a different inhaled corticosteroid before pregnancy, it seems reasonable to continue that medication during pregnancy. All inhaled corticosteroids are currently labeled U.S. Food and Drug Administration pregnancy class C except budesonide, which is class B.

Inhaled Beta$_2$-Agonists

Inhaled β_2-agonists are currently recommended for all degrees of asthma during pregnancy (37, 46). Albuterol has the advantage of a rapid onset of effect in the relief of acute bronchospasm by way of smooth muscle relaxation, and is an excellent bronchoprotective agent for pretreatment before exercise. Salmeterol and formoterol are long-acting preparations. Beta$_2$-agonists are associated with tremor, tachycardia, and palpitations. They do not block the development of airway hyperresponsiveness (47). Indeed, a comparison of an inhaled glucocorticoid, budesonide, with the inhaled terbutaline, raised the question whether routine use of terbutaline could result in increased airway hyperresponsiveness (40). An increased frequency of bronchodilator use could be an indicator of the need for additional antiinflammatory therapy; chronic use of short acting β_2-agonists has been associated with an increased risk of death (46, 48). Beta$_2$-agonists seem to be safe, based on a National Asthma Education and Prevention Program review of six published studies with 1,599 women with asthma who took β_2-agonists during pregnancy (37). Additionally, in a large prospective study, no significant relationship was found between the use of inhaled β_2-agonists (N = 1,828) and adverse pregnancy outcomes (30).

Cromolyn

Cromolyn sodium is virtually devoid of significant side effects; it blocks both the early and late phase pulmonary response to allergen challenge as well as prevents the development of airway hyperresponsiveness (47). Cromolyn does not have any intrinsic bronchodilator or antihistaminic activity. Compared with inhaled corticosteroids, the time to maximal clinical benefit is longer for cromolyn. Cromolyn seems to be less effective than inhaled corticosteroids in reducing objective and subjective manifestations of asthma. Cromolyn seems to be safe during pregnancy (30) and is an alternative treatment for mild persistent asthma (37).

Theophylline

Theophylline is an alternative treatment for mild persistent asthma and an adjunctive treatment for the management of moderate and severe persistent asthma during pregnancy (38). Subjective symptoms of adverse theophylline effects, including insomnia, heartburn, palpitations, and nausea, may be difficult to differentiate from typical pregnancy symptoms. High doses have been observed to cause jitteriness, tachycardia, and vomiting in mothers and neonates (49). New treatment guidelines have recommended that serum theophylline concentrations be maintained at 5–12 mcg/mL during pregnancy

(37). Theophylline can have significant interactions with other drugs, which can cause decreased clearance with resultant toxicity. For instance, cimetidine can cause a 70% increase in serum levels, while erythromycin use can increase theophylline serum levels by 35% (50). The main advantage of theophylline is the long duration of action, 10–12 hours with the use of sustained-release preparations, which is especially useful in the management of nocturnal asthma (51). Theophylline is only indicated for chronic therapy and is not effective for the treatment of acute exacerbations during pregnancy (52). Theophylline has antiinflammatory actions (53) that may be mediated from inhibition of leukotriene production and its capacity to stimulate prostaglandin E$_2$ production (54). Theophylline may potentiate the efficacy of inhaled corticosteroids (55).

The National Asthma Education and Prevention Program reviewed eight human studies that had a total of 660 women with asthma who took theophylline during pregnancy (37). These studies and clinical experience confirm the safety of theophylline at a serum concentration of 5–12 mcg/mL during pregnancy. In a recent randomized controlled trial, there where no differences in asthma exacerbations or perinatal outcomes in a cohort receiving theophylline compared with the cohort receiving inhaled beclomethasone (56, 57). However, the theophylline cohort had significantly more reported side effects and discontinuation of study medication and an increased proportion of those with an FEV$_1$ less than 80% predicted.

Leukotriene Moderators

Leukotrienes are arachidonic acid metabolites that have been implicated in transducing bronchospasm, mucous secretion, and increased vascular permeability (58). Bronchoconstriction associated with aspirin ingestion can be blocked by leukotriene receptor antagonists (59). Treatment with leukotriene receptor antagonist montelukast has been shown to improve pulmonary function significantly as measured by FEV$_1$ (58). The leukotriene receptor antagonists zafirlukast and montelukast are both labeled U.S. Food and Drug Administration pregnancy class B. It should be noted that there are minimal data regarding the efficacy or safety of these agents during human pregnancy. Leukotriene receptor antagonists are an alternative treatment for mild persistent asthma and an adjunctive treatment for the management of moderate and severe persistent asthma during pregnancy (37).

Oral Corticosteroids

The National Asthma Education and Prevention Program Working Group reviewed eight human studies, including one report of two meta-analyses (37). Most participants in these studies did not take oral corticosteroids for asthma, and the length, timing, and dose of exposure to the drug were not well described. The panel concluded that findings from the current evidence review are conflicting. Oral corticosteroid use during the first trimester of pregnancy is associated with a threefold increased risk for isolated cleft lip, with or without cleft palate, with a background incidence of about 0.1%, thus the excess risk attributable to oral steroids would be 0.2–0.3% (60). Oral corticosteroid use during pregnancy in patients who have asthma has been associated with an increased incidence of preeclampsia, preterm delivery, and low birth weight (14, 19, 27, 30, 60). A recent prospective study found that systemic corticosteroids resulted in a deficit of about 200 g in birth weight compared with controls and those exclusively treated with β_2-agonists (61). However, it is difficult to separate the effects of the oral corticosteroids on these outcomes from the effects of severe or uncontrolled asthma.

Because of the uncertainties in these data and the definite risks of severe uncontrolled asthma to the mother and fetus, the National Asthma Education and Prevention Program Working Group recommends the use of oral corticosteroids when indicated for the long-term management of severe asthma or exacerbations during pregnancy (37). For the treatment of acute exacerbations, methylprednisolone or other corticosteroids may be given up to 120–180 mg/d in three or four divided doses; once the PEFR reaches 70% of personal best, the daily dosage of parenteral or oral corticosteroid, such as prednisone, could be decreased to 60–80 mg/d (37).

Management of Allergic Rhinitis

Rhinitis, sinusitis, and gastroesophageal reflux may exacerbate asthma symptoms, and their management should be considered an integral aspect of asthma care. Intranasal corticosteroids are the most effective medications for control of allergic rhinitis. Loratadine or cetirizine are recommended second-generation antihistamines. Oral decongestant ingestion during the first trimester has been associated with gastroschisis; therefore, inhaled decongestants or inhaled corticosteroids should be considered before use of oral decongestants (37). Immunotherapy is considered safe during pregnancy but, because of the risk of anaphylaxis, initiation of immunotherapy is not recommended during pregnancy.

Antenatal Management

Patients with moderate and severe asthma should be considered to be at risk for pregnancy complications. Adverse outcomes can be increased by underestimation of asthma severity and undertreatment of asthma. The first prenatal visit should include a detailed medical history, with attention to medical conditions that could complicate the management of asthma, including active pulmonary disease. The patient should be questioned about smoking history and the presence and severity of symptoms, episodes of nocturnal asthma, the number of days of work missed, and emergency care visits because of asthma. Asthma severity should be determined. The type and amount of asthma medications, including the number of puffs of β_2-agonists used each day, should be noted.

The scheduling of prenatal visits for pregnant women with moderate or severe asthma should be based on clinical judgment. In addition to routine care, monthly or more frequent evaluations of asthma history (emergency visits, hospital admissions, symptom frequency, severity, nocturnal symptoms, medications, dosages, and compliance) and pulmonary function (FEV_1 or PEFR) are recommended. Patients should be instructed on the proper dosage and administration of their asthma medications.

Daily peak flow monitoring should be considered for patients with moderate to severe asthma, and especially for patients who have difficulty perceiving signs of worsening asthma (37). It may be helpful to maintain an asthma diary containing daily assessment of asthma symptoms, including peak flow measurements, symptom and activity limitations, indication of any medical contacts initiated, and a record of regular and as-needed medications taken. Identifying and avoiding asthma triggers can lead to improved maternal well-being, with less need for medications. Specific recommendations can be made for appropriate environmental controls based on the patient's history of exposure and, when available, skin test reactivity to asthma triggers.

Women who have moderate or severe asthma during pregnancy also may benefit from additional fetal surveillance in the form of ultrasound examinations and antenatal fetal testing. Because asthma has been associated with intrauterine growth restriction and preterm birth, it is useful to establish pregnancy dating accurately by first-trimester ultrasonography where possible. In the opinion of the National Asthma Education and Prevention Program Working Group (37), the evaluation of fetal activity and growth by serial ultrasound examinations may be considered for women who have suboptimally controlled asthma, who have moderate to severe asthma (starting at 32 weeks of gestation), and who have recovered from a severe asthma exacerbation. The intensity of antenatal surveillance of fetal well-being should be considered on the basis of the severity of the asthma as well as any other high-risk features of the pregnancy that may be present. All patients should be instructed to be attentive to fetal activity.

Home Management of Asthma Exacerbations

An asthma exacerbation that causes minimal problems for the mother may have severe sequelae for the fetus. Indeed, abnormal fetal heart rate tracing may be the initial manifestation of an asthmatic exacerbation. A maternal PO_2 less than 60 or hemoglobin saturation less than 90% may be associated with profound fetal hypoxia. Therefore, asthma exacerbations in pregnancy should be aggressively managed. Patients should be given an individualized guide for decision making and rescue management and educated to recognize signs and symptoms of early asthma exacerbations, such as coughing, chest tightness, dyspnea, or wheezing, or by a 20% decrease in their PEFR. This is important so that prompt home rescue treatment may be instituted to avoid maternal and fetal hypoxia. In general, patients should use inhaled albuterol, 2–4 puffs every 20 minutes up to 1 hour (Box 4-2). A response is considered good if symptoms are resolved or become subjectively mild, normal activities can be resumed, and the PEFR is more than 70% of personal best. The patient should seek further medical attention if the response is incomplete or if fetal activity is decreased.

BOX 4-2

HOME MANAGEMENT OF ACUTE ASTHMA EXACERBATIONS*

Poor response—PEFR less than 50% predicted, or severe wheezing and shortness of breath, or decreased fetal movement, repeat albuterol, 2–4 puffs by MDI, and obtain emergency care

Incomplete response—PEFR is 50–80% predicted or, if persistent wheezing and shortness of breath, repeat albuterol treatment, 2–4 puffs MDI at 20-minute intervals up to two more times. If repeat PEFR is 50–80% predicted or if decreased fetal movement, contact caregiver or seek emergency care

Good response—PEFR more than 80% predicted, no wheezing or shortness of breath, and fetus is moving normally. May continue inhaled albuterol, 2–4 puffs MDI every 3–4 hours as needed.

*Use albuterol metered-dose inhaler, 2–4 puffs, and measure peak expiratory flow rate.

Abbreviations: MDI, metered-dose inhaler; PEFR, peak expiratory flow rate.

Dombrowski MP. Asthma and pregnancy. Obstet Gynecol 2006;108:667–81.

Hospital and Clinic Management

The principal goal should be the prevention of hypoxia. Measurement of oxygenation by pulse oximetry is essential; arterial blood gas assessments should be obtained if oxygen saturation remains less than 95%, but chest X-rays are commonly not needed. Continuous electronic fetal monitoring should be initiated if gestation has advanced to the point of potential fetal viability. Albuterol (2.5–5 mg every 20 minutes for three doses, then 2.5–10 mg every 1–4 hours as needed or 10–15 mg/h, continuously) should be delivered by nebulizer driven with oxygen (37). Occasionally, nebulized treatment is not effective because the patient is moving air poorly. In such cases, terbutaline, 0.25 mg, can be administered subcutaneously every 15 minutes for three doses. The patient should be assessed for general level of activity, color, pulse rate, use of accessory muscles, and airflow obstruction determined by auscultation and FEV_1, PEFR, or both before and after each bronchodilator treatment. Guidelines for the management of asthma exacerbations are presented in Box 4-3.

Labor and Delivery Management

Asthma medications should not be discontinued during labor and delivery. Although asthma is usually quiescent during labor, consideration should be given to assessing PEFRs upon admission and at 12-hour intervals. The patient should be kept hydrated and should receive adequate analgesia to decrease the risk of bronchospasm. If systemic corticosteroids have been used in the previous 4 weeks, then intravenous corticosteroids (eg, hydrocortisone, 100 mg every 8 hours) should be administered during labor and for the 24-hour period after delivery to prevent adrenal crisis (37). An elective delivery should be postponed if the patient is having an exacerbation.

It is rarely necessary to perform a cesarean delivery for an acute asthma exacerbation. Usually, maternal and fetal compromise will respond to aggressive medical management. Occasionally, delivery may improve the respiratory status of a patient with unstable asthma who has a mature fetus. Prostaglandin E_2 or E_1 can be used for cervical ripening, the management of spontaneous or induced abortions, or postpartum hemorrhage, although the patient's respiratory status should be monitored (62). Carboprost (15-methyl $PGF_{2\alpha}$), ergonovine, and methylergonovine can cause bronchospasm (63). Magnesium sulfate is a bronchodilator, but indomethacin can induce bronchospasm in the aspirin-sensitive patient. There are no reports of the use of calcium channel blockers for tocolysis among patients with asthma, although an association with bronchospasm has not been observed with wide clinical use.

BOX 4-3

EMERGENCY DEPARTMENT AND HOSPITAL-BASED MANAGEMENT OF ASTHMA EXACERBATION

Initial assessment and treatment
- History and examination (auscultation, use of accessory muscles, heart rate, respiratory rate), PEFR or FEV_1, oxygen saturation, and other tests as indicated.
- Initiate fetal assessment (consider fetal monitoring or biophysical profile or both if fetus is potentially viable)
- If severe exacerbation (FEV_1 or PEFR less then 50% with severe symptoms at rest) then high-dose albuterol by nebulization, every 20 minutes or continuously for 1 hour, and inhaled ipratropium bromide and systemic corticosteroid
- Albuterol by metered-dose inhaler or nebulizer, up to three doses in first hour
- Oral corticosteroid if no immediate response or if patient recently treated with systemic corticosteroid
- Oxygen to maintain saturation more than 95%
- Repeat assessment: symptoms, physical examination, PEFR, oxygen saturation
- Continue albuterol every 60 minutes for 1–3 hours, provided there is improvement

Repeat assessment
- Symptoms, physical examination, PEFR, oxygen saturation, other tests as needed
- Continue fetal assessment

Good response
- FEV_1 or PEFR 70% or more
- Response sustained 60 minutes after last treatment
- No distress
- Physical examination is normal
- Reassuring fetal status
- Discharge

Incomplete response
- FEV_1 or PEFR 50% or more but less than 70%
- Mild or moderate symptoms

- Continue fetal assessment until patient is stabilized
- Monitor FEV_1 or PEFR, oxygen saturation, pulse
- Continue inhaled albuterol and oxygen
- Inhaled ipratropium bromide
- Systemic (oral or intravenous) corticosteroid
- Individualize decision for hospitalization

Poor response
- FEV_1 or PEFR less than 50%
- Pco_2 more than 42 mm Hg
- Physical examination: severe symptoms, drowsiness, confusion
- Continue fetal assessment
- Admit to intensive care unit

Impending or actual respiratory arrest
- Admit to intensive care unit
- Intubation and mechanical ventilation with 100% oxygen
- Nebulized albuterol plus inhaled ipratropium bromide
- Intravenous corticosteroid

Intensive care unit
- Inhaled albuterol, hourly or continuously, plus inhaled ipratropium bromide
- Intravenous corticosteroid
- Oxygen
- Possible intubation and mechanical ventilation
- Continue fetal assessment until patient stabilized

Discharge home
- Continue treatment with albuterol
- Oral systemic corticosteroid if indicated
- Initiate or continue inhaled corticosteroid until review at medical follow-up
- Patient education
  —Review medicine use
  —Review and initiate action plan
  —Recommend close medical follow-up

Abbreviations: FEV_1, forced expiratory volume in 1 second; PEFR, peak expiratory flow rate.
Dombrowski MP. Asthma and pregnancy. Obstet Gynecol 2006;108:667–81.

Lumbar anesthesia has the benefit of reducing oxygen consumption and minute ventilation during labor (64). Fentanyl may be a better analgesic than meperidine, which causes histamine release, but meperidine is rarely associated with the onset of bronchospasm during labor. A 2% incidence of bronchospasm has been reported with regional anesthesia (65). Ketamine is useful for induction of general anesthesia because it can prevent bronchospasm (66). Communication between the obstetric,

anesthetic, and pediatric care providers is important for optimal care.

Breastfeeding

In general, only small amounts of asthma medications enter breast milk. Prednisone, theophylline, antihistamines, beclomethasone, β_2-agonists, and cromolyn are not considered to be contraindications for breastfeeding (37, 67). However, among sensitive individuals, theophylline may cause toxic effects in the neonate, including vomiting, feeding difficulties, jitteriness, and cardiac arrhythmias.

Summary

Asthma is an increasingly common problem during pregnancy. Mild and moderate asthma can be associated with excellent maternal and perinatal pregnancy outcomes, especially if patients are managed according to contemporary National Asthma Education and Prevention Program recommendations. Severe and poorly controlled asthma may be associated with increased prematurity, need for cesarean delivery, preeclampsia, and growth restriction. Severe asthma exacerbations can result in maternal morbidity and mortality and can have commensurate adverse pregnancy outcomes. The management of asthma during pregnancy should be based on objective assessment, trigger avoidance, patient education, and step-therapy. Asthma medications should be continued during pregnancy and while breastfeeding.

References

1. Schatz M, Zeiger RS, Hoffman CP. Intrauterine growth is related to gestational pulmonary function in pregnant asthmatic women. Kaiser-Permanente Asthma and Pregnancy Study Group. Chest 1990;98:389–92.
2. Alexander S, Dodds L, Armson BA. Perinatal outcomes in women with asthma during pregnancy. Obstet Gynecol 1998;92:435–40.
3. Kwon HL, Belanger K, Bracken M. Asthma prevalence among pregnant and childbearing-aged women in the United States: estimates from national health surveys. Ann Epidemiol 2003;13:317–24.
4. Schatz M, Dombrowski MP, Wise R, Thom EA, Landon M, Mabie W, et al. Asthma morbidity during pregnancy can be predicted by severity classification. J Allergy Clin Immunol 2003;112:283–8.
5. Gordon M, Niswander KR, Berendes H, Kantor AG. Fetal morbidity following potentially anoxigenic obstetric conditions. VII. Bronchial asthma. Am J Obstet Gynecol 1970;106:421–9.
6. Bahna SL, Bjerkedal T. The course and outcome of pregnancy in women with bronchial asthma. Acta Allergol 1972;27:397–406.
7. Wen SW, Demissie K, Liu S. Adverse outcomes in pregnancies of asthmatic women: results from a Canadian population. Ann Epidemiol 2001;11:7–12.
8. Dombrowski MP, Bottoms SF, Boike GM, Wald J. Incidence of preeclampsia among asthmatic patients lower with theophylline. Am J Obstet Gynecol 1986;155:265–7.
9. Stenius-Aarniala B, Piirila P, Teramo K. Asthma and pregnancy: a prospective study of 198 pregnancies. Thorax 1988;43:12–18.
10. Demissie K, Breckenridge MB, Rhoads GG. Infant and maternal outcomes in the pregnancies of asthmatic women. Am J Respir Crit Care Med 1998;158:1091–5.
11. Liu S, Wen SW, Demissie K, Marcoux S, Kramer M. Maternal asthma and pregnancy outcomes: a retrospective cohort study. Am J Obstet Gynecol 2001;184:90–6.
12. Mihrshahi S, Belousova E, Marks GB, Peat JK; Childhood Asthma Prevention Team. Pregnancy and birth outcomes in families with asthma. J Asthma 2003;40:181–7.
13. Rudra CB, Williams MA, Frederick IO, Luthy DA. Maternal asthma and risk of preeclampsia, a case-control study. J Reprod Med 2006;51:94–100.
14. Perlow JH, Montgomery D, Morgan MA, Towers CV, Porto M. Severity of asthma and perinatal outcome. Am J Obstet Gynecol 1992;167:963–7.
15. Kallen B, Rydhstroem H, Aberg A. Asthma during pregnancy—a population based study. Eur J Epidemiol 2000;16:167–71.
16. Sorensen TK, Dempsey JC, Xiao R, Frederick IO, Luthy DA, Williams MA. Maternal asthma and risk of preterm delivery. Ann Epidemiol 2003;13:267–72.
17. Lao TT, Huengsburg M. Labour and delivery in mothers with asthma. Eur J Obstet Gynecol Reprod Biol 1990;35:183–90.
18. Mabie WC, Barton JR, Wasserstrum N, Sibai BM. Clinical observations on asthma in pregnancy. J Matern Fetal Med 1992;1:45–50.
19. Schatz M, Zeiger RS, Hoffman CP, Harden K, Forsythe A, Chilingar L, et al. Perinatal outcomes in the pregnancies of asthmatic women: a prospective controlled analysis. Am J Respir Crit Care Med 1995;151:1170–4.
20. Minerbi-Codish I, Fraser D, Avnun L, Glezerman M, Heimer D. Influence of asthma in pregnancy on labor and the newborn. Respiration 1998;65:130–5.
21. Stenius-Aarniala BS, Hedman J, Teramo KA. Acute asthma during pregnancy. Thorax 1996;51:411–4.
22. Olesen C, Thrane N, Nielsen GL, Sorensen HT, Olsen J; EuroMAP Group. A population-based prescription study of asthma drugs during pregnancy: changing the intensity of asthma therapy and perinatal outcomes. Respiration 2001;68: 256–61.
23. Norjavaara E, de Verdier MG. Normal pregnancy outcomes in a population-based study including 2,968 pregnant women exposed to budesonide. J Allergy Clin Immunol 2003;111:736–42.
24. Doucette JT, Bracken MB. Possible role of asthma in the risk of preterm labor and delivery. Epidemiology 1993; 4:143–50.
25. Jana N, Vasishta K, Saha SC, Khunnu B. Effect of bronchial asthma on the course of pregnancy, labour and perinatal outcome. J Obstet Gynaecol 1995;21:227–32.
26. Lehrer S, Stone J, Lapinski R, Lockwood CJ, Schachter BS, Berkowitz R, et al. Association between pregnancy-induced hypertension and asthma during pregnancy. Am J Obstet Gynecol 1993;168:1463–6.
27. Bracken MB, Triche EW, Belanger K, Saftlas A, Beckett WS, Leaderer BP. Asthma symptoms, severity, and drug therapy: a prospective study of effects on 2205 pregnancies. Obstet Gynecol 2003;102:739–52.

28. Dombrowski MP, Schatz M, Wise R, Momirova V, Landon M, Mabie W, et al. Asthma during pregnancy. Obstet Gynecol 2004;103:5–12.

29. Triche EW, Saftlas AF, Belanger K, Leaderer BP, Bracken MB. Association of asthma diagnosis, severity, symptoms, and treatment with risk of preeclampsia. Obstet Gynecol 2004;104:585–93.

30. Schatz M, Dombrowski MP, Wise R, Momirova V, Landon M, Mabie W, et al. The relationship of asthma medication use to perinatal outcomes. J Allergy Clin Immunol 2004; 113:1040–5.

31. Schatz M, Dombrowski MP, Wise R, Momirova V, Landon M, Mabie W, et al. Spirometry is related to perinatal outcomes in pregnant women with asthma. Am J Obstet Gynecol 2006;194:120–6.

32. National Institutes of Health, National Heart, Lung, and Blood Institute. National Asthma Education Program. Report of the Working Group on Asthma and Pregnancy: management of asthma during pregnancy. 1993 Available at: http://www.nhlbi.nih.gov/health/prof/lung/asthma/astpreg.txt. Retrieved June 28, 2006.

33. National Institutes of Health, National Heart, Lung, and Blood Institute, National Asthma Education and Prevention Program. Expert panel report 2. Guidelines for the diagnosis and management of asthma. 1997 Available at: http://www.nhlbi.nih.gov/guidelines/asthma/asthgdln.pdf. Retrieved June 28, 2006.

34. Schatz M, Dombrowski M. Asthma and allergy during pregnancy: outcomes of pregnancy in asthmatic women. Immunol Asthma Clin N America 2000;20:1–13.

35. Fitzsimons R, Greenberger PA, Patterson R. Outcome of pregnancy in women requiring corticosteroids for severe asthma. J Allergy Clin Immunol 1986;78:349–53.

36. Greenberger PA, Patterson R. The outcome of pregnancy complicated by severe asthma. Allergy Proc 1988;9: 539–43.

37. National Institutes of Health, National Heart, Lung, and Blood Institute, National Asthma Education and Prevention Program. Working group report on managing asthma during pregnancy: recommendations for pharmacologic treatment, update 2004. Available at: http://www.nhlbi.nih.gov/health/prof/lung/asthma/astpreg.htm. Retrieved June 28, 2006.

38. Nolten WE, Rueckert PA. Elevated free cortisol index in pregnancy: possible regulatory mechanisms. Am J Obstet Gynecol 1981;139:492–8.

39. Bailey K, Herrod HG, Younger R, Shaver D. Functional aspects of T-lymphocyte subsets in pregnancy. Obstet Gynecol 1985;66:211–5.

40. Haahtela T, Jarvinen M, Kava T, Kiviranta K, Koskinen S, Lehtonen K, et al. Comparison of beta 2-agonist, terbutaline, with an inhaled corticosteroid, budesonide, in newly detected asthma. N Engl J Med 1991;325:338–92.

41. Ernst P, Spitzer WO, Suissa S, Cockcroft D, Habbick B, Horwitz RI, et al. Risk of fatal and near-fatal asthma in relation to inhaled corticosteroid use. JAMA 1992;268: 3462–4.

42. Kraan J, Koeter GH, van der Mark TW, Boorsma M, Kukler J, Sluiter HJ, et al. Dosage and time effects of inhaled budesonide on bronchial hyperactivity. Am Rev Respir Dis 1988;137:44–8.

43. Lowhagen O, Rak S. Modification of bronchial hyperreactivity after treatment with sodium cromoglycate during pollen season. J Allergy Clin Immunol 1985;75:460–7.

44. Woolcock AJ, Jenkins C. Corticosteroids in the modulation of bronchial hyperresponsiveness. Immunol Allergy Clin North Am 1990;10:543–57.

45. Kallen B, Rydhstroem H, Aberg A. Congenital malformations after the use of inhaled budesonide in early pregnancy. Obstet Gynecol 1999;93:392–5.

46. Sears MR, Taylor DR, Print CG, Lake DC, Li QQ, Flannery EM, et al. Regular inhaled beta-agonist treatment in bronchial asthma. Lancet 1990;336:1391–6.

47. Cockcroft DW, Murdock KY. Comparative effects of inhaled salbutamol, sodium cromoglycate, and beclomethasone dipropionate on allergen-induced early asthmatic responses, late asthmatic responses, and increased bronchial responsiveness to histamine. J Allergy Clin Immunol 1987;79:734–40.

48. Spitzer WO, Suissa S, Ernst P, Horwitz RI, Habbick B, Cockcroft D, et al. The use of beta-agonists and the risk of death and near death from asthma. N Engl J Med 1992; 326:501–6.

49. Arwood LL, Dasta JF, Friedman C. Placental transfer of theophylline: two case reports. Pediatrics 1979;63:844–6.

50. Hendeles L, Jenkins J, Temple R. Revised FDA labeling guideline for theophylline oral dosage forms. Pharmacotherapy 1995;15:409–27.

51. Joad JP, Ahrens RC, Lindgren SD, Weinberger MM. Relative efficacy of maintenance therapy with theophylline, inhaled albuterol, and the combination for chronic asthma. J Allergy Clin Immunol 1987;79:78–85.

52. Wendel PJ, Ramin SM, Barnett-Hamm C, Rowe TF, Cunningham FG. Asthma treatment in pregnancy: a randomized controlled study. Am J Obstet Gynecol 1996; 175:150–4.

53. Pauwels R, Van Renterghem D, Van der Straeten M, Johannesson N, Persson CG. The effect of theophylline and enprofylline on allergen-induced bronchoconstriction. J Allergy Clin Immunol 1985;76:583–90.

54. Juergens UR, Degenhardt V, Stober M, Vetter H. New insights in the bronchodilatory and anti-inflammatory mechanisms of action of theophylline. Arzneimittelforschung 1999;49:694–8.

55. Evans DJ, Taylor DA, Zetterstrom O, Chung KF, O'Connor BJ, Barnes PJ. A comparison of low-dose inhaled budesonide plus theophylline and high-dose inhaled budesonide for moderate asthma. N Engl J Med 1997;337: 1412–8.

56. Dombrowski MP, Schatz M, Wise R, Thom EA, Landon M, Mabie W, et al. Randomized trial of inhaled beclomethasone dipropionate versus theophylline for moderate asthma during pregnancy. Am J Obstet Gynecol 2004;190:737–44.

57. Schatz M, Zeiger RS, Harden KM, Hoffman CP, Forsythe AB, Chilingar LM, et al. The safety of inhaled beta-agonist bronchodilators during pregnancy. J Allergy Clin Immunol 1988;82:686–95.

58. Knorr B, Matz J, Bernstein JA, Nguyen H, Seidenberg BC, Reiss TF, et al. Montelukast for chronic asthma in 6- to 14-year-old children: a randomized, double-blind trial. Pediatric Montelukast Study Group. JAMA 1998;279:1181–6.

59. Wenzel SE. New approaches to anti-inflammatory therapy for asthma. Am J Med 1998;104:287–300.

60. Park-Wyllie L, Mazzotta P, Pastuszak A, Moretti ME, Beique L, Hunnisett L, et al. Birth defects after maternal exposure to corticosteroids: prospective cohort study and meta-analysis of epidemiological studies. Teratology 2000;62:385–92.

61. Bakhireva LN, Jones KL, Schatz M, Johnson D, Chambers CD, Organization Of Teratology Information Services Research Group. Asthma medication use in pregnancy and fetal growth. J Allergy Clin Immunol 2005;116:503–9.

62. Towers CV, Briggs GG, Rojas JA. The use of prostaglandin E2 in pregnant patients with asthma. Am J Obstet Gynecol 2004;190:1777–80.

63. Crawford JS. Bronchospasm following ergometrine. Anesthesiology 1980;35:397–8.

64. Hagerdal M, Morgan CW, Sumner AE, Gutsche BB. Minute ventilation and oxygen consumption during labor with epidural analgesia. Anesthesiology 1983;59:425–7.

65. Fung DL. Emergency anesthesia for asthma patients. Clin Rev Allergy 1985;3:127–41.

66. Hirshman CA, Downes H, Farbood A, Bergman NA. Ketamine block of bronchospasm in experimental canine asthma. Br J Anaesth 1979;51:713–8.

67. American Academy of Pediatrics Committee on Drugs: transfer of drugs and other chemicals into human milk. Pediatrics 1989;84:924–36.

CHAPTER 5

Chronic Hypertension in Pregnancy

Baha M. Sibai

According to data from the Third National Health and Nutrition Examination Survey, 1988–1991, the prevalence of chronic hypertension among women of childbearing age increased from 0.6–2% for women aged 18–29 years to 4.6–22.3% for women aged 30–39 years. The lower prevalence rates are reported for white women, and higher prevalence rates are reported for black women (1). Because of the current trend of childbearing at an older age, it is expected that the incidence of chronic hypertension in pregnancy will continue to increase. During the new millennium and estimating a prevalence of chronic hypertension during pregnancy of 3%, at least 120,000 pregnant women with chronic hypertension (3% of 4 million pregnancies) will be seen per year in the United States.

Definition and Diagnosis

In pregnant women, chronic hypertension is defined as elevated blood pressure that is present and documented before pregnancy. In women whose prepregnancy blood pressure is unknown, the diagnosis is based on the presence of sustained hypertension before 20 weeks of gestation. Sustained hypertension is defined as either systolic blood pressure of at least 140 mm Hg or diastolic blood pressure of at least 90 mm Hg on at least two occasions measured at least 4 hours apart. The diagnosis may be difficult in women with previously undiagnosed chronic hypertension who begin prenatal care after 16 weeks of gestation because a physiologic decrease in blood pressure usually begins at that time. This decrease may result in normal blood pressure findings at that time, which will eventually increase again during the third trimester. These women are more likely to be erroneously diagnosed with gestational hypertension (2).

Women with chronic hypertension are at increased risk of superimposed preeclampsia. The development of superimposed preeclampsia is associated with high rates of adverse maternal and perinatal outcomes (3). Super-

imposed preeclampsia should be diagnosed in the presence of any of the following findings:

1. In women with chronic hypertension and without proteinuria early in pregnancy (less than 20 weeks of gestation), preeclampsia is diagnosed if there is new-onset proteinuria (0.5 g of protein or more in a 24-hour specimen).

2. In women with chronic hypertension and preexisting proteinuria before 20 weeks of gestation, the diagnosis is confirmed if there is an exacerbated increase in blood pressure to the severe range (systolic pressure of 160 mm Hg or more or diastolic pressure of 110 mm Hg or more) in a woman whose hypertension has previously been well controlled with antihypertensive drugs, particularly if associated with headaches, blurred vision, or epigastric pain, or if there is a significant increase in liver enzymes (unrelated to methyldopa), or if the platelet count is less than 100,000/mm^3 (4).

Etiology and Classification

The etiology and severity of chronic hypertension are important considerations in the management of pregnancy. Chronic hypertension is subdivided into two categories: primary (essential) and secondary. Primary hypertension is by far the most common cause of chronic hypertension seen during pregnancy (90%). In 10% of the cases, chronic hypertension is secondary to one or more underlying disorders such as renal disease (glomerulonephritis, interstitial nephritis, polycystic kidneys, renal artery stenosis), collagen vascular disease (lupus, scleroderma), endocrine disorders (diabetes mellitus with vascular involvement, pheochromocytoma, thyrotoxicosis, Cushing's disease, hyperaldosteronism), or coarctation of the aorta (4, 5).

Chronic hypertension during pregnancy can be subclassified as either mild or severe, depending on the systolic and diastolic blood pressure readings. Systolic and diastolic (Korotkoff sound, phase V) blood pressures of at least 160 mm Hg and 110 mm Hg, respectively, constitute severe hypertension (4, 5).

For management and counseling purposes, chronic hypertension in pregnancy also is categorized as either low risk or high risk, as described in Figure 5-1. The patient is considered to be at low risk when she has mild essential hypertension without any organ involvement. Blood pressure criteria are based on blood pressure measurements at the initial visit regardless of whether patients are on antihypertensive medications. For example, if the patient's a blood pressure is 140/80 mm Hg while she is taking antihypertensive drugs, she is still classified as low risk. The medications should be discontinued and her blood pressure should be monitored very closely. If it reaches severe levels, she then would be classified as high risk, and treated as such. A patient who initially is classified as low risk early in pregnancy may become high risk if she later develops severe hypertension or if she develops preeclampsia, or fetal growth restriction.

Maternal–Perinatal Risks

Women with pregnancies complicated by chronic hypertension are at increased risk for the development of superimposed preeclampsia and abruptio placentae. The reported rates of preeclampsia with mild hypertension range from 10% to 25% (Table 5-1) (2, 3, 6, 7). The rate of preeclampsia in women with severe chronic hypertension is approximately 50% (7, 8). One study examined the rate of superimposed preeclampsia among 763 women with chronic hypertension who were observed prospectively at several medical centers in the United States (3). The overall rate of superimposed preeclampsia was 25%. The rate was not affected by maternal age, race, or presence of proteinuria early in pregnancy. However, the rate was significantly greater in women who had hypertension for at least 4 years (31% versus 22%), in those who had had preeclampsia during a previous pregnancy (32% versus 23%), and in those whose diastolic blood pressure was 100–110 mm Hg when compared with those whose diastolic blood pressure was below 100 mm Hg at baseline (42% versus 24%) (3).

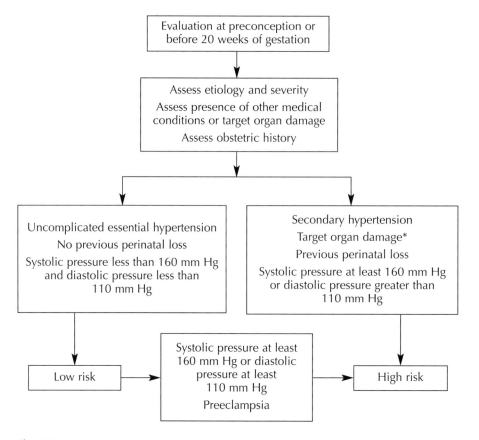

Fig. 5-1. Initial evaluation of women with chronic hypertension. *Left ventricular dysfunction, retinopathy, dyslipidemia, maternal age older than 40 years, microvascular disease, and stroke. (Sibai BM. Chronic hypertension in pregnancy. Obstet Gynecol 2002;100:369–377.)

The reported rate of abruptio placentae in women with mild chronic hypertension ranges from 0.7% to 1.5% (Table 5-1). The rate in those with severe or high-risk hypertension may be 5–10% (8). In the recent multicenter study that included 763 women with chronic hypertension, the overall rate of abruptio placentae was reported at 1.5%, and the rate was significantly higher in those who developed superimposed preeclampsia than in those without this complication (3% versus 1%, $P = .04$) (3). However, the rate was not influenced by either maternal age, race, or duration of hypertension (4). In addition, the results of a systematic review of nine observational studies revealed that the rate of abruptio placentae is double (odds ratio [OR] 2.1, 95% confidence interval [CI] 1) in women with chronic hypertension compared with either the normotensive or the general obstetric population (1, 3, 9).

In addition to preeclampsia and abruptio placentae, women with high-risk chronic hypertension are at an increased risk for life-threatening maternal complications such as pulmonary edema, hypertensive encephalopathy, retinopathy, cerebral hemorrhage, and acute renal failure (4). These risks are particularly increased in women with uncontrolled severe hypertension, in those with significant renal dysfunction early in pregnancy, and in those with left ventricular dysfunction before conception (10, 11).

Fetal and neonatal complications also are increased in women with chronic hypertension. The risk of perinatal mortality is increased three to four times compared with the general obstetric population (OR, 3.4; 95% CI, 3–3.7) (9). The rates of premature deliveries and small for gestational age (SGA) infants also are increased in women with chronic hypertension (Table 5-1). In women with severe chronic hypertension in the first trimester, the reported rates of preterm deliveries were 62–70% and the rates of SGA infants were 31–40% (7–8). Recently, risk factors for adverse perinatal outcome among 763 women with mild chronic hypertension who were enrolled in a multicenter trial comparing

low-dose aspirin to a placebo were reported (3). The authors found that the development of superimposed preeclampsia was associated with higher rates of preterm delivery (OR, 3.9; 95% CI, 2.7–5.4), higher rates of neonatal intraventricular hemorrhage (OR, 4.5; 95% CI, 1.5–14.2), and higher rates of perinatal death (OR, 2.3; 95% CI, 1.4–4.8). In addition, the presence of proteinuria early in pregnancy was also an independent risk factor associated with higher rates of preterm delivery (OR 3.1; 95% CI, 1.8–5.3), higher rates of SGA infants (OR, 2.8; 95% CI, 1.6–5), and higher rates of neonatal intraventricular hemorrhage (OR, 3.9; 95% CI, 1.3–11.6) (3).

Goals of Antihypertensive Therapy

In nonpregnant individuals, long-term blood pressure control can lead to significant reductions in the rates of stroke and cardiovascular morbidity and mortality (12). In those with mild to moderate hypertension, the benefit is achieved after at least 5 years of treatment (12). The side effects of therapy are restricted to the treated individual. Hypertension in pregnancy is different because the duration of therapy is shorter, the benefits to the mother may not be obvious during the short time of treatment, and the exposure to drugs will include both mother and fetus. In this respect, one must balance the potential short-term maternal benefits against possible short- and long-term benefits and risks to the fetus and infant (9, 13).

Most women with chronic hypertension during pregnancy have mild essential uncomplicated hypertension and are at minimal risk for cardiovascular complications within the short time frame of pregnancy (9, 13). Several retrospective and prospective studies have been conducted to determine whether antihypertensive therapy in these women would improve pregnancy outcome (2, 3, 6, 7, 14–17). A summary of the results of these studies revealed that, regardless of the antihypertensive therapy used, maternal cardiovascular and renal complications were minimal or absent (9, 13). Based on the available data, there is no compelling evidence that short-

Table 5-1. Rates of Adverse Pregnancy Outcome in Observational Studies Describing Mild Chronic Hypertension in Pregnancy

Study	Preeclampsia (%)	Abruptio Placentae (%)	Delivery at Less Than 37 Weeks of Gestation (%)	Small for Gestational Age Fetuses (%)
Sibai et al (2) (n = 211)	10	1.4	12	8
Rey and Couturier (6) (n = 337)	21	0.7	34.4	15.5
McCowan et al (7) (n = 142)	14	NR	16	11
Sibai et al (3) (n = 763)	25	1.5	33.3	11.1

Abbreviation: NR, not reported

term antihypertensive therapy benefits women with low-risk hypertension in pregnancy, with the exception of reducing the rate of exacerbation of hypertension (18, 19).

There are no placebo-controlled trials examining the benefits of antihypertensive therapy in women with severe hypertension in pregnancy, and none are likely to be performed because of the potential risks of untreated severe hypertension (8). Antihypertensive therapy is necessary in these women to reduce the acute risk of stroke, congestive heart failure, or renal failure. In addition, control of severe hypertension also may permit pregnancy prolongation and thereby improve perinatal outcome. However, there is no evidence that control of severe hypertension reduces the rates of either superimposed preeclampsia or abruptio placentae (7, 8).

There are no trials examining the treatment of women with chronic hypertension and other risk factors, such as preexisting renal disease, diabetes mellitus, or cardiac disease (9). However, there is evidence from retrospective and observational studies that uncontrolled mild to moderate hypertension may exacerbate target organ damage during pregnancy in women with renal disease, in those with diabetes mellitus with vascular disease, and in those with left ventricular dysfunction (20, 21). Therefore, some authors recommend aggressive treatment of mild hypertension in these women because of the belief that such management may reduce both short- and long-term cardiovascular complications (20, 21).

There are many retrospective and prospective studies examining the potential fetal–neonatal benefits of pharmacologic therapy in women with mild essential uncomplicated hypertension (low risk) (9, 19). Some investigators compared treatment with no treatment or with a placebo, others compared two different antihypertensive drugs, and others used a combination of drugs. In addition, the gestational age at time of treatment, the level of blood pressure achieved during treatment, and the duration of therapy were highly variable. Only four of these studies were randomized trials that included women enrolled before 20 weeks of gestation (14–17). Only two of the trials had a moderate sample size to evaluate the risks of superimposed preeclampsia and abruptio placentae (16, 17). The findings of these two trials revealed contradictory results regarding the effects of antihypertensive therapy on the rates of superimposed preeclampsia and abruptio placentae. Antihypertensive therapy did not affect gestational age at the time of delivery in any of the four trials; only one small trial demonstrated a significantly lower average birth weight and significantly higher rate of SGA infants in the atenolol-treated group (5). The total number of women enrolled in these trials was only 450, and the largest trial included 263 women (16). In addition, in one study there was an imbalance in the number of women with risk factors for preeclampsia and abruptio placentae (17). This imbalance favored the treated arm of the study. Therefore, none of these trials had a sample size with adequate power to detect moderate (20–30%) reductions or increases in rates of preeclampsia, SGA infants, or abruptio placentae (9).

Safety of Antihypertensive Drugs

The potential adverse effects for most commonly prescribed antihypertensive agents are either poorly established or unclearly quantified (9). Most of the evidence on adverse effects associated with antihypertensive drugs in pregnancy is limited to case reports. The interpretation of these reports is difficult because it is impossible to ascertain the exact number of women exposed to antihypertensive drugs during pregnancy (9). Also, it is likely that the number of published case reports is an underestimate of the actual number of women experiencing the reported adverse reaction. This limitation is amplified by the fact that information related to previous exposure and previous use during pregnancy are nonexistent. Furthermore, the condition for which pregnant women are treated with antihypertensive drugs can be partially responsible for the adverse fetal and neonatal outcomes.

In general, available information about teratogenicity, except in laboratory animals, is limited and selective. All available data have been obtained from registries such as state medical registry data (22). Because of the lack of multicenter randomized trials in women with chronic hypertension, there are no placebo-controlled evaluations regarding the safety of these drugs when used at the time of conception and throughout pregnancy. Currently, there are few data to help the clinician evaluate the benefits or risks of most antihypertensive drugs when used in pregnancy. Nevertheless, the limited data suggest that there are potential adverse fetal effects such as oligohydramnios and fetal–neonatal renal failure when angiotensin-converting enzyme inhibitors are used in the second or third trimesters (9, 22). Similar effects are to be expected with the use of angiotensin II receptor blockers. Therefore, these agents should be avoided, if possible, in the second and third trimesters (13, 22).

The use of atenolol during the first and second trimesters is associated with significantly reduced fetal growth along with decreased placental growth and weight (15, 23). However, no such effects on fetal or placental growth were reported with other β-blockers, such as metoprolol, pindolol, and oxprenolol, but data on the use of these agents in early pregnancy are very scarce (9). Prospective trials that studied the effect of either methyldopa or labetalol in women with mild chronic hypertension revealed no adverse maternal or fetal outcome with the use of these medications (9, 13). In a large and unique trial in which methyldopa or labetalol was started between 6 weeks and 13 weeks of gestation in patients with chronic hypertension, none of the exposed newborns had major congenital anomalies (16).

There is large clinical experience with the use of thiazide diuretics during pregnancy. The available data suggest that the use of diuretics in the first trimester and throughout gestation is not associated with an increased risk of major fetal anomalies or adverse fetal–neonatal events (9, 13). However, the use of these drugs was associated with reduced plasma volume expansion. There is little information regarding the use of calcium channel blockers in women with mild chronic hypertension. The available evidence suggests that the use of calcium channel blockers, particularly nifedipine in the first trimester, was not associated with increased rates of major birth defects (22, 24). The effects of nifedipine on fetal–neonatal outcome were evaluated in a prospective randomized trial of 283 women with mild to moderate hypertension in pregnancy in which 47% of the participants had chronic hypertension (25). Sixty-six of these women were enrolled between 12 weeks and 20 weeks of gestation. In this study, the use of slow-release nifedipine was not associated with adverse fetal–neonatal outcomes (25).

Information regarding the long-term effects on children of maternal exposure to antihypertensive drugs during pregnancy is lacking, except for limited information concerning the use of methyldopa and nifedipine (26, 27). A follow-up study of infants after 7.5 years showed no long-term adverse effects on development among those exposed to methyldopa in utero compared with infants not exposed to such treatment (26). Results of a similar study examining the effects of slow-release nifedipine after 1.5 years of follow-up demonstrated no adverse effects on development (27).

Management

The primary objective in the management of pregnancies complicated by chronic hypertension is to reduce maternal risks and achieve optimal perinatal survival. This objective can be achieved by formulating a rational approach that includes preconception evaluation and counseling, early antenatal care, frequent antepartum visits to monitor both maternal and fetal well-being, timely delivery with intensive intrapartum monitoring, and proper postpartum management.

Evaluation and Classification

Management of chronic hypertension should ideally begin before pregnancy, whereby extensive evaluation

and a complete workup are undertaken to assess the cause, severity, and presence of other medical illnesses and to rule out the presence of target organ damage of long-standing hypertension. An in-depth history should delineate in particular the duration of hypertension, the use of antihypertensive medications, the type of medications used, and the response to these medications. Also, attention should be given to the presence of cardiac or renal disease, diabetes, thyroid disease, and a history of cerebrovascular accident or congestive heart failure. A detailed obstetric history should include maternal as well as neonatal outcome of previous pregnancies, with stresses on history of development of abruptio placentae, superimposed preeclampsia, preterm delivery, SGA infants, intrauterine fetal death, and neonatal morbidity and mortality.

Laboratory studies are obtained to assess the function of different organ systems that are likely to be affected by chronic hypertension and to establish a baseline for future assessments. These studies should include the following tests for all patients: urine analysis, urine culture and sensitivity, 24-hour urine evaluations for protein and electrolyte levels, complete blood count, and glucose tolerance test.

Women who have had long-standing hypertension for several years, particularly those with histories of poor compliance with antihypertensive therapy or poor blood pressure control, should be evaluated for target organ damage, including left ventricular hypertrophy, retinopathy, and renal injury. These women should receive an electrocardiography examination (echocardiography if the electrocardiography results are abnormal), ophthalmologic evaluation, and creatinine clearance.

Certain tests should be done selectively to identify secondary causes of hypertension such as pheochromocytoma, primary hyperaldosteronism, or renal artery stenosis. These conditions require selective biochemical testing and are amenable to diagnosis with either computed tomography or magnetic resonance imaging (4, 5). Pheochromocytoma should be suspected in women with paroxysmal severe hypertension, hyperglycemia, and sweating. Primary aldosteronism is extremely rare in pregnancy and should be considered in women with severe hypertension and marked hypokalemia. Based on this evaluation, the patient is then classified as having low- or high-risk chronic hypertension and treated accordingly (Fig. 5-2).

Low-Risk Hypertension

Women with low-risk chronic hypertension without superimposed preeclampsia usually have a pregnancy outcome similar to that of the general obstetric population (2, 6, 16). In addition, discontinuation of antihyper-

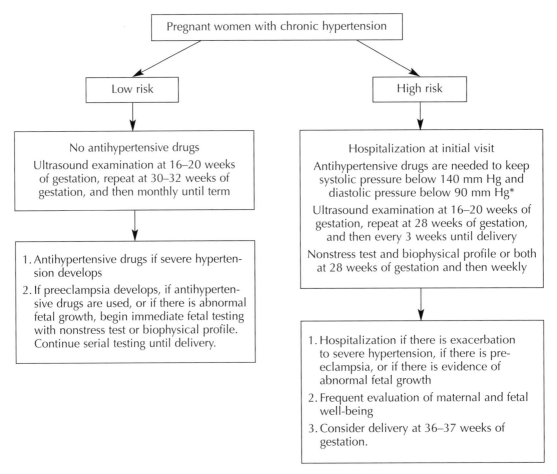

Fig. 5-2. Antepartum management of chronic hypertension. *For women with target organ damage. (Sibai BM. Chronic hypertension in pregnancy. Obstet Gynecol 2002;100:369–377.)

tensive therapy early in pregnancy does not affect the rates of preeclampsia, abruptio placentae, or preterm delivery in these women (2, 16). Antihypertensive treatment should be discontinued at the first prenatal visit because most of these women will have good pregnancy outcomes without such therapy (2). Although these women do not require pharmacologic therapy, careful management is still essential (Fig. 5-2). At the time of initial and subsequent visits, the patient should be educated about nutritional requirements, weight gain, and sodium intake (maximum of 2.4 g/d). She also should be counseled that consumption of alcohol and smoking during pregnancy can aggravate maternal hypertension and are associated with adverse effects, such as fetal growth restriction and abruptio placentae. During each subsequent visit patients should be observed very closely for early signs of preeclampsia and fetal growth restriction.

Fetal evaluation should include an ultrasound examination at 16–20 weeks of gestation, to be repeated at 32–34 weeks of gestation, and monthly thereafter until term. Ultrasound examinations for fetal growth also may

be indicated if there is poor weight gain or evidence of poor fetal growth. Antihypertensive medications with either nifedipine or labetalol should be initiated if the patient develops severe hypertension before term. The development of severe hypertension, preeclampsia, or abnormal fetal growth requires immediate fetal testing with a nonstress test or biophysical profile. Women who develop severe hypertension, have fetal growth restriction documented by ultrasound examination, and superimposed preeclampsia at or beyond 37 weeks of gestation require hospitalization and delivery. In the absence of these complications, the pregnancy may be continued until 40 weeks of gestation.

High-Risk Hypertension

Women with high-risk chronic hypertension are at increased risk for adverse maternal and perinatal complications. The frequency and the maternal–fetal effects of these complications will depend on the cause of the hypertension as well as the degree of target organ damage. Women with significant renal insufficiency (serum creatinine levels greater than 1.4 mg/dL), diabetes mellitus with vascular involvement (retinal or renal involvement), severe collagen vascular disease, cardiomyopathy, or coarctation of the aorta should receive thorough counseling before conception regarding the adverse effects of pregnancy. Women with high-risk hypertension should be advised that pregnancy may exacerbate their condition, with the potential for congestive heart failure, acute renal failure requiring dialysis, and even death. In addition, perinatal loss and neonatal complications are markedly increased in these women. These women should be treated by or in consultation with a subspecialist in maternal–fetal medicine, as well as other medical specialists as needed. In addition, they must be observed and give birth in a tertiary care center with adequate maternal–neonatal care facilities.

Women with high-risk hypertension should be hospitalized at the time of their first prenatal visit for evaluation of cardiovascular and renal status and for regulation of antihypertensive medications, as well as other prescribed medications (insulin, cardiac drugs, thyroid drugs), if needed. Women receiving atenolol, angiotensin-converting enzyme inhibitors, or angiotensin II receptor antagonists should discontinue using these medications, if possible, under close observation. Antihypertensive therapy with one or more of the drugs listed in Table 5-2 is used subsequently in all women with systolic blood pressure of 160 mm Hg or greater or diastolic blood pressure of 110 mm Hg or greater. In women without target organ damage, the goal of antihypertensive therapy is to keep systolic blood pressure between 140 mm Hg and 150 mm Hg and diastolic blood pressure between 90 mm Hg and 100 mm Hg. In addition, antihypertensive therapy is indicated for women with mild hypertension plus target organ damage because there are short-term maternal benefits from lowering blood pressure. In these women, it is recommended that systolic blood pressure be kept below 140 mm Hg and diastolic blood pressure below 90 mm Hg. In some women, blood pressure may be difficult to control initially, demanding the use of intravenous therapy with hydralazine or labetalol or oral short-acting nifedipine with doses as described in Table 5-2. For maintenance therapy, oral methyldopa, labetalol, slow-release nifedipine, or a diuretic may be chosen (25–27). Methyldopa is the drug most commonly recommended to treat hypertension during pregnancy (4, 5). However, it is rarely used in nonpregnant hypertensive women. Therefore, it is not practical to switch medications for hypertensive women to methyldopa because of pregnancy. In addition, methyldopa is associated with dry mouth and drowsiness in many pregnant women. Other side effects include liver function abnormalities. The drug of choice for control of hypertension in pregnancy is labetalol, starting at 100 mg, twice daily, and increasing to a maximum of 2,400 mg/d. If maternal blood pressure is not controlled with maximum doses of labetalol, a second drug such as a thiazide diuretic or nifedipine may be added. For women with diabetes mellitus and vascular disease, the preferred drug is oral nifedipine or nicardipine. Oral nifedipine or a thiazide diuretic is the drug of choice for young African-American women with hypertension because these women often manifest a low-renin or salt-sensitive hypertension (12, 13). If maternal blood pressure is adequately controlled with these medications, the patient can continue taking the same drug after delivery.

Diuretics are commonly prescribed in women with essential hypertension before conception (12, 13). The use of diuretics throughout pregnancy is controversial. The primary concern relates to the fact that women who

Table 5-2. Drugs Used to Treat Hypertension in Pregnancy

Drug	Starting Dose	Maximum Dose
Acute treatment of severe hypertension		
Hydralazine	5–10 mg IV every 20 min	30 mg*
Labetalol[†]	20–40 mg IV every 10–15 min	220 mg*
Nifedipine	10–20 mg orally every 30 min	50 mg*
Long-term management of hypertension		
Methyldopa	250 mg, twice daily	4 g/d
Labetalol[†]	100 mg, twice daily	2,400 mg/d
Nifedipine	10 mg, twice daily	120 mg/d
Thiazide diuretic	12.5 mg, twice daily	50 mg/d

Abbreviation: IV, intravenously.

*If desired blood pressure levels are not achieved, switch to another drug.

[†]Avoid in women with asthma or congestive heart failure.

use diuretics early in pregnancy do not have an increase in plasma volume to the degree of plasma volume in normal pregnancy (14). However, this reduction in plasma volume was not shown to be associated with an adverse effect on fetal outcome (14, 28). Therefore, it is appropriate to start diuretics as a single agent during pregnancy or to use them in combination with other agents, particularly in women with excessive salt retention (4). However, diuretics should be discontinued immediately if superimposed preeclampsia develops or if there is evidence of suspected fetal growth restriction because of the potential of reduced uteroplacental blood flow secondary to reduced plasma volume in women with such complications (14).

Early and frequent prenatal visits are the key for successful pregnancy outcome in women with high-risk chronic hypertension. These patients need close observation throughout pregnancy and may require serial evaluation of 24-hour urine protein excretion and a complete blood count with metabolic profile at least once every trimester. Further laboratory testing can be performed, depending on the clinical progress of the pregnancy. During each visit, the woman should be advised about the adverse effects of smoking and alcohol abuse and should receive nutritional advice regarding diet and salt intake.

Fetal evaluation should include an ultrasound examination at 16–20 weeks of gestation, to be repeated at 28 weeks of gestation and subsequently every 3 weeks until delivery. A nonstress test or biophysical profile testing usually is started at 28 weeks of gestation and then repeated weekly. The development of uncontrolled severe hypertension, preeclampsia, or evidence of fetal growth restriction requires maternal hospitalization for more frequent evaluation of maternal and fetal well-being. The development of any of these complications at or beyond 34 weeks of gestation should be considered an indication for delivery. In all other women, delivery should be considered at 36–37 weeks of gestation after fetal lung maturity is documented.

Postpartum Management

Women with high-risk chronic hypertension are at risk for postpartum complications such as pulmonary edema, hypertensive encephalopathy, and renal failure (10, 11). These risks are particularly increased in women with target organ involvement, superimposed preeclampsia, or abruptio placentae (11). In these patients, blood pressure must be closely controlled for at least 48 hours after delivery. Intravenous labetalol or hydralazine can be used as needed, and diuretics may be appropriate in women with circulatory congestion and pulmonary edema (10). Loop diuretics such as furosemide are very useful in patients with congestive heart failure or pulmonary edema. In case of acute pulmonary edema, the usual dose of furosemide is 20–40 mg extended intravenous bolus, to be repeated as needed based on maternal response. Side effects of chronic use of furosemide include hypokalemia. This therapy is usually needed in those who develop exaggerated and sustained severe hypertension in the first week postpartum.

Oral therapy may be needed to control blood pressure after delivery. In some women, it often is necessary to switch to a new agent such as an angiotensin-converting enzyme inhibitor, particularly in those with pregestational diabetes mellitus and those with cardiomyopathy. Some patients may wish to breastfeed their infants. All antihypertensive drugs are found in the breast milk, although differences have been found in the milk/plasma ratio of these drugs (22). Additionally, the long-term effect of maternal antihypertensive drugs on breastfeeding infants has not been specifically studied. Milk concentrations of methyldopa appear to be low and are considered to be safe. The β-blocking agents (atenolol and metoprolol) are concentrated in breast milk, whereas labetalol or propanolol has a low concentration (21, 29). Concentrations of diuretic agents in breast milk are low; however, they may induce a decrease in milk production (22).

There is little information about the transfer of calcium channel blockers to breast milk, but there are no apparent side effects. Angiotensin-converting enzyme inhibitors and angiotensin II receptor antagonists should be avoided because of their effects on neonatal renal function, even though their concentrations appear to be low in breast milk.

In women who are breastfeeding, the use of methyldopa as first-line oral therapy is reasonable. If methyldopa is contraindicated, labetalol may be used.

Summary

Many important clinical issues faced by clinicians who care for pregnant women with preexisting chronic hypertension remain unresolved. There is a lack of agreement regarding the blood pressure levels at which to initiate antihypertensive therapy, and there is a lack of information regarding the optimal blood pressure to be achieved during antihypertensive therapy. The evidence regarding benefits and risks of antihypertensive drugs remains scant and provides little direction to clinicians. There are no studies assessing the costs, benefits, or risks of various fetal evaluation techniques (ultrasound examinations, serial nonstress testing, or biophysical profile testing) in women with chronic hypertension. Various international and national societies recommend different guidelines and different antihypertensive agents as the treatment of choice (4, 5, 30, 31). These recommendations are based on consensus rather than on solid scientific evidence. Therefore, until multicenter trials are performed in this area, management of chronic hypertension in pregnancy will continue to be based on expert opinion.

References

1. Burt VL, Whelton P, Rochella EJ, Brown C, Cutler JA, Higgins M, et al. Prevalence of hypertension in the US adult population: results from the third national health and nutrition examination survey, 1988-1991. Hypertension 1995;23:305–13.

2. Sibai BM, Abdella TN, Anderson GD. Pregnancy outcome in 211 patients with mild chronic hypertension. Obstet Gynecol 1983;61:571– 6.

3. Sibai BM, Lindheimer M, Hauth J, Caritis S, VanDorsten P, Klebanoff M, et al. Risk factors for preeclampsia, abruptio placentae, and adverse neonatal outcomes among women with chronic hypertension. N Engl J Med 1998; 339:667–71.

4. Report of the National High Blood Pressure Education Program Working Group on High Blood Pressure in Pregnancy. Am J Obstet Gynecol 2000;183:S1–22.

5. Chronic hypertension in pregnancy. ACOG practice bulletin No. 29. American College of Obstetricians and Gynecologists. Obstet Gynecol 2001;98:177–85.

6. Rey E, Couturier A. The prognosis of pregnancy in women with chronic hypertension. Am J Obstet Gynecol 1994;171:410–6.

7. McCowan LM, Buist RG, North RA, Gamble G. Perinatal morbidity in chronic hypertension. Br J Obstet Gynaecol 1996;103:123–9.

8. Sibai BM, Anderson GD. Pregnancy outcome of intensive therapy in severe hypertension in first trimester. Obstet Gynecol 1986;67:517–22.

9. Ferrer RL, Sibai BM, Murlow CD, Chiquette E, Stevens KR, Cornell J. Management of mild chronic hypertension during pregnancy: a review. Obstet Gynecol 2000;96: 849–60.

10. Mabie WC, Ratts TE, Ramanathan KB, Sibai BM. Circulatory congestion in obese hypertensive women: a subset of pulmonary edema in pregnancy. Obstet Gynecol 1988;72:553–8.

11. Sibai BM, Villar MA, Mabie BC. Acute renal failure in hypertensive disorders of pregnancy: pregnancy outcome and remote prognosis in thirty-one consecutive cases. AmJ Obstet Gynecol 1990;162:777– 83.

12. The sixth report of the Joint National Committee on prevention, detection, evaluation, and treatment of high blood pressure. Arch Intern Med 1997;157:2413–46.

13. Umans JG, Lindheimer MD. Antihypertensive treatment. In: Lindheimer MD, Roberts JM, Cunningham FG, editors. Chesley's hypertensive disorders in pregnancy. 2nd ed. Norwalk (CT): Appleton and Lange; 1998. p. 581–604.

14. Sibai BM, Grossman RA, Grossman HG. Effects of diuretics on plasma volume in pregnancies with long-term hypertension. Am J Obstet Gynecol 1984;150:831–5.

15. Butters L, Kennedy S, Rubin PC. Atenolol in essential hypertension during pregnancy. BMJ 1990;301:587–9.

16. Sibai BM, Mabie WC, Shamsa F, Villar MA, Anderson GD. A comparison of no medication versus methyldopa or labetalol in chronic hypertension during pregnancy. Am J Obstet Gynecol 1990;162:960–6.

17. Steyn DW, Odendaal HJ. Randomized controlled trial of ketanserin and aspirin in prevention of pre-eclampsia. Lancet 1997;350:1267–71.

18. Magee LA, Ornstein MP, von Dadelszen P. Management of hypertension in pregnancy. BMJ 1999;318:1332–6.

19. Magee LA, Duley L. Oral beta-blockers for mild to moderate hypertension during pregnancy. Cochrane Database Syst Rev 2001;4:CD002863.

20. Jones DC, Hayslett JP. Outcome of pregnancy in women with moderate or severe renal insufficiency. N Engl J Med 1996;335:226–32.

21. Easterling TR, Carr DB, Brateng D, Diederichs C, Schumucker B. Treatment of hypertension in pregnancy: effect of atenolol on maternal disease, preterm delivery and fetal growth. Obstet Gynecol 2001,98:427–33.

22. Briggs GG, Freeman RK, Yaffee SJ. Drugs in pregnancy and lactation: a reference guide to fetal and neonatal risk. 5th ed. Baltimore (MD): Williams & Wilkins; 1998.

23. Easterling TR, Brateng D, Schmucker B, Brown Z, Millard SP. Prevention of preeclampsia: a randomized trial of atenolol in hyperdynamic patients before onset of hypertension. Obstet Gynecol 1999;93:725–33.

24. Magee LA, Schick B, Donnenfeld AE, Sage SR, Conover B, Cook L, et al. The safety of calcium channel blockers in human pregnancy: a prospective, multicenter cohort study. Am J Obstet Gynecol 1996;174:823–8.

25. Gruppo di Studio Ipertensione in Gravidanza. Nifedipine versus expectant management in mild to moderate hypertension in pregnancy. Br J Obstet Gynaecol 1998;105: 718–22.

26. Cockburn J, Moar VA, Ounsted M, Redman LW. Final report of study on hypertension during pregnancy: the effects of specific treatment on the growth and development of the children. Lancet 1982;1:647–9.

27. Bartolus R, Ricci E, Chatenoud L, Parazzini F. Nifedipine administration in pregnancy: effect on the development of children at 18 months. Br J Obstet Gynaecol 2000;107: 792–4.

28. Collins R, Yusuf S, Peto R. Overview of randomized trials of diuretics in pregnancy. Br Med J 1985;290:17–23.

29. White WB. Management of hypertension during lactation. Hypertension 1984;6:297–300.

30. Rey E, Lelorier J, Burgess E, Lange IR, Leduc L. Report of the Canadian Hypertension Society Consensus Conference: 3. Pharmacologic treatment of hypertensive disorders in pregnancy. CMAJ 1997;157:1245–54.

31. Brown MA, Hague WM, Higgins J, Lowe S, McCowan L, Peek MJ. The detection, investigation and management of hypertension in pregnancy. Full consensus statement. Aust N Z J Obstet Gynaecol 2000;40:139–55.

CHAPTER 6

Antiphospholipid Syndrome

D. Ware Branch and Munther A. Khamashta

Antiphospholipid antibodies are a family of autoantibodies that bind to negatively charged phospholipids, phospholipid-binding proteins, or a combination of the two. Clinicians first recognized that antiphospholipid antibodies were associated with hypercoagulability 50 years ago. An association with pregnancy loss was established in the mid-1970s. The term "antiphospholipid syndrome" was introduced in 1986 to formalize the association of antiphospholipid antibodies with these clinical features. Over a decade of subsequent international laboratory and clinical experience led to the development of an international consensus statement on preliminary criteria for definite antiphospholipid syndrome, first published in 1999 (1) and revised in 2005 (2). There is widespread recognition, however, that refining the diagnostic criteria of antiphospholipid syndrome is an ongoing process (3). In this regard, no area has generated more controversy than obstetric antiphospholipid syndrome. Recent studies even bring the treatment of some women with antiphospholipid antibodies into question. This review involves the pathogenesis, diagnosis, and management of the obstetric aspects of antiphospholipid syndrome and addresses controversies that have emerged in obstetric antiphospholipid syndrome.

Historically, the first antiphospholipid autoantibody detected was the false-positive Wassermann reaction, found especially in patients with systemic lupus erythematosus. Lupus anticoagulant was first described in the early 1950s as prolonging certain clotting assays. A few years later, lupus anticoagulant was found to be associated with the false-positive test result for syphilis and (paradoxically) thrombosis. The key antigenic component of the Wassermann reaction was cardiolipin, a phospholipid found in mitochondrial membranes, and a much more sensitive immunoassay was developed in the early 1980s using cardiolipin as the solid phase antigen. Anticardiolipin antibodies identified in this assay proved strongly correlated with lupus anticoagulant and thrombosis. In the early 1990s, anticardiolipin autoantibodies were found to require the presence of the plasma phospholipid-binding protein β_2-glycoprotein I to bind to cardiolipin (4). In contrast, anticardiolipin antibodies from patients with syphilis or other infections are β_2-glycoprotein I independent, binding directly to cardiolipin without requiring a cofactor. As a result of these findings, antiphospholipid autoantibody research has recently focused on phospholipid-binding proteins, rather than phospholipids themselves, with regard to pathophysiology and antibody specificity (4).

The association of antiphospholipid antibodies with thrombosis and pregnancy loss is now well established. With regard to thrombosis, antiphospholipid syndrome is an important diagnosis because the high recurrence risk of thrombosis requires consideration of long-term anticoagulation (5). With regard to pregnancy loss, antiphospholipid syndrome is an important diagnosis because treatment may improve subsequent pregnancy outcomes and because of potential maternal risks, including thrombosis in pregnancy (6, 7). Clinicians should recognize, however, that detectable antiphospholipid antibodies are found in up to 5% of apparently healthy controls and up to 35% of patients with systemic lupus erythematosus (3). The prospective risks of positive test results for antiphospholipid antibodies in otherwise healthy individuals are unknown.

Pathogenesis of Obstetric Features of Antiphospholipid Syndrome

Whether antiphospholipid antibodies per se are the cause of adverse obstetric outcomes associated with the antibodies remains a subject of debate. Working with mice, some investigators found administration of human antiphospholipid antibodies results in clinical manifestations of antiphospholipid syndrome, including fetal loss (8, 9). The induction of fetal loss in this model is, however, variable. One group has used a mouse venous thrombosis model to show that circulating human and mouse antiphospholipid antibodies are associated with larger and more persistent thrombi than in mice treated with control antibodies (10).

A variety of mechanisms by which antiphospholipid antibodies may cause pregnancy loss and thrombosis have been suggested. Antiphospholipid antibodies may interfere with the normal in vivo function of phospholipids or phospholipid-binding proteins that are crucial to the regulation of coagulation. Candidate molecules or pathways that might be adversely affected include β_2-glycoprotein I (which has anticoagulant properties), prostacyclin, prothrombin, protein C, and tissue factor. Antiphospholipid antibodies also might promote local thrombosis via interference with trophoblastic annexin V (11), which is abundant in the human placenta. Antiphospholipid antibodies may activate endothelial cells, as indicated by increased expression of adhesion molecules, secretion of cytokines, and production of arachidonic acid metabolites (12). Other evidence suggests that antiphospholipid antibodies cross-react with oxidized low-density lipoprotein and bind only to oxidized cardiolipin (13), implying that antiphospholipid antibodies may participate in oxidant-mediated injury of the vascular endothelium. Finally, antiphospholipid antibodies might cause placental damage or dysfunction by impairing trophoblastic hormone production or invasion (14). The in vivo target(s) of antiphospholipid antibodies remain unknown. Normal, living cells do not express phospholipids bound by antiphospholipid antibodies on their surface. The antibodies do, however, bind to phospholipids expressed by perturbed cells, such as activated platelets or apoptotic cells. Contemporary studies show that the dimerization of β_2-glycoprotein I by anti–β_2-glycoprotein I antibodies results in a 100-fold increase in the affinity of β_2-glycoprotein I for phospholipids (12). The binding of the high affinity autoantibody–β_2-glycoprotein I dimer complex to phospholipids is now thought to play a major role in antiphospholipid antibody mediated interference with phospholipid surface function in vivo. This concept is supported by the finding that monoclonal anti–β_2-glycoprotein I antibodies, but not isolated anti–β_2-glycoprotein I specific Fab fragments, induce increased thrombus formation in a rodent model.

Contemporary work also emphasizes the complement system as having a major role in antiphospholipid syndrome-related pregnancy loss, showing that C3 activation is required for fetal loss in a mouse model (9, 12). Not only does blocking the complement cascade abrogate antiphospholipid-induced pregnancy loss, but genetically engineered mice deficient in either C3 or C5 are resistant to antiphospholipid antibody-induced pregnancy loss and thrombosis after passive administration of antiphospholipid antibodies. Heparin may prevent pregnancy loss by blocking activation of complement, rather than primarily via an anticoagulant effect. In association with pregnancy loss, antiphospholipid antibodies administered to pregnant mice induce increased expression of both decidual and systemic tumor necrosis factor-alpha (TNF-α). Both TNF-α deficiency and blockade are protective against pregnancy loss in this murine model.

Ultimately, the negative effect of antiphospholipid syndrome on pregnancy is most likely tied to abnormal placental function (15). The immediate cause of fetal death in antiphospholipid syndrome appears to be related to abnormalities in the decidual spiral arteries. Some investigators have found narrowing of the spiral arterioles, intimal thickening, acute atherosis, and fibrinoid necrosis in cases of fetal loss associated with antiphospholipid syndrome (15). Others have found extensive placental necrosis, infarction, and thrombosis.

A current model, albeit somewhat speculative, for antiphospholipid antibody-associated pregnancy loss is that the pathogenic autoantibodies bind β_2-glycoprotein I, which in turn facilitates β_2-glycoprotein I binding to cell membrane phospholipids or phospholipid-associated receptors or both (Fig. 6-1). It may be that perturbed membranes are particularly rich sites of such binding. Cell surface binding of the autoantibody–β_2-glycoprotein I complex then results in cell activation with increased expression of cellular adhesion and prothrombotic molecules. Local complement activation then occurs, introducing increased levels of C3a-, C5a-, C5b-membrane attack complex and other products of the complement cascade that potentiate endothelial, monocyte, and platelet cell activation. Some of these are potent chemotactic molecules that promote infiltration with neutrophils and monocytes. The result of this local inflammation, cellular activation, and thrombosis is poor placentation marked by inadequate trophoblast invasion and spiral arteriolar vasculopathy.

Diagnostic Approach to Antiphospholipid Syndrome

The diagnosis of antiphospholipid syndrome is first and foremost clinical—the patient must have one or more thrombotic or obstetric features of the condition. Laboratory testing for antiphospholipid antibodies is used to confirm or refute the diagnosis. The international consensus statements on preliminary classification criteria for definite antiphospholipid syndrome (1, 2) provide simplified criteria for the classification of antiphospholipid syndrome (Box 6-1).

A patient with antiphospholipid syndrome must manifest at least one of two clinical criteria: 1) vascular thrombosis, or 2) pregnancy morbidity; and at least one of three laboratory criteria: 1) positive lupus anticoagulant, 2) medium to high titer β_2-glycoprotein I-depend-

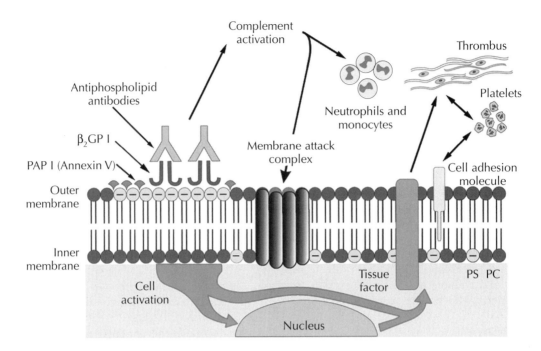

Fig. 6-1. Proposed mechanisms leading to fetal death in antiphospholipid syndrome. Beta$_2$-glycoprotein I binds to syncytial, externalized phosphatidylserine and, in turn, antiphospholipid antibodies bind to β$_2$-glyco-protein I dimers. Complement activation initiates a signaling cascade that attracts neutrophils and monocytes and induces cell surface tissue factor expression and adhesion molecules, causing platelets to aggregate and initiate thrombosis. Local complement activation then occurs, introducing increased levels of C3a-, C5a-, C5b-membrane attack complex and other products of the complement cascade that potentiate endothelial, monocyte, and platelet cell activation, as well as damage or destroy cells. Antiphospholipid antibodies also may disrupt the protective "anticoagulant shield" of the trophoblast by competing with the natural anticoagulant placental anticoagulant protein I, also know as annexin V, at the cell surface for phosphatidylserine. The result of this local inflammation, cellular activation, and thrombosis is poor placentation marked by inadequate trophoblast invasion and spiral arteriolar vasculopathy. Abbreviations: β$_2$GP I, β$_2$-glycoprotein I; PAP I, placental anticoagulant protein I; PC, phosphatidylcholine; PS, phosphatidylserine. Illustration: Jerrald Roberts.

ent immunoglobulin (Ig) G or IgM isotype anticardi-olipin antibodies, or 3) medium to high titer anti–β$_2$-glycoprotein I-IgG or IgM isotype antibodies.

Clinical Criteria

Vascular thrombosis can occur in any organ or tissue and can involve vessels of any size (including capillary networks), within either the arterial or venous systems. Pregnancy morbidity, which includes features of both the preembryonic–embryonic and the fetal–neonatal periods, is divided into three categories, one encompassing early pregnancy loss and the other two relating primarily to complications in the second or third trimesters. "Primary" antiphospholipid syndrome occurs in patients without clinical evidence of another autoimmune disease, whereas "secondary" antiphospholipid syndrome occurs in patients with autoimmune or other diseases.

Laboratory Criteria

The most commonly detected antiphospholipid antibodies, and the only three currently recognized by the 2005 international consensus statement, are lupus anticoagulant, anticardiolipin antibodies, and anti–β$_2$-glycoprotein I antibodies. Lupus anticoagulant is identified by in vitro coagulation assays, in which the antibodies prolong clotting times. Published laboratory criteria for the diagnosis of lupus anticoagulant should be followed (3). Both anticardiolipin and anti–β$_2$-glycoprotein I antibodies are detected by enzyme-linked immunosorbent assays. Positive antibody test results must be confirmed on two separate occasions, at least 12 weeks apart.

Whereas lupus anticoagulant is reported as being positive or negative, anticardiolipin and anti–β$_2$-glycoprotein I antibodies are most commonly reported in terms of international units (designated GPL for IgG binding and MPL for IgM binding). In most laboratories there is substantial concordance between lupus anticoagulant activity and anticardiolipin and anti–β$_2$-glycoprotein I antibodies. However, these antibodies may not be identical, either because they detect different epitopes altogether or because they have different affinities to various epitopes in different test systems. The anticardio-

BOX 6-1

INTERNATIONAL CONSENSUS STATEMENT ON PRELIMINARY CRITERIA FOR THE CLASSIFICATION OF THE ANTIPHOSPHOLIPID SYNDROME*

Clinical criteria

1. Vascular thrombosis

   One or more clinical episodes of arterial, venous, or small vessel thrombosis, occurring within any tissue or organ. Thrombosis must be confirmed by imaging, Doppler ultrasound examination, or histopathology, with the exception of superficial venous thrombosis for which clinical diagnosis is allowed. For histopathological confirmation, thrombosis should be present without significant evidence of inflammation in the vessel wall.

2. Pregnancy morbidity[†]

   a. One or more unexplained deaths of a morphologically normal fetus at or beyond 10 weeks of gestation, with normal fetal morphology documented by ultrasonography or by direct examination of the fetus, or

   b. One or more premature births of a morphologically normal neonate before 34 weeks of gestation because of eclampsia or severe preeclampsia defined according to standard definitions, or recognized features of placental insufficiency[‡], or

   c. Three or more unexplained consecutive spontaneous abortions before 10 weeks of gestation, with maternal anatomic or hormonal abnormalities and paternal and maternal chromosomal causes excluded.

Laboratory criteria[§]

1. Anticardiolipin antibodies

   Anticardiolipin antibodies of immunoglobulin G or immunoglobulin M isotype or both in blood, present in medium or high titer[||], on two or more occasions, at least 12 weeks apart, measured by a standardized enzyme-linked immunosorbent assay for β_2-glycoprotein I-dependent anticardiolipin antibodies

2. Anti–β_2-glycoprotein I antibodies

   Anticardiolipin antibodies of immunoglobulin G or immunoglobulin M isotype or both in blood, present in medium or high titer[¶], on two or more occasions, at least 12 weeks apart, measured by a standardized enzyme-linked immunosorbent assay for β_2-glycoprotein I antibodies

3. Lupus anticoagulant antibodies

   Lupus anticoagulant present in plasma, on two or more occasions, at least 12 weeks apart, detected according to the guidelines of the International Society on Thrombosis and Hemostasis (2)

*Definite antiphospholipid syndrome may be diagnosed if at least one of the clinical criteria and at least one of the laboratory criteria are met. The current International Consensus holds that no more than 5 years separate the clinical event and the positive laboratory findings (2).

[†]In studies of populations of patients who have more than one type of pregnancy morbidity, investigators are strongly encouraged to stratify groups of subjects according to a, b, or c as described above.

[‡]Generally accepted features of placental insufficiency include: abnormal or nonreassuring fetal surveillance test results (eg, a nonreactive nonstress test, suggestive of fetal hypoxemia), abnormal Doppler flow velocimetry waveform analysis suggestive of fetal hypoxemia (eg, absent end-diastolic flow in the umbilical artery), oligohydramnios (eg, an amniotic fluid index of 5 cm or less), or a postnatal birth weight less than the 10th percentile for the gestational age.

[§]The following antiphospholipid antibodies currently are not included in the laboratory criteria: anticardiolipin antibodies of the immunoglobulin A isotype, anti–β_2-glycoprotein I antibodies of the immunoglobulin A isotype, and antiphospholipid antibodies directed against phospholipids other than cardiolipin (eg, phosphatidylserine, phosphatidylethanolamine) or against phospholipid-binding proteins (eg, prothrombin, annexin V, protein C, protein S).

[||]The threshold used to distinguish "medium or high titer" from "low titer" anticardiolipin antibodies has not been standardized and may depend on the population under study. Many laboratories use 15 or 20 international phospholipid units as the threshold separating low from medium titer anticardiolipin antibodies. Others define the threshold as 2 or 2.5 times the median titer of anticardiolipin antibodies or as the 99th percentile of anticardiolipin antibody titers within a normal population. The current international consensus suggests more than 40 GPL or MPL units or greater than the 99th percentile (2).

[¶]These guidelines include the following steps: 1) prolonged phospholipid-dependent coagulation demonstrated on a screening test (eg, activated partial thromboplastin time , kaolin clotting time, dilute Russell's viper venom time, dilute prothrombin time, Textarin time), 2) failure to correct the prolonged coagulation time on the screening test by mixing with normal, platelet-poor plasma, 3) shortening or correcting the prolonged coagulation time on the screening test by the addition of excess phospholipid, 4) exclusion of other coagulopathies (eg, factor VIII inhibitor, or heparin, as appropriate.

Modified from Levine JS, Rauch J, Branch DW. Anti-phospholipid syndrome. N Engl J Med 2002;346:752–63; Copyright © 2002 Massachusetts Medical Society. All rights reserved. Adapted with permission 2007. and Wilson WA, Gharavi AE, Koike T, Lockshin MD, Branch DW, Piette JC, et al. International consensus statement on preliminary classification criteria for definite antiphospholipid syndrome. Report of an international workshop. Arthritis Rheum 1999;42:1309–11; Copyright © 1999 John Wiley & Sons, Inc.

lipin antibody enzyme-linked immunosorbent assay is the more sensitive test for antiphospholipid syndrome, whereas lupus anticoagulant and anti–β_2-glycoprotein I antibodies may be more specific. For both anticardiolipin and anti–β_2-glycoprotein I antibodies, specificity for antiphospholipid syndrome increases with an increasing antibody titer. Low positive antibody results should be viewed with suspicion—they may be found in up to 5% of normal individuals and should not be used to diagnose antiphospholipid syndrome. Only medium- to high-titer anticardiolipin antibodies should be considered in the classification of definite antiphospholipid syndrome. The threshold used to distinguish "medium- or high-titer" from "low-titer" anticardiolipin or anti–β_2-glycoprotein I antibodies has not been standardized. Many laboratories use 15 or 20 international phospholipid units as the threshold separating low from medium titer antibody levels. Others define the threshold as 2 or 2.5 times the median titer or as the 99th percentile of titers within a normal population. The specificity also is higher for anticardiolipin or anti–β_2-glycoprotein I antibodies of the IgG versus IgM isotype. In spite of well-intentioned efforts at standardization and the availability of positive standard sera, substantial interlaboratory variation when testing the same sera remains a serious problem.

Clinicians should recognize that the international consensus criteria were developed primarily for research purposes to ensure more uniform characterization, as well as subcategorization, of patients included in studies. We view this objective as crucial for credible investigative efforts and for appreciation of subtleties of treatment. The consensus criteria also serve to emphasize standardization of laboratory testing, an area of proven concern in antiphospholipid antibodies. As with other autoimmune conditions, such as systemic lupus erythematosus, there are individuals who present with one or more clinical or laboratory features suggestive of antiphospholipid syndrome but in whom the diagnosis cannot be determined based on the relatively strict international consensus criteria. In such cases, experienced clinical judgment is required for best care.

Therapeutic Approach to Antiphospholipid Syndrome in Pregnancy

The ideal treatment for antiphospholipid syndrome during pregnancy would improve maternal and fetal–neonatal outcome by preventing pregnancy loss, preeclampsia, placental insufficiency, and preterm birth and reduce or eliminate the maternal thrombotic risk of antiphospholipid syndrome during pregnancy. Treatment of anti-

phospholipid syndrome in pregnancy to improve fetal outcome has evolved considerably. Early enthusiasm for corticosteroids waned when a small, randomized trial found maternally administered heparin to be as effective as prednisone (16). Maternally administered heparin is widely considered the treatment of choice at present (17). As shown in Box 6-1, pregnant women with antiphospholipid syndrome can be viewed as falling into one of three groups for treatment purposes: 1) women with antiphospholipid syndrome diagnosed because of recurrent preembryonic or embryonic losses but without prior thrombosis, 2) women with antiphospholipid syndrome diagnosed because of prior fetal death or early delivery because of severe preeclampsia or severe placental insufficiency but without prior thrombosis, and 3) women with antiphospholipid syndrome who have had a thrombosis. In the first two groups, heparin treatment is usually initiated in the early first trimester after ultrasonographic demonstration of a live embryo. Most women in the third group (those with prior thrombosis) will be taking long-term warfarin therapy prior to conception. In such cases, warfarin may be continued up until the fifth week of gestation, and the patient then is switched to full anticoagulation with heparin. Alternatively, the patient may be switched to full anticoagulation with heparin prior to conception.

The suggested doses of heparin required for safe and effective treatment in groups one and two differ very little. In one trial of nearly 100 women, two thirds of whom had recurrent preembryonic and embryonic pregnancy loss and none of whom had a history of thromboembolic disease, a heparin dose of 5,000 units, twice daily, was associated with a 71% live-birth rate (18). Another study of similar patients achieved a similarly high live birth rate also using twice daily heparin, but the dose was adjusted to keep the midinterval activated partial thromboplastin time approximately 1.5 times the control mean (19). The optimal dose of heparin for women whose antiphospholipid syndrome is diagnosed because of prior fetal loss or neonatal death after delivery at less than 34 weeks of gestation for severe preeclampsia or placental insufficiency has not been established in adequate clinical trials. These women are at risk for thromboembolic disease (20), and it is our opinion that these cases should receive sufficient thromboprophylaxis as suggested in Box 6-2. For patients in group three, those with a prior thrombosis, the recommended heparin doses are considerably higher, and full anticoagulation is urged by many experts (21). In most case series and trials, daily low-dose aspirin is included in the treatment regimen.

In Europe, low molecular weight heparins are widely used for the treatment of antiphospholipid syndrome in pregnancy, whereas cost considerations limit

BOX 6-2

SUBCUTANEOUS HEPARIN REGIMENS USED IN THE TREATMENT OF ANTIPHOSPHOLIPID SYNDROME DURING PREGNANCY

Prophylactic Regimens

Recurrent (three or more) preembryonic and embryonic loss; no history of thrombotic events

- Standard heparin—5,000–7,500 units every 12 hours in the first trimester, 5,000–10,000 units every 12 hours in the second and third trimesters
- Low molecular weight heparin
  —Enoxaparin, 40 mg once daily or dalteparin, 5,000 units once daily, or
  —Enoxaparin, 30 mg every 12 hours or dalteparin, 5,000 units every 12 hours*

Prior fetal death or early delivery because of severe preeclampsia or severe placental insufficiency, with no history of thrombotic events

- Standard heparin—7,500–10,000 units every 12 hours in the first trimester, 10,000 units every 12 hours in the second and third trimesters
- Low molecular weight heparin
  —Enoxaparin, 40 mg once daily or dalteparin, 5,000 units once daily, or
  —Enoxaparin, 30 mg every 12 hours or dalteparin, 5,000 units every 12 hours*

Anticoagulation Regimens (recommended in women with a history of thrombotic events)

- Standard heparin—7,500 units every 8–12 hours adjusted to maintain the midinterval heparin levels[†] in the therapeutic range
- Low molecular weight heparin
  —Weight adjusted (eg, enoxaparin, 1 mg/kg every 12 hours or dalteparin, 200 units/kg every 12 hours)[‡]
  —Intermediate dose (eg, enoxaparin, 40 mg once daily or dalteparin, 5,000 units once daily until 16 weeks of gestation and every 12 hours from 16 weeks of gestation)[‡]

*Two regimens are described because some expert clinicians believe that twice daily dosing provides better thromboprophylactic coverage than once daily dosing. The two regimens have not been compared in clinical studies.

[†]Heparin levels equal anti-Factor Xa levels. Women without a lupus anticoagulant in whom the activated partial thromboplastin time is normal can be monitored using the activated partial thromboplastin time.

[‡]The authors recommend testing the peak (3 hours after the dose) and trough (just before the next dose) heparin levels approximately once each month to assess for pregnancy-related changes in low molecular weight heparin activity.

Modified from Branch DW, Khamashta MA. Antiphospholipid syndrome: obstetric diagnosis, management, and controversies. Obstet Gynecol 2003;101:1333–44.

the use of low molecular weight heparins in the United States. There is little reason to suspect that one preparation would be better than the other if used in regimens that provide equivalent anticoagulant effects over 24 hours. However, a direct comparison of standard heparin versus low molecular weight heparin in pregnancy is lacking.

In women with antiphospholipid syndrome who are fully anticoagulated during pregnancy with low molecular weight heparin, pregnancy-induced changes in heparin metabolism or clearance would suggest that peak (3 hours after the dose) and trough (just before the next dose) heparin (anti-Factor Xa) levels should be checked approximately once each month and the dose adjusted accordingly. Clinical experience with standard heparin would suggest that peak and trough heparin levels should be monitored somewhat more frequently, perhaps every 2 or 3 weeks. In women with antiphospholipid syndrome who are negative for lupus anticoagulant, midinterval activated partial thromboplastin times may be used.

Compared with standard heparin, there appears to be an increased risk of neuraxial hematoma in patients taking low molecular weight heparin who undergo epidural or spinal anesthesia, and guidelines for safety have been created by the American Society of Regional Anesthesia (22). Thus, in women treated with low molecular weight heparin, some clinicians prefer to switch to standard heparin at 34–36 weeks of gestation in an effort to lower the risk of neuraxial hematoma associated with epidural or spinal anesthesia in patients taking low molecular weight heparin.

Women with particularly egregious thrombotic histories, such as recurrent thrombotic events or cerebral thrombotic events, are understandably viewed as being at very high risk for thrombosis during pregnancy. In such selected cases, we recommend anticoagulation with warfarin in the second and early third trimesters, switching to heparin in the first trimester (from 5 weeks to 12 weeks of gestation) and near the time of delivery (from 34–36 weeks of gestation).

Intravenous immune globulin also has been used during pregnancy, usually in conjunction with heparin and low-dose aspirin, especially in women with particularly poor histories or recurrent pregnancy loss during heparin treatment (23). However, two randomized, controlled, studies of intravenous immune globulin treatment during pregnancy in unselected antiphospholipid syndrome cases found no benefit to this expensive therapy relative to heparin and low-dose aspirin (24, 25).

Clinicians should realize that otherwise healthy women with recurrent pregnancy loss and low titers of antiphospholipid antibodies do not require treatment. One controlled trial included a majority of such women and found no difference in live-birth rates using either low-dose aspirin or a placebo (26).

Given the array of potential complications of antiphospholipid syndrome in pregnancy, appropriate obstetric care calls for frequent prenatal visits, at least every 2–4 weeks before midgestation and perhaps more often thereafter, depending on the clinical status of the patient. The objectives are close observation for maternal hypertension and other features of preeclampsia, periodic patient evaluation and obstetric ultrasonography to assess fetal growth and amniotic fluid volume, and appropriate fetal surveillance testing. The latter should

begin at 32 weeks of gestation, or earlier if the clinical situation indicates placental insufficiency may be present, and continue at least weekly until delivery. Rheumatologic consultation and concurrent care is recommended for women with antiphospholipid syndrome and a history thrombosis or evidence other autoimmune disease, such as systemic lupus erythematosus. An algorithm for the management of antiphospholipid syndrome in pregnancy is shown in Figure 6-2.

Anticoagulant coverage of the postpartum period in women with antiphospholipid syndrome and prior thrombosis is critical (20). We prefer switching the

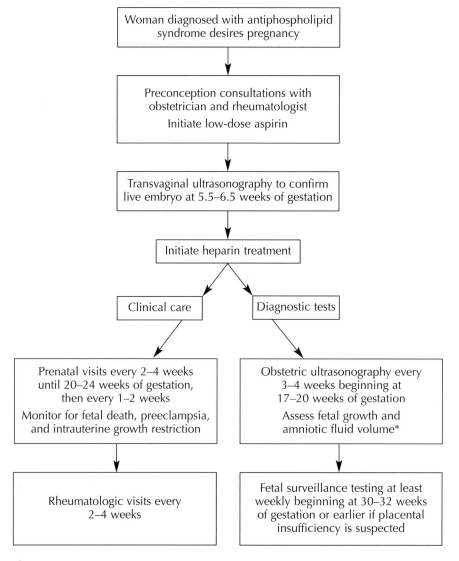

Fig. 6-2. Suggested algorithm for the management of antiphospholipid syndrome in pregnancy. *In the United Kingdom, Doppler ultrasound assessment of the uterine arteries is commonly used at 20–24 weeks of gestation for the prediction of preeclampsia and placental insufficiency risks. This is not commonly done in the United States. (Branch DW, Khamashta MA. Antiphospholipid syndrome: obstetric diagnosis, management, and controversies. Obstet Gynecol 2003;101:1333–44.)

patient to warfarin thromboprophylaxis as soon as she is clinically stable after delivery. In most cases, an international normalized ratio (INR) of 2–2.5 is desirable (27). In switching from heparin to warfarin, it is prudent to continue heparin until the INR is in an acceptable range.

There is no international consensus regarding the postpartum management of those women without prior thrombosis in whom antiphospholipid syndrome is diagnosed because of either recurrent preembryonic or embryonic losses or prior fetal loss or neonatal death after delivery at or before 34 weeks of gestation for severe preeclampsia or placental insufficiency. Postpartum thromboprophylaxis using heparin for 3–5 days, especially in the event of cesarean delivery, is recommended in the United Kingdom. The recommendation in the United States is anticoagulant therapy for 6 weeks after delivery, although whether to use prophylactic therapy (eg, 40 mg of enoxaparin, once daily) versus full anticoagulation doses of medication (eg, warfarin to achieve an INR of 2–2.5) is debated. Both heparin and warfarin are safe for use by nursing mothers.

Complications of Antiphospholipid Syndrome in Pregnancy

The potential complications of pregnancy in women with antiphospholipid syndrome include recurrent pregnancy loss (including fetal death), preeclampsia, placental insufficiency, maternal thrombosis (including stroke), and complications caused by treatment. In women with systemic lupus erythematosus, the potential complications also include lupus exacerbation.

In case series of antiphospholipid syndrome in pregnancies that included women with systemic lupus erythematosus and prior thrombosis, the median rate of gestational hypertension–preeclampsia is 32–50% (6, 7 28–30). Placental insufficiency requiring delivery also is relatively frequent in some of these case series (6, 7, 29). Not surprisingly, the rate of preterm birth in these series ranges from 32% to 65% (6, 7, 29–31). In contrast to the high rate of preeclampsia observed in some case series of women previously diagnosed with antiphospholipid syndrome, antiphospholipid antibodies are not found in a statistically significant proportion of a general obstetric population presenting with preeclampsia (32) or in women at moderate risk to develop preeclampsia because of conditions such as underlying chronic hypertension or preeclampsia in a prior pregnancy (33).

The potential complications of heparin treatment during pregnancy include hemorrhage, osteoporosis with fracture, and heparin-induced thrombocytopenia. Fortunately, the reported rate of osteoporosis and associated fracture is low (probably less than 1%), although

cases have occurred even with low molecular weight heparin (7). It is likely that the risk is higher in women with underlying autoimmune disease who have required corticosteroid treatment. It is reasonable and prudent to recommend calcium supplementation, 1,500–2,000 mg of calcium carbonate daily, in addition to prenatal vitamins.

Heparin-induced thrombocytopenia, which may be lethal and occurs in some nonpregnant individuals, also is fortunately infrequent in pregnant women, probably occurring in less than 1% of treated cases (34). It has been recommended that platelet counts be checked on day 5 and then periodically for the first 2 weeks of heparin therapy.

Controversies in Obstetric Antiphospholipid Syndrome

Laboratory Testing for Antiphospholipid Antibodies

Despite international efforts to standardize laboratory testing for antiphospholipid antibodies (3), significant variation in the performance of antiphospholipid antibody assays (and hence the results) remains a critical problem. Large interlaboratory variation in anticardiolipin antibody testing has been amply documented (35). Agreement among commercially available kits also is poor (36). It is not surprising that the prevalence of antiphospholipid antibodies varies from center to center. This variation contributes to the controversies in our current understanding of antiphospholipid syndrome. Indeed, the authors believe that substantial further progress in antiphospholipid syndrome testing can only be made when well-characterized and well-standardized assays and calibrators are widely available and used in periodic interlaboratory comparisons.

The important issue of interlaboratory variation in antiphospholipid antibody testing aside, there are currently three other areas of controversy in the laboratory testing for antiphospholipid antibodies: 1) the definition and relevance of low positive IgG antiphospholipid antibodies, 2) the relevance of isolated IgM or IgA antiphospholipid antibodies (without either lupus anticoagulant or IgG anticardiolipin antibodies), and 3) the relevance of antiphospholipid antibodies other than lupus anticoagulant and anticardiolipin antibodies (eg, antiphosphatidylserine).

Many studies of patients with recurrent pregnancy loss and antiphospholipid antibodies have included patients with low levels of IgG antiphospholipid antibodies (18, 26, 37). Two groups (38, 39) have found that a significant proportion of women with recurrent pregnancy loss had normalized values indicating low levels of IgG anticardiolipin antibodies (defined as more than the 95th percentile or the 99th percentile). One of these studies showed marked differences between the low levels of anticardiolipin antibodies in the recurrent pregnancy loss population and the much higher levels found in a population of women with antiphospholipid syndrome characterized by fetal death or thrombosis (39). One study found that women with low positive IgG anticardiolipin antibodies had no greater risk for antiphospholipid antibody–related events than women who tested negative (40). Currently, low levels of antiphospholipid antibodies should be considered of questionable clinical significance, and treatment should not be initiated.

Isolated IgM or IgA antiphospholipid antibodies also are of uncertain clinical significance. Early criteria did not recognize isolated IgM anticardiolipin antibodies in the diagnosis of antiphospholipid syndrome. Women with isolated IgM anticardiolipin antibodies have been found to have no greater risk for antiphospholipid antibody-related events than women who tested negative (41). More recently, patients with isolated IgM antiphospholipid antibodies have been entered into treatment trials (18, 19, 26, 37), but their outcomes were not separately analyzed. The 2005 international consensus statement recognizes IgM anticardiolipin antibody levels in medium to high titer for the diagnosis of the antiphospholipid syndrome, but we would urge caution in making a diagnosis of or initiating treatment for antiphospholipid syndrome on the basis of isolated IgM antiphospholipid antibodies less than 40 MPL units.

Isolated IgA anticardiolipin antibodies are viewed by many experts with the same suspicion as isolated IgM. Immunoglobulin A anticardiolipin antibodies were not measured or compared with IgG and IgM isotypes until recently, in part because reference sera for IgA anticardiolipin antibodies were not available until 1994. Studies of the significance of IgA anticardiolipin antibodies are mixed, with some experts finding them to be of little additional diagnostic significance compared with IgG and IgM anticardiolipin antibodies, and the 2005 international consensus statement does not recognize IgA anticardiolipin antibodies in the diagnosis of the antiphospholipid syndrome. Immunoglobulin A anti–β_2-glycoprotein I antibodies have been associated with thrombosis in patients with systemic lupus erythematosus, although they may not add to the diagnosis of antiphospholipid syndrome when compared with testing for lupus anticoagulant or IgG or IgM isotypes (42).

Some investigators have attempted to link antiphospholipid antibodies other than lupus anticoagulant, anticardiolipin antibodies, or anti–β_2-glycoprotein I anti-bodies to recurrent pregnancy loss, including antibodies to phosphatidylserine, phosphatidylethanolamine, phosphatidylinositol, phosphatidylglycerol, phosphatidylcholine, and phosphatidic acid (38, 43). Others remain skeptical, finding that these antibodies are not associated with recurrent pregnancy loss once patients with test results that are positive for lupus anticoagulant or anticardiolipin antibodies are excluded (39). Similarly, another experienced group found that multiple antiphospholipid antibody tests do not increase the diagnostic yield in antiphospholipid syndrome (44). Indeed, substituting negatively charged phospholipids, such as phosphatidylserine or phosphatidylinositol, for cardiolipin in the immunoassay system yields comparable results. Also, no assays other than the anticardiolipin and anti–β_2-glycoprotein I antibody assays have been subjected to international standardization efforts, a persuasive argument against using alternative phospholipid assays for the diagnosis of antiphospholipid syndrome.

Low levels of antiphospholipid antibodies, including low levels of IgG antiphospholipid antibodies, should not be used to diagnose antiphospholipid syndrome or to initiate treatment in pregnancy. Likewise, isolated IgM antiphospholipid antibodies less than 40 MPL units and isolated IgA antiphospholipid antibodies of any titer should be viewed with caution and are not used to diagnose the syndrome. Using alternative phospholipid assays for the diagnosis of antiphospholipid syndrome also is not recommended.

Clinical Features and Diagnosis

Initially, "fetal loss" was proposed as the obstetric criterion for antiphospholipid syndrome. Indeed, obstetric histories detailed in some case series of women with antiphospholipid syndrome suggest that 40% or more of pregnancy losses reported by women with lupus anticoagulant or medium to high positive IgG anticardiolipin antibodies occurred in the fetal period (at least 10 menstrual weeks of gestation). This contrasts sharply with unselected populations of women with sporadic or recurrent pregnancy loss, for whom loss of the pregnancy occurs far more commonly in the preembryonic (less than 6 menstrual weeks of gestation) or embryonic (6–9 menstrual weeks of gestation) periods. In addition to a high rate of fetal death, prospectively followed pregnancies in several large case series that included women with systemic lupus erythematosus, prior thrombosis, and other medical conditions have demonstrated high rates of premature delivery for gestational hypertension–preeclampsia and uteroplacental insufficiency as manifested by fetal growth restriction, oligohydramnios, and nonreassuring fetal surveillance (6, 7, 31).

More recent work focusing on women with recurrent preembryonic and embryonic pregnancy loss without significant medical histories has shown that 10–20% of these more typical cases of recurrent miscarriage have detectable antiphospholipid antibodies (39). Six of the seven prospective treatment trials (16, 18, 19, 26, 37, 45) have included most of these cases—otherwise healthy women with recurrent early miscarriage—and found relatively low rates of adverse second- or third-trimester outcomes. The median rates of fetal death, preeclampsia, and preterm birth in these trials were 4.5% (range 0–15%), 10.5% (range 0–15%), and 10.5% (range 5–40%), respectively. Among all six trials, comprising more than 300 patients, only one woman experienced a thrombotic event, and there were no neonatal deaths caused by complications of prematurity. It would appear, then, that women identified in the clinical setting of recurrent early pregnancy loss, particularly recurrent preembryonic and embryonic losses, without other important medical histories represent a different population from those identified because of thromboembolic disease, systemic lupus erythematosus, or adverse second- or third-trimester obstetric outcomes.

The relationship between antiphospholipid syndrome cases resulting in complications during the fetal period (fetal death or premature delivery caused by obstetric complications) and those during the preembryonic and embryonic periods (identified by recurrent pregnancy loss) is seen as a continuum by some (46) and questioned by others (47). The former view would hold that the same underlying mechanism (eg, antiphospholipid antibody-mediated hypercoagulability) could operate along the continuum of gestation to cause either predominantly first-trimester or predominantly second- and third-trimester complications. Certainly it is easy to envisage a common mechanism for fetal death and preterm birth resulting from severe preeclampsia or placental insufficiency—hypercoagulability causing a defective uteroplacental circulation and, in turn, diminished intervillous blood flow. The question remains whether the same mechanism would also be responsible for recurrent preembryonic and embryonic losses and be associated with relatively low rates of second- and third-trimester complications in treated patients, even those treated with low-dose aspirin alone.

The alternative view holds that women presenting with recurrent preembryonic and embryonic losses and antiphospholipid antibodies represent a largely different patient population. Their pregnancy losses are likely to be caused by different mechanisms than later pregnancy complications, perhaps relating to different antiphospholipid antibody specificities or antiphospholipid antibodies operating on a fundamentally different pathophysiologic background.

Pregnancy Treatment in Different Patient Groups

Women with antiphospholipid syndrome without a history of thromboembolic disease fall into the two categories: 1) those with recurrent preembryonic and embryonic pregnancy loss and 2) those with one or more prior fetal losses or neonatal deaths after delivery at less than 34 weeks of gestation because of severe preeclampsia or placental insufficiency. Regarding the group with adverse pregnancy outcomes during the fetal period, most authorities recommend heparin during pregnancy, based on the widely held perception that anticoagulant therapy is likely to benefit both the mother and fetus. It must be said, however, that this particular group has never been singled out for a randomized treatment trial to determine if heparin is efficacious and at what dose. In a small randomized treatment trial (24), more than 80% of those included had one or more prior fetal loss (women with systemic lupus erythematosus and prior thromboembolic disease also were included). Using doses of heparin between 17,000 units and 20,000 units/d in divided doses, all women had a live birth, and none had a thrombotic event.

In contrast, there are six published treatment trials that included women whose antiphospholipid syndrome was diagnosed in most cases because of recurrent pregnancy loss in the first trimester (16, 18, 19, 26, 37, 45). Five were randomized, and one (19) alternated treatments with every other patient. Substantial differences in patients included in these trials deserve mention. The proportion of women who had one or more prior fetal losses in these trials ranged from 11% (19) to 47% (45). One trial (45) included women with thromboembolic disease, although only two patients (6%) actually had such a history. Two trials did not specifically exclude women with systemic lupus erythematosus, although neither recruited any (16, 45). The other four trials specifically excluded women with systemic lupus erythematosus and prior thromboembolic disease (18, 19, 26, 37) and one specifically excluded women with lupus anticoagulant (19). Low positive IgG anticardiolipin antibody results and isolated IgM results were allowed in five trials (16, 18, 26, 37, 45), and one trial included women with antibodies to phosphatidylserine (19).

Given these substantial differences in patient selection, one might expect equally substantial differences in study pregnancy outcomes. In the trial in which prednisone and low-dose aspirin were compared with heparin and low-dose aspirin, the live-birth rates were the same in each group (75%) (16). Two trials found low-dose aspirin to be as efficacious as the study treatment (37, 45), and one found placebo as effective as low-dose aspirin (26).

The live-birth rates in each arm of these three trials, including two low-dose aspirin arms and a placebo arm, exceeded 75%. Two trials (18, 19) found that a combination of heparin and low-dose aspirin was more effective than low-dose aspirin alone for achieving live births, reporting 71% and 80% live-birth rates, respectively, in patients treated with aspirin and heparin versus live-birth rates less than 50% in patients treated with aspirin alone. Different doses of heparin were used in each of these two trials, with only 10,000 units of heparin per day used in one (18).

The clinician is bound to be confused by the discrepant results from these trials. At the heart of the problem is patient selection, both clinical and laboratory. The obvious differences in patient selection and subsequent obstetric outcomes with a variety of treatments have led three groups to call for subcategorization of obstetric antiphospholipid syndrome patients (46–48). Moreover, the 2005 international consensus statement specifically calls for stratification of populations that include more than one type of pregnancy morbidity. Based on existing data, the most important obstetric subcategorization would distinguish women with prior thromboembolic events from those without and women with recurrent preembryonic or embryonic losses from those with fetal losses. Also, women with low levels of antiphospholipid antibodies or isolated IgM antiphospholipid antibodies should be distinguished from those with lupus anticoagulant or medium to high levels of IgG antiphospholipid antibodies.

Treatment of Antiphospholipid Syndrome in Pregnancy in "Refractory" Cases

Despite treatment with heparin, recurrent pregnancy losses occur in 20–30% of cases in most case series and trials. The best approach to such cases in subsequent pregnancies is unknown, although clinicians and patients understandably feel as if they should try an alternative therapy or add another drug to their regimen in a next pregnancy attempt. In the early 1990s, experts were often inclined to use corticosteroids, often in substantial doses. This approach may have merit in refractory cases, but it is untested in clinical trials. By the mid-1990s, intravenous immune globulin, usually used in conjunction with heparin and low-dose aspirin, was touted as beneficial, based on selected cases (23). As with a combination of corticosteroids and heparin, this intravenous immune globulin use in refractory antiphospholipid syndrome cases has never been studied in a properly designed trial.

Hydroxychloroquine has been shown to diminish the thrombogenic properties of antiphospholipid antibodies in a murine thrombosis model. Past concerns about ocular damage or defects in exposed embryos and fetuses have been allayed to some degree by a series of recent reports (49). There are few case reports and no trials of patients with antiphospholipid syndrome being treated during pregnancy with hydroxychloroquine.

Because there are no properly designed trials evaluating treatments of "refractory" antiphospholipid syndrome, we can only offer speculative opinion as to promising and acceptable treatment alternatives. In women whose treated pregnancy failure occurred on a prophylactic regimen, full anticoagulation in the next pregnancy would seem rational. If the treated pregnancy failed while the patient was taking full anticoagulation therapy, we would be inclined to add an immunomodulatory agent such as glucocorticoids, immune globulin, or hydroxychloroquine to the anticoagulation regimen.

References

1. Wilson WA, Gharavi AE, Koike T, Lockshin, MD, Branch DW, Piette J C, et al. International consensus statement on preliminary classification criteria for definite antiphospholipid syndrome. Report of an international workshop. Arthritis Rheum 1999;42:1309–11.

2. Miyakis S, Lockshin MD, Atsumi T, Branch DW, Brey RL, Cervera R, et al. International consensus statement on an update of the classification criteria for definite antiphospholipid syndrome (APS). J Thromb Haemost 2006;4: 295–306.

3. Levine JS, Rauch J, Branch DW. Anti-phospholipid syndrome. N Engl J Med 2002;346:752–63.

4. Roubey RAS. Autoantibodies to phospholipid-binding plasma proteins: a new view of lupus anticoagulants and other "antiphospholipid" antibodies. Blood 1994;84: 2854–67.

5. Khamashta MA, Cuadrado MJ, Mujic F, Taub NA, Hunt BJ, Hughes GRV. The management of thrombosis in the antiphospholipid-antibody syndrome. N Eng J Med 1995;332:993–7.

6. Branch DW, Silver RM, Blackwell JL, Reading JC, Scott JR. Outcome of treated pregnancies in women with antiphospholipid syndrome: an update of the Utah experience. Obstet Gynecol 1992;80:614–20.

7. Lima F, Khamashta MA, Buchanan NM, Kerslake S, Hunt BJ, Hughes GR. A study of sixty pregnancies in patients with the antiphospholipid syndrome. Clin Exp Rheumatol 1996;14:131–6.

8. Branch DW, Dudley DJ, Mitchell MD, Creighton KA, Abbott TM, Hammond EH, et al. Immunoglobulin G fractions from patients with antiphospholipid antibodies cause fetal death in BALB/c mice: a model for autoimmune fetal loss. Am J Obstet Gynecol 1990;163:210–16.

9. Holers VM, Girardi G, Mo L, Guthridge JM, Molina H, Pierangeli SS, et al. Complement C3 activation is required for antiphospholipid antibody-induced fetal loss. J Exp Med 2002;195:211–220.

10. Pierangeli SS, Gharavi AE, Harris EN. Experimental thrombosis and antiphospholipid antibodies: new insights. J Autoimmunity 2000;15:241–7.

11. Rand JH, Wu S, Andree HAM, Lockwood CJ, Guller S, Scher J, et al. Pregnancy loss in the antiphospholipid antibody syndrome—a possible thrombogenic mechanism. N Engl J Med 1997;337:154–160.

12. Branch DW, Grosvenor Eller A. Antiphospholipid syndrome and thrombosis. Clin Obstet Gynecol 2006;49: 861–74.

13. Hörkkö S, Miller E, Dudl E, Reaven P, Curtiss LK, Zvaifler NJ, et al. Antiphospholipid antibodies are directed against epitopes of oxidized phospholipids: recognition of cardiolipin by monoclonal antibodies to epitopes of oxidized low density lipoprotein. J Clin Invest 1996;98:815–25.

14. di Simone N, Meroni PL, Del Papa N, Raschi E, Caliandro D, De Carolis S, et al. Antiphospholipid antibodies affect trophoblast gonadotropin secretion and invasiveness by binding directly and through adhered beta2-glycoprotein I. Arthritis Rheum 2000;43:140–50.

15. Van Horn JT, Craven C, Ward K, Branch DW, Silver RM. Histologic features of placentas and abortion specimens from women with antiphospholipid and antiphospholipid-like syndromes. Placenta 2004;25:642–8.

16. Cowchock FS, Reece EA, Balaban D, Branch DW, Plouffe L. Repeated fetal losses associated with antiphospholipid antibodies: a collaborative randomized trial comparing prednisone with low-dose heparin treatment. Am J Obstet Gynecol 1992;166:1318–23.

17. Lassere M, Empson M. Treatment of antiphospholipid syndrome in pregnancy—a systematic review of randomized therapeutic trials. Thromb Res 2004;114:419–26.

18. Rai R, Cohen H, Dave M, Regan L. Randomised controlled trial of aspirin and aspirin plus heparin in pregnant women with recurrent miscarriage associated with phospholipid antibodies. Brit Med J 1997;314:253–7.

19. Kutteh WH. Antiphospholipid antibody-associated recurrent pregnancy loss: treatment with heparin and low-dose aspirin is superior to low-dose aspirin alone. Am J Obstet Gynecol 1996;174:1584–9.

20. Erkan D, Merrill JT, Yazici Y, Sammaritano L, Buyon JP, Lockshin MD. High thrombosis rate after fetal loss in antiphospholipid syndrome: effective prophylaxis with aspirin. Arthritis Rheum 2001;44:1466–7.

21. Bates SM, Greer IA, Hirsh J, Ginsberg JS. Use of antithrombotic agents during pregnancy: the Seventh ACCP Conference on Antithrombotic and Thrombolytic Therapy. Chest 2004;126(3 Suppl):627S–644S.

22. Horlocker TT, Wedel DJ, Benzon H, Brown DL, Enneking FK, Heit JA, et al. Regional anesthesia in the anticoagulated patient: Defining the risks (the second ASRA Consensus Conference on Neuraxial Anesthesia and Anticoagulation). Reg Anesth Pain Med 2003;28:172–97.

23. Clark AL, Branch DW, Silver RM, Harris EN, Pierangeli S, Spinnato JA. Pregnancy complicated by the antiphospholipid syndrome: Outcomes with intravenous immunoglobulin therapy. Obstet Gynecol 1999;93:437–41.

24. Branch DW, Peaceman AM, Druzin M, Silver RK, El-Sayed Y, Silver RM, et al. A multicenter, placebo-controlled pilot study of intravenous immune globulin treatment of antiphospholipid syndrome during pregnancy. The Pregnancy Loss Study Group. Am J Obstet Gynecol 2000;182:122–7.

25. Triolo G, Ferrante A, Ciccia F, Accardo-Palumbo A, Perino A, Castelli A, et al. Randomized study of subcutaneous low molecular weight heparin plus aspirin versus intravenous immunoglobulin in the treatment of recurrent fetal loss associated with antiphospholipid antibodies. Arthritis Rheum 2003;48:728–31.

26. Pattison NS, Chamley LW, Birdsall M, Zanderigo AM, Liddell HS, McDougall J. Does aspirin have a role in improving pregnancy outcome for women with the antiphospholipid syndrome? A randomized controlled trial. Am J Obstet Gynecol 2000;183:1008–12.

27. Lim W, Crowther MA, Eikelboom JW. Management of antiphospholipid antibody syndrome: a systematic review. JAMA 2006;295:1050–7.

28. Pauzner R, Dulitzki M, Langevitz P, Livneh A, Kenett R, Many A. Low molecular weight heparin and warfarin the treatment of patients with antiphospholipid syndrome during pregnancy. Thromb Haemost 2001;86:1379–84.

29. Lockshin MD, Druzin ML, Qamar T. Prednisone does not prevent recurrent fetal death in women with antiphospholipid antibody. Am J Obstet Gynecol 1989;160:439–43.

30. Caruso A, de Carolis S, Ferrazzani S, Valesini G, Caforio L, Mancuso S. Pregnancy outcome in relation to uterine artery flow velocity waveforms and clinical characteristics in women with antiphospholipid syndrome. Obstet Gynecol 1993;82:970–7.

31. Huong DLT, Wechsler B, Bletry O, Vauthier-Brouzes D, Lefebvre G, Piette J-C. A study of 75 pregnancies in patients with antiphospholipid syndrome. J Rheumatol 2001;28:2025–30.

32. Dreyfus M, Hedelin G, Kutnahorsky R, Lehmann M, Viville B, Langer B, et al. Antiphospholipid antibodies and preeclampsia: a case-control study. Obstet Gynecol 2001; 97:29–34.

33. Branch DW, Porter TF, Rittenhouse L, Caritis S, Sibai B, Hogg B, et al. Antiphospholipid antibodies in women at risk for preeclampsia. Am J Obstet Gynecol 2001;184: 825–32.

34. Fausett MB, Vogtlander M, Lee RM, Esplin MS, Branch DW, Rodgers GM, et al. Heparin-induced thrombocytopenia is rare in pregnancy. Am J Obstet Gynecol 2001; 185:148–52.

35. Favaloro EJ, Silvestrini R, Mohammed A. Clinical utility of anticardiolipin antibody assays: high inter-laboratory variation and limited consensus by participants of external quality assurance programs signals a cautious approach. Pathology 1999;31:142–7.

36. Reber G, Arvieux J, Comby E, Degenne D, de Moerloose P, Sanmarco M, et al. Multicenter evaluation of nine commercial kits for the quantitation of anticardiolipin antibodies. The Working Group on Methodologies in Haemostasis from the GEHT (Groupe d'Etudes sur l'Hemostase et la Thrombose). Thromb Haemost 1995; 73:444–52.

37. Farquharson RG, Quency S, Greaves M. Antiphospholipid syndrome in pregnancy: a randomised controlled trial of treatment. Obstet Gynecol 2002;100:408–13.

38. Aoki K, Hayashi Y, Hirao Y, et al: Specific antiphospholipid antibodies as a predictive variable in patients with recurrent pregnancy loss. Am J Reprod Immunol 1993; 29:82–7.

39. Branch DW, Silver R, Pierangeli S, van Leeuwen I, Harris EN. Antiphospholipid antibodies other than lupus anticoagulant and anticardiolipin antibodies in women with recurrent pregnancy loss, fertile controls, and antiphospholipid syndrome. Obstet Gynecol 1997;89:549–55.

40. Silver RM, Porter TF, van Leeuween I, Jeng G, Scott JR, Branch DW. Anticardiolipin antibodies: clinical consequences of "low titers." Obstet Gynecol 1996;87:494–500.

41. Silver RM, Draper ML, Scott JR, Lyon JL, Reading J, Branch DW. Clinical consequences of antiphospholipid antibodies: an historic cohort study. Obstet Gynecol 1994;83:372–7.

42. Bertolaccini ML, Atsumi T, Escudero CA, Khamashta MA, Hughes GR. The value of IgA antiphospholipid testing for diagnosis of antiphospholipid (Hughes) syndrome in systemic lupus erythematosus. J Rheumatol 2001;28: 2637–43.

43. Yetman DL, Kutteh WH. Antiphospholipid antibody panels and recurrent pregnancy loss: prevalence of anticardiolipin antibodies compared with other antiphospholipid antibodies. Fertil Steril 1996;66:540–6.

44. Bertolaccini ML, Roch B, Amengual O, Atsumi T, Khamashta MA, Hughes GR. Multiple antiphospholipid tests do not increase the diagnostic yield in antiphospholipid syndrome. Br J Rheumatol 1998;37:1229–32.

45. Silver RK, MacGregor SN, Sholl JS, Hobart JM, Neerhof MG, Ragin A. Comparative trial of prednisone plus aspirin versus aspirin alone in the treatment of anticardiolipin antibody-positive obstetric patients. Am J Obstet Gynecol 1993;169:1411–7.

46. Clark CA, Spitzer KA, Laskin CA. The spectrum of the antiphospholipid syndrome: a matter of perspective. J Rheumatol 2001;28:1939–41.

47. Sullivan A, Branch DW. Can you manage antiphospholipid syndrome during pregnancy? Cont Obstet Gynecol 2001;46:100–22.

48. Derksen RH, Khamashta MA, Branch DW. Management of the obstetric antiphospholipid syndrome. Arthritis Rheum 2004;50:1028–39.

49. Levy RA, Vilela VS, Cataldo MJ, Ramos RC, Duarte JL, Tura BR, et al. Hydroxychloroquine (HCQ) in lupus pregnancy: double-blind and placebo-controlled study. Lupus 2001;10:401–4.

CHAPTER 7

Inherited Thrombophilias in Pregnant Patients

CHARLES J. LOCKWOOD

*T*hromboembolic disease is the leading cause of maternal mortality in the United States (1). Stillbirth, severe (third percentile) intrauterine growth restriction (IUGR), abruption, and severe early-onset preeclampsia complicate 0.2–3% of pregnancies and are leading causes of perinatal morbidity and mortality. Histologic examination of uteroplacental vessels and intervillous architecture from such pathologic pregnancies typically display increased fibrin deposition, thrombosis, and hypoxia-associated endothelial and trophoblast changes (2). These findings suggest that thrombosis of the uteroplacental circulation underlies these obstetric conditions. The presence of inherited and acquired thrombophilias has recently been linked to most cases of maternal venous thrombotic events as well as a number of these adverse obstetric outcomes (1, 3).

The most common inherited thrombophilias are heterozygosity for the factor V Leiden and prothrombin G20210A mutations, homozygosity for the *4G/4G* mutation in the plasminogen activator inhibitor *(PAI-1)* gene, and the methylenetetrahydrofolate reductase C677T and A1298C polymorphisms, the most common causes of hyperhomocysteinemia. Rarer thrombophilias include autosomal-dominant deficiencies of antithrombin, protein C, and protein S. The principal acquired thrombophilia is antiphospholipid antibody syndrome (3). During pregnancy, the maternal thrombogenic potential of all these disorders is enhanced (3, 4). Not including *PAI-1* and methylenetetrahydrofolate reductase polymorphisms, thrombophilias are collectively present in approximately 15% of white European populations, are responsible for more than 80% of maternal thromboembolic events, and have been convincingly linked to a twofold to threefold increased risk of fetal loss and abruption (1, 3–6). However, there are conflicting reports on the association between thrombophilias and recurrent early (less than 10 weeks) spontaneous abortions (1, 3, 7–12). Moreover, there is no convincing link between thrombophilias and either preeclampsia or IUGR (13, 14). Although there is consensus on the diagnosis and treatment of antiphospholipid antibody syndrome in pregnancy (3), the proper approach to the detection and management of inherited thrombophilias in pregnancy remains shrouded in confusion. This review attempts to define a practical approach to screening for the disorder and treating affected patients.

Physiologic Initiation and Control of Hemostasis

The primary initiator of coagulation is tissue factor, a cell membrane-bound glycoprotein expressed by perivascular cells throughout the body but not by cells in contact with the circulation (ie, endothelial cells) (Fig. 7-1). After vascular disruption, perivascular, cell membrane-bound tissue factor complexes with plasma-derived factor VII. The complex of tissue factor and factor VII bound to negatively charged (anionic) phospholipids in the presence of ionized calcium initiates clotting. Factor VII is the only zymogenic (ie, precursor) form of a clotting factor to exhibit activity and allows for "on-demand" clotting. Once clotting begins, factor VII is fully activated by thrombin and other activated clotting factors to form factor VIIa, which is 100-fold more active. The tissue factor–VIIa complex directly converts factor X to Xa (extrinsic pathway), or indirectly generates Xa by converting factor IX to IXa, which, in turn, complexes with its cofactor, factor VIIIa, to convert X to Xa (intrinsic pathway).

This initial clotting reaction is quickly inhibited by the tissue factor pathway inhibitor, which binds to the tissue factor–VIIa–Xa complex to rapidly stop tissue factor-mediated clotting. However, factor XIIa-activated factor XIa sustains the clotting reaction by serving as an alternative activator of factor IX on the surface of newly aggregated platelets. In any case, factor Xa, once generated, complexes with its cofactor, Va, to convert prothrombin (factor II) to thrombin (IIa). Thrombin then cleaves fibrinogen to generate fibrin monomers, which spontaneously polymerize and are cross-linked by thrombin-activated factor XIIIa to form a stable clot (Fig. 7-1).

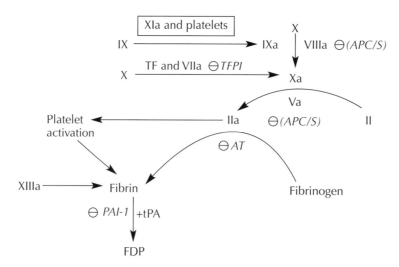

Fig. 7-1. The coagulation, anticoagulation, and fibrinolytic pathways. ⊖ = inhibitor; II = prothrombin; IIa = thrombin. Abbreviations: *APC/S*, activated protein C and protein S; AT, antithrombin; TFPI, tissue factor pathway inhibitor; TPA, tissue-type plasminogen activator. (Lockwood CJ. Inherited thrombophilias in pregnant patients: detection and treatment paradigm. Obstet Gynecol 2002;99:333–41.)

Because the anticoagulant effects of the tissue factor pathway inhibitor can be short-circuited by factor XIa, effective inhibition of the clotting cascade requires inhibition of subsequent factor IXa and Xa activity. This is accomplished by the complex of activated protein C and protein S. Protein C is activated by the complex of thrombomodulin and thrombin residing on damaged endothelial cells. The activated protein C and protein S complex inactivates factors VIIIa and Va, the requisite cofactors for factors IXa and Xa, respectively.

Both protein C and protein S are hepatocyte products that depend on vitamin K-dependent enzymes to γ-carboxylate their glutamine-rich plasma membrane-binding domains (1). Protein C and protein S have plasma half-lives of 6–8 hours and 42 hours, respectively. Circulating protein S exists in both free (40%) and bound (60%) forms. The complement 4b-binding protein serves as a carrier protein for protein S. Because only free protein S complexes with activated protein C, any condition that increases the complement 4b-binding protein (eg, pregnancy, inflammation, and surgical stress) will reduce protein S activity.

The most crucial endogenous anticoagulant system involves antithrombin. In addition to its thrombin inhibitory properties, antithrombin can inactivate factors Xa, IXa, and VIIa (1). The anticoagulant activity of antithrombin is increased 5,000-fold to 40,000-fold by heparin.

Finally, fibrinolysis serves to prevent excess clotting by breaking down the fibrin clot. Fibrinolysis is mediated by tissue-type plasminogen activator, which binds to fibrin where it activates plasmin. Plasmin, in turn,

degrades fibrin but can be inactivated by α-2-antiplasmin embedded in the fibrin clot. Fibrinolysis is primarily inhibited by *PAI-1*, the fast inactivator of tissue-type plasminogen activator.

Pregnancy-Associated Changes in Hemostasis and Fibrinolysis

The net effect of pregnancy-associated changes in hemostatic, anticoagulant, and fibrinolytic proteins is to enhance the risk of thromboembolism and, thus, exacerbate the clinical effects of the inherited thrombophilias (1). Pregnancy is associated with a 20–200% increase in levels of fibrinogen and factors II, VII, VIII, X, and XII, whereas concentrations of factors V and IX are unchanged. In contrast, endogenous anticoagulant levels increase minimally (tissue factor pathway inhibitor), remain constant (antithrombin and protein C), or significantly decrease (protein S) in pregnancy. Moreover, levels of immunoreactive and functionally active *PAI-1* increase up to threefold in pregnancy. Thus, the net effect of these pregnancy-induced changes is to promote clot formation, extension, and stability.

Pathophysiology of the Inherited Thrombophilias

Factor V Leiden Mutation

The factor V Leiden mutation is present in 5–9% of white European populations, but is rare in Asian and African populations. (1, 15). It arises from a (G to A) mutation in nucleotide 1691 of the factor V gene's 10th exon, resulting in a substitution of a glutamine for an arginine at position 506 in the factor V polypeptide (factor V Q506). The resultant amino acid substitution impairs the activated protein C and protein S complex inactivation of factor Va. This defect is termed the factor V Leiden mutation and is primarily inherited in an autosomal-dominant fashion (1, 16). Heterozygosity for the factor V Leiden mutation is present in 20–40% of nonpregnant patients with thromboembolic disease (1). Homozygosity for the mutation, although rare, confers a far higher (more than 100-fold) risk of thromboembolism (1).

Pregnancy-induced reductions in protein S enhance factor V Leiden prothrombotic effects. The proportion of pregnant patients with thromboembolic events attributable to the factor V Leiden mutation has been reported to be approximately 40% (11–78%) (1, 4, 17). Despite this high occurrence rate, given the low prevalence of thromboembolism in pregnancy, the actual risk of thromboembolism in asymptomatic pregnant patients without a personal or strong family history (ie, first degree relative) of thromboembolism is only 0.2% (17). In contrast, the risk of thromboembolism in pregnancy may be at least 10% among those with a personal or strong family history (18).

Although there is no consensus on the association between the factor V Leiden mutation and early (less than 10 weeks of gestation) pregnancy loss, the evidence suggests a twofold to threefold increased risk of late first-, second-, and third-trimester fetal loss (1, 6, 7, 10, 19–21). There is a complex association between factor V Leiden and other latter adverse pregnancy events, including abruption, severe preeclampsia, and IUGR. An association between factor V Leiden and abruption (odds ratio [OR], 4.9; 95% confidence interval [CI], 1.4–17.4), and severe preeclampsia (OR, 5.3; 95% CI, 1.8–15.6) has been observed but not IUGR (less than fifth percentile) (20). However, subsequent studies have demonstrated no link between factor V Leiden and moderate and severe preeclampsia, (22–24) or IUGR (14, 24). An evaluation of 19 studies involving 2,742 hypertensive women and 2,403 controls concluded that factor V Leiden increased the OR of hypertensive disease in pregnancy by 2.25-fold (95% CI, 1.5–3.38) but noted that, while studies published up to 2000 showed an OR of 3.16 (CI, 2.04–4.92), no association was seen in studies published after that time (OR 0.97; 95% CI, 0.61–1.54), suggesting publication bias toward reports showing a positive association (25). In contrast, another meta-analysis found strong associations between placental abruption and both homozygosity and heterozygosity for the factor V Leiden mutation with ORs of 16.9 (95% CI, 2.0–141.9) and 6.7 (95% CI, 2.0–21.6), respectively (26). Similar findings have been noted by others (10). Thus, there appears to be

a consistent although modest association between factor V Leiden and fetal loss after 10 weeks of gestation as well as abruption; however, the link between this common inherited thrombophilia and preeclampsia and IUGR is unproved. Finally, factor V Leiden homozygosity is associated with an increase in the risk of developing spastic quadriplegia (OR, 9.12; 95% CI, 0.86–53.71) among children born at less than 32 weeks of gestation (27).

Prothrombin Gene Mutation

Heterozygosity for a mutation in the promoter of the prothrombin gene (G20210A), present in 2–3% of white European populations, leads to increased (150–200%) circulating levels of prothrombin and an increased risk of thromboembolism (1, 15). This mutation accounts for 17% of thromboembolism in pregnancy (17). However, the actual risk of clotting in an asymptomatic pregnant carrier without a personal or strong family history of thromboembolism is only 0.5% (17). By contrast, the risk of venous thromboembolism in pregnant heterozygous women with a personal or strong family history may be more than 10% (17, 18). Homozygosity for the prothrombin mutation confers a risk of thrombosis, equivalent to that of factor V Leiden homozygosity (1).

The prothrombin (G20210A) mutation has been associated with an increased risk of fetal loss and abruption (1, 6, 10, 28). In one study, 7 of 80 recurrent pregnancy loss patients and 2 of 100 controls were carriers of the prothrombin (G20210A) mutation ($P = .04$ [OR, 4.6; 95% CI, 0.9–23.2]) (9). However, no link has been found between the prothrombin (G20210A) mutation and other inherited thrombophilias and early (less than 10 weeks of gestation) pregnancy loss (10). There are conflicting reports of the link between this thrombophilia and preeclampsia (24, 29, 30) and no clear association with IUGR (14).

4G/4G PAI-1 Mutation

The *PAI-1* gene's promoter region contains at least two alleles producing either a *4G* or *5G* base-pair region. The *5G* allele permits the binding of transcription factor inhibitors that suppress gene transcription. In contrast, the *4G* allele is too small to permit the binding of gene repressors. Therefore, individuals homozygous for the *4G/4G* allele have a threefold to fivefold higher level of circulating *PAI-1* compared with those bearing the *5G/5G* or *5G/4G* alleles (31). The prevalence of homozygosity for the *4G/4G* genotype is high, ranging from 23.5% to 32.3% (32, 33). Moreover, most studies have not found a consistent, independent relationship between this polymorphism and either thromboembolism (34) or adverse pregnancy outcomes (35–37).

Antithrombin Deficiency

Antithrombin deficiency, also known as antithrombin III deficiency, is the most thrombogenic of the inherited thrombophilias with a 70–90% lifetime risk of thromboembolism (1, 4). Deficiencies in antithrombin result from numerous (more than 250) point mutations, deletions, and insertions, and are usually inherited in an autosomal-dominant fashion (38). The two classes of antithrombin deficiency are: 1) type I, the most common deficiency, characterized by concomitant reductions in both antigenic protein levels and activity; and 2) type II deficiency, characterized by normal antigenic levels but decreased activity. The type II deficiency is further classified by the site of the mutation (eg, reactive site, heparin binding site, and pleiotropic functional defects) (1, 22). Because the prevalence of antithrombin deficiency is low, one in 1,000 in 5,000, it is only present in 1% of patients with thromboembolism (4). The risk of venous thromboembolism in pregnancy among patients with antithrombin deficiency who are without a personal or family history is 3–7% and among those with such a history it is 11–40% (18).

Adjusted ORs for miscarriage and stillbirth of 1.7 (95% CI, 1.0–2.8) and 5.2 (95% CI, 1.5–18.1), respectively have been reported (7). However, because of its low prevalence compared with that of fetal loss, severe preeclampsia, IUGR, and abruption, antithrombin deficiency is rarely the cause of these disorders (1, 6).

Protein C and Protein S Deficiencies

Deficiencies of protein C result from numerous (more than 160) mutations, although two primary types are recognized: 1) type I, in which both immunoreactive and functionally active protein C levels are reduced; and 2) type II, in which immunoreactive levels are normal, but activity is reduced (1). More than 130 mutations have been linked to protein S with most affected patients characterized as having both a low total and free protein S antigen level (type I) or by having only a low free protein S antigen level because of enhanced binding to the complement 4b-binding protein (type IIa). Type IIb, characterized by normal free immunoreactive levels but reduced activated protein C cofactor activity is rare. Different mutations have highly variable procoagulant sequelae making it extremely difficult to predict which patients with protein C or protein S deficiencies will develop thromboembolism. The prevalence of protein C and protein S deficiencies is 0.2–0.5% and 0.08%, respectively (1), and inheritance is autosomal dominant.

The reported pregnancy and puerperal risk of thromboembolism with either protein C or protein S deficiency appears less than 1% in the absence of a personal or strong family history of clotting, but increases with such a history (18). The risk of stillbirth is modestly increased with both protein C and protein S deficiencies (adjusted OR, 2.3; 95% CI, 0.6–8.3 and adjusted OR, 3.3; 95% CI, 1.0–11.3, respectively) (7). In contrast, the risk of miscarriage does not appear to be increased with either protein C and protein S deficiency (OR, 1.4; 95% CI, 0.9–2.2 and OR, 1.2; 95% CI, 0.7–1.9, respectively) (7). This may reflect admixture of embryonic and fetal losses in such spontaneous loss studies (10). Although rates of severe preeclampsia, abruption, and IUGR appear increased in affected patients, the paucity of affected patients suggests caution should be exercised in concluding that such an association exists (1, 6, 20). Patients who are homozygous for protein C or protein S deficiency present with neonatal purpura fulminans and extensive necrosis and are unlikely to be encountered during pregnancy.

Hyperhomocysteinemia

Homocysteine is generated from the metabolism of the amino acid methionine. It normally circulates in the plasma at concentrations of 5–16 micromole/L (1). Inherited hyperhomocysteinemia can be exacerbated by nutritional deficiencies in folic acid. Hyperhomocysteinemia can be diagnosed by measuring fasting homocysteine levels by gas–chromatography–mass spectrometry or other sensitive biochemical means. The disorder is classified into three categories according to the extent of the fasting homocysteine elevation: 1) severe (more than 100 micromole/L), 2) moderate (25–100 micromole/L), or 3) mild (16–24 micromole/L). Methionine loading can improve diagnostic sensitivity.

The severe form has a prevalence of 1 in 200,000 to 1 in 355,000 and presents with neurologic abnormalities, premature atherosclerosis, and recurrent thromboembolism. The mild and moderate forms of hyperhomocysteinemia generally result from autosomal-dominant (heterozygote) deficiencies in cystathionine β-synthase (0.3–1.4% of population) or, most commonly, from homozygosity for methylenetetrahydrofolate reductase mutants (1). Homozygosity for the methylenetetrahydrofolate reductase C677T and A1298C polymorphisms is present in 10–16% and 4–6% of all Europeans, respectively (39). These latter mutations do not increase the risk of venous thrombosis in the absence of hyperhomocysteinemia (40, 41). These findings suggest that screening should be limited to fasting homocysteine levels rather than mutation analysis.

Although there are conflicting data on the link between hyperhomocysteinemia and recurrent spontaneous abortions (1, 9, 10, 12), meta-analyses have suggested a link between elevated fasting homocysteine levels and recurrent fetal loss at less than 16 weeks of gestation (42). A number of investigators have linked hyperhomocysteinemia with severe preeclampsia, stillbirths, and severe IUGR (less than the fifth percentile), respectively (1, 6, 43). A 26% prevalence of hyperhomocysteinemia has been reported among patients with placental abruption (43). Meta-analyses also have found that patients with hyperhomocysteinemia had a larger pooled OR for abruption (OR, 5.3; 95% CI, 1.8–15.9) than did homozygosity for the methylenetetrahydrofolate reductase mutation (OR, 2.3; 95% CI, 1.1–4.9) (44). Patients with mild and moderate hyperhomocysteinemia also are at risk for atherosclerosis and thromboembolism as well as fetal neural tube defects and recurrent abortion (1). In a case–control study, it was found that fetal homozygosity for the methylenetetrahydrofolate reductase C677T mutation was associated with an increased risk of developing cerebral palsy (OR, 2.55; 95% CI, 1.12–5.74), whereas the heterozygous state conferred a lesser risk (OR, 1.91; 95% CI, 1.01–3.66) (27). Paradoxically, heterozygosity for methylenetetrahydrofolate reductase A1298C was associated with a reduced risk of diplegia developing at 32–36 weeks of gestation (OR, 0.16; 95% CI, 0.02–0.70). These findings raise concerns about ascertainment biases or confounding by the presence or absence of concomitant hyperhomocysteinemia. Heterozygous prothrombin (G20210A) gene mutation and homozygous methylenetetrahydrofolate reductase C677T when combined were associated with quadriplegia following birth at any gestational ages (OR, 5.33; 95% CI, 1.06–23.25) (27).

Diagnosis

Taken as a group, inherited thrombophilias clearly increase the risk of maternal thromboembolism. However, there does not appear to be a strong link between the inherited thrombophilias and early (less than 10 weeks of gestation) pregnancy loss (10); thrombophilias appear to be modestly linked to subsequent fetal loss and abruption. The link between inherited thrombophilias and severe preeclampsia and IUGR remains unproved and unlikely.

Who Should Be Tested?

Information on the presence of either inherited or acquired (ie, antiphospholipid antibody syndrome) thrombophilias plays a crucial role in determining the need for anticoagulation therapy in pregnancy. Therefore, all patients with a history of venous thrombotic events who are pregnant or planning to conceive should be tested. Given the strong evidence of an association between thrombophilias and fetal loss and abruption, it would appear to be prudent to test women with such a history as well. However, it is unclear whether patients with a history of recurrent early (less than 10 weeks of gestation) embryonic losses, preeclampsia, and IUGR should be evaluated for inherited thrombophilias. Our most recent data would suggest that such testing is not required.

How Should Patients Be Tested?

The prevalence, inheritance, thrombogenic potential, and diagnostic tests for the major inherited thrombophilias are presented in Table 7-1. The workup should begin with the most common disorders (ie, genotyping to rule out heterozygosity for the factor V Leiden or prothrombin [G20210A] mutations). If the patient is not pregnant, the factor V Leiden mutation can be ruled out

Table 7-1. Inheritance, Diagnosis, Prevalence, and Relative Pathogenicity of the Inherited Thrombophilias

Disorder	Genetics	Assays	Prevalence	Risk of Venous Thrombotic Event
Factor V Leiden	AD	DNA	2–15%	Threefold to eightfold
Prothrombin G20210A	AD	DNA	2–3%	Threefold
Antithrombin	AD	Activity assay	0.02%	25- to 50-fold
Protein C	AD	Activity assay	0.2–0.3%	10- to 15-fold
Protein S	AD	Activity assay if low, assess total and free antigen	0.1–2.1%	Twofold
Hyperhomocysteinemia	AR	Fasting homocysteine level	Less than 2%	2.5-fold (levels greater than 18.5 micromole/L) and threefold to fourfold (greater than 20 micromole/L)
PAI-1	AR	DNA	High	Unknown

Lockwood CJ. Inherited thrombophilias in pregnant patients: detection and treatment paradigm. Obstet Gynecol 2002;99:333–41.

with a functional assay for actual protein C resistance. Assays for functionally active antithrombin and protein C also should be obtained using diagnostic cutoffs of 60% and 50%, respectively. Screening for protein S deficiency with a functional activity assay is subject to very high interassay and intraassay variability because of fluctuations in levels of complement 4b-binding protein. Therefore, detection of free protein S antigen levels of less than 55% in nonpregnant women and less than 45% in pregnant patients, on two separate occasions, appears to be the optimal screening test (45). Fasting plasma homocysteine levels should also be assessed in lieu of, or in addition to, the methylenetetrahydrofolate reductase mutation. Although there is no consensus on the proper cutoff value for the diagnosis of hyperhomocysteinemia, we employ more than 12 micromole/L to define an elevated homocysteine level in pregnancy and more than or equal to 16 micromole/L to define elevations in nonpregnant patients.

All coagulation activity testing should be performed remote from the thrombotic event and while the patient is not taking heparin or other anticoagulant therapy. Heparin induces a decrease in antithrombin levels, and warfarin decreases protein C and protein S concentrations. The charges for this standard screen for inherited thrombophilias appear to range from $800 to $1,800.

Treatment

Pregnant patients with antithrombin deficiency or compound heterozygotes for the factor V Leiden and prothrombin (G20210A) mutations are at higher risk for maternal thromboembolic disorders and require therapeutic unfractionated or therapeutic low molecular weight heparin therapy throughout pregnancy (1). The latter regimen has several advantages, including less need for monitoring antifactor Xa activity and lower risks of osteopenia, thrombocytopenia, and hemorrhage. This therapy should be continued throughout the antepartum period until labor. We would suggest that among pregnant patients with these two highly thrombogenic thrombophilias and those homozygous for factor V Leiden or the prothrombin (G20210A) mutation, who are without a personal or strong family history of venous thrombosis or other thrombotic risks, "high" prophylactic doses may be considered, targeting peak antifactor Xa levels between 0.4 units/mL and 0.6 units/mL. Because low molecular weight heparin has a longer half-life than unfractionated heparin and its use has been associated with epidural hematoma formation; neuroaxial anesthesia should not be used within 18–24 hours of the last dose of low molecular weight heparin. Alternatively, we replace low molecular weight heparin with unfraction-

ated heparin at 36–37 weeks of gestation to facilitate the use of epidural anesthesia in labor. In any case, 6–12 hours after delivery, heparin therapy should be resumed and warfarin therapy begun. Heparin should be continued for at least 5 days after the initiation of warfarin and not discontinued until the International Normalized Ratio (INR) has been in the therapeutic range (ie, 2–3) for 2 consecutive days. Premature cessation of heparin may cause a paradoxical thrombosis because warfarin decreases protein C levels before that of the vitamin K-dependent clotting factors (1). In patients who are antithrombin deficient, antithrombin concentrates can be used during labor and delivery or when there are obstetric complications in which the risks of bleeding from anticoagulation are increased (eg, placenta previa and abruptions). Warfarin should be continued for at least 6 weeks and longer (3–6 months or life long) if there have been prior thromboembolic events.

Women with or without the other lesser thrombogenic inherited or acquired thrombophilias who develop venous thrombotic disorders during pregnancy require full therapeutic heparinization with either unfractionated or low molecular weight heparin for at least 4 months. This can be followed by prophylactic therapy with either the unfractionated or low molecular weight heparin throughout the remainder of the pregnancy. Low molecular weight heparin can be switched to unfractionated heparin at 36–37 weeks of gestation to permit epidural anesthesia. The heparin should be resumed 6–12 hours after delivery and warfarin initiated. The heparin should be continued during the postpartum period for at least 5 days or for at least 48 hours after the patient has achieved a therapeutic INR on warfarin (1). The latter therapy should be maintained for 6–18 weeks with the precise duration dependent on the site of the thromboembolism (eg, longer for pulmonary emboli and iliofemoral thromboses, shorter for distal leg thromboses) (1).

The issue of whether prophylactic heparin therapy should be offered to all pregnant patients with a history of prior venous thrombotic events has recently been examined. In a prospective study of 125 pregnant women with a single previous episode of venous thromboembolism, 95 were tested for laboratory evidence of thrombophilia (46). Antepartum heparin was withheld, but anticoagulant therapy was given for 4–6 weeks postpartum. Although 3 of the 125 women (2.4%) had an antepartum recurrence of venous thromboembolism (95% CI, 0.2–6.9), there were no recurrences among the 44 women without evidence of thrombophilia and whose previous thrombosis was associated with a temporary risk factor (eg, oral contraceptives, fracture-induced immobilization). In contrast, 3 of 51 (5.9%) women with a thrombophilia or whose prior thrombotic episode was not associated with a temporary thrombotic risk factor had an antepartum recurrence of venous thromboembolism. Thus, it would appear that prophylactic heparin is not required among women without a detectable inherited or acquired thrombophilia in whom a previous venous thrombotic event was associated with a nonrecurring risk factor. However, such therapy should be employed in the postpartum period when the risk of thrombosis is highest (Fig. 7-2). In contrast, antepartum and postpartum prophylaxis appears warranted in patients with a personal history or first-degree relative with a history of thromboembolic disease and who have an identifiable thrombophilia or whose prior thrombosis occurred in the absence of a nonrecurring risk factor (Fig. 7-2).

The management of patients in whom inherited thrombophilias are identified is presented in Figure 7-3. With the exception of pregnant patients with antithrombin deficiency or those who are homozygotes or compound heterozygotes for the factor V Leiden or prothrombin (G20210A) mutations, there does not appear to be any justification for antenatal heparin treatment in asymptomatic patients incidentally found to

have an inherited thrombophilia but who are without a personal or strong family history of prior venous thrombosis or characteristic adverse pregnancy outcomes. Their risks of thromboembolism or adverse pregnancy outcomes are likely less than 1%. In contrast, patients with such a history should receive antenatal prophylaxis. Postpartum prophylaxis appears warranted among such patients if they have a personal or family history, or other risk factors for thrombosis (eg, cesarean delivery) (Fig. 7-3).

Patients with a personal or strong family history of thromboembolic events and lesser thrombogenic thrombophilias should receive prophylactic heparin therapy in the antepartum period. Warfarin can be started in the immediate postpartum period with the heparin continued for at least 5 days or until the INR has been therapeutic for 48 hours. Warfarin is continued for 4–6 weeks (Fig. 7-3).

There is no consensus on the need for treatment among asymptomatic women without a personal or family history of clotting with an inherited thrombophilia of lower thrombogenic potential and only a history of characteristic adverse pregnancy outcomes. However, an argument can be made that the recurrence risk of women with prior fetal loss or abruption (10) is high enough to justify treatment (Fig. 7-3). A randomized clinical trial evaluated anticoagulation in women with one unexplained fetal loss at more than 10 weeks of gestation who were heterozygous for factor V Leiden, the prothrombin G20210A mutation, or protein S deficiency (47). Patients were all given 5 mg of folic acid daily, begun before conception, and once pregnant were randomized to receive either low-dose aspirin (100 mg) daily or the low molecular weight heparin, enoxaparin, 40 mg daily starting at the eighth week. Live births were noted in only 28.8% of the aspirin alone group but in 86.2% of the enoxaparin group ($P < 0.0001$) (OR, 15.5; 95% CI, 7–34). Such patients should be offered postpartum anticoagulation prophylaxis if they have an affected first-degree relative or thrombotic risk (eg, cesarean delivery).

If hyperhomocysteinemia is the sole coagulation defect, consideration should be given to adding folic acid supplementation (4 mg/d) before and throughout the pregnancy. Although there are no randomized clinical trials to support such an approach, the toxicity of this therapy is minimal, and folic acid has proven value in reducing the occurrence of fetal neural tube defects. Prophylactic heparin should be considered among hyperhomocysteinemic patients with a history of thromboembolism or characteristic adverse pregnancy outcomes, whose elevated homocysteine levels are unresponsive to such vitamin therapy.

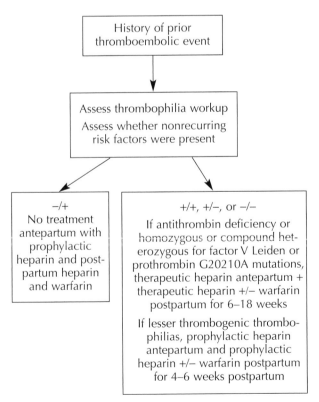

Fig. 7-2. The management of patients with a prior venous thromboembolic event. (Lockwood CJ. Inherited thrombophilias in pregnant patients: detection and treatment paradigm. Obstet Gynecol 2002;99:333–41.)

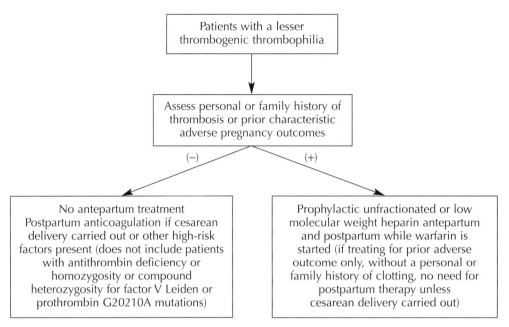

Fig. 7-3. The management of patients with a lesser thrombogenic thrombophilia. (Modified from Lockwood CJ. Inherited thrombophilias in pregnant patients: detection and treatment paradigm. Obstet Gynecol 2002;99:333–41.)

References

1. Lockwood CJ. Inherited thrombophilias in pregnant patients. Prenat Neonat Med 2001;6:3–14.

2. Kingdom JC, Kaufmann P. Oxygen and placental villous development: Origins of fetal hypoxia. Placenta 1997;18:613–21.

3. Lockwood CJ, Rand J. The immunobiology and obstetrical consequences of antiphospholipid antibodies. Obstet Gynecol Survey 1994;49:432–41.

4. Girling J, de Swiet M. Inherited thrombophilia and pregnancy. Curr Opin Obstet Gynecol 1998;10:135–44.

5. Gris J-C, Quere I, Monpeyroux F, Mercier E, Ripart-Neveu S, Tailland ML, et al. Case-control study of the frequency of thrombophilic disorders in couples with late foetal loss and no thrombotic antecedent. The Nimes Obstetricians and Haematologists Study (NOHA). Thromb Haemost 1999;81:891–9.

6. Kupferminc MJ, Eldor A, Steinman N, Many A, Bar-Am A, Jaffa A, et al. Increased frequency of genetic thrombophilia in women with complications of pregnancy. N Engl J Med 1999;340:9–13.

7. Preston FE, Rosendaal FR, Walker ID, Briet E, Berntorp E, Conard J, et al. Increased fetal loss in women with heritable thrombophilia. Lancet 1996;348:913–6.

8. Ridker PM, Miletich JP, Buring JE, Ariyo AA, Price DT, Manson JE, et al. Factor V Leiden mutation as a risk factor for recurrent pregnancy loss. Ann Intern Med 1998;128:1000–3.

9. Foka ZJ, Lambropoulos AF, Saravelos H, Karas GB, Karavida A, Agorastos T, et al. Factor V Leiden and prothrombin G20210A mutations, but not methylenetetrahydrofolate reductase C677T, are associated with recurrent miscarriages. Hum Reprod 2000;15:458–62.

10. Roque H, Paidas M, Rebarber A, Khan S, Kuczynski E, Lockwood CJ. There is no association between maternal thrombophilia and recurrent first-trimester loss. Am J Obstet Gynecol 2001;184:S15.

11. Kutteh WH, Park VM, Deitcher SR. Hypercoagulable state mutation analysis in white patients with early first trimester recurrent pregnancy loss. Fertil Steril 1999;71:1048–53.

12. Murphy RP, Donoghue C, Nallen RJ, D'Mello M, Regan C, Whitehead AS, et al. Prospective evaluation of the risk conferred by factor V Leiden and thermolabile methylenetetrahydrofolate reductase polymorphisms in pregnancy. Arterioscler Thromb Vasc Biol 2000;20:266–70.

13. Kosmas IP, Tatsioni A, Ioannidis JP. Association of Leiden mutation in factor V gene with hypertension in pregnancy and pre-eclampsia: a meta-analysis. J Hypertens. 2003;21:1221–8.

14. Infante-Rivard C, Rivard GE, Yotov WV, Genin E, Guiguet M, Weinberg C, et al. Absence of association of thrombophilia polymorphisms with intrauterine growth restriction. New Engl J Med. 2002;347:19–25.

15. Ridker PM, Miletich JP, Hennekens CH, Buring JE. Ethnic distribution of factor V Leiden in 4047 men and women. Implications for venous thromboembolism screening. JAMA 1997;277:1305–7.

16. Voorberg J, Roeise J, Koopman R, Buller H, Berends F, ten Cate JW, et al. Association of idiopathic venous thromboembolism with single point-mutation at Arg 506 of factor V. Lancet 1994;343:1535–6.

17. Gerhardt A, Scharf RE, Beckman MW, Struve S, Bender HG, Pillny M, et al. Prothrombin and factor V mutations in women with a history of thrombosis during pregnancy and the puerperium. N Engl J Med 2000;342:374–80.

18. Zotz RB, Gerhardt A, Scharf RE. Inherited thrombophilia and gestational venous thromboembolism. Best Pract Res Clin Haematol 2003;16:243–59.

19. Brenner B, Mandel H, Lanir N, Younis J, Rothbart H, Ohel G, et al. Activated protein C resistance can be associated with recurrent fetal loss. Br J Haematol 1997;97:551–4.

20. Kupferminc MJ, Fait G, Many A, Gordon D, Eldor A, Lessing JB. Severe preeclampsia and high frequency of genetic thrombophilic mutations. Obstet Gynecol 2000;96:45–9.

21. Blumenfeld Z, Brenner B. Thrombophilia-associated pregnancy wastage. Fertil Steril 1999;72:765–74.

22. Currie L, Peek M, McNiven M, Prosser I, Mansour J, Ridgway J. Is there an increased maternal-infant prevalence of Factor V Leiden in association with severe preeclampsia? BJOG 2002;109:191–6.

23. van Pampus MG, Wolf H, Koopman MM, van den Ende A, Buller HR, Reitsma PH. Prothrombin 20210 G: a mutation and Factor V Leiden mutation in women with a history of severe preeclampsia and (H)ELLP syndrome. Hypertens Pregnancy 2001;20:291–8.

24. D'Elia AV, Driul L, Giacomello R, Colaone R, Fabbro D, Di Leonardo C, et al. Frequency of factor V, prothrombin and methylenetetrahydrofolate reductase gene variants in preeclampsia. Gynecol Obstet Invest 2002;53:84–7.

25. Kosmas IP, Tatsioni A, Ioannidis JP. Association of Leiden mutation in factor V gene with hypertension in pregnancy and pre-eclampsia: a meta-analysis. J Hypertens 2003;21:1221–8.

26. Alfirevic Z, Roberts D, Martlew V. How strong is the association between maternal thrombophilia and adverse pregnancy outcome? A systematic review. Eur J Obstet Gynecol Reprod Biol 2002;101:6–14.

27. Gibson CS, MacLennan AH, Hague WM, Haan EA, Priest K, Chan A, et al. South Australian Cerebral Palsy Research Group. Associations between inherited thrombophilias, gestational age, and cerebral palsy. Am J Obstet Gynecol 2005;193:1437.

28. Martinelli I, Taioli E, Cetin I, Marinoni A, Gerosa S, Villa MV, et al. Mutations in coagulation factors in women with unexplained late fetal loss. N Engl J Med 2000;343:1015–8.

29. Morrison ER, Miedzybrodzka ZH, Campbell DM, Haites NE, Wilson BJ, Watson MS, Greaves M, Vickers MA. Prothrombotic genotypes are not associated with pre-eclampsia and gestational hypertension: results from a large population-based study and systematic review. Thromb Haemost 2002;87:779–85.

30. Alfirevic Z, Roberts D, Martlew V. How strong is the association between maternal thrombophilia and adverse pregnancy outcome? A systematic review. Eur J Obstet Gynecol Reprod Biol 2002;101:6–14.

31. Kohler HP, Grant PJ. Plasminogen-activator inhibitor type-1 and coronary artery disease. New Engl J Med 2000;342:1792–801.

32. Buchholz T, Lohse P, Rogenhofer N, Kosian E, Pihusch R, Thaler CJ. Polymorphisms in the ACE and PAI-1 genes are associated with recurrent spontaneous miscarriages. Hum Reprod 2003;18:2473–7.

33. Varela ML, Adamczuk YP, Forastiero RR, Martinuzzo ME, Cerrato GS, Pombo G, et al. Major and potential pro-thrombotic genotypes in a cohort of patients with venous thromboembolism. Thromb Res 2001;104:317–24.

34. Gubric N, Stegnar M, Peternel P, Kaider A, Binder BR. A novel G/A and the 4G/5G polymorphism within the promoter of the plasminogen activator inhibitor-1 gene in patients with deep vein thrombosis. Thromb Res 1996;84:431–43.

35. Wolf CE, Haubelt H, Pauer HU, Hinney B, Krome-Cesar C, Legler TJ, et al. Recurrent pregnancy loss and its relation to FV Leiden, FII G20210A and polymorphisms of plasminogen activator and plasminogen activator inhibitor. Pathophysiol Haemost Thromb 2003;33:134–7.

36. Dossenbach-Glaninger A, van Trotsenburg M, Dossenbach M, Oberkanins C, Moritz A, Krugluger W, et al. Plasminogen activator inhibitor 1 4G/5G polymorphism and coagulation factor XIII Val34Leu polymorphism: impaired fibrinolysis and early pregnancy loss. Clin Chem 2003;49:1081–6.

37. Glueck CJ, Phillips H, Cameron D, Wang P, Fontaine RN, Moore SK, et al. The 4G/4G polymorphism of the hypofibrinolytic plasminogen activator inhibitor type 1 gene: An independent risk factor for serious pregnancy complications. Metabolism 2000;49:845–52.

38. Lane DA, Bayston T, Olds RJ, Fitches AC, Cooper DN, Millar DS, et al. Antithrombin mutation database: 2nd (1997) update. For the Plasma Coagulation Inhibitors Subcommittee of the Scientific and Standardization Committee of the International Society on Thrombosis and Haemostasis. Thromb Haemost 1997;77:197–211.

39. Peng F, Labelle LA, Rainey BJ, Tsongalis GJ. Single nucleotide polymorphisms in the methylenetetrahydrofolate reductase gene are common in US Caucasian and Hispanic American populations. Int J Mol Med 2001;8:509–11.

40. McColl MD, Ellison J, Reid F, Tait RC, Walker ID, Greer IA. Prothrombin 20210 G—>A, MTHFR C677T mutations in women with venous thromboembolism associated with pregnancy. BJOG 2000;107:565–9.

41. Morelli VM, Lourenco DM, D'Almeida V, Franco RF, Miranda F, Zago MA, et al. Hyperhomocysteinemia increases the risk of venous thrombosis independent of the C677T mutation of the methylenetetrahydrofolate reductase gene in selected Brazilian patients. Blood Coagul Fibrinolysis 2002;13:271–5.

42. Nelen WL, Blom HJ, Steegers EA, den Heijer M, Eskes TK. Hyperhomocysteinemia and recurrent early pregnancy loss: A meta-analysis. Fertil Steril 2000;74:1196.

43. de Vries JI, Dekker GA, Huijgens PC, Jakobs C, Blomberg BM, van Geijn HP. Hyperhomocysteinaemia and protein S deficiency in complicated pregnancies. Br J Obstet Gynaecol 1997;104:1248–54.

44. Ray JG, Laskin CA. Folic acid and homocyst(e)ine metabolic defects and the risk of placental abruption, pre-eclampsia and spontaneous pregnancy loss: A systematic review. Placenta 1999;20:519–29.

45. Goodwin AJ, Rosendaal FR, Kottke-Marchant K, Bovill EG. A review of the technical, diagnostic, and epidemiologic considerations for protein S assays. Arch Pathol Lab Med 2002;126:1349–66.

46. Brill-Edwards P, Ginsberg JS, Gent M, Hirsh J, Burrows R, Kearon C, et al. Safety of withholding heparin in pregnant women with a history of venous thromboembolism. Recurrence of clot in this pregnancy study group. N Engl J Med 2000;343:1439–44.

47. Gris JC, Mercier E, Quere I, Lavigne-Lissalde G, Cochery-Nouvellon E, Hoffet M, et al. Low-molecular-weight heparin versus low-dose aspirin in women with one fetal loss and a constitutional thrombophilic disorder. Blood 2004;103:3695–9

CHAPTER 8

Management of Obesity in Pregnancy

PATRICK M. CATALANO

Obesity is an epidemic not only in the United States and developed countries but also in the developing world. "Indeed, it is now so common that it (obesity) is replacing the more traditional public health care concerns including undernutrition and infectious disease as one of the most significant contributors to ill health" (1). The World Health Organization and the National Institutes of Health define normal weight as a body mass index (BMI, weight [kg]/height [m^2]) of 18.5–24.9, overweight as a BMI of 25–29.9, and obesity as a BMI of 30 or greater. Obesity is further characterized by BMI into class I (30–34.9), class II (35–39.9), and class III (greater than 40) (1). In women of reproductive age in the United States, the prevalence of obesity was 30.2%, while the prevalence of overweight was 56.7% in the latest Centers for Disease Control and Prevention (CDC) reports. The problem of obesity is greatest among non-Hispanic black women (48.8%), as compared with Mexican-American (38.9%) and non-Hispanic white women (31.3%). Potentially more important, the prevalence of obesity in children as young as 2 years old and adolescents has increased by 11.3% between 1994 and 2000 (2). Again, the increased prevalence has been especially notable among Mexican–American and non-Hispanic black adolescents.

The problems relating to the management of obesity in pregnancy are many. There are both short- and long-term complications and implications for both mother and fetus. This issue has recently been addressed by the American College of Obstetricians and Gynecologists (ACOG) in Committee Opinion No. 315, "Obesity in Pregnancy" (3). I will attempt to first comment on the Committee Opinion, and secondarily discuss the potential implications of obesity for women and their offspring.

Obesity is a risk factor for a number of pregnancy complications. Therefore, as recommended by ACOG in Committee Opinion No. 315, obese women should be encouraged to decrease weight before considering pregnancy. Also recently, ACOG Committee Opinion No. 319, "The Role of the Obstetrician–Gynecologist in the Assessment and Management of Obesity," offers obstetrician–gynecologists practical guidelines on how to assess and manage obesity in the nonpregnant woman (4). Included are primers on the assessment of a patient's readiness to make behavioral changes. Lifestyle measures of calorie-restricted diets and exercise, when employed together, are potentially more beneficial than either modality alone. As noted in ACOG Committee Opinion No. 319, fad diets, even those with a potential physiological basis such as low-glycemic diets, are controversial at best with respect to long-term efficacy. Also included is information regarding approved weight-loss medications and guidelines for referral for bariatric surgery evaluation, which will be discussed later.

Although preconception weight loss is certainly a laudable goal for obese women, many, if not most, pregnancies are not planned. The limited success in normalization of pregravid glucose control in women with pregestational diabetes to decrease the risk of congenital malformations is an analogous example of the limitation of preconception management of lifestyle issues. Long-term public health programs addressing awareness of the problems of obesity, like those programs in recent decades that promoted smoking cessation programs and legislation, hold promise for success in the future. In the meantime we need not give up hope because some obese patients with the proper counseling can achieve meaningful weight loss before conception.

Pregravid Obesity Versus Weight Gain In Pregnancy

The obstetric complications of maternal obesity are generally related to issues of maternal pregravid obesity rather than excessive weight gain during gestation that results in a nonobese woman becoming obese. Weight gain in pregnancy is generally considered to be the difference between a woman's weight at the last antenatal visit and her pregravid weight or her weight at the first antenatal visit. However, the concept of "net maternal weight gain" has gathered more interest because this takes into account the fact that, on average, 4–5 kg of weight at term represents the fetus (3.5 kg), the placenta (0.5 kg), and amniotic fluid (0.5–1.0 kg). Therefore, one could easily express net maternal weight gain as the difference between a woman's weight at her last antenatal visit and the combination of her pregravid weight and fetal weight.

The recommendations for weight gain in pregnancy have been based on the Institute of Medicine (IOM) guidelines that were published in 1990 (5). The suggested weight gains are a weight gain of 11.2–15.9 kg (25–35 lb) for women with a normal BMI, 6.8–11.2 kg (15–25 lb) for overweight women, and less than 6.8 kg (15 lb) for obese women. These guidelines were initially intended to help decrease the risk of fetal growth restriction. In a report by Schieve et al (6) from the CDC Pregnancy Nutrition Surveillance System, in more than 266,000 women, the mean maternal weight gain and net weight gain, even when adjusted for week of gestation, both decrease with increasing BMI. Moreover, overweight and obese women had mean weight gains greater than the IOM guidelines. Based on these and other data, including the increasing prevalence of obesity in the population, the IOM currently is reviewing the recommendations for weight gain in pregnancy.

The components of weight gain have been previously estimated to be approximately 1 kg of protein and 4 kg of fat, with the remainder being water (7). Prospective studies initiated before pregnancy in women with a wide range of BMIs, reported a wide range of incremental accretion of fat, depending on a subject's pregravid BMI (8). The net accrual of fat mass was 5.3 kg in women with low BMIs, 4.6 kg in women with normal BMIs, and 8.4 kg in the high BMI group. However, there was a wide range in increased fat mass within each group. In our own prospective studies, we found no significant difference in gain of fat mass in lean compared with obese women (4.7 ± 3.2 kg versus 4.2 ± 3.5 kg, $P = .58$), nor lean body mass (7.6 ± 3.9 kg versus 8.8 ± 2.6 kg, $P = .18$), although the increase in percentage of body fat was significantly greater in the lean compared with the obese women (3.3 ± 3.8% versus 0.1 ± 3.3%, $P = .004$) (9). The increase in subcutaneous fat was in a central distribution (ie, between the midthorax through the upper thigh). Interestingly, there was no significant difference in accretion of fat mass in women with normal glucose tolerance compared with women with gestational diabetes mellitus (GDM) matched for pregravid body composition. There are limited data about the relative changes in visceral fat, which potentially may be of more metabolic significance. An increase in both preperitoneal and subcutaneous fat layers by the third trimester of pregnancy, as well as an increase in the ratio of peritoneal to subcutaneous fat,

have been reported (10), suggesting intraabdominal fat increases during pregnancy. Hence, the accrual of fat mass in pregnancy is variable and may depend on a woman's pregravid metabolic status and other lifestyle variables such as diet and physical activity.

Obstetric Risks Associated With Maternal Obesity: Early Gestation

Obese women are at an increased risk of myriad obstetric problems in early pregnancy. There is an increased risk of early miscarriage (odds ratio [OR], 1.2; 95% confidence interval [CI], 1.01–1.46, $P = .04$) and recurrent miscarriage (OR, 3.5; 95% CI, 1.03–12.01, $P = .04$) in obese women compared with normal weight controls after natural conception (11). In overweight women conceiving after in vitro fertilization or intracytoplasmic sperm injection, there was an increase in the abortion rate during the first 6 weeks of gestation (22% versus 12%) compared with lean or average weight women (12). The relative risk of spontaneous abortion was 1.77 (95% CI, 1.05–2.97). Therefore, particularly in obese women considering assisted reproductive therapy, weight loss before conception should be strongly considered and measures initiated by the patient's health care provider.

As early as 1994, it was thought that offspring of obese women were at increased risk of neural tube defects (OR, 1.8; 95% CI, 1.1–3.0), especially spina bifida (OR, 2.6; 95% CI, 1.5–4.5) (13). These results have been confirmed in subsequent studies and also have implicated maternal obesity with increased risks of heart defects (OR, 1.18; 95% CI, 1.09–1.27) (14) and omphalocele (OR, 3.3; 95% CI, 1.0–10.3) (15). Because these types of congenital anomalies are often seen with pregestational diabetes, some investigators have suggested that many of these obese women may have had undiagnosed type 2 diabetes (14). Additionally, because neural tube defects are associated with folic acid deficiencies, in one study it was found that after controlling for intake of folate in food and nutritional supplements, increased BMI was associated with lower serum folate concentrations ($P < .001$) (16). This finding suggested that women with a BMI greater than 30 would need to increase their folate consumption by 350 mcg/d to achieve the same folate levels as women with BMIs less than 20. In contrast, a study in a Canadian population estimated whether the risk of neural tube defects was lower after flour was fortified with folic acid (17). Before fortification of flour, increased maternal weight was associated with a modest increased risk of neural tube defects (OR, 1.4; 95% CI, 1.0–1.8). After flour fortification, the risk actually increased (OR, 2.8; 95% CI, 1.2–6.6). Therefore, although the evidence implicated maternal obesity with an increased risk of congenital anomalies, particularly neural tube defects, the mechanisms are not well understood. Practically, short of preconception weight loss in the management of obese pregnant women, one should consider glucose screening of obese women in early pregnancy to rule out undiagnosed pregestational diabetes. Folate supplementation of cereal products was initiated in this country in 1998, and whether additional folate supplementation should be offered to obese women before conception or in early pregnancy is speculative at this point. Obviously, more research must be done, but recognition of obesity as a risk factor for congenital anomalies remains an important factor for the clinician to consider in the management of obese pregnant women.

If, indeed, obese women are at increased risk of neural tube defects and other congenital anomalies, how then does maternal obesity affect our diagnostic abilities in this population? There is a significant correlation between maternal serum alpha-fetoprotein (AFP) and maternal weight ($r = 0.24$, $P < .001$), with lighter women having greater amounts of maternal serum AFP than heavier women (18). This is generally believed to be a result of the proportionally greater plasma volume in obese compared with nonobese women. Therefore, standard adjustments of maternal AFP values for maternal weights up to 200 lb have been implemented (19). Additionally, the use of cell-free DNA in the diagnosis of chromosomal abnormalities may be affected by a woman's degree of obesity. In one study, it was reported that in the first trimester there was no significant association between maternal weight and plasma-free DNA levels (20). However, in the second trimester there was a significant inverse correlation between maternal weight and serum-free DNA ($r = -0.26$, $P = .007$), particularly if the woman weighed more than 170 lb.

The other modality commonly used in early pregnancy to identify congenital anomalies is ultrasonography. A significant impairment of adequate ultrasound visualization of fetal anatomy has been shown to occur when BMI was greater than 36; visualization decreased by 14.5% (21). A decrease in visualization was most marked for the fetal heart and spine. Subsequently, in more than 11,000 pregnancies in which 38.6% of the patients were obese, the rate of suboptimal visualization of fetal anatomy was 37.3% in obese women compared with 18.7% in nonobese women ($P < .001$) (22). Increased severity of obesity was again noted for both cardiac and craniospinal structures. The use of advanced ultrasound equipment may be able to improve suboptimal visualization of the outflow tracts in obese women after 18 weeks of gestation but not of the four-chamber view (23).

Although obese women may be at increased risk of neural tube defects, interpretation of serum markers is more difficult because of the changes in the volume of distribution of these markers, and care needs to be taken so as not to increase the number of false-negative results. The use of population-specific values may aid in the interpretation of results. Similarly, the ability of ultrasonography to detect fetal cardiac and craniospinal abnormalities is significantly limited in obese women compared with nonobese women. The use of advanced ultrasound equipment and delaying evaluation until after 18 weeks may be of some value, although overall maternal obesity still limits visibility of fetal structures.

Obstetric Risks Associated With Maternal Obesity in Late Gestation: Maternal Pregnancy Metabolic Dysfunction

The obese nonpregnant woman is at significant risk for what has variously been termed the metabolic syndrome or insulin resistance syndrome. This syndrome has as its metabolic core obesity (ie, central obesity as estimated by an elevated waist-to-hip ratio) and insulin resistance. The clinical manifestations of the metabolic syndrome include hypertension, glucose intolerance, and elevated cholesterol and triglycerides. Maternal obesity in pregnancy also is associated with an increased risk of "metabolic syndromelike complications" in late pregnancy, for example, gestational hypertension and preeclampsia. In retrospective studies, a significant increase in the risk of preeclampsia in women with increased BMI has been reported (24). Based on a prospective multicenter study of 16,102 women, initially evaluated at 10–14 weeks of gestation, 85% were controls (BMI less than 30), 9% were obese (BMI 30–34.9), and 6% were morbidly obese (BMI 35 or greater). Obese women and morbidly obese women were 2.5 and 3.2 times, respectively, more likely to develop gestational hypertension than the control group. Similarly, preeclampsia was 1.6 and 3.3 times more likely to develop in obese and morbidly obese women, respectively (25). The increase in preeclampsia in obese compared with average weight women extends to women with GDM as well. In women with well-controlled GDM, there is a significant increased risk of preeclampsia in obese women (10.8%) compared with average BMI women (8.2%) (26). The risk of preeclampsia also is increased in obese women with GDM with poor control (14.9%). Furthermore, the Australian Carbohydrate Intolerance Study in Pregnant Women showed that the risk of preeclampsia in the intervention group for GDM was 12%, whereas in the routine care group the risk was 18% ($P < .02$) (27). Although currently there are no known proven therapies to prevent the development of preeclampsia in obese women (eg, aspirin or calcium supplementation), there are data suggesting that tight glucose control in obese women with GDM may decrease the risk. Additionally, the use of antioxidants for the prevention of preeclampsia in obese women has a theoretical benefit because of the increase in oxidative stress generated from maternal adipose tissue. Two recent randomized controlled trials, however, have reported no benefit of antioxidants (1,000 mg of vitamin C and 400 international units of vitamin E) in the reduction of preeclampsia in treatment compared with placebo-controlled groups (28, 29). In the Vitamins in Preeclampsia trial, the investigators examined the risk of preeclampsia in primiparous women with a BMI greater than 30 at enrollment. In the subgroup, there was no benefit of antioxidants in decreasing the risk of preeclampsia: risk ratio 0.87 (range 0.59–1.30). The Vitamins in Preeclampsia trial also reported an increase in low birth weight babies in the supplemented groups compared with the placebo-control groups (29). Despite these data, after review by the data safety monitoring committee, the Maternal–Fetal Medicine Units Network has decided to continue ongoing recruitment. To date, the results of clinical trials of the use of antioxidants to prevent preeclampsia are not definitive as to their efficacy, and the Maternal–Fetal Medicine Units Network Study is currently in progress.

Gestational diabetes mellitus is the clinical manifestation of glucose intolerance in pregnancy. The pathophysiology of GDM involves both decreased insulin sensitivity and inadequate insulin response, resulting in hyperglycemia. In general, obese women are more insulin resistant (or have decreased insulin sensitivity) compared with nonobese women, whether pregravid or during pregnancy, when there are already significant 50–60% decreases in maternal insulin sensitivity by the end of the third trimester. Decreased insulin sensitivity is the limited ability of insulin to transport glucose from the intravascular into the peripheral tissues, primarily skeletal muscle. Therefore, it is not surprising that obese women also are at significantly greater risk for the development of GDM because they have decreased insulin sensitivity compared with nonobese women (Fig. 8-1). In the First and Second Trimester Evaluation of Risk trial, after adjusting for potential covariables, it was reported that the adjusted OR for the risk of GDM was 2.6 (95% CI, 2.1–3.4; P <.001) for obese and 4.0 (95% CI, 3.1–5.2; P <.01) for morbidly obese women (25). Therefore, in the management of obese pregnant women, consideration should be given to early glucose screening rather than waiting until the 24–28-week standard screening period. This would be helpful in women with other risk factors for GDM, such as a previous history of GDM, a family history of type 2 diabetes (particularly maternal), or a history of a macrosomic fetus.

Increasing non–insulin-mediated glucose disposal is of theoretical benefit in the prevention of GDM. Therefore, exercise with increased use of large skeletal muscles, such as walking or swimming, may be beneficial. Although the use of insulin sensitizers such as metformin and thiazolidinediones may be theoretically useful to increase insulin sensitivity, these agents cross the placenta and their fetal safety has not been documented. High fiber and complex carbohydrate–low glycemic diets may decrease the need for a large insulin response to a meal and theoretically decrease β cell failure, but the data on efficacy are again controversial. Glyburide, which has recently been introduced into the armamentarium of the treatment of GDM, helps restore euglycemia by enhancing insulin response. Therefore, because obese women may have decreased insulin sensitivity relative to nonobese women even in early gestation, in addition to early testing for GDM, lifestyle measures such as moderate physical activity and nutritional counseling may be beneficial in obese women with normal glucose tolerance.

Because obese women have an increased risk of developing or having preexisting manifestations of the metabolic syndrome with, for example, hypertension, proteinuria, dyslipidemia, and diabetes, we also are experiencing an increase in medical problems previously assumed to be diagnosed primarily in an older nonpregnant population, for example, sleep apnea, nonalcoholic fatty liver disease, and chronic renal and cardiac dysfunction. As such, consideration should be given to obtaining data, for example, electrocardiography to evaluate cardiac function and further cardiac evaluation, such as maternal echocardiography, depending on clinical history and physical and laboratory evaluation of obese women with chronic hypertension. Because these women also are at increased risk for the development of preeclampsia, assessment of renal function and degree of proteinuria in early gestation may assist in distinguishing the chronic renal dysfunction secondary to maternal chronic hypertension or diabetes or both from pregnancy-associated hypertension or preeclampsia. Similarly, elevated liver function test results may be an indication of nonalcoholic fatty liver disease rather than a manifestation of severe preeclampsia. To date, there are no published studies evaluating the prevalence of nonalcoholic fatty liver disease in pregnancy (PubMed research of the literature, English language, 1990–2006, key words: "non-alcoholic steatohepatitis," "NASH," "pregnancy"). We have seen an increasing number of obese women in pregnancy after extensive workup in the past 5 years. This is not surprising, given that obesity is recognized as the most common factor associated with nonalcoholic fatty liver disease in the nonpregnant population. Other common risk factors, such as increased estrogen concentrations, elevated lipids,

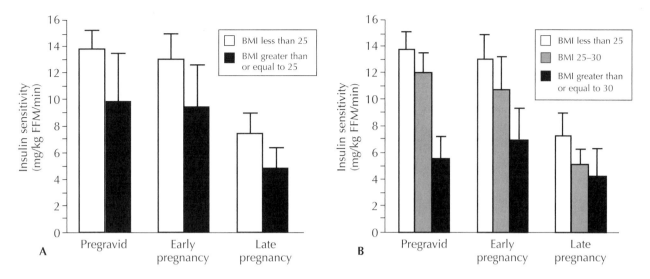

Fig. 8-1. A. The longitudinal changes in insulin sensitivity in women whose pregravid body mass index was less than 25 (n = 6) and in those with a body mass index of 25 or more (n = 9) as estimated using the hyperinsulinemic-euglycemic clamp. There is a significant decrease in insulin sensitivity over time (P <.001) and between groups (P = .007). **B.** The women with a body mass index of 25 or more before conception were separated into body mass index overweight (body mass index 25–30, n = 6) and obese (body mass index 30 or more, n = 3). There is a significant difference among groups (P <.001) and a group–time interaction (P = .002). Abbreviations: BMI, body mass index; FFM, fat-free mass. (Catalano PM. Management of obesity in pregnancy. Obstet Gynecol 2007;109:419–33 and Catalano PM, Ehrenberg HM. The short- and long-term implications of maternal obesity on the mother and her offspring. BJOG 2006;113:1126–33. Copyright © 2006, with permission from Blackwell Publishing, Ltd.)

and increased insulin resistance (all present in obese pregnant women), have been recognized as contributing factors (31). Therefore, as we have observed in our own population, we anticipate that nonalcoholic fatty liver disease will become a more common diagnosis in obese pregnant women with abnormal liver function studies. Unfortunately, there are no simple laboratory tests to screen for maternal sleep apnea. However, a history of daytime somnolence and a partner's complaint of loud snoring should increase suspicion of sleep apnea. Consideration of referral of these patients to the appropriate pulmonary specialist to diagnose obstructive sleep apnea and initiate treatment, such as nighttime continuous positive airway pressure, may be helpful because these women will have an increased risk of cesarean delivery.

Preterm Delivery

In reviewing the literature relating preterm birth to maternal pregravid BMI or weight gain during gestation, most investigators have reported both low pregravid weight and poor weight gain in women with low BMIs as risk factors for preterm birth. One study showed that the greatest risk of a preterm delivery was in women with a low pregravid BMI and weight gain less than 0.10 kg/wk (32). In a follow-up study, the same investigators (33) reported that, compared with women of average BMI and average pregnancy weight gain, the risk of preterm deliv-

ery increased progressively with decreasing pregravid BMI and weight gain of less than 0.5 lb/wk; BMI greater than 26 (OR, 1.6; 95% CI, 0.7–3.5), BMI 19.8–26 (OR, 3.6; 95% CI, 1.6–8.0), and BMI less than 19.8 (OR, 6.7; 95% CI, 1.1–40.6). Because as many as 25% of preterm births are indicated because of maternal medical or obstetric problems rather than the spontaneous births resulting from preterm labor or preterm rupture of membranes, many of the preterm births in the obese women may relate to indicated preterm delivery because of underlying medical or obstetric issues or both. Morbidly obese women have a significantly increased risk (OR, 1.5; 95% CI, 1.1–2.1) of preterm delivery in comparison with a normal weight control group (25). Because the initial goal of the IOM guidelines for weight gain in pregnant women was decreasing the risk of preterm and growth-restricted neonates, the issue of weight gain among pregnant women relative to these issues is being reconsidered.

Intrauterine Fetal Death

There has been an increasing awareness in the past decade of the role of maternal obesity in the risk of unexplained antepartum fetal death. In a Canadian population, examination of factors related to 196 unexplained fetal deaths, 25% of the fetal deaths in their population, revealed that the factor most strongly associated with unexplained fetal death was increased prepregnancy weight (34). Maternal pregravid weight greater than 68 kg increased the risk of unexplained fetal death (OR, 2.77; 95% CI, 1.85–4.68), even after adjusting for maternal age and excluding maternal diabetes and hypertensive disorders. Factitious postdate pregnancies were eliminated because of early ultrasound dating. Not unexpectedly, there was an increase in unexplained fetal deaths when the birth weight ratios were greater than average (ie, more than 1.15 [OR, 2.36; 95% CI, 1.26–4.44]). These results were confirmed in a recent Danish National Birth Cohort study among 54,000 births from 1998 to 2001 (35). Compared with normal weight women, the fetal death rate among obese women increased with increasing gestational age: from 28 weeks to 36 weeks the hazard rate was 2.1 (95% CI, 1.0–4.4), at 37–39 weeks the hazard rate was 3.5 (95% CI, 1.9–6.4), and at 40 weeks or more the hazard rate was 4.6 (95% CI, 1.6–13.4). A similar trend was observed in overweight women. In contrast to the Canadian study, the birth weights of the unexplained fetal deaths among obese women were lower than the median birth weights of the live births, suggesting intrauterine growth restriction. Consistent with this finding was the fact that obesity was associated with a fivefold increase in the rate of stillbirth with histological placental dysfunction. At this time, we can only speculate as to the pathophysiology of unexplained intrauterine fetal death in obese women. However, because these women are at increased risk for gestational hypertensive disorders and glucose intolerance, increased vigilance for these problems, known to be associated with increased perinatal mortality, is warranted. Given that maternal obesity may be associated with an increased risk of stillbirth, how should we manage these pregnancies? Women with obesity-related problems such as hypertension and diabetes need to be monitored closely, as would nonobese women, including assessment of fetal wellbeing and growth, which is all the more difficult, however, as noted previously in obese women. In women without medical or obstetric complications, the increase in stillbirths in overweight women was twice that of normal weight women, whereas the increase in stillbirth in obese women was 240% greater than that in normal weight women (36). Certainly, close fetal monitoring with assessments such as fetal kick counts in these women is prudent, but the cost/potential benefit ratio of more extensive evaluation is again speculative at this time.

Obstetric Risks Associated With Maternal Obesity: Peripartum

In addition to the increased risk of antenatal obstetric problems in obese women, there is an increased risk of cesarean delivery and associated morbidities. Both regional and general anesthesia are concerns in this population. There can be difficulty with placement of epidural or spinal anesthesia in obese women, requiring multiple attempts. Additionally, general anesthesia carries the risk of difficult intubation, and the increased incidence of sleep apnea postpartum. Therefore, obtaining an anesthesiology consultation before the onset of labor should be encouraged. In the multicenter study (25), the cesarean delivery rate for nulliparous women was 20.7% for women with a BMI of 29.9 or less, 33.8% for women with a BMI of 30–34.9, and 47.7% for women with a BMI of 35–39.9. Similar data were reported in women attempting vaginal birth after one prior cesarean delivery (VBAC) (37). Of 510 women attempting a trial of labor, 337 (66%) were successful and 173 (34%) required repeat cesarean delivery. The greatest success rate for VBAC was in underweight (BMI less than 19.8) women (84.7%) as compared with normal weight women ($P = .04$). Decreased VBAC success was observed in obese women (54.6%), but not in overweight women (65.5%) compared with normal weight women (70.5%), $P = .003$ and $P = .36$, respectively. Additionally, normal weight women who gained weight between pregnancies to become overweight during their attempted VBAC had decreased success rates compared with those women whose BMI remained average, (56.6% versus 74.2%, $P = .006$). Unfortunately, the converse was not true, in that weight loss resulting in a status change from overweight to average did not significantly improve the VBAC success (64.0% versus 58.4%, $P = .67$). The increased cesarean delivery rate in overweight and obese women also is associated with an increase in postoperative complications such as wound infection or breakdown, excessive blood loss, deep vein thrombophlebitis, and postpartum endometritis. Therefore, if an obese patient requires cesarean delivery, she should receive preoperative antibiotics even if the surgery is elective.

In obese women there are no prospective randomized trials to determine the optimal type of skin incision (ie, vertical or horizontal) to decrease the risk of wound disruption or infection. The vertical incision may afford greater exposure and room to deliver a macrosomic fetus and avoid an incision in a thick pannus, but this incision may result in increased postoperative pain and risk of evisceration because of lateral tension. In contrast, the Pfannenstiel incision may offer more postoperative comfort but, if there is a wound breakdown, management may be difficult because of exposure. Therefore, the decision regarding the type of incision to be used for cesarean delivery in obese patients will be made at the time of surgery based on maternal anthropometry and the experience of the individual surgeon. Because obese women are at increased risk for wound breakdown, attempts to obviate these complications have included closure of the subcutaneous layers or placement of subcutaneous drains or both. As noted in ACOG Committee Opinion No. 315, suture closure of the subcutaneous layer after cesarean delivery may lead to a significant decrease in wound disruption (3). However, the efficacy of subcutaneous drains to prevent morbidity of wound breakdown is less clear. Obese women also are at increased risk for postoperative deep vein thrombosis (DVT). The use of early ambulation and compression stockings may be of benefit if used properly. The use of postoperative heparin therapy is of value in the obese high-risk patient (eg, a patient with a history of DVT). The data on the use of postoperative heparin in all obese women to prevent DVT are insufficient to make any general recommendations regarding risk benefit. Overweight and obese women are at risk of increased medical and obstetric problems in pregnancy, which in turn increase their risk of preterm delivery, cesarean delivery, and attendant operative morbidities.

Bariatric Surgery for Obese Women: Gestational Considerations

As discussed previously, the best way to decrease the risk of medical and obstetric problems in obese women planning pregnancy is weight loss before conception. Given that lifestyle measures and medical treatments have had limited long-term success to date, more obese women of reproductive age are seeking bariatric surgery as an alternative. It is estimated that there are 150,000 bariatric surgical procedures performed in the United States each year. Bariatric surgery may be considered in patients with class III obesity (ie, BMI greater than 40 or BMI greater than 35 with comorbid conditions) if nonsurgical modalities have failed. Bariatric surgical procedures can be categorized into two primary types: 1) malabsorptive procedures such as Roux-en-Y gastric bypass, and 2) restrictive procedures such as laparoscopic adjustable gastric banding. The previously performed malabsorptive procedures were associated with complications during pregnancy, such as small bowel ischemia (38), as well as nutrient deficiencies, such as iron, folate, and B_{12} deficiencies (39). There also were reports of fetal abnormalities, small for gestational age infants, and premature births (35, 40). In one report (41), 298 patients who became pregnant after bariatric surgery underwent either malabsorptive or restrictive procedures. Compared with the general population, there was an increase in premature rupture of membranes (OR, 1.4; 95% CI, 1.3–2.7. $P = .001$), labor induction (OR, 2.1; 95% CI, 1.6–2.7; $P = .001$), birth weight more than 4 kg (OR, 2.1; 95% CI, 1.4–3.0; $P = .001$), and cesarean delivery 25.2% versus 12.2% (OR, 2.4; 95% CI, 1.9–3.1 $P < .001$). The increased risk of cesarean delivery in women with previous bariatric surgery remained significant after

adjusting for possible confounders. Of note, there were no significant differences between groups regarding other morbidities such as placental abruption, placenta previa, labor dystocia, or perinatal complications.

Although restrictive procedures, including laparoscopic adjustable gastric banding, are becoming more common, they are not without potential morbidity, including gastric ulcer perforation (42), intragastric band migration and balloon defect (43), and gastrointestinal hemorrhage resulting from erosion of a synthetic graft from a vertical banded gastroplasty (44). However, the early reported results from laparoscopic adjustable gastric banding studies are encouraging. In two separate Australian studies, it was reported that maternal weight gain during pregnancy was significantly reduced in women who underwent laparoscopic adjustable gastric banding in comparison with control groups, without significant differences in birth weights (45, 46). The incidence of gestational diabetes and pregnancy hypertensive disorders also were significantly reduced in women after laparoscopic adjustable gastric banding (Table 8-1). One report showed no decreased folate or B_{12} levels in the women with laparoscopic adjustable gastric banding, but some women who were not taking multivitamins regularly had elevated homocysteine concentrations (45).

Based on the available data, which does not include any randomized prospective trials or long-term follow-up of offspring of obese women who underwent bariatric surgery before pregnancy (PubMed search, English language, 1990–2006, key words: "bariatric surgery," "pregnancy"), the following recommendations of ACOG Committee Opinion No. 315 (3) are endorsed and expanded:

1. Patients with laparoscopic adjustable gastric banding should be advised that they are at risk of becoming pregnant unexpectedly after weight loss following surgery and should use appropriate contraceptive methods.

2. All patients undergoing laparoscopic adjustable gastric banding should delay pregnancy for 12–18 months to avoid the rapid weight loss phase of the procedure until their weight stabilizes and they are no longer catabolic. This will allow for a greater weight loss before conception and possibly decrease the risk of pregnancy-related complications such as hypertension and GDM.

3. Women with laparoscopic adjustable gastric banding should be monitored by their obstetricians and bariatric surgeons during pregnancy. Adjustments of gastric bands may reduce nausea and vomiting in pregnancy, but prophylactic removal or elimination of all the gastric band fluid may decrease the effectiveness of the treatment and result in excessive weight gain.

4. All women should have adequate supplementation of folate, calcium, and B_{12} after any bariatric surgical procedure because this may decrease the risk of subclinical nutritional deficiencies. Additional nutritional supplementation and close monitoring of fetal growth is necessary in women who have undergone diversionary or malabsorptive procedures.

Fetal Growth

Maternal obesity is a well-recognized risk factor for fetal macrosomia, more specifically, obesity and long-term risks of adolescent components of the metabolic syndrome. The incidence of fetal macrosomia, defined as birth weight greater than 4,000 g, has been reported as 8.3% in nonobese women, 13.3% in obese women, and 14.6% in the infants of the morbidly obese women (25). However, just as there has been an increase in obesity in the adult and adolescent populations in the past decade, neonatal birth weights have increased significantly. Recent studies from both North America and Europe have reported an increase in mean birth weights, particularly those infants either greater than the 90th percentile in weight for gestational age (large for gestational age) or macrosomic (birth weight more than 4 kg) (47, 48). In Denmark, the percentage of macrosomic newborns

increased from 16.7% in 1990 to 20.0% in 1999 (49). Factors such as decreased maternal smoking, an increased incidence of diabetes, and increasing maternal BMI have all been implicated.

In our own population, we have observed a mean increase of 116 g in term singleton birth weight over the past 30 years (Fig. 8-2). There was a mean 116-g increase in birth weight at term (37–41 weeks) from 1975 to 2003 (3,204 ± 477 versus 3,320 ± 488 g). The increase in birth weight was significant at the 5th, 10th, 50th, 90th, and 95th percentiles (range 85–173 g), with no significant difference among the percentiles (Fig. 8-3). From 1987 to 2003, the percentage of women who weighed less than 150 lb at delivery decreased from 33% to 16%, and the percentage of women who weighed more than 200 lb increased from 17% to 34%, with no change in the group between 150 lb and 200 lb (50%). Mean maternal age increased from 23.8 years to 25.3 years. The percentage of white women decreased from 49.4% to 39.1%, while the percentage of Hispanic (6.8–16.2%) and Asian (0.6–2.3%) women increased. The percentage of women with diabetes increased from 4% to 5.7%, while the percentage of women who smoked decreased from 34.4% to 18.4%. There was no significant change in parity or gestational age at delivery. Using a stepwise regression analysis, 8% of the variance in the increase in birth weight was related to the increase in maternal weight, while African-American

Table 8-1. Changes in Maternal Weight Gain, Neonatal Birth Weight, and Obesity-Related Complications in Obese Women With Laparoscopic Adjustable Gastric Banding and Historical Controls

	LAGP (n = 79)	Control (n = 79)	P Value
Dixon et al (45)			
Weight gain (kg)	9.6 ± 9	15.5 ± 9	<.05
Neonatal birth weight (g)	3,397 ± 545	3,297 ± 814	NS
Pregnancy-induced hypertension (%)	10	38	<.05
Gestational diabetes (%)	6.3	19	<.05
Skull, et all (46)			
Weight gain (kg)	3.7 (0.6–6.9)	15.6 (12.4–18.7)	.0001
Neonatal birth weight (kg)	3.31 (3.14–3.49)	3.53 (3.35–3.72)	0.19
Diabetes mellitus (%)	8.2	25.8	.048
Hypertension (%)	8	22.5	.06

Data for the Dixon et al (45) study (laparoscopic adjustable gastric banding: n = 79) are expressed as mean + standard deviation, and data for Skull et al (46) study (laparoscopic adjustable gastric banding: n = 49; Control: n = 31) are expressed as mean (95% confidence interval), except where otherwise indicated.

Abbreviations: LAGP, laparoscopic adjustable gastric banding; NS, not significant.

Modified from Dixon JB, Dixon ME, O'Brien PE. Birth outcomes in obese women after laparoscopic adjustable gastric banding. Obstet Gynecol 2005;106:965–72 and Skull AJ, Slater GH, Duncombe JE, Fielding GA. Laparoscopic adjustable banding in pregnancy: safety, patient tolerance and effect on obesity-related pregnancy outcomes. Obes Surg 2004;14:230–5.

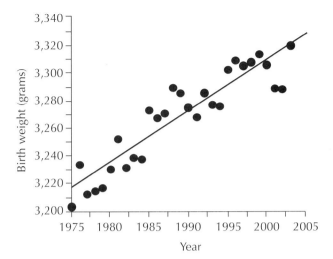

Fig. 8-2. Term singleton birth weight in grams from 37 weeks to 41 weeks from 1975 to 2003 at MetroHealth Medical Center, P <.001. (Catalano PM. Management of obesity in pregnancy. Obstet Gynecol 2007;109:419–33.)

race and female gender of the neonate accounted for an additional negative 4% of the variance in birth weight. None of the remaining demographic variables that were considered were found to be significant contributors to the change in birth weight.

Maternal anthropometric variables are important factors relating to fetal growth. Maternal pregravid weight has a very strong correlation with birth weight (50). Although maternal height also is associated with an increase in birth weight, when adjusted for weight, there was no longer a significant correlation between maternal height and birth weight (51). Maternal weight gain during gestation is positively correlated with birth weight (52). The correlation is stronger in nulliparous women ($r = 0.26$) compared with parous women ($r = 0.16$). In a study of the interaction of maternal pregravid weight and weight gain (53), there was a progressively stronger correlation between maternal weight gain and birth weight in moderately overweight, ideal body weight, and underweight women. In women weighing 135% of ideal weight for height before conception, there was no correlation between weight gain during pregnancy and birth weight. Lastly, maternal age and parity have independently been reported to have a positive correlation with birth weight. However, when maternal age was adjusted for parity, there was no longer a significant correlation between maternal age and birth weight (54). Parity has been shown to be associated with a mean 100–150 g increase in birth weight in subsequent pregnancies (55). However, the additional effect of parity on birth weight is diminished with increasing parity.

Relative to maternal factors, paternal anthropometric factors have limited impact on fetal growth. In half-

siblings with the mother as the common parent, the correlation between birth weight and the half siblings was $r = 0.58$ (56). In contrast, the correlation of birth weight in half siblings with the father as the common parent was only $r = 0.10$. Animal crossbreeding studies support these findings. In a crossbreed of Shetland ponies with Shire horses, the size of the foals was roughly the same as the foals of the maternal pure breed (57). Thus, maternal regulation was more important in determining intrauterine growth than were paternal factors. Using a Danish population registry, paternal birth weight, adult height, and adult weight together explained approximately 3% of the variance in birth weight, compared with 9% for the corresponding maternal factors (58). In summary, maternal factors, most importantly maternal pregravid weight, have the strongest correlations with birth weight.

In our studies of fetal overgrowth and macrosomia, we have elected to concentrate on measures of body composition (ie, fat and fat free or lean body mass). The rationale for this approach stems from work done in the previous century. As early as 1923, the variability in weight within mammalian species was explained by the amount of adipose tissue, whereas the amount of lean body mass was relatively constant and changed in a consistent manner over time (59). In the human fetus, autopsy data and chemical analysis in 169 stillborns disclosed a relatively comparable rate of accretion of lean body mass in small for gestational age, average for gestational age, and large for gestational age fetuses but considerable variation in the accretion of fetal fat (60). Fat accretion in the small for gestational age fetuses was considerably less than in the average for gestational age fetuses, which in turn was less than that of the large for gestational age fetuses. The term human fetus at birth has the greatest percentage of body fat (approximately 12%) compared with other mammals (61). For these reasons, we have elected to assess fetal growth in our studies, using estimates of body composition. The methodologies we have employed include anthropometric, stable isotope, and total body electrical conductivity. These methods have been previously described (62–64).

The utility of using body composition in understanding fetal growth is exemplified by a previous study evaluating the proportion of the variance in birth weight explained by body composition analysis of the fetus, and particularly fat and fat free mass. The mean birth weight of the population was $3,553 \pm 462$ g and the mean percentage of body fat was $13.7 \pm 4.2\%$. Fat free mass, which accounted for approximately 86% of mean birth weight, accounted for 83% of the variance in birth weight. In contrast, body fat, which accounted for only approximately 14% of birth weight, explained 46% of the variance in birth weight (65).

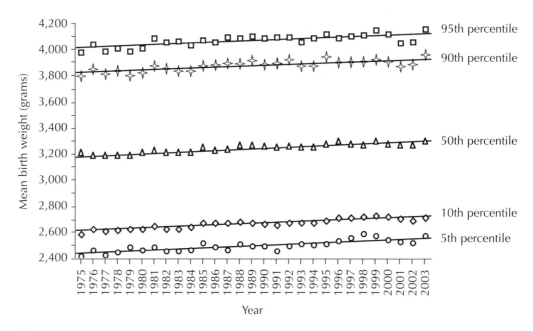

Fig. 8-3. Mean term singleton (37–41 weeks) birth weight in grams for the 5th, 10th, 50th, 90th, and 95th percentiles from 1975 to 2003 at Metro-Health Medical Center. (Catalano PM. Management of obesity in pregnancy. Obstet Gynecol 2007;109:419–33.)

In an effort to better understand the potential independent effect of maternal obesity on fetal growth in infants of women with normal glucose tolerance, we performed a stepwise logistic regression analysis of body composition on 220 infants of women with normal glucose tolerance (Table 8-2) previously published (66). Although maternal weight gain and height had the strongest correlations with birth weight and lean body mass, respectively, maternal pregravid weight had the strongest correlation with estimates of neonatal fat and percentage of body fat. Using the same data set, the increase in birth weights between infants of women with a BMI of 25 or greater, compared with those having a BMI of less than 25, was explained by an increase in fat mass rather than lean body mass (Table 8-3) (66). This was the case despite significantly less weight gain (13.8 ± 7.5 versus 15.2 ± 5.3 lb, $P = .001$) in the overweight–obese women compared with the lean–average weight women.

What is the relative contribution of maternal obesity and GDM to the risk of fetal overgrowth in the population? Ehrenberg et al (67) reported that the risk of having a larger than gestational age neonate was greatest for women with a history of diabetes (OR, 4.4) when compared with maternal obesity (OR, 1.6). However, there was a fourfold greater number of large for gestational age infants born of obese women than women with diabetes because the relative prevalence of overweight and obesity to diabetes was 47% and 5%, respectively. Therefore, at least in our population, maternal obesity and not diabetes

appears to be the more important factor contributing to the population's increase in mean birth weight.

Relative to obstetric management, again a decrease in maternal pregravid weight appears to be the most important factor relating to fetal overgrowth, defined as an increase in adipose tissue rather than lean body mass. However, limiting weight gain in obese women may prove beneficial in the decreased accretion of fat mass in the infants of overweight and obese women. In one study, weight gain in overweight and obese women (BMI of 25 or greater) had the strongest correlation with percentage of body fat ($r^2 = 0.13$, $P = .002$), whereas weight gain was not significantly related to fat mass in the lean and average weight women (66). However, optimal weight gain in average weight women, let alone obese women, has yet to be defined. Obviously, total caloric intake is importantly related to fetal growth, but so is the composition of the diet, ie, the percentage and types of fat as well as carbohydrate and protein. The other end of the energy equation, of course, is energy expenditure, ie, physical activity. A sedentary lifestyle only increases the tendency for weight gain. There are not enough evidence-based data, and it is beyond the scope of this review to speculate about the optimal diet in pregnancy for obese women. However, the problems related to maternal pregravid obesity and weight gain in pregnancy are not improving and will only worsen unless appropriate research studies and trials begin to address these issues because the consequences, as will be discussed, have far-reaching implications.

Table 8-2. Stepwise Regression Analysis of Factors Related to Body Composition of Neonates (n = 220) of Women With Normal Glucose Tolerance

	r^2	ΔDr^2	*P* Value
Birth weight			
Maternal pregravid weight	0.029	—	.01
Maternal weight gain	0.07	0.041	<0.001
Maternal age	0.098	0.028	<0.001
Lean body mass			
Maternal height	0.025	—	.02
Fat mass			
Maternal weight gain	0.044	—	.002
Pregravid weight	0.10	0.056	<.001
Percentage of body fat			
Maternal weight gain	0.031	—	.012
Maternal pregravid weight	0.073	0.042	<.001

Catalano PM. Management of obesity in pregnancy. Obstet Gynecol 2007;109:419-33.

Table 8-3. Neonatal Body Composition of Infants of Women With Pregravid Body Mass Index Less Than 25 Compared With Women With A Body Mass Index of 25 or More

	Pregravid Body Mass Index		
	Less Than 25 (n = 144)	25 or more (n = 76)	*P* Value
Birth weight (g)	3,284 ± 534	3,436 ± 567	.051
Body composition (TOBEC) lean body mass	2,951 ± 406	3,023 ± 410	.22
Fat mass (g)	331 ± 179	406 ± 221	.008
Body fat (%)	9.6 ± 4.3	11 ± 4.7	.006

Data are expressed as mean ± standard deviation.

Abbreviation: TOBEC, total body electrical conductivity.

Modified from Sewell, Huston-Presley L, Super DM, Catalano PM. Increased neonatal fat mass, and not lean body mass, is associated with maternal obesity. Am J Obstet Gynecol 2006;195:1100–3. Copyright © 2006, with permission from Elsevier.

Long-Term Risks for the Fetus of the Obese Mother

Although much has been written about the increased risk of the metabolic syndrome (obesity, hypertension, insulin resistance, and dyslipidemia) in infants born small for gestational age, recent evidence points toward an increase in adolescent and adult obesity in infants born either large for gestational age or macrosomic (68). There is abundant evidence linking higher birth weights to increased obesity in adolescents as well as adults for at least 25 years (69, 70). Large cohort studies such as the Nurses Health Study (71) and the Health Professional Follow-up Study (72) report a J-shaped curve (ie, a slightly greater BMI) among subjects born small but a much greater prevalence of overweight and obesity in those

born large (73). The increased prevalence of adolescent obesity is related to an increased risk of the metabolic syndrome. The increased incidence of obesity accounts for much of the 33% increase in type 2 diabetes, particularly among the young. Fifty to ninety percent of adolescents with type 2 diabetes have a BMI greater than 27 (74), and 25% of obese children 4–10 years of age have impaired glucose tolerance (75). Hence, the epidemic of obesity and subsequent risk of diabetes and components of the metabolic syndrome may begin in utero with fetal overgrowth and adiposity rather than undergrowth.

A recent retrospective cohort study in more than 8,400 children in the United States in the early 1990s reported that children who were born to obese mothers (based on BMI in the first trimester) were twice as likely to be obese by 2 years of age (76). If a woman had a BMI of 30 or more in the first trimester, the prevalence of childhood obesity (BMI greater than the 95th percentile based on CDC criteria) at ages 2, 3, and 4 years was 15.1%, 20.6%, and 24.1%, respectively. This was between 2.4 and 2.7 times the prevalence of obesity observed in children of mothers whose BMI was in the normal range (18.5–24.9). This effect was only slightly modified by birth weight.

There is an independent effect of maternal pregravid weight and diabetes not only on birth weight but also on the adolescent risk of obesity. In obese women with GDM whose glucose was well controlled on diet alone, the odds of fetal macrosomia (birth weight greater than 4,000 g) is significantly increased (OR, 2.12) compared with women with a well controlled (diet only) GDM with normal BMI (77). Similar results were reported in women with GDM whose condition was poorly controlled with diet or insulin. In well-controlled insulin-requiring GDM, there was no significant increased risk of macrosomia with increasing pregravid BMI. Additionally, the mean adolescent BMI has been reported to be 2.6 greater in sibling offspring of diabetic pregnancies compared with the index siblings born when the mother had previously had normal glucose tolerance (78). Hence, both maternal pregravid obesity and the presence of maternal diabetes may independently affect the risk of adolescent obesity in the offspring.

This risk of developing the metabolic syndrome in adolescents was recently addressed in a longitudinal cohort study of average for gestational age and large for gestational age infants of women with normal glucose tolerance and GDM (79). The metabolic syndrome was defined as the presence of two or more of the following components: obesity, hypertension, glucose intolerance, and dyslipidemia. Maternal obesity was defined as a pregravid BMI greater than 27.3. Children who were large for gestational age at birth had an increased hazard rate for metabolic syndrome (2.19; 95% CI, 1.25–3.82; $P = .01$) by 11 years of age, as did children of obese women (1.81; 95% CI, 1.03–3.19; $P = .04$). The presence of maternal GDM was not independently significant, but the risk of the development of metabolic syndrome was significantly different between large for gestational age and average for gestational age offspring of women with GDM by age 11 years (relative risk 3.6).

Summary

The primary objective in the management of obesity during pregnancy is prevention. Having obese women lose weight with lifestyle changes and achieve a normal BMI before conception would be the ideal goal, but realistically it is quite difficult to achieve. Once an obese woman does conceive, management should be directed at increased surveillance for these risks: 1) in early gestation, the risks of spontaneous abortion and congenital anomalies; 2) in later gestation, gestational hypertension and diabetes-related problems, as well as the increased risk of unexplained stillbirths; and 3) at parturition, the increased risk of cesarean delivery and attendant complications of anesthesia, wound disruption, infection, and deep vein thrombosis (Box 8-1). Limiting weight gain in pregnancy to IOM guidelines (currently under review) (5), and tight glucose control in women with GDM may improve maternal and neonatal outcomes. Therefore, prevention rather than treatment may offer the best hope of breaking the vicious cycle of obesity during pregnancy. Until we attain a better understanding of the underlying genetic predispositions, physiology, and mechanisms relating to maternal and fetoplacental interactions and how these, in turn, relate to fetal growth and development, all treatments must, by necessity, be empiric.

BOX 8-1

KEY MEDICAL AND OBSTETRIC COMPLICATIONS IN OBESE PREGNANT WOMEN

Early Pregnancy
- Spontaneous abortion
- Congenital anomalies—neural tube defects

Late Pregnancy
- Gestational hypertension or preeclampsia
- Gestational diabetes
- Preterm delivery—related to maternal medical and obstetric conditions?
- Intrauterine fetal demise

Peripartum
- Cesarean delivery—failed vaginal birth after cesarean delivery
- Operative morbidities
  —Anesthesia complications
  —Postpartum endometritis
  —Wound breakdown
  —Postpartum thrombophlebitis

Fetus or neonate
- Macrosomia
- Fetal obesity
- Childhood obesity

Catalano PM. Management of obesity in pregnancy. Obstet Gynecol 2007;109:419–33.

References

1. World Health Organization. Obesity: preventing and managing a global epidemic. World Health Organ Tech Rep Ser 2000;894:1–4.

2. Ogden CL, Flegal KM, Carroll MD, Johnson CL. Prevalence and trends in overweight among US children and adolescents. JAMA 2002;288:1728–32.

3. Obesity in pregnancy. ACOG Committee Opinion No. 315. American College of Obstetricians and Gynecologists. Obstet Gynecol 2005;106:671–5.

4. The role of the obstetrician–gynecologist in the assessment and management of obesity. ACOG Committee Opinion No. 319. American College of Obstetricians & Gynecologists. Obstet Gynecol 2005;106:895–9.

5. Institute of Medicine. Nutritional status and weight gain. In: Nutrition during pregnancy. Washington, DC: National Academies Press; 1990. p. 27–233.

6. Schieve LA, Cogswell ME, Scanlon KS. Maternal weight gain and preterm delivery: differential effects by body mass index. Epidemiology 1999;10:141–7.

7. Hytten FE. Weight gain in pregnancy. In: Hytten FE, Chamberlain G, editors. Clinical physiology in obstetrics. 2nd ed. Oxford: Blackwell Scientific Publications; 1990. p. 173–203.

8. Butte NF, Wong WW, Treuth MS, Ellis KJ, O'Brian Smith E. Energy requirements during pregnancy based on total energy expenditure and energy deposition. Am J Clin Nutr 2004;79:1078–87.

9. Ehrenberg HM, Huston-Presley L, Catalano PM. The influence of obesity and gestational diabetes mellitus on accretion and the distribution of adipose tissue in pregnancy. Am J Obstet Gynecol 2003;189:944–8.

10. Kinoshita T, Itoh M. Longitudinal variance of fat mass deposition during pregnancy evaluated by ultrasonography: the ratio of visceral fat to subcutaneous fat in the abdomen. Gynecol Obstet Invest 2006;61:115–8.

11. Lashen H, Fear K, Sturdee DW. Obesity is associated with increased first trimester and recurrent miscarriage: matched case-control study. Hum Reprod 2004;19:1644–6.

12. Fedorcsak P, Storeng R, Dale PO, Tanbo T, Abyholm T. Obesity is a risk factor for early pregnancy loss after IVF or ICSI. Acta Obstet Gynecol Scand 2000;79:43–8.

13. Waller DK, Mills JL, Simpson JL, Cunningham GC, Conley MR, Lassman ML, et al. Are obese women at higher risk for producing malformed offspring? Am J Obstet Gynecol 1994;170:541–8.

14. Cedergren MI, Kallen BA. Maternal obesity and infant heart defects. Obes Res 2003;11:1065–71.

15. Watkins ML, Rasmussen SA, Honeru MA, Botto LD, Moore CA. Maternal obesity and risk for birth defects. Pediatrics 2003;111:1152–8.

16. Mojtabai R. Body mass index and serum folate in childbearing women. Eur J Epidemiol 2004;19:1029–36.

17. Ray JG, Wyatt PR, Vermeulen MJ, Meir C, Cole DE. Greater maternal weight and the ongoing risk of neural tube defects after folic acid flour fortification. Obstet Gynecol 2005;105:261–5.

18. Wald N, Cuckle H, Boreham J, Terzian E, Redman C. The effect of maternal weight on maternal serum alpha-fetoprotein levels. Br J Obstet Gynecol 1981;88:1094–6.

19. Drugan A, Dvorin E, Johnson MP, Uhlmann WR, Evans MI. The inadequacy of the current correction for maternal weight in maternal serum alpha-fetoprotein interpretation. Obstet Gynecol 1989;74:698–701.

20. Wataganara T, Peter I, Messerlian GM, Borgatta L, Bianchi DW. Inverse correlation between maternal weight and second trimester circulating cell-free DNA levels. Obstet Gynecol 2004;104:545–50.

21. Wolfe HM, Sokol RJ, Martier SM, Zador IE. Maternal obesity: a potential source of error in sonographic prenatal diagnosis. Obstet Gynecol 1990;76:339–42.

22. Hendler I, Blackwell SC, Bujold E, Treadwell MC, Wolfe HM, Sokol RJ, et al. The impact of maternal obesity on mid trimester sonographic visualization of fetal cardiac and cranio-spinal structures. Int J Obstet Relat Metab Disord 2004;28:1607–11.

23. Hendler I, Blackwell SC, Treadwell MC, Bujold E, Sokol RJ, Sorokin Y. Does advanced ultrasound equipment improve the adequacy of ultrasound visualization of fetal cardiac structures in the obese gravid women? Am J Obstet Gynecol 2004;190:1616–20.

24. Sibai BM, Ewell M, Levine RJ, Klebanoff MA, Esterlitz J, Catalano PM, et al. Risk factors associated with subsequent preeclampsia in healthy nulliparous women. Am J Obstet Gynecol 1997;177:1003–10.

25. Weiss JL, Malone FD, Emig D, Ball RH, Nyberg DA, Comstock CH, et al. Obesity, obstetric complications and cesarean delivery rate: a population based screening study. Am J Obstet Gynecol 2004;190:1091–7.

26. Yogev Y, Xenakis EM, Langer O. The association between preeclampsia and the severity of gestational diabetes: the impact of glycemic control. Am J Obstet Gynecol 2004; 191:1655–60.

27. Crowther CA, Hiller JE, Moss JR, McPhee AJ, Jeffries WS, Robinson JS, et al. Effect of treatment of gestational diabetes on pregnancy outcomes. N Engl J Med 2005;352: 2477–86.

28. Rumbold AR, Crowther CA, Haslam RR, Dekker GA, Robinson JS; ACTS Study Group. Vitamins C and E and the risks of preeclampsia and perinatal complications. N Engl J Med 2006;354:1796–806.

29. Poston L, Briley AL, Seed PT, Kelly FJ, Shennan AH; the Vitamins in Pre-eclampsia (VIP) trial consortium. Vitamin C and Vitamin E in pregnant women at risk for pre-eclampsia (VIP Trial): randomized placebo controlled trial. Lancet 2006;367:1145–54.

30. Catalano PM, Ehrenberg HM. The short- and long-term implications of maternal obesity on the mother and her offspring. BJOG 2006;113:1126–33.

31. Utzschneider KM, Kahn SE. The role of insulin resistance in nonalcoholic fatty liver disease. J Clin Endocrinol Metab 2006;91:4753–61.

32. Schieve LA, Cogswell ME, Scanlon KS. Maternal weight gain and preterm delivery: differential effects of body mass index. Epidemiology 1999;10:141–7.

33. Schieve LA, Cogswell ME, Scanlon KS, Perry G, Ferre C, Blackmore-Prince C, et al. Prepregnancy body mass index and pregnancy weight gain: associations with preterm delivery. The NMIHS Collaborative Study Group. Obstet Gynecol 2000;96:194–200. 34. Huang DY, Usher RH, Kramer MS, Yang H, Morin L, Fretts RC. Determinants of unexplained antepartum fetal deaths. Obstet Gynecol 2000;95:215–21.

35. Ingardia CJ, Fischer JR. Pregnancy after jejunoileal bypass and SGA infant. Obstet Gynecol 1978;52:215–8.

36. Nohr EA, Bech BH, Davies MJ, Frydenberg M, Henriksen TB, Olsen J. Prepregnancy obesity and fetal death: a study within the Danish National Birth Cohort. Obstet Gynecol 2005;106:250–9.

37. Durnwald CP, Ehrenberg HM, Mercer BM. The impact of maternal obesity and weight gain on vaginal birth after cesarean section success. Am J Obstet Gynecol 2004;191:954–7.

38. Charles A, Domingo S, Goldfadden A, Fader J, Lampmann R, Mazzeo R. Small bowel ischemia after Roux-en-Y gastric bypass complicated by pregnancy: a case report. Am J Surg 2005;71:231–4.

39. Gurewitsch ED, Smith-Levitin M, Mack J. Pregnancy following gastric bypass surgery for morbid obesity. Obstet Gynecol 1996;88:658–61.

40. Knudsen LB, Kallen B. Intestinal bypass operation and pregnancy outcome. Acta Obstet Gynecol Scand 1986;65:831–4.

41. Sheiner E, Levy A, Silverberg D, Menes TS, Levy I, Katz M, et al. Pregnancy after bariatric surgery is not associated with adverse perinatal outcome. Am J Obstet Gynecol 2004;190:1335–40.

42. Erez O, Maymon E, Mazor M. Acute gastric ulcer perforation in a 35 weeks' nulliparous patient with gastric banding. Am J Obstet Gynecol 2004;191:1721–2.

43. Weiss HG, Nehoda H, Labeck B, Hourmont K, Marth C, Aigner F. Pregnancies after gastric banding. Obes Surg 2001;11:303–6.

44. Ramirez MM, Turrentine MA. Gastrointestinal hemorrhage during pregnancy in a patient with a history of vertical banded gastroplasty. Am J Obstet Gynecol 1995;173:1630–1.

45. Dixon JB, Dixon ME, O'Brien PE. Birth outcomes in obese women after laparoscopic adjustable gastric banding. Obstet Gynecol 2005;106:965–72.

46. Skull AJ, Slater GH, Duncombe JE, Fielding GA. Laparoscopic adjustable banding in pregnancy: safety, patient tolerance and effect on obesity-related pregnancy outcomes. Obes Surg 2004;14:230–5.

47. Surkan PJ, Hsieh CC, Johansson AL, Dickman PW, Cnattingius S. Reasons for increasing trends in large for gestational age births. Obstet Gynecol 2004;104:720–6.

48. Ananth CV, Wen SW. Trends in fetal growth among singleton gestations in the United States and Canada, 1985 through 1998. Semin Perinatol 2002;26:260–7.

49. Orskou J, Kesmodel U, Henriksen TB, Secher NJ. An increasing proportion of infants weigh more than 4000 grams at birth. Acta Obstet Gynecol Scand 2001;80:931–6.

50. Eastman NJ, Jackson E. Weight relationships in pregnancy. I. The bearing of maternal weight gain and pre-pregnancy weight on birth weight in full term pregnancies. Obstet Gynecol Surv 1968;23:1003–25.

51. Love EJ, Kinch RA. Factors influencing the birth weight in normal pregnancy. Am J Obstet Gynecol 1965;91:342–9.

52. Humphreys RC. An analysis of the maternal and foetal weight factors in normal pregnancy. J Obstet Gynecol Br Emp 1954;61:764–71.

53. Abrams BF, Laros RK. Prepregnancy weight, weight gain, and birth weight. Am J Obstet Gynecol 1986;154:503–9.

54. McKeown T, Gibson JR. Observations on all births (23,970) in Birmingham, 1947. II. Birth weight. Br J Soc Med 1951;5:98–112.

55. Thomson AM, Billewicz WZ, Hytten FE. The assessment of fetal growth. J Obstet Gynaecol Br Commonw 1968;75:903–16.

56. Morton NE. The inheritance of human birth weight. Ann Hum Genet 1955;20:125–34.

57. Walton A, Hammond S. Maternal effects on growth and conformation in Shire horse–Shetland pony crosses. Proc R Soc Lond B Biol Sci 1938;125B:311–35.

58. Klebanoff MA, Mednick BR, Schulsinger C, Secher NJ, Shiono PH. Father's effect on infant birth weight. Am J Obstet Gynecol 1998;178:1022–6.

59. Moulton CR. Age and chemical development in mammals. J Biol Chem 1923;57:79–97.

60. Sparks JW. Human intrauterine growth and nutrient accretion. Semin Perinatol 1984;8:74–93.

61. Girard J, Ferre P. Metabolic and hormonal changes around birth. In: Jones CT, editor. Biochemical development of the fetus and neonate. New York (NY): Elsevier Biomedical Press; 1982. p. 517.

62. Fiorotto ML, Klish WJ. Total body electrical conductivity measurements in the neonate. Clin Perinatol 1991;18:611–27.

63. Catalano PM, Thomas AJ, Avallone DA, Amini SB. Anthropometric estimation of neonatal body composition. Am J Obstet Gynecol 1995;173:1176–81.

64. Fiorotto ML, Cochran WJ, Runk RC, Sheng HP, Klish WJ. Total body electrical conductivity measurements: effects of body composition and geometry. Am J Physiol 1987;252:R798–800.

65. Catalano PM, Tyzbir ED, Allen SR, McBean JH, McAuliffe TL. Evaluation of fetal growth by estimation of body composition. Obstet Gynecol 1992;79:46–50.

66. Sewell MF, Huston-Presley L, Super DM, Catalano PM. Increased neonatal fat mass, and not lean body mass, is associated with maternal obesity. Am J Obstet Gynecol 2006;195:1100–3.

67. Ehrenberg HM, Mercer BM, Catalano PM. The influence of obesity and diabetes on the prevalence of macrosomia. Am J Obstet Gynecol 2004;191:964–8.

68. Oken E, Gillman MW. Fetal origins of obesity. Obes Res 2003;11:496–506.

69. Garn SM, Clark DC. Trends in fatness and the origins of obesity. Pediatrics 1976;57:443–56.

70. Garn SM, Cole PE, Bailey SM. Living together as a factor in family line resemblances. Hum Biol 1979;51:565–87.

71. Curhan GC, Cherton GM, Willet WC, Spiegelman D, Colditz GA, Manson JE, et al. Birth weight and adult hypertension and obesity in women. Circulation 1996;94:1310–15.

72. Curhan GC, Willett WC, Rimm EB, Spiegelman D, Ascherio AL, Stampfer MJ. Birth weight and adult hypertension, diabetes mellitus and obesity in U.S. men. Circulation 1996;94:3246–50.

73. Martorell R, Stein AD, Schroeder DG. Early nutrition and adiposity. J Nutr 2001;131:874S–80S.

74. Mokdad AH, Ford ES, Bowman BA, Nelson DE, Engelmau MM, Vinicor F, et al. Diabetes trends in the U.S. 1990–1998. Diabetes Care 2000;23:1278–83.

75. Sinha R, Fisch G, Teague B, Tamborlane WV, Banyas B, Allen K, et al. Prevalence of impaired glucose tolerance among children and adolescents with marked obesity [published erratum in N Engl J Med 2002;346:1756]. N Engl J Med 2002;346:802–10.

76. Whitaker RC. Predicting preschooler obesity at birth: the role of maternal obesity in early pregnancy. Pediatrics 2004;114:e29–36.

77. Langer O, Yogev Y, Xenakis EM, Brustman L. Overweight and obese in gestational diabetes: the impact on pregnancy outcome. Am J Obstet Gynecol 2005;192:1368–76.

78. Dabelea D, Hanson RL, Lindsay RS, Pettitt DJ, Imperatore G, Gabir MM, et al. Intrauterine exposure to diabetes conveys risks for type 2 diabetes and obesity: a study of discordant sibships. Diabetes 2000;49:2208–11.

79. Boney CM, Verma A, Tucker R, Vohr BR. Metabolic syndrome in childhood: association with birth weight, maternal obesity and gestational diabetes mellitus. Pediatrics 2005;115:e290–6.

CHAPTER 9

Management of Diabetes Mellitus Complicating Pregnancy

Steven G. Gabbe and Cornelia R. Graves

$\mathcal{D}$iabetes mellitus complicates the lives of millions of women in the United States and is observed in 3–5% of all pregnancies (1–2). Type 2 diabetes mellitus, the most common form of diabetes mellitus in this country, is characterized by onset later in life, peripheral insulin resistance, relative insulin deficiency, obesity, and vascular, renal, and neuropathic complications. The incidence of type 2 diabetes mellitus is increasing rapidly, related in part to increasing obesity in the U.S. population. More than one half of the women who develop gestational diabetes mellitus (GDM), which represents approximately 90% of all cases of diabetes complicating pregnancy, will develop type 2 diabetes mellitus later in life.

Type 1 diabetes mellitus occurs early in life, is characterized by an autoimmune process that destroys the insulin-producing cells of the pancreas and, therefore, must be treated with insulin replacement. Like type 2 diabetes mellitus, type 1 diabetes can result in serious or even life-threatening complications. Care of patients with type 1 diabetes mellitus, particularly in the presence of vasculopathy and nephropathy, is a significant challenge for the obstetrician and patient health care team.

When developing a plan of management for the patient with a medical complication of pregnancy, obstetricians must ask two important questions: 1) How will the pregnancy affect this medical condition? and 2) How will this medical disorder affect pregnancy outcome? Pregnancy is characterized by increased insulin resistance and reduced sensitivity to insulin action. These changes are largely a result of the placental production of human placental lactogen and progesterone. Other hormones that may contribute include prolactin and cortisol. Early in pregnancy, relatively higher levels of estrogen enhance insulin sensitivity and, when associated with nausea and vomiting, increase the risk for maternal hypoglycemia. Insulin resistance is most marked in the third trimester. It is at this time that GDM most often occurs, and the risk of ketoacidosis is greatest for patients with type 1 and type 2 diabetes mellitus.

Diabetes mellitus increases the risk of adverse outcomes of pregnancy. In women with type 1 diabetes mellitus that is poorly controlled at the time of conception and during the early weeks of gestation, the incidence of spontaneous abortion and major congenital malformations is increased (3). Glucose crosses the placenta by facilitated diffusion and, therefore, the concentration in maternal blood determines the level in the fetus. Insulin does not cross the placenta. In the second trimester, maternal hyperglycemia produces fetal hyperglycemia, causing stimulation of the fetal β cells and fetal hyperinsulinemia. Insulin is the major fetal growth hormone and produces excessive fetal growth particularly in fat, the most insulin-sensitive tissue. The fetus of a woman with poorly controlled type 1 diabetes mellitus is not only more likely to weigh more than 4,000 g but also to have a disproportionately large chest and shoulders, more than doubling the risk for shoulder dystocia at vaginal delivery (Fig. 9-1). These large fetuses also are at greater risk for intrauterine fetal death during the last 4–6 weeks of gestation (4). Hyperinsulinemia can contribute to a significantly higher rate of respiratory distress syndrome, thwarting attempts to reduce the risk of a stillborn fetus by elective early delivery. The rate of preeclampsia is doubled in pregnancies complicated by diabetes mellitus, especially when maternal nephropathy exists. In the setting of hypertension and nephropathy, the rate of fetal growth restriction is more than doubled (Fig. 9-1). For the infant, long-term adverse outcomes associated with intrauterine hyperglycemia and hyperinsulinemia include obesity and carbohydrate intolerance.

Gestational Diabetes Mellitus

Gestational diabetes mellitus has been defined as "carbohydrate intolerance of variable severity with onset or first recognition during pregnancy. The definition applies regardless of whether insulin is used for treatment or the condition persists after pregnancy. It does not exclude the possibility that unrecognized glucose intolerance may

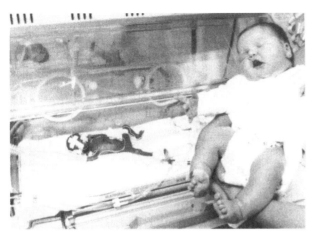

Fig. 9-1. Two extremes of growth abnormalities seen in infants of diabetic mothers. The small growth-restricted infant on the left weighed 470 grams and is the offspring of a woman with nephropathy, hypertension, and severe preeclampsia delivered at 28 weeks of gestation. The neonate on the right is the 5,100-gram baby of a woman with suboptimally controlled diabetes. (Reprinted from Landon MB, Catalano PM, Gabbe SG. Diabetes mellitus. In: Gabbe SG, Niebyl JR, Simpson JL, editors. Obstetrics: normal and problem pregnancies. Philadelphia (PA): Churchill Livingstone; 2002. p. 1099–100. Copyright © 2002 with permission from Elsevier, Inc.)

have antedated the pregnancy" (5). As obesity increases in this country and our population becomes more diverse, the rate of gestational diabetes mellitus will increase. Gestational diabetes mellitus complicates 2–5% of all pregnancies and is especially common in populations with a higher rate of type 2 diabetes mellitus, such as African Americans, Asian Americans, Hispanic Americans, and Native Americans (6). Gestational diabetes mellitus is characterized in most cases by postprandial hyperglycemia, resulting from impaired insulin release and an exaggeration of the insulin resistance seen in normal pregnancies. These patients can be treated with diet therapy and have not been found to be at increased risk for intrauterine fetal death. In contrast, when fasting glucose levels are elevated not only will insulin therapy be required but such hyperglycemia also places these women at greater risk for a stillbirth. Although there is controversy regarding which diagnostic standards to use for GDM, there is agreement that excellent blood glucose control, with diet and when necessary with insulin, will result in an improved perinatal outcome.

The identification of women with GDM is improved when an organized screening program is implemented. Should all patients be screened for GDM? Although the U.S. Preventive Services Task Force concludes that "...the evidence is insufficient to recommend for or against screening for gestational diabetes" (7), such screening is believed to be important for two reasons. First, identifi-

cation of women with GDM, followed by appropriate treatment and monitoring, will reduce fetal macrosomia and identify women who are at greater risk for fetal death. Second, given the likelihood that women who manifest GDM will develop type 2 diabetes mellitus, identification of these patients will permit interventions after delivery that might delay or prevent the onset of type 2 diabetes mellitus. Therefore, all pregnant women should be screened for GDM, starting with a complete medical history at the first prenatal visit.

The American Diabetes Association has proposed that women at low risk for GDM—that is, women who have all of the following characteristics: younger than 25 years, normal body weight, no first-degree relatives with diabetes mellitus, not a member of an ethnic group at increased risk for type 2 diabetes mellitus, no history of abnormal glucose metabolism, and no history of poor obstetric outcome—need not be screened (8). However, the difficulty in selecting these patients in a busy practice might make this approach impractical and, therefore, screening all women appears to be a better choice.

For most women, glucose screening should be conducted at 24–28 weeks of gestation, with use of a 50-g oral glucose load, without regard to the time of day or the time of the last meal (5). A venous plasma glucose measurement is taken 1 hour later, and a value of 140 mg/dL or greater necessitates a full diagnostic 100-g oral glucose tolerance test (GTT). Testing at this time not only enables the obstetrician to assess glucose tolerance in the presence of the insulin-resistant state of pregnancy but, should GDM be diagnosed, permits treatment to begin before excessive fetal growth has occurred. Using a cutoff of 140 mg/dL will detect 80–90% of women with GDM and will require that a GTT be performed in 15% of patients. Lowering the cutoff to 130 mg/dL will increase the sensitivity to nearly 100% but will require GTTs in nearly 25% of all patients (6). A value of 200 mg/dL on screening is so likely to be associated with the diagnosis of GDM that the GTT need not be performed, and treatment can be started.

Women who seem to be at high risk for GDM based on their own history of GDM, a strong family history of type 2 diabetes mellitus, or marked obesity should be tested as soon as possible (5). If the results of the initial screening are negative, the patient should be retested at 24–28 weeks of gestation. If a patient is found to have GDM before 20 weeks of gestation, she might have had diabetes mellitus antedating pregnancy. An elevated glycosylated hemoglobin level supports this conclusion and indicates that the fetus is at greater risk for major fetal malformations. Observed in approximately 2% of singleton pregnancies, glycosuria correlates poorly with blood glucose levels (9). However, women with repetitive glycosuria should be screened for GDM (10). As mentioned previously, an abnormal screening test result necessitates a 100-g oral GTT, performed after an overnight fast but with the patient consuming her usual unrestricted daily diet in the days preceding the test. A fasting plasma level is taken first, followed by samples at 1, 2, and 3 hours. If two or more values are met or exceeded, the diagnosis of GDM is established (Table 9-1). Most capillary glucose meters lack the precision needed for screening. If a meter is used, its precision should be known, and the relationship between venous blood samples taken simultaneously and capillary blood samples should be determined (6). Meters should not be used to diagnose GDM (11). Two sets of cutoff values currently are in use: 1) values proposed by the National Diabetes Data Group in 1979, and 2) a modification of these values by Carpenter and Coustan in 1982 (Table 9-1) (12, 13). The latter values have been endorsed by the American Diabetes Association (8). Use of these lower values will increase the number of GDM diagnoses from approximately 3% to 5% (14). However, research has demonstrated that this approach will identify women whose risk for perinatal morbidity, insulin treatment, and the subsequent development of type 2 diabetes mellitus is comparable to that of patients detected by the National Diabetes Data Group criteria. What should be done for patients who have a single abnormal value? Women with one abnormal value on the oral GTT have insulin resistance comparable to patients with GDM and are more likely to give birth to a macrosomic infant (15, 16). Although it has been recommended that these patients be treated as though they had GDM, it also is reasonable to repeat the oral GTT in 4 weeks.

Once the diagnosis of GDM has been established, the patient should be evaluated every 1–2 weeks until 36 weeks of gestation and then weekly thereafter. Dietary therapy is the key element in treating patients with GDM (17). The diet generally will consist of 2,000–2,200 calories per day and will emphasize the use of complex, high-fiber carbohydrates with the exclusion of concentrated

sweets. The caloric prescription is based on the patient's ideal prepregnancy body weight with 30 kcal/kg for the average patient, 35 kcal/kg for the underweight patient, and 25 kcal/kg for the obese patient. Some diets with a caloric content as low as 1,600–1,800 calories have been advocated for obese women in an effort to reduce weight gain and maternal hyperglycemia. If that approach is followed, the patient should be instructed to check her morning urine for ketones to determine whether the caloric content of the diet needs to be increased (8). Patients should be encouraged to exercise daily for 20–30 minutes per session. Brisk walking is ideal.

Once patients have started dietary therapy, it is important that capillary glucose levels be monitored to determine the efficacy of this treatment. Patients should check their fasting glucose and 1-hour or 2-hour postprandial glucose levels after each meal, for a total of four determinations each day. If, after several days of testing, the patient is maintaining good glucose control on this regimen, the frequency of monitoring may be decreased. If the fasting capillary glucose values are 95 mg/dL or more, the 1-hour values 130–140 mg/dL or more, or the 2-hour values 120 mg/dL or more, additional intervention will be required (5). First, the patient's diet and her adherence to this regimen should be reviewed. If the patient is adhering to her diet and if more than one half of her fasting or postprandial values or both are elevated, insulin therapy should be initiated. Most women can be instructed in the use of insulin. The starting insulin dose can be calculated based on the patient's weight; the recommended dose is 0.8 units/kg of actual body weight per day in the first trimester, 1 unit/kg/d in the second trimester, and 1.2 units/kg/d in the third trimester of pregnancy (18). The total dose is divided, with two thirds administered in the fasting state as two thirds insulin isophane suspension and one third rapid-acting insulin and the remaining one third of the total dose given as one half rapid acting insulin at dinner and one half at bedtime as insulin isophane suspension. Regular insulin or insulin lispro may be used. Appropriate increases in the insulin dosage are made on the basis of monitoring not only fasting glucose but also levels before and after each meal and at bedtime.

An alternative to insulin therapy is the oral hypoglycemic agent glyburide. This second-generation sulfonylurea does not cross the placenta. It has its onset of action in approximately 4 hours and has a duration of action of approximately 10 hours. In a study of 404 women, glyburide was found to be comparable to insulin in improving glucose control, with less than 10% of patients randomized to glyburide requiring insulin (19). Although there was no difference noted in maternal complications or neonatal outcomes, the rate of maternal hypoglycemia was significantly lower with glyburide

Table 9-1. Diagnosis of Gestational Diabetes Mellitus With 100-Gram Oral Glucose Load*

	National Diabetes Data Group (mg/dL)	Carpenter and Coustan Conversion (mg/dL)
Fasting	105	95
1 h	190	180
2 h	165	155
3 h	145	140

*Two or more of the venous plasma concentrations must be met or exceeded to establish the diagnosis of gestational diabetes mellitus.

use. In our experience, glyburide has become the first choice of our patients with GDM who require therapy beyond diet. We begin with a starting dose of 2.5 mg, twice daily, and increase the dose as necessary. Most patients will require, on average, 5 mg, twice daily. The maximum dose is 10 mg, twice daily. Studies of the pharmacodynamics of glyburide in pregnancy are currently being conducted, and results of these studies should assist us in prescribing doses.

Patients with GDM treated with diet are monitored until 40–41 weeks of gestation. At 40 weeks of gestation, they begin a program of fetal assessment with twice weekly nonstress tests (NSTs) (20). Patients with GDM who have had a stillborn fetus or have hypertension begin twice-weekly NST testing at 32 weeks of gestation. Clinical estimation of fetal size and ultrasound images are used to detect fetal macrosomia, most often reflected as accelerated growth of the fetal abdominal circumference. If the fetal weight is estimated to be 4,500 g or more, cesarean delivery should be considered to reduce the risk of shoulder dystocia. Of course, the patient's obstetric history and clinical pelvimetry are used when counseling the patient about the method of delivery (6). Patients who require insulin or glyburide as well as dietary therapy to maintain normoglycemia are observed with a program of antepartum fetal monitoring that is identical to that used for women with pregestational diabetes (twice-weekly NSTs). If the GDM is well controlled, these patients may be allowed to progress to their due dates. In patients with poorly controlled GDM, an elective delivery may be considered at 38–39 weeks of gestation. If delivery is scheduled before 39 weeks of gestation, amniocentesis is performed to assess fetal lung maturity. While in labor, patients with GDM who have been treated with insulin or glyburide should have their capillary glucose levels checked at the bedside every 1–2 hours. They will rarely require insulin therapy to maintain a glucose level of no more than 110 mg/dL. After birth, the infant of a patient with GDM should be observed closely for hypoglycemia, hypocalcemia, and hyperbilirubinemia. Breastfeeding should be encouraged.

It is essential that the patient be evaluated postpartum to determine whether she has returned to a state of normal carbohydrate tolerance. Obese women in whom GDM has been diagnosed early in gestation and have required insulin or glyburide therapy are most likely to have persistent glucose intolerance or diabetes mellitus (21). Approximately 15% of women who have had GDM will remain glucose intolerant or will demonstrate overt diabetes in the postpartum state. The American Diabetes Association recommends that a 75-g oral GTT, administered under the conditions described for the 100-g oral GTT, be performed 6–8 weeks after delivery (Table 9-2) (8). Patients also may continue to monitor their fasting and postprandial glucose levels. If these levels remain normal during the first 6 weeks postpartum, it is unlikely that the patient will have an abnormal GTT result. If the patient's postpartum GTT result is normal, she should be evaluated at no less than 3-year intervals with a fasting glucose test. Should the patient have glucose intolerance documented in the postpartum period, she should be treated with dietary therapy and exercise and be monitored annually. All patients who have had GDM should be encouraged to exercise and lose weight if they are obese, to reduce the likelihood of developing type 2 diabetes mellitus (22). They should be evaluated for glucose intolerance or diabetes mellitus before a subsequent pregnancy and treated, if necessary, to decrease the likelihood of having an infant with a major congenital malformation. Patients who have had GDM may use combination low-dose estrogen and progestogen oral contraceptives for family planning, without concerns that these medications will cause deterioration of carbohydrate tolerance.

Type 1 and Type 2 Diabetes Mellitus

Preconception Counseling

Major congenital anomalies are the leading cause of perinatal mortality in pregnancies complicated by diabetes mellitus, occurring in 6–12% of all infants (3). One study examined 835 consecutive infants of women with diabetes and compared them with 1,212 infants of women without diabetes (23). Fatal malformations and malformations involving more than one organ system were six times more frequent in the infants of women without

Table 9-2. Evaluation for Postpartum Carbohydrate Intolerance*

Normal	Impaired Fasting Glucose or Impaired Glucose Tolerance	Diabetes Mellitus
Fasting less than 100 mg/dL	100–125 mg/dL	Greater than or equal to 126 mg/dL
2 h less than 140 mg/dL	2 h greater than or equal to 140–199 mg/dL	2 h greater than or equal to 200 mg/dL

*Requires a 75-gram oral glucose load

diabetes. Poor glucose control during the critical weeks of organogenesis, 5–8 weeks after the last menstrual period, is thought to be the key etiologic factor (3). The glycosylated hemoglobin level, which reflects average glucose control over the preceding 2–3 months, can be closely correlated with the frequency of anomalies. One study demonstrated that when the glycosylated hemoglobin levels were no more than 8.5%, the fetal malformation rate was 3.4%. However, when the glycosylated hemoglobin level was greater than 9.5%, the rate of fetal malformations approached 22% (24). Complex cardiac defects, central nervous system anomalies such as anencephaly and spina bifida, and skeletal malformations, including sacral agenesis, are most common (Box 9-1) (Fig. 9-2) (23). Studies also have linked an increased rate of spontaneous abortion to poor preconception control (25). Most major anomalies can be detected by a targeted ultrasound examination, which includes a carefully performed assessment of fetal cardiac structure, including the great vessels at 18–20 weeks of gestation (26).

Both major malformations and spontaneous abortion can be reduced when prepregnancy and early postconception diabetic control are achieved. It is, therefore, imperative that patients with diabetes mellitus be encouraged to seek preconception care. However, in the United States, less than one third of women with diabetes mellitus receive preconception counseling. For a woman with diabetes mellitus, any visit to a health care provider should be an opportunity to review the patient's plans for pregnancy. The discussion should focus on obtaining glucose control and achieving a healthy lifestyle before conception. Glucose levels should be stabilized and a glycosylated hemoglobin level less than 1% above the normal range achieved (27). Angiotensin-converting enzyme inhibitors should be discontinued, and patients with type 2 diabetes who are using oral agents should be converted to insulin because they will invariably require insulin when they become pregnant. In addition, an evaluation for vasculopathy should be accomplished. Family planning also should be discussed (2). Low-dose combination oral contraceptives may be used by women without vasculopathy, whereas progestin-only formulations can be prescribed for women with vascular disease. Barrier methods, although less effective, will not affect glucose control or vascular disease. The intrauterine device can be used by multiparous women in a monogamous relationship. Sterilization should be considered for

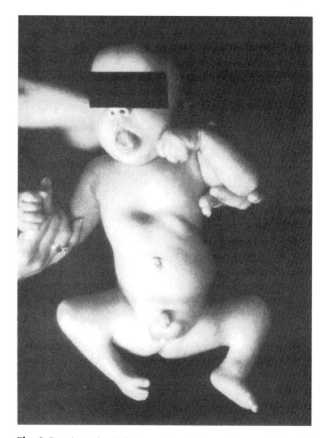

Fig. 9-2. Infant of a diabetic mother with sacral agenesis (caudal regression syndrome). The mother of this infant presented for her first prenatal visit at 26 weeks of gestation with previously undiagnosed nephropathy and poor glycemic control. Ultrasound examination revealed absent lower lumbar spine and sacrum and hypoplastic lower extremities. (Reprinted from Landon MB, Catalano PM, Gabbe SG. Diabetes mellitus. In: Gabbe SG, Niebyl JR, Simpson JL, editors. Obstetrics: normal and problem pregnancies. Philadelphia (PA): Churchill Livingstone; 2002. p. 1099–100. Copyright © 2002 with permission from Elsevier, Inc.)

BOX 9-1

CONGENITAL MALFORMATIONS IN INFANTS OF DIABETIC MOTHERS

Cardiovascular
- Atrial septal defect
- Ventricular septal defect
- Hypoplastic left heart
- Transposition of the great vessels
- Tetralogy of Fallot
- Truncus arteriosis

Central nervous system
- Anencephaly
- Encephalocele
- Meningomyelocele
- Holoprosencephaly

Skeletal
- Sacral agenesis

Genitourinary
- Renal agenesis
- Polycystic kidneys

women with serious vasculopathy or for those who have completed their families.

Retinopathy

Diabetic retinopathy, the leading cause of blindness in patients 24–64 years old, includes a wide spectrum of lesions: background retinopathy, including retinal microaneurysms and dot–blot hemorrhages; preproliferative changes, including cotton wool infarcts; and proliferative retinopathy with marked neovascularization. The presence and severity of retinopathy can be attributed to poor glycemic control. The rapid institution of strict glycemic control during pregnancy has been associated with short-term progression of retinopathy. Worsening of retinopathy also is more likely to occur in hypertensive patients (28). Few long-term studies have examined the effect of pregnancy on retinopathy. However, two reports have shown no difference in retinopathy between parous and nulliparous women (29, 30). These findings suggest that although pregnancy might accelerate the short-term progression of retinopathy, it has no long-term effect on the disease process. Active proliferative retinopathy might worsen in pregnancy and should ideally be controlled with laser therapy before conception. All patients should undergo screening with retinal examinations at their first prenatal visit. If retinopathy is present, then follow-up examinations during the pregnancy and postpartum are recommended.

Nephropathy

Diabetic nephropathy eventually will appear in 30–40% of patients with type 1 diabetes and is the most common cause of end-stage renal disease in the United States. Its prevalence during pregnancy has been estimated to range from 5% to 10% (31). There is an increased risk for maternal and fetal morbidity and perinatal mortality when pregnancies are complicated by nephropathy. Diabetic nephropathy significantly increases the risk of maternal hypertensive complications, including preeclampsia, preterm birth because of worsening maternal disease, and fetal growth restriction. Renal dysfunction as measured by decreased creatinine clearance and proteinuria is the best predictor of poor perinatal outcome. Although proteinuria will increase during gestation, most studies have failed to demonstrate a permanent worsening in pregnancy. However, in a small subset of women with advanced renal disease, those with a serum creatinine level exceeding 1.5 mg/dL, pregnancy might accelerate progression to end-stage renal disease (31). All patients with a history of microalbuminuria or those with diabetes for longer than 10 years should be screened for total protein and creatinine with a 24-hour urine collection before pregnancy or at the initial prenatal visit.

Coronary Artery Disease

Women with diabetes mellitus are at increased risk for coronary artery disease. Patients with long-standing disease who have developed hypertension and nephropathy are at the highest risk (32). The hemodynamic changes associated with pregnancy increase myocardial stress. Furthermore, epinephrine released in response to hypoglycemia might exacerbate the risk for myocardial injury. Coronary artery disease is a potential contraindication to pregnancy. These patients should undergo preconception counseling and be informed of these risks before attempting pregnancy. Baseline studies, including an electrocardiography and echocardiography, should be considered.

Other Maternal Complications

Diabetic neuropathy, either peripheral or autonomic, has not been well studied in pregnancy. However, nausea and vomiting, commonly seen during pregnancy, might be worsened in patients with gastroparesis (33). Peripheral neuropathy should be assessed at the preconception visit or early in gestation by a careful examination of the patient's feet for sensory loss. Instructions on safe foot care should be provided for all women with diabetes.

Management

The management of diabetes in pregnancy includes a careful combination of diet, exercise, and insulin therapy. During pregnancy in patients with a singleton fetus, caloric requirements are increased approximately 300 kcal above basal needs (17). New guidelines advocate the use of carbohydrate counting to increase dietary flexibility. Carbohydrate counting is extremely useful in pregnancy as long as one considers overall daily caloric intake to avoid excessive weight gain. For women with a normal body weight, the diet is usually 30–35 kcal/kg of actual weight, with an increase to 30–40 kcal/kg in women who are less than 90% of desirable body weight and 24 kcal/kg in those who are more than 120% of desirable body weight. Caloric composition includes 40–50% from complex, high-fiber carbohydrates, 20% from protein, and 30–40% from primarily unsaturated fats. The calories may be distributed 10–20% at breakfast, 20–30% at lunch, 30–40% at dinner, and 30% with snacks, especially a bedtime snack to reduce nocturnal hypoglycemia.

In the women with pregestational diabetes, insulin is the mainstay of therapy. Metformin has been used as a treatment for infertility in women with polycystic ovary disease. Although metformin is a category B drug, its use in pregnancy has not been well studied, and it is has been recommended that the drug be stopped once pregnancy has been established (34, 35).

Currently, most insulin used in the treatment of diabetes is biosynthetic human insulin. Insulin requirements will increase throughout pregnancy, most markedly in the period between 28 weeks and 32 weeks of gestation. As noted previously, insulin needs increase from 0.8 units/kg body weight per day in the first trimester, to 1 unit/kg/d in the second trimester, and 1.2 units/kg/d in the third trimester (18). Maintaining capillary glucose levels as close to normal as possible is the goal of therapy, including a fasting glucose level of no more than 95 mg/dL, premeal values of no more than 100 mg/dL, 1-hour postprandial levels of no more than 140 mg/dL, and 2-hour postprandial values of no more than 120 mg/dL (36). During the night, glucose levels should not decrease below 60 mg/dL. Mean capillary glucose levels should be maintained at an average of 100 mg/dL, with a glycosylated hemoglobin level no higher than 6%. The ability to achieve physiologic glucose control will depend on the patient's motivation, her ability to understand the complex interactions between diet, insulin, and exercise, the support she receives from the health care team, including the obstetrician or maternal–fetal medicine specialist, nutritionist, and teaching nurse, and her ability to recognize hypoglycemia.

Short- or rapid-acting insulins (prandial insulins) are administered before meals to reduce glucose elevations associated with eating and allow use of consumed fuels (37, 38). Longer-acting insulins are basal insulins, used to restrain hepatic glucose production between meals and in the fasting state (Table 9-3). The two most commonly used rapid-acting insulins are regular and insulin lispro. Although, insulin lispro may be used in place of regular insulin, they are not interchangeable. Regular insulin has its peak effect at 2–3 hours with a long duration of action, 4–6 hours, giving it features of a basal insulin. Regular insulin should be administered approximately 30 minutes before eating. Insulin lispro has its peak effect in 1–2 hours, with a duration of 4 hours. Because of its rapid onset of action, 15–20 minutes, it

should be given immediately before eating. Although its rapid onset of action improves compliance, insulin lispro can cause significant hypoglycemia in the unprepared patient. It also is more expensive than regular insulin. Patients who were treated with insulin lispro had lower predelivery glycosylated hemoglobin levels and a higher level of patient satisfaction (39). There has been some concern regarding the progression of diabetic retinopathy in patients who use insulin lispro. However, this has not been supported by recent studies (40).

Intermediate-acting insulin (insulin isophane suspension or insulin zinc suspension) has its peak effect in approximately 8 hours, with a duration of approximately 12–24 hours. This insulin usually is given before breakfast with a short-acting insulin and before the evening meal or at bedtime (Fig. 9-3). Bedtime dosing is preferred because an injection given with the evening meal might increase the risks of nocturnal hypoglycemia. Long-acting insulins include ultralente and glargine. Ultralente has an onset of action of 1–2 hours, with a peak at approximately 16–18 hours and may be administered once or twice daily. Its prolonged duration of action might make it difficult to determine the timing of its effect, especially if it is given twice daily. Glargine is a recently developed human insulin analog produced with recombinant deoxyribonucleic acid by the addition of two arginines to the C-terminus of the insulin β chain and replacement of asparagine with glycine at position 21 of the insulin α chain (41). This alteration delays insulin absorption and creates a basal insulin with no peak and a 24-hour duration. Experience with glargine use in pregnancy has been limited.

In patients who are highly insulin resistant, regular U-500 (concentrated) insulin might be valuable. Although it has a rapid onset, its duration of action is more like that of an intermediate-acting insulin. Regular U-500 insulin is recommended for patients who require more than 200 units of insulin per day. It can be given in three equally divided doses before breakfast, lunch, and

Table 9-3. Action Profile of Commonly Used Insulins

Insulin	Onset of Action	Peak of Action	Duration of Action
Lispro	1–15 min	1–2 h	4–5 h
Regular	30–60 min	2–4 h	6–8 h
Insulin isophane suspension	1–3 h	5–7 h	13–18 h
Insulin zinc suspension	1–3 h	4–8 h	13–20 h
Extended insulin zinc suspension	2–4 h	8–14 h	18–30 h
Glargine	1 h	No peak	24 h

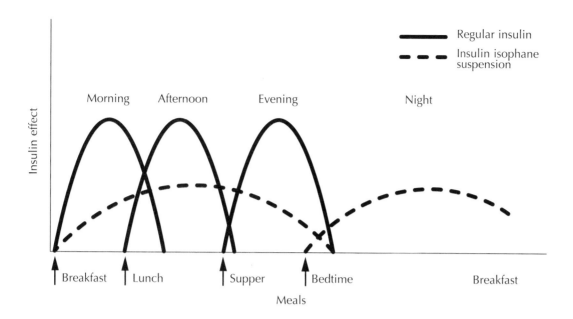

Fig. 9-3. A combination of rapid-acting and longer-acting insulins (regular insulin and insulin isophane suspension, respectively) is used to control maternal glucose levels. An injection of regular insulin is used with each meal. Insulin lispro also may be substituted. Insulin isophane suspension is administered to control glucose levels in the basal state between meals. The insulin isophane suspension dose in the morning is usually larger because this period is associated with a greater insulin resistance. Administration of the second injection of insulin isophane suspension at bedtime delays its peak effect until early morning and reduces the risk for nocturnal hypoglycemia.

dinner in conjunction with a dose of insulin isophane suspension at bedtime. Regular U-500 insulin is five times more concentrated than regular insulin. This must be emphasized to the patient.

Continuous subcutaneous insulin infusion therapy—the insulin pump—is used to deliver insulin in a pattern that closely resembles physiologic insulin secretion (37). A short-acting insulin, most often regular or insulin lispro, is used. Usually 50–60% of the total daily dose is administered as a continuous basal rate, with boluses before meals and snacks making up 40–50% of the total daily dose (Fig. 9-4). Patients who use an insulin pump must be highly motivated and compliant. The advantages of the pump include more lifestyle flexibility (making it ideal for physicians and nurses with diabetes), improved patient satisfaction, decreased severe hypoglycemia, and better control of early morning hyperglycemia caused by the "dawn phenomenon" (42). Disadvantages include the increased cost of the pump itself and pump supplies. In addition, should the administration of insulin be interrupted or impaired by a battery failure or infection at the infusion site, diabetic ketoacidosis might develop rapidly. A recent study has noted that women who initiate pump therapy during pregnancy are highly likely to continue with the pump after they give birth. They maintain better glucose con-

trol than do patients using multiple insulin injections (42).

Frequent capillary blood glucose monitoring is imperative to achieve euglycemia without significant hypoglycemia during pregnancy. A glucose meter with a memory should be used to check capillary glucose levels in the fasting state, before and after each meal, and before bedtime. Insulin and diet should be adjusted in response to trends of hyperglycemia or hypoglycemia. In selected patients, especially those using insulin pumps, determinations at 2:00–3:00 AM might help detect nocturnal hypoglycemia or pump failure. In general, insulin doses are changed, plus or minus 20%, in response to this information. It also is helpful to provide general guidelines on insulin use and carbohydrate intake; for example, 1) for most patients, 1 unit of rapid-acting insulin will decrease blood glucose 30 mg/dL, 2) 10 g of carbohydrate will increase blood glucose 30 mg/dL, and 3) one unit of rapid-acting insulin is enough for the consumption of 10 g of carbohydrate. A glycosylated hemoglobin test in each trimester of pregnancy will provide an overview of glucose control.

Even with meticulous monitoring, hypoglycemia is more frequent in pregnancy. An incidence of 71% for moderate hypoglycemia requiring assistance and 34% for severe hypoglycemia with loss of consciousness was

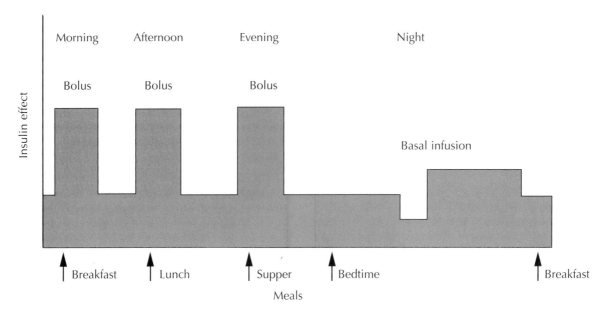

Fig. 9-4. Profile of insulin administration in a patient using an insulin pump. The basal infusion is maintained at a constant rate during most of the day but is lowered late in the evening and the hours after midnight to reduce the risk of nocturnal hypoglycemia. The basal infusion rate is increased in the early morning hours in response to the dawn phenomenon, which heightens insulin resistance. Boluses are administered with meals or snacks.

reported in one study (43). Intensively treated pregnant women with type 1 diabetes mellitus seem to have impaired counterregulatory responses to hypoglycemia, with diminished release of epinephrine and glucagon (44). Maternal glucose levels decrease more rapidly overnight because of placental and fetal glucose consumption while the mother is fasting. This "accelerated starvation" might further increase the risk for nocturnal hypoglycemia. In response to hypoglycemia, the patient and her health care team should carefully review her diet, insulin regimen, and exercise program. The patient and her family must be taught how to respond appropriately to hypoglycemia (eg, with a glass of milk for moderate hypoglycemia and glucagon for severe cases).

Antepartum Management

Antepartum fetal assessment has been proved to be a valuable approach to safely prolonging the pregnancies of women with type 1 and type 2 diabetes. The NST has become the most widely applied technique. In 1981, a stillborn fetus rate of 4% in patients with a reactive NST within 1 week of delivery was reported (45). In response to this study, twice weekly testing has been widely adopted. More recently, a biophysical profile (BPP) score of 8 out of 10 has been shown to be as reliable as a reactive NST in predicting fetal well-being. Daily fetal movement counting is a simple technique for antepartum assessment that also should be considered. In our institution, patients with type 1 and type 2 diabetes are moni-

tored twice weekly with an alternating BPP and NST beginning at 32 weeks of gestation. Doppler velocimetry of the umbilical artery might be useful in monitoring pregnancies with vascular complications and poor fetal growth (46).

The likelihood of an abnormal test result is increased in patients who have had poor glucose control or have vasculopathy with a growth-restricted fetus. If there is a combination of abnormal test results, such as decreased fetal movement, a nonreactive NST, and an abnormal BPP or contraction stress test, delivery should be considered. In a preterm gestation, an amniocentesis to assess fetal lung maturity might help in the decision-making process. In this setting, if corticosteroids are administered to accelerate lung maturation, an increased insulin requirement over the next 5 days should be anticipated, and the patient's glucose levels must be closely monitored (47).

Intrapartum and Postpartum Management

Optimal timing of delivery relies on careful balancing of the risks of intrauterine fetal death and excessive fetal growth if pregnancy is continued versus the risks of prematurity. If delivery is to be performed before 39 weeks of gestation, an amniocentesis is recommended to assess fetal lung maturity. The obstetrician should be familiar with the test used in his or her institution and how it has performed in the pregnancy complicated by diabetes because falsely mature test results might occur more frequently. Patients with well-controlled diabetes may be allowed to progress to their expected date of delivery with reassuring twice-weekly testing. To prevent traumatic birth injury, it is recommended that cesarean delivery be considered if the estimated fetal weight is greater than 4,500 g. During induction of labor, maternal glycemia can be controlled with an intravenous infusion of regular insulin titrated to maintain hourly readings of capillary blood glucose of less than 110 mg/dL. Five percent dextrose is recommended as the intravenous infusion. Avoiding maternal hyperglycemia intrapartum will prevent fetal hyperglycemia and reduce the likelihood of subsequent neonatal hypoglycemia.

Insulin requirements decrease rapidly after delivery. One half of the predelivery dose may be reinstituted before starting regular food intake (36). For patients who have cesarean deliveries, rapid-acting insulin may be used to treat glucose values greater than 140–150 mg/dL until a regular meal pattern has been established. Breastfeeding should be encouraged for women with type 1 and type 2 diabetes mellitus. Women with diabetes mellitus are as likely as women without diabetes mellitus to choose breastfeeding, recognizing that separation, should the newborn need to go to the neonatal intensive care unit, may make the initiation of breastfeeding more difficult (48, 49). It is important that caloric intake (30–32 kcal/kg) be maintained to support breastfeeding and avoid hypoglycemia (50).

Summary

Diabetes mellitus is one of the most common medical complications of pregnancy, affecting more than 200,000 women in the United States each year. Gestational diabetes mellitus represents approximately 90% of these cases and results from heightened insulin resistance during gestation. The detection of GDM requires a carefully developed plan for screening. Most women with GDM will respond to dietary therapy. The greatest perinatal risk in such cases is fetal macrosomia, which has been associated with a higher rate of cesarean delivery. Women with GDM are at considerable risk for the development of type 2 diabetes mellitus later in life and will require careful follow-up. Women with type 1 and type 2 diabetes mellitus are at greater risk for maternal morbidity and perinatal morbidity and mortality (Fig. 9-5). These risks are greatest in women who have poor glucose control and vasculopathy. When the patient has diabetic vasculopathy, the obstetrician, maternal–fetal medicine specialist, endocrinologist, and other members of the health care team must perform a challenging balancing act that promotes fetal health while minimizing maternal risk. The leading cause of perinatal mortality in pregnancies complicated by type 1 and type 2 diabetes mellitus is the major congenital malformation. These anomalies can be prevented by control of maternal glycemia before gestation and during the early weeks of pregnancy.

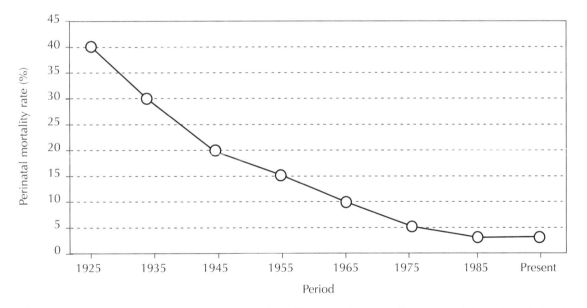

Fig. 9-5. Perinatal mortality rate in pregnancies complicated by type 1 diabetes mellitus. Perinatal deaths have declined dramatically since the discovery of insulin in 1921, a result of improved control of maternal glucose levels, advances in neonatal care, and reliable techniques for antepartum fetal monitoring, which have allowed safe prolongation of gestation and delivery at term. (Reprinted from Landon MB, Catalano PM, Gabbe SG. Diabetes mellitus. In: Gabbe SG, Niebyl JR, Simpson JL, editors. Obstetrics: Normal and problem pregnancies. Philadelphia (PA): Churchill Livingstone; 2002. p. 1099–100. Copyright © 2002 with permission from Elsevier, Inc.)

Currently, women with diabetes mellitus who receive comprehensive medical care can look forward to a pregnancy outcome similar to that of women without diabetes mellitus. Finally, the goal of our educational programs should be not only to improve pregnancy outcome but also to promote healthy lifestyle changes for the mother that will last long after delivery.

References

1. Engelgau MM, Herman WH, Smith PJ, German RR, Aubert RE. The epidemiology of diabetes and pregnancy in the U.S., 1988. Diabetes Care 1995;18(7):1029–33.

2. American Diabetes Association. Economic costs of diabetes in the U.S. in 2002. Diabetes Care 2003;26:917–32.

3. Kitzmiller JL, Buchanan TA, Kjos S, Combs CA, Ratner RE. Pre-conception care of diabetes, congenital malformations, and spontaneous abortions. Diabetes Care 1996;19: 514–40.

4. Lauenborg J, Mathiesen E, Ovesen P, Westergaard JG, Ekbom P, Molsted-Pedersen L, et al. Audit on stillbirths in women with pregestational type 1 diabetes. Diabetes Care 2003;26:1385–9.

5. Metzger BE, Coustan DR, and the Organizing Committee. Summary and recommendations of the 4th International Workshop Conference on gestational diabetes. Diabetes Care 1998;21(Suppl 2):B161–7.

6. Gestational diabetes. ACOG practice bulletin No. 30. American College of Obstetricians and Gynecologists 2001;98:525–538.

7. U.S. Preventive Services Task Force. Screening for gestational diabetes mellitus: Recommendations and rationale. Obstet Gynecol 2003;101(2):393–4.

8. American Diabetes Association. Gestational diabetes mellitus. Diabetes Care 2003;26(Suppl 1):S103–5.

9. Chen WW, Sese L, Tantakasen P, Tricomi V. Pregnancy associated with renal glucosuria. Obstet Gynecol 1976;47: 37–40.

10. Gordon MC. Maternal physiology in pregnancy. In: Gabbe SG, Niebyl JR, Simpson JL, editors. Obstetrics: Normal and problem pregnancies. Philadelphia (PA): Churchill Livingstone; 2002. p. 78.

11. Sacks DB, Bruno DE, Goldstein DE, Maclaren NK, McDonald JM, Parrott M. Guidelines and recommendations for laboratory analysis in the diagnosis and management of diabetes mellitus. Clin Chem 2002;48:436–72.

12. Eastman RC, Vinicor F, The Expert Committee on the Diagnosis and Classification of Diabetes Mellitus. Report of the expert committee on the diagnosis and classification of diabetes mellitus. Diabetes Care 1997;20:1183–97.

13. Carpenter MW, Coustan DR. Criteria for screening tests for gestational diabetes. Am J Obstet Gynecol 1982;144: 768–73.

14. Ferrara A, Hedderson MM, Quesenberry CP, Selby JV. Prevalence of gestational diabetes mellitus detected by the National Diabetes Data Group or the Carpenter and Coustan plasma glucose thresholds. Diabetes Care 2002; 25(9):1625–30.

15. Ergin T, Lembet A, Duran H, Kuscu E, Bagis T, Saygili E, et al. Does insulin secretion in patients with one abnormal glucose tolerance test value mimic gestational diabetes mellitus? Am J Obstet Gynecol 2002;186:204–9.

16. Langer O, Anyaegbunam A, Brustman L, Divon M. Management of women with one abnormal oral glucose tolerance test value reduces adverse pregnancy outcome. Am J Obstet Gynecol 1989;161:593–9.

17. American Diabetes Association. Evidence-based nutrition principles and recommendations for the treatment and prevention of diabetes and related complications. Diabetes Care 2003;26(Suppl 1):S51–61.

18. Langer O, Anyaebunam A, Brustman L. Pregestational diabetes: Insulin requirements throughout pregnancy. Am J Obstet Gynecol 1988;159:616–62.

19. Langer O, Conway DL, Berkus MD, Xenakis EMJ, Gonzales O. A comparison of glyburide and insulin in women with gestational diabetes mellitus. N Engl J Med 2000;343:1134–8.

20. Gabbe SG, Mestman JH, Freeman RK, Anderson GV, Lowensohn RI. Management and outcome of Class A diabetes mellitus. Am J Obstet Gynecol 1977;127:465–9.

21. Kjos SL, Buchanan TA, Greenspoon JS, Montoro M, Bernstein GS, Mestman JH. Gestational diabetes mellitus: The prevalence of glucose intolerance and diabetes mellitus in the first two months postpartum. Am J Obstet Gynecol 1990;163:93–8.

22. American Diabetes Association and National Institute of Diabetes, Digestive and Kidney Diseases. The prevention or delay of type 2 diabetes. Diabetes Care 2002;25(4):742–9.

23. Molsted-Pedersen L, Tygstrup I, Pederson J. Congenital malformations in newborn infants of diabetic women. Lancet 1964;i:1124–6.

24. Miller E, Hare JW, Cloherty JP, Dunn PJ, Gleason RE, Soeldner JS, et al. Elevated maternal hemoglobin A1c in early pregnancy and major congenital anomalies in infants of diabetic mothers. N Engl J Med 1981;304:1331–4.

25. Mills JL, Simpson JL, Driscoll SG, Jovanovic-Peterson L, Van Allen M, Aarons JH, et al. Diabetes in early pregnancy study: Incidence of spontaneous abortion among normal women and insulin-dependent diabetic women whose pregnancies were identified within 21 days of conception. N Engl J Med 1988;319:1617–23.

26. Albert TJ, Landon MB, Wheller JJ, Samuels P, Cheng RF, Gabbe SG. Prenatal detection of fetal anomalies in pregnancies complicated by insulin-dependent diabetes mellitus. Am J Obstet Gynecol 1996;174:1423–8.

27. American Diabetes Association. Preconception care of women with diabetes. Diabetes Care 2003;26(Suppl 1): S91–3.

28. Rosenn B, Miodovnik M, Kranias G, Khoury J, Combs CA, Mimouni F, et al. Progression of diabetic retinopathy in pregnancy: association with hypertension in pregnancy. Am J Obstet Gynecol 1992;166:1214–8.

29. Lovestam AM, Agardh CD, Aberg A, Agardh E. Pre-eclampsia is a potent risk factor for deterioration of retinopathy during pregnancy in type 1 diabetic patients. Diabetic Med 1997;14:1059–65.

30. Miodovnik M, Rosenn B, Berk M, Kranias G, Khoury J, Lipman M, et al. The effect of pregnancy on microvascular complications of insulin dependent diabetes (IDDM): A prospective study. Am J Obstet Gynecol 1998;178:S53.

31. Gordon M, Landon MB, Samuels P, Hissrich S, Gabbe SG. Perinatal outcome and long-term follow-up associated with modern management of diabetic nephropathy. Obstet Gynecol 1996;87:401–9.

32. Gordon MC, Landon MB, Boyle J, Stewart K, Gabbe SG. Coronary artery disease in insulin-dependent diabetes mellitus of pregnancy (Class H): A review of the literature. Obstet Gynecol Surv 1996;51:437–44.

33. Airaksinei KEJ, Anttila LM, Linnaluoto MK, Jouppila PI, Takkunen JT, Salmela PI. Autonomic influence on pregnancy outcome in IDDM. Diabetes Care 1990;13:756–61.

34. Harborne L, Fleming R, Lyall H, Norman J, Sattar N. Descriptive review of the evidence for the use of metformin in polycystic ovary syndrome. Lancet 2003;361: 1894–901.

35. Heard MJ, Pierce A, Carson SA, Buster JE. Pregnancies following use of metformin for ovulation induction in patients with polycystic ovary syndrome. Fertil Steril 2002;77:669–73.

36. Landon MB, Catalano PM, Gabbe SG. Diabetes mellitus. In: Gabbe SG, Niebyl JR, Simpson JL, editors. Obstetrics: Normal and problem pregnancies. Philadelphia (PA): Churchill Livingstone; 2002. p. 1099–100.

37. DeWitt DE, Hirsch IB. Outpatient insulin therapy in type 1 and type 2 diabetes mellitus. JAMA 2003;289(17):2254–64.

38. DeWitt DE, Dugdale DC. Using new insulin strategies in the outpatient treatment of diabetes. JAMA 2003;289(17): 2265–9.

39. Bhattacharyya A, Brown S, Hughes S, Vice PA. Insulin lispro and regular insulin in pregnancy. Q J Med 2001;94: 255–60.

40. Loukovaara S, Immonen I, Teramo KA, Kaaja R. Pro-gression of retinopathy during pregnancy in type 1 diabetic women treated with insulin lispro. Diabetes Care 2003; 26(4):1193–8.

41. Owens DR, Zinman B, Bolli GB. Insulins today and beyond. Lancet 2001;358:739–46.

42. Gabbe SG, Holing E, Temple P, Brown ZA. Benefits, risks, costs, and patient satisfaction associated with insulin pump therapy for the pregnancy complicated by type 1 diabetes mellitus. Am J Obstet Gynecol 2000;182:1283–91.

43. Rosenn BM, Miodovnik M, Holcberg G, Khoury JC, Siddiqi T. Hypoglycemia: the price of intensive insulin therapy for pregnant women with insulin dependent diabetes mellitus. Obstet Gynecol 1995;85:417–22.

44. Diamond MP, Reece EA, Caprio S, Jones TW, Amiel S, DeGennaro N, et al. Impairment of counterregulatory hormone responses to hypoglycemia in pregnant women with insulin-dependent diabetes mellitus. Am J Obstet Gynecol 1992;166:70–7.

45. Barrett JM, Salyer SL, Boehm F. The nonstress test: An evaluation of 1,000 patients. Am J Obstet Gynecol 1981; 141:153–8.

46. Landon MB, Langer O, Gabbe SG, Schick C, Brustman L. Fetal surveillance in pregnancies complicated by insulin dependent diabetes mellitus. Am J Obstet Gynecol 1992; 167:617–21.

47. Mathiesen ER, Christensen A-BL, Hellmuth E, Hornnes P, Stage E, Damm P. Insulin dose during glucocorticoid treatment for fetal lung maturation in diabetic pregnancy: Test of an algorithm. Acta Obstet Gynecol Scand 2002;81: 835–9.

48. Johnston M, Graves C, Arbogast PG, Cooper WO. Feeding attitudes of pregnant women with diabetes. Diabetes Care 2006;29(6)1457–8.

49. Ferris AM, Neubauer SH, Bendel RB, Green KW, Ingardia CJ, Reece EA. Perinatal lactation protocol and outcome in mothers with and without insulin-dependent diabetes mellitus. Am J Clin Nutr 1993;58:43–8.

50. Ferris AM, Dalidowitz CK, Ingardia CM, Reece EA, Fumia FD, Jensen RG, et al. Lactation outcome in insulin-dependent diabetic women. J Am Diet Assoc 1988;88(3):317–22.

PART III

OBSTETRIC COMPLICATIONS

CHAPTER 10

Intrauterine Growth Restriction

ROBERT RESNIK

*B*efore the early 1960s, it was assumed that a newborn with a birth weight less than 2,500 g was "premature." It was not until 1963 that obstetricians and pediatricians recognized that there exists a cohort of newborns who do not achieve their growth potential and that their failure to do so imparts a significant burden of an increased rate of perinatal mortality as well as short- and long-term childhood morbidity (1). One study demonstrated that for any given gestational age at birth, a weight below the 10th percentile increased the mortality risk dramatically (1). This distinction has more recently been brought into sharper focus by the observation that rates of perinatal morbidity and mortality increase markedly as birth weight decreases from the 10th to the first percentile (Fig. 10-1) (2). Overall, infants born between 38 weeks and 42 weeks of gestation whose weights are between 1,500 g and 2,500 g have perinatal morbidity and mortality rates 5–30 times that of infants whose weights are between the 10th percentile and the 90th percentile and substantially higher if the birth weight is less than 1,500 g (3). An infant with a weight of 1,250 g at 38–40 weeks of gestation has a greater perinatal mortality risk than one born of similar weight at 32 weeks of gestation.

Consequently, it becomes the challenge of the obstetrician to optimize the outcome of these at-risk infants by identifying when inadequate growth occurs, determining its cause and severity, counseling the parents, consulting with their neonatal colleagues, and selecting the appropriate time and mode of delivery.

Definitions and Standards

There has been considerable debate about what limits should be used to define the fetus or newborn that is small for gestational age (SGA). The most commonly used definition of SGA in the United States is a birth weight less than the 10th percentile for gestational age. However, it is important to emphasize that some SGA infants may be constitutionally small, part of the lower end of a normal distribution, and have none of the clini-

cal stigmata of the growth-restricted fetus that has not achieved its growth potential.

Additionally, numerous standard curves for fetal growth have been published, and it is well recognized that growth may be influenced by factors such as race, gender, socioeconomic environment, and altitude. For example, the Denver Intrauterine Growth Curves, widely used in the 1960s and 1970s, were obtained from a relatively small sample size (n = 5,635) of predominately white and Hispanic neonates born at altitude (1). In contrast, growth and weight curves derived from California birth data, U.S. national data using more than 4 million births, and fetal growth curves from Japanese and Chinese populations demonstrate disparate weight cutoffs at the 10th

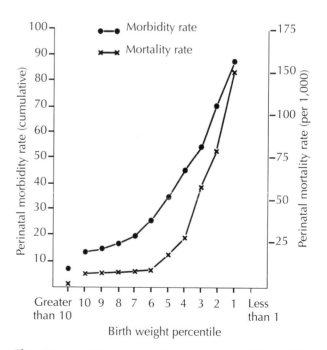

Fig. 10-1. Morbidity and mortality rates among 1,560 small for gestational age fetuses. (Manning FA. Intrauterine growth retardation. In: Manning FA, editor. Fetal medicine: Principles and practice. Norwalk (CT): Appleton and Lange; 1995. Copyright © 1995. Reproduced with permission of The McGraw-Hill Companies)

percentile (3–6). Consequently, it would seem prudent to use an individualized standard that takes into account both ethnic and geographical differences.

It also is important to recognize that a fetus may have a weight in the "normal" range (between the 10th percentile and the 90th percentile) but may not have achieved its true growth potential because of maternal illness or behaviors (eg, hypertension, smoking). It is not unusual for such neonates to have a birth weight appropriate for gestational age but manifest complications at birth similar to those observed in growth-restricted infants. In contrast, many infants have constitutional "smallness," have achieved their full growth potential, and are entirely normal (7).

It is helpful for the clinician to be cognizant of the normal variation in rates of growth across gestation. Fetal growth accelerates from approximately 5 g/d at 14–15 weeks of gestation to 10 g/d at 20 weeks of gestation, peaking at 30–35 g/d at 32–34 weeks of gestation, after which time growth rates decrease. The growth rates for normal singleton and multifetal pregnancies are shown in Figure 10-2 (3).

Pathophysiology

Intrauterine growth restriction (IUGR) is not a specific disease entity but rather a manifestation of many possible fetal and maternal disorders. Because clinical man-

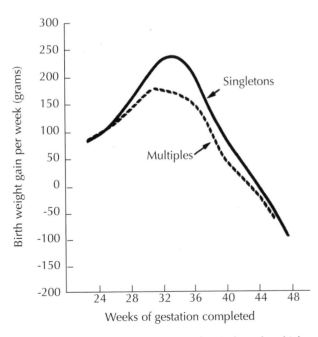

Fig. 10-2. Median growth rate curves for single and multiple births in California, 1970–1976. (RL Williams, RK Creasy, GC Cunningham, WE Hawes, FD Norris, M Tashiro. Fetal growth and perinatal viability in California. Obstet Gynecol 1982;59:624–32.)

agement, counseling, and ultimate outcome are largely dependent on the cause, it is important for the clinician to ascertain the specific cause of growth failure.

There is a strong association between IUGR, chromosomal disorders, and congenital malformations. Fetuses with chromosomal disorders, including trisomy 13, 18, and 21 are frequently growth restricted, and newborns with other autosomal abnormalities (various deletions and ring chromosome structure alterations) also have suboptimal growth. Although sex chromosome disorders are frequently lethal, fetuses that survive may be growth restricted at birth. The impact of aneuploidy on fetal growth is illustrated by the findings of a study that performed fetal blood karyotyping on 458 fetuses between 17 weeks and 39 weeks of gestation of women referred for the evaluation of IUGR (8). Eighty-nine fetuses (19%) had chromosomal defects, most commonly trisomy 18. Another study observed a 22% frequency of IUGR among 13,000 infants born with major structural malformations (9). Those abnormalities, most commonly associated with poor growth, were trisomy 18 and anencephaly.

Overall, chromosomal disorders and multifactorial congenital malformations are responsible for approximately 20% of the cases of IUGR in fetuses, and that percentage is substantially higher if growth failure is detected before 26 weeks of gestation or is associated with polyhydramnios. One study reported that among 39 fetuses with IUGR and polyhydramnios, 36 (92%) had major abnormalities and 15 (38%) had aneuploidy (10).

Maternal vascular disease, with an associated decrease in uteroplacental perfusion, is believed to account for 25–30% of all infants with IUGR. It is the most common cause of IUGR in the nonanomalous infant. Early onset, severe preeclampsia, and chronic hypertension with superimposed preeclampsia usually have the most profound effect on fetal growth. It is well established that these disorders are associated with the failure to augment plasma volume and have significant and specific placental pathology. The findings of one study comparing 370 preeclamptic pregnancies with normotensive pregnancies noted a 12% decrease in birth weight with severe disease and 23% with early onset disease (11).

The contribution of the thrombophilic disorders to IUGR is also under intensive investigation, and most current evidence derived from case–control studies suggests that the thrombophilia polymorphisms are not associated with intrauterine growth restriction (12–16). The antiphospholipid syndrome, an acquired coagulopathy caused by lupus anticoagulant and anticardiolipin antibodies, has been associated with a wide spectrum of pregnancy complications, including thromboembolic disease, abortion, late fetal loss, and preeclampsia, as well as IUGR.

Maternal nutritional abnormalities also may lead to poor fetal growth if substrate deprivation is severe. Birth weights of infants born during the Nazi occupation of Holland in World War II, when pregnant women were exposed to profound caloric restriction, were significantly lower than that of their siblings. Poor fetal growth also has been observed in pregnant women with incapacitating inflammatory bowel disease. Lower fetal weights also may result from a low prepregnancy weight or inadequate gain in asthenic women. It is uncommon to observe IUGR in heavier women (greater than 150 lb, prepregnant weight) whose pregnancies are otherwise normal.

The placentae of fetuses with IUGR frequently will be abnormal in size, function, or both. In one study, 1,569 chromosomally normal infants with IUGR were evaluated for placental weight, birth weight, and their ratio and compared with infants of normal weight. The infants with IUGR had a 24% smaller placenta when gestational age was used as a covariant (17). One study used electron microscopy to study anatomic placental morphology in the placentae of fetuses with IUGR that had absent umbilical end-diastolic flow. Researchers found significant abnormalities in the terminal villous compartment, which would serve to explain the vascular impedance observed clinically using laser-Doppler velocimetry (18). Also, IUGR has been reported with circumvallate placentae and those with chorioangiomas.

Fetal infections also may cause IUGR, although they are a less frequent cause and usually are related to a primary cytomegalovirus infection before 20 weeks of gestation. Fetal infections with rubella and parvovirus early in gestation also have been reported to impair fetal growth.

Maternal smoking has been known to decrease fetal weight by 135–300 g. A recent study of 170,254 pregnant women demonstrated a 2.4-fold increase in the risk of IUGR among smokers (19–20). Cessation of smoking during pregnancy appears to have a beneficial effect and may be the only current correctable cause of suboptimal fetal growth (21–22). Drugs such as cocaine, heroin, and alcohol as well as prescribed medications, including the anticonvulsants and the warfarin derivates, may influence fetal growth and development.

Multiple gestations are associated with both preterm delivery and IUGR. The growth curve of twins deviates from that of singletons after 32 weeks of gestation, and 15–30% of twin gestations may be growth restricted. This is more commonly observed in monochorionic twins with fetal transfusion syndrome, but discordant growth also may be observed in dichorionic twins, depending on the trophoblastic surface area available to each.

There has been considerable interest in the role of the assisted reproductive technologies and pregnancy outcome. Although assisted reproductive technology is associated with a number of pregnancy complications, it is not clear whether IUGR is observed more commonly, with one large study suggesting an increased risk and another suggesting no increased risk in singleton pregnancies (23, 24).

It is apparent that the causes of IUGR are varied, and the differential diagnosis requires ultrasound evaluation to delineate fetal anatomy in all cases. Depending on the maternal history and ultrasound findings, further diagnostic evaluation may require any or all of the following assessments:

* Fetal karyotyping
* Maternal serum studies for evidence of seroconversion when there is suspicion of viral infection, and specific amniotic fluid viral DNA testing when indicated
* Careful observation for early detection of preeclampsia
* Evaluation of the acquired thrombophilic disorders, particularly if a previous pregnancy was complicated by early and severe preeclampsia

A summary of risk factors for IUGR is shown in Table 10-1.

Diagnosis

Currently, ultrasound evaluation of the fetus is considered the standard approach for establishing a diagnosis of IUGR. It offers the advantages of reasonably precise estimates of fetal weight as well as the ability to follow interval growth and the pattern of growth abnormality (symmetric versus asymmetric). Reliability of the diagnosis requires knowledge of the gestational age, and it is helpful if the clinician has performed a crown–rump length measurement in the first trimester. However, it also is clear that the clinician first must have an index of suspicion that IUGR exists or may develop before further testing even is considered.

The clinical diagnosis of IUGR by physical examination alone is inaccurate, with the diagnosis being incorrectly made approximately 50% of the time. Tape measurement of the uterine fundus is helpful in documenting continued growth when performed by the same examiner but, because maternal habitus is highly variable, the classic hallmarks for gestational age are unreliable as are clinical estimates of fetal weight. Nevertheless, these indicators, combined with information obtained from maternal history and specific aspects of the patient's risk factors, may serve to initiate additional ultrasound evaluation. The appropriate ultrasound evaluation has been well standardized and is based on ample

Table 10-1. Risk Factors Associated With Fetal Intrauterine Growth Restriction

Fetal	Placental	Maternal
Chromosomal abnormalities	Small placenta	Extremes of malnutrition
Multifactorial congenital malformations	Circumvallate placenta	Vascular and renal disease
Multiple gestations	Chorioangiomata	Acquired thrombophilic disorder
Infection	Velamentous cord insertion	Smoking, drugs, and lifestyle
		High altitude or significant hypoxic disorder

clinical studies (19, 25–27). The following standard measurements should be obtained:

1. Fetal abdominal circumference
2. Head circumference
3. Biparietal diameter
4. Femur length

These parameters are converted to fetal weight estimates, using various published equations and formulae. The measurements for each morphologic parameter and computed weight are then plotted on a standard growth curve, which relates the measurements to gestational age at the appropriate percentiles. This information allows the clinician to determine when the actual weight is below the 10th percentile and to follow growth velocity at 2–4 week intervals. If the fetus is somewhat small but anatomically normal, with an appropriate amniotic fluid volume and growth rate, the outcome usually will be a normal, constitutionally small neonate.

It is of some clinical importance to distinguish between these two patterns of growth abnormality. Symmetrical growth restriction, characterized by smaller dimensions in skeletal and head size as well as abdominal circumference, has been considered to be indicative of an early intrinsic insult impairing fetal growth, such as chromosomal abnormalities and congenital malformations, exposure to drugs or other chemical agents, or infection. Growth is symmetrically impaired because the insult happens at a time when fetal growth occurs primarily by cell division. In contrast, asymmetric growth restriction is the consequence of extrinsic factors, usually resulting from the inadequate availability of substrates for fetal metabolism. In this pattern, the musculoskeletal dimensions and head circumference are spared, and the abdominal circumference is decreased because of subnormal liver size and a paucity of subcutaneous fat. Most commonly, the disorders that limit fetal metabolic substrate availability are maternal vascular disease and decreased uteroplacental perfusion. These generally present later in pregnancy at a time when fetal growth occurs primarily by an increase in cell size rather than cell number.

Because the causes of symmetric and asymmetric growth restriction are disparate, it is possible that distinguishing between them might provide useful information for diagnostic and counseling purposes. For example, a diagnosis of symmetric IUGR early in pregnancy suggests a poor prognosis when one considers the various causes. Conversely, asymmetric IUGR observed in the third trimester, particularly in conjunction with new onset maternal hypertension, carries a more optimistic prognosis with careful medical management. However, the clinician should exercise caution in interpreting these aberrant growth patterns because they may merge, as is the case of long-standing maternal vascular disease or severe nutritional disorders occurring early in pregnancy. Further, symmetric IUGR with a normal interval rate of growth may simply represent a constitutionally small and otherwise normal fetus.

The ultrasound examination also should include a careful analysis of amniotic fluid volume, fetal anatomy, and placentation. Although fluid volume is variable in pregnancies complicated by fetal aneuploidy and certain anomalies, it usually is diminished in asymmetric IUGR because of maternal disorders associated with decreased available substrates for metabolism (eg, maternal hypertensive diseases, small placenta, small twin with discordant growth). Conversely, the presence of normal fluid volume in a small fetus with normal growth velocity is most often indicative of a constitutionally small but normal fetus.

Management

Because fetuses with IUGR are at increased risk of hypoxia and metabolic acidosis during labor and death, it is necessary for the obstetrician to provide meticulous surveillance of fetal growth and well-being (28). The appropriate timing of delivery is determined by the gestational age and fetal condition. In some instances, the presence of fetal lung maturity in a preterm fetus will facilitate the decision.

Delivery may be indicated for fetuses with IUGR at term or near term, particularly if there is little or no growth observed over time or if the mother is hypertensive. When remote from term, management is more challenging, and different modalities have been used to monitor fetal well-being, including the biophysical profile (BPP), nonstress test, amniotic fluid volume measurement, and laser-Doppler velocimetry of fetal vessels.

The BPP is attractive because it provides an evaluation of multiple fetal physiologic parameters, is relatively easy to perform, and because fetal death within 1 week of a normal score is extremely rare (29). Its application in fetuses remote from term with IUGR may be less reliable inasmuch as the preterm fetus may have decreased fetal heart rate variability as well as a delay in well-defined behavioral states. Furthermore, although the number of fetuses studied and reported with the BPP is large, there is a paucity of evidence derived from prospective randomized trials (30). Observational studies have shown that IUGR pregnancies complicated by oligohydramnios, defined as a single vertical pocket less than 2 cm or an amniotic fluid index less than 6 cm, have a sharply increased risk of perinatal mortality. Conversely, normal amniotic fluid volume is less frequently associated with either IUGR or fetal demise, unless the cause is a congenital malformation or aneuploidy. The BPP, of which amniotic fluid volume measurement and the nonstress tests are components, remains a useful tool in the screening evaluation of well-being in the fetus with IUGR.

In the past few years, attention has been directed toward the evaluation of flow impedance through selected vessels in the fetal circulation by laser-Doppler velocimetry as an indicator of fetal condition. It is now well established, by numerous randomized trials, that the use of this modality can significantly reduce perinatal death as well as unnecessary induction of labor in the preterm fetus with IUGR (31). Although absence or reversal of end-diastolic flow in the umbilical artery is suggestive of poor fetal condition, normal or diminished umbilical flow (normal or elevated systolic/diastolic ratio) is rarely associated with significant morbidity. A large meta-analysis of randomized trials has shown that umbilical artery laser-Doppler velocimetry will reduce the risk of perinatal death in fetuses suspected of having IUGR and decrease unnecessary obstetric interventions (32, 33).

Moreover, the fetus with IUGR seems to be at even greater risk of imminent demise when abnormalities in the venous circulation (ductus venosus and umbilical vein) are observed with laser-Doppler velocimetry (34). Recently, one study has shown that abnormal flow through the ductus venosus (absence or reversal of atrial systolic flow velocity) and pulsatile flow through the umbilical vein may more accurately predict the risk of asphyxia and stillbirth in fetuses with severe IUGR with absent or reversed end-diastolic flow through the umbilical artery (35).

Findings and guidelines for the evaluation and management of IUGR are summarized in Table 10-2. Several reasonable conclusions regarding practical clinical management may be drawn from existing evidence:

- The term or near-term fetus with IUGR should be delivered if there is evidence of maternal hypertension; failure of apparent growth over a 2–4 week period; or a low BPP score (less than 6) or absence or reversal of flow revealed by umbilical arterial laser-Doppler velocimetry.
- If delivery is not elected or indication for delivery is not certain, the patient should undergo antenatal monitoring of fetal condition by BPP, umbilical laser-Doppler velocimetry, or both twice weekly. Evidence of fetal lung maturity by phospholipid analysis may provide sufficient reassurance to proceed with delivery in many instances.
- Remote from term, evidence of normal umbilical artery flow by laser-Doppler velocimetry is reassuring with regard to immediate neonatal outcome. However, absence or reversal of flow is an ominous finding, which frequently will indicate the need for delivery. Changes in the venous circulation, including evidence of flow aberrations in the ductus venosus or pulsatile umbilical venous flow, may help to more accurately define fetal condition when umbilical arterial abnormalities are observed.
- Intrapartum management requires detailed attention to fetal status because of increased risks of hypoxia. If oligohydramnios is present, the umbilical cord may be more vulnerable to compression. Although the specificity of an abnormal fetal heart rate tracing is low, a normal heart rate with adequate beat-to-beat variability and accelerations is indicative of normal fetal acid base status. Cesarean delivery should be performed early if there is any concern regarding fetal condition.

Treatment

There is a paucity of evidence from randomized trials that indicates that any specific antenatal treatment for fetuses with IUGR is beneficial. Numerous approaches have been used, including nutritional supplementation, plasma volume expansion, low-dose aspirin, and maternal oxygen therapy. None has consistently been shown to be of value, although one meta-analysis of the use of low-dose aspirin started early in pregnancy demonstrated a reduction in the risk of IUGR (36). Nutritional supplements such as vitamin C and vitamin E have not

Table 10-2. Evaluation and Management of Intrauterine Growth Restriction

	Constitutionally Small Fetus	Fetus With Structural or Chromosomal Abnormality or Fetal Infection	Substrate Deprivation or Uteroplacental Insufficiency
Growth rate and pattern	Usually below but parallel to normal, symmetric	Markedly below normal, symmetric	Variable, usually asymmetric
Anatomy	Normal	Usually abnormal	Normal
Amniotic fluid volume	Normal	Normal or hydramnios, decreased in the presence of renal agenesis or urethral obstruction	Low
Additional evaluation	None	Karyotype, specific testing for viral DNA in amniotic fluid as indicated	Fetal lung maturity testing as indicated
Additional laboratory evaluation of fetal well-being	Normal BPP, UAV findings	BPP variable, normal	BPP score decreases, UAV evidence of vascular resistance
Continued surveillance and timing of delivery	None, anticipate term delivery	Dependent on cause	BPP and UAV, delivery timing requires balance of gestational age and BPP and UAV findings, fetal lung maturity testing often helpful

Abbreviations: BPP, biophysical profile; UAV, umbilical artery velocimetry.

been shown to be effective in reducing the risk of IUGR (37). Short-term, maternal hyperoxia may improve fetal acid-base status at the time of delivery. Although the long-term use of maternal hyperoxia has been reported to lower the perinatal mortality rate compared with controls, the differences may be attributed to more advanced gestational age in the oxygen-treated group (38).

The efficacy of antenatal corticosteroids in the treatment of preterm fetuses with IUGR remains controversial, with two large studies showing conflicting results (39, 40). Until more information is available, it is reasonable to treat preterm fetuses with IUGR with antenatal steroids to decrease neonatal pulmonary and central nervous system morbidity.

Neonatal Complications and Long-Term Sequelae

Given the multiple causes of IUGR, it is not surprising that the outcomes of fetuses with IUGR will be varied and related to the specific cause of growth failure. Excluding those with aneuploidy, congenital malformations, and fetal infection, the remainder of fetuses may exist in a state of mild to moderate chronic oxygen and substrate deprivation, which may result in antepartum, intrapartum, or neonatal hypoxia and neonatal ischemic encephalopathy, meconium aspiration, polycythemia, hypoglycemia, and other metabolic abnormalities. Consequently, it is imperative to optimize the timing of

delivery, avoid progressive hypoxia during labor, and provide immediate skilled neonatal care.

Infants with IUGR have a higher risk of neonatal morbidity and mortality, particularly among those born very preterm (41, 42). With respect to long-term outcome, studies have shown outcomes ranging from normal to small decreases (which are statistically but not clinically significant) in intelligence quotients to a sharply increased risk of cerebral palsy (43, 44). One recent report suggested that IUGR has a negative impact on intellectual outcome even in the presence of catch-up growth (45). As might be anticipated, the worst outcomes have been observed in the more severely growth-restricted infants who are preterm and who exhibit the most overt evidence of impaired umbilical flow (46, 47). The prognosis for intact neurologic function is quite favorable in fetuses with IUGR when the cause is related to substrate deprivation, the timing of delivery is carefully selected, the fetus remains well oxygenated intrapartum, and the fetus receives skilled neonatal care.

References

1. Lubchenco LO, Hansman C, Boyd E. Intrauterine growth as estimated from live born birth-weight data at 24–42 weeks of gestation. Pediatrics 1963;32:793.

2. Manning FA. Intrauterine growth retardation. In: Manning FA, editors. Fetal medicine: Principles and practice. Norwalk (CT): Appleton and Lange; 1995.

3. Williams RL, Creasy RK, Cunningham GC, Hawes WE, Norris FD, Tashiro M. Fetal growth and perinatal viability in California. Obstet Gynecol 1982;59:624–32.

4. Zhang J, Bowes WA Jr. Birth-weight-for-gestational-age patterns by race, sex, and parity in the United States population. Obstet Gynecol 1995;86:200–8.

5. Shinozuka N, Masda H, Taketani Y. Standard values of fetal ultrasonographic biomtery. Japanese Journal of Medical Ultrasonics 1996;12:877–888.

6. Fok TF, Lam TK, Lee N, Chow CB, Au Yeung HC, Leung NK, et al. A prospective study on the intrauterine growth of Hong Kong Chinese babies. Biol Neonate 1987;51: 312–323.

7. Gardosi J. New definition of small for gestational age based upon fetal growth potential. Horm Res 2006;65 (suppl 3): 15–18.

8. Snijders RJM, Sherrod C, Gosden CM, Nicolaides KH. Fetal growth retardation: associated malformations and chromosome abnormalities. Am J Obstet Gynecol 1993; 168:547–55.

9. Khoury MJ, Erickson D, Cordero JE, McCarthy BJ. Congenital malformations and intrauterine growth retardation: a population study. Pediatrics 1988;82:83–90.

10. Sickler GK, Nyberg DA, Sohaey R, Luthy DA. Poly-hydramnios and fetal intrauterine growth restriction: ominous combination. J Ultrasound Med 1997;16:609–14.

11. Odegard RA, Vatten LJ, Nilsen ST, Salvesen KA, Austgulen R. Preeclampsia and fetal growth. Obstet Gynecol 2000; 96:950 –5.

12. Infante-Rivard C, Rivard GE, Yotov WV, Genin E, Guiguet M, Weinberg C, et al. Absence of association of thrombophilia polymorphisms with intrauterine growth restriction. N Eng J Med 2002;347:19–25.

13. Salomon O, Seligsohn U, Steinberg DM, Zalel Y, Lerner A, Rosenberg N, et al. The common prothrombotic factors in nulliparous women do not compromise blood flow in the feto-maternal circulation and are not associated with preeclampsia or intrauterine growth restriction. Am J Obstet Gynecol 2004;191:2002–2009.

14. Franchi F, Cetin I, Todros T, Antonazzo P, Nobile de Santis MS, Cardaropoli S, et al. Intrauterine growth restriction and genetic predisposition to thrombophilia. Haematologica 2004;89:444–449

15. Infante-Rivard C, Rivard GE, Guiguet M, Gauthier R. Thrombophilic polymorphisms and intrauterine growth restriction. Epidemiology 2005;16:281–287.

16. Dizon-Townson D, Miller C, Sibai B, Spong CY, Thom E, Wendel Jr G, et al. The relationship of the factor V Leiden mutation and pregnancy outcomes for the mother and fetus. Obstet Gynecol 2005;106:517–524.

17. Heinonen S, Taipale P, Saarikoski S. Weights of placentae from small-for-gestational age infants revisited. Placenta 2001;22:399–404.

18. Krebs C, Macara LM, Leiser R, Bowman AW, Greer IA, Kingdom JC. Intrauterine growth restriction with absent end-diastolic flow velocity in the umbilical artery is associated with maldevelopment of the placental terminal villous tree. Am J Obstet Gynecol 1996;175:1534–42.

19. American College of Obstetricians and Gynecologists. Intrauterine growth restriction. ACOG Practice Bulletin 12. Washington, DC: ACOG; 2000.

20. Hammoud AO, Bujold E, Sorokin Y, Schild C, Krapp M, Baumann P. Smoking in pregnancy revisited: findings from a large population-based study. Am J Obstet Gynecol 2005;192:1856–1862.

21. Malchodi CS, Oncken C, Dornelas EA, Caramanica L, Gregonis E, Curry SL. The effects of peer counseling on smoking cessation and reduction. Obstet Gynecol 2003; 101:504–510.

22. Bernstein IM, Mongeon JA, Badger GJ, Soloman L, Heil SH, Higgins ST. Maternal smoking and its association with birth weight. Obstet Gynecol 2005;106:986–991.

23. Jackson RA, Gibson KA, Wu YW, Croughan MS. Perinatal outcomes in singletons following in vitro fertilization: a meta-analysis. Obstet Gynecol 2004;103:551–563.

24. Shevell T, Malone FD, Vidaver J, Porter TF, Luthy DA, Comstock CH, et al. Assisted reproductive technology and pregnancy outcome. Obstet Gynecol 2005;106:1039–1045.

25. Harding K, Evans S, Newnham J. Screening for the small fetus: A study of the relative efficacies of ultrasound biometry and symphysiofundal height. Aust N Z J Obstet Gynaecol 1995;35:160–4.

26. Hadlock FB, Deter RL, Harrist RB, Park SK. Estimating fetal age: Computer-assisted analysis of multiple fetal growth parameters. Radiology 1984;152:497–501.

27. Warsof SL, Cooper DJ, Little D, Campbell R. Routine ultrasound screen for antenatal detection of intrauterine growth restriction. Obstet Gynecol 1986;67:33–9.

28. Low JA, Austin RW, Pancham SR. Fetal asphyxia during the antepartum period in intrauterine growth retarded infants. Am J Obstet Gynecol 1972;113:351.

29. Dayal AK, Manning FA, Berck DJ, Mussalli GM, Avila C, Harman CR, et al. Fetal death after normal biophysical profile score: An eighteen year experience. Am J Obstet Gynecol 1999;181:1231.

30. Alfirevic Z, Neilson JP. Biophysical profile for fetal assessment in high-risk pregnancies. Cochran Database Syst Rev 2000;2:CD00038.

31. Alfirevic Z, Neilson JP. Doppler ultrasonography in high-risk pregnancies: Systematic review with meta analysis. Am J Obstet Gynecol 1995;172:1379–87.

32. Ott WJ. Intrauterine growth restriction and Doppler ultrasonography. J Ultrasound Med 2000;19:661–5.

33. Westergaard HB, Langhoff-Roos J, Lingman G, Marsal K, Kreiner S. A critical appraisal of the use of umbilical artery Doppler ultrasound in high-risk pregnancies: use of meta-analyses in evidence-based obstetrics. Ultrasound Obstet Gynecol 2001;17:464.

34. Baschat AA, Harman CR. Antenatel assessment of the growth restricted fetus. Current Opinion Obstet Gynecol 2001;13:161–8.

35. Baschat AA, Gembruch U, Weiner CP, Harman CR. Qualitative venous Doppler waveform analysis improves prediction of critical perinatal outcomes in premature growth-restricted fetuses. Ultrasound Obstet Gynecol 2003;22:240–245.

36. Leitich H, Egarter C, Husslein P, Kaider A, Schemper M. A meta-analysis of low dose aspirin for the prevention of intrauterine growth retardation. Br J Obstet Gynecol 1997;104:450–459.

37. Rumbold AR, Crowther CA, Haslam RR, Dekker GA, Robinson JS. ACTS Study Group. N Engl J Med 2006;354: 1796–1806.

38. Gulmezoglu AM, Hofmeyr GJ. Maternal oxygen administration for suspected and impaired fetal growth. Cochran Database Syst Rev 2000;2:CD000137.

39. Elimian A, Verma U, Canterino J, Shah J, Visintainer P, Tejani N. Effectiveness of antenatal steroids in obstetrics subgroups. Obstet Gynecol 1999;93:174–9.

40. Schaap AH, Wolf H, Bruinse HW, Smolders-DeHaas H, Van Ertbruggen I, Treffers EE. Effects of antenatal corticosteroid administration on mortality and long-term morbidity in early preterm growth restricted infants. Obstet Gynecol 2001;97:954–60.

41. Bernstein IM, Horbar JD, Badger GJ, Ohlsson A, Golan A. Morbidity and mortality among very low birth weight infants with intrauterine growth restriction. The Vermont Oxford Network. Am J Obstet Gynecol 2000;182:198.

42. Simchen MJ, Beiner ME, Strauss-Liviathan N, Dulitzky M, Kuint J, Maschiach S, et al. Neonatal outcome and growth-restricted versus appropriately grown preterm infants. Am J Perinat 2000;17:187–92.

43. Paz I, Laor A, Gale R, Harlap S, Stevenson DK, Seidman DS. Term infants with fetal growth restriction are not at increased risk for low intelligence scores at age 17 years. J Pediat 2001;138:87–91.

44. Blair E, Stanley F. Intrauterine growth and spastic cerebral palsy. I. Association with birth weight for gestational age. Am J Obstet Gynecol 1990;162:229.

45. Puga B, Ferrandez LA, Garcia Romero R, Mayayo E, Labarta JL. Psychomotor and intellectual development of children born with intrauterine growth retardation (IUGR). J Pediatr Endocrinol Metab 2004;(suppl 3):445–450.

46. Wienerroither H, Steinder H, Tomaselli J, Lobendanz M, Thun-Hohenstein L. Intrauterine blood flow and long-term intellectual, neurologic and social development. Obstet Gynecol 2001;97:449–53.

47. Vossbeck S, deCamargo OK, Grab D, Bode H, Pohlandt F. Neonatal neuro developmental outcome in infants born before 30 weeks gestation with absent or reversed end-diastolic flow velocities in the umbilical artery. European J Pediat 2001;160:128–34.

CHAPTER 11

Fetal Death

Robert M. Silver

$\mathcal{P}$regnancy loss is one of the most common obstetric complications, affecting more than 30% of conceptions (1). Most of these occur early in gestation, are caused by problems with implantation, and may not be clinically apparent. However, 12–15% of conceptions result in clinically recognized pregnancy loss. Most of these losses are first trimester miscarriages, and fewer than 5% of pregnancies are lost after 10 weeks of gestation. These later losses (fetal deaths) are particularly emotionally devastating for families and clinicians, yet relatively little is known about second and third trimester pregnancy loss. This chapter will review the epidemiology, causes, management, and evaluation of fetal death.

Overview

Nomenclature of Pregnancy Loss

The terminology of pregnancy loss is confusing and could potentially benefit from revision. Historically, pregnancy losses before 20 weeks of gestation are referred to as abortions, whereas those after 20 weeks of gestation are termed fetal deaths or stillbirths. These definitions are somewhat arbitrary, inconsistent with advances in our understanding of reproductive biology, and not clinically helpful. Instead, it may be more useful to classify pregnancy losses in terms of stages of gestational development. Pregnancy losses could be defined in terms of developmental biology, as preembryonic (anembryonic), embryonic, or fetal. The expression "blighted ovum" should be abandoned and replaced with anembryonic or preembryonic pregnancy loss. The preembryonic period begins from conception and lasts through 5 weeks of gestation (based on menstrual dating). The embryonic period lasts from 6 weeks through 9 weeks of gestation. At 10 weeks of gestation, the fetal period begins, extending through delivery. Alternatively, losses less than 20 weeks of gestation could be described as early (eg, less than 10 weeks of gestation) compared with late (more than 10 weeks of gestation) abortions.

Increased specificity regarding the timing in gestation of pregnancy loss has important clinical implications. First, the causes of losses are different across gestational ages. For example, losses before the development of an embryo (anembryonic losses) are more likely to be associated with genetic problems than those later in gestation (2). In contrast, losses after 10 weeks of gestation are more strongly associated with disorders that may affect placental blood flow, such as antiphospholipid syndrome or heritable thrombophilias, when compared with early pregnancy losses (3, 4). The timing in gestation of pregnancy losses also has considerable influence on the recurrence risk and timing in gestation of subsequent losses (5). Too often, details regarding the timing in gestation of pregnancy losses are lacking, with patients and physicians simply reporting a "miscarriage" based on the interval between menses and the onset of vaginal bleeding. However, failure of growth or death of the conceptus often precedes clinical symptoms of miscarriage, sometimes by several weeks. Clinicians are strongly encouraged to document ultrasound findings, pathologic examinations, and other data pertinent to distinguishing among types of pregnancy losses.

Nomenclature regarding stillbirth also is controversial. The World Health Organization defines stillbirth as pregnancy lost after 20 completed weeks of gestation. If gestational age is unknown, a birth weight of 500 g or more is considered to be a stillbirth (6). However, others advocate the use of 24 weeks or 28 weeks of gestation to define stillbirth (7). The rationale behind the use of these latter definitions is to focus on fetal deaths after viability outside of the womb and is limited in clinical relevance by changes in the limit of viability over time and according to survival potential in different countries and regions.

A distinction also must be made between sporadic and recurrent early pregnancy loss and fetal death. Sporadic pregnancy loss is common in normal couples and is usually caused by de novo nondisjunctional events. Recurrent pregnancy loss is variably defined, most often as three or more losses with no more than one live birth. Up to 1% of couples suffer recurrent pregnancy loss. This is more common than would be expected by chance alone, suggesting that some couples have underlying conditions increasing the probability of pregnancy loss. Both with early miscarriage and fetal death, recurrent cases substantially increase the odds of an underlying predisposing medical or genetic condition. In turn, this influences the prognosis for subsequent pregnancies.

Epidemiology

The rate of stillbirth has decreased substantially from the 1950s (20 per 1,000 births) through the 1980s with improved care for conditions such as diabetes, red cell alloimmunization, and preeclampsia. However, stillbirth rates have been relatively stable over the past 20 years, reaching a plateau in the United States of approximately 6.4 per 1,000 births in 2002. In contrast, infant mortality has decreased by more than 30% in the last 20 years. In the United States in 2001, 26,373 fetal deaths were recorded compared with 27,568 infant deaths. Thus, fetal death currently accounts for approximately 50% of all perinatal deaths. As with other perinatal morbidity, there is considerable racial disparity in fetal death rates. In 2001, African Americans suffered a stillbirth rate of 12.1 per 1,000 births compared with 5.5 per 1,000 for whites.

Diagnosis

Fetal death may be associated with a cessation of previously perceived fetal movements or a decrease in pregnancy-related symptoms such as nausea. In some cases, women will present with bleeding, cramping, or labor. However, many patients with fetal death have no bleeding or contractions, and fetal death may precede clinical symptoms by a variable and often extended period of time. A definitive diagnosis is made by real-time ultrasonography confirming the presence of a fetus and the absence of fetal heart pulsations. If the ultrasonographer is inexperienced, the diagnosis should be confirmed by someone with appropriate expertise.

Classification of Fetal Death

It is often difficult to determine a "certain" cause of fetal death. First, many risk factors that are associated with fetal death in epidemiologic studies are present in numerous, apparently normal, women with uncomplicated pregnancies. Second, most studies of fetal death do not include controls, making it difficult to ascertain the contribution of a potential abnormality to the stillbirth. For example, heritable thrombophilias often are present in women who give birth to liveborn infants. Accordingly, a positive test result for thrombophilia in a case of fetal death, especially without evidence of placental insufficiency, does not prove causality. Third, several conditions may be present simultaneously. If a stillborn fetus with trisomy 13 has evidence of group B streptococcal infec-

tion, is the death caused by infection or fetal aneuploidy? Sometimes fetal death may be caused by the interaction or additive effect of two or more disorders. Even after an extensive evaluation, it may not be possible to determine a cause of fetal death. Such unexplained losses are common, especially in third trimester stillbirth.

There have been numerous attempts to catalog causes of fetal death, typically greater than 20 weeks of gestation, using classification systems. None has been universally accepted, and all have advantages and disadvantages. Further confusion arises from the use of different definitions of fetal death among systems and the inclusion of neonatal deaths in some but not all classification schemes. Popular classifications schemes include the Aberdeen clinicopathologic classification (8) and the Wigglesworth classification (9) scheme that is probably most commonly used today. Recently, a new system that substantially decreased the proportion of unexplained stillbirths compared with traditional classification schemes has been developed (10). However, this system ascribed a very large proportion (43%) of deaths to fetal growth restriction, which may be an association rather than a cause of fetal death. There is ongoing dialogue among investigators throughout the world to agree on a uniform system to facilitate comparison of fetal death rates and research into causes and prevention of fetal death.

It is important to distinguish between conditions that clearly and unequivocally cause fetal death and those that are associated with the condition. These latter conditions are present in many cases of live births and do not always cause the unavoidable death of the fetus. This distinction is not merely academic; it has important implications for clinical practice and counseling of couples with fetal death.

Risk Factors and Causes

Maternal Conditions

DEMOGRAPHICS

Consistent demographic factors for fetal death include race, low socioeconomic status, inadequate prenatal care, less education, and advanced maternal age (11, 12). African-American women have rates of fetal death that are more than twice the rate for white women. In part, this may be caused by secondary risk factors such as socioeconomic status and a lack of prenatal care. However, African Americans have higher fetal death rates than whites even among women receiving prenatal care (13). This may be because of higher rates of medical and obstetric complications in African Americans (13). It is unclear whether improved use of obstetric care would reduce the fetal death rate in African-American women, but it seems likely.

MATERNAL AGE

Increasing maternal age after 35 years is associated with an increased risk for fetal death (14). These findings have been confirmed in numerous studies, and the association persists when adjusting for potential confounding variables such as genetic problems, birth defects, medical problems, and maternal weight. A large inpatient-based study in the United States estimated the odds ratio for stillbirth to be 1.28 (95% confidence interval [CI], 1.24 –1.32) in women aged 35–39 years and 1.72 (95% CI, 1.6–1.81) in women aged 40 years or older compared with 20–34-year-old women (15).

OBESITY

The rate of fetal death also is increased in obese women. Numerous studies have shown a consistent doubling in the risk for fetal death in cases of maternal obesity (body mass index of 30 or more) (16). Increased body mass index increases the risk for several conditions known to increase the risk of stillbirth, such as diabetes, hypertensive disorders, including preeclampsia, socioeconomic status, and smoking. Nonetheless, obesity remains associated with fetal death after controlling for these confounders. The association between obesity and fetal death is of particular concern given the dramatic and persistent increase in the rate of maternal obesity.

MEDICAL DISORDERS

Several maternal medical disorders are associated with an increased risk for fetal death. It is debatable as to whether these conditions are causal or risk factors because most affected women give birth to liveborn infants. Perinatal outcome is influenced by obstetric management and decreased morbidity, and mortality from maternal diseases such as diabetes and hypertension are responsible for much of the improvement in fetal death rates over the past half century. It is estimated that maternal diseases play a role in 10% of fetal deaths.

Despite improved care, women with diabetes mellitus (type 1 and 2) have a 2.5-fold increase in the risk for fetal death (17). Conversely, true gestational diabetes (type 2 diabetes may be first recognized during pregnancy) is not associated with an increased risk for fetal death. In part, fetal death in diabetic women is caused by increased fetal anomalies and comorbid conditions such as high blood pressure and obesity. The increased risk of fetal death persists after controlling for these factors. Maternal hyperglycemia and disorders of fetal growth, metabolism, and possible acidosis contribute to fetal death, and treating women with diabetes mellitus with insulin during pregnancy decreases the risk (18).

Fetal death has been attributed to numerous other maternal diseases, including hypertension, thyroid disease, kidney disease, asthma, cardiovascular disease, and systemic lupus erythematosus. Pregnancy loss in the setting of these conditions typically occurs in women with clinically apparent and severe disease. Asymptomatic disease (such as mild glucose intolerance or abnormal thyroid function) has been proposed as a cause of fetal death. Although of interest, the theory remains unproved.

Antiphospholipid syndrome is an autoimmune disorder characterized by the presence of specified levels of antiphospholipid antibodies and one or more clinical features, including pregnancy loss, thrombosis, or autoimmune thrombocytopenia (19). The histologic findings of placental infarction, necrosis, and vascular thrombosis in some cases of pregnancy loss associated with antiphospholipid antibodies have led to the hypothesis that thrombosis in the uteroplacental circulation may lead to placental infarction and ultimately, pregnancy loss (Fig. 11-1). Numerous retrospective and prospective studies have linked recurrent pregnancy loss, especially fetal death, with antiphospholipid syndrome (3). The two best characterized antiphospholipid antibodies are lupus anticoagulant and anticardiolipin antibodies.

THROMBOPHILIAS

Fetal death also has been associated with heritable thrombophilias. These disorders typically involve deficiencies or abnormalities in anticoagulant proteins or an increase in procoagulant proteins, and like antiphospholipid syndrome, have been associated with a risk for vascular thrombosis and pregnancy loss. Several case series and retrospective studies reported an association between the factor V Leiden mutation (associated with abnormal factor V resistance to the anticoagulant effects of protein C), the G20210A mutation in the promoter of the prothrombin gene, deficiencies of the anticoagulant proteins antithrombin III, protein C, and protein S, and fetal death (19).

In most studies, thrombophilias are more strongly associated with losses after 10 weeks of gestation as opposed to early pregnancy losses. A recent meta-analysis indicated an odds ratio of 2 for "early" and 7.8 for "late" recurrent pregnancy loss for women with the factor V Leiden mutation, and an odds ratio of 2.6 for "early" recurrent fetal loss in those with the prothrombin gene mutation (4). Protein S deficiency, but not the methylenetetrahydrofolate mutation associated with hyperhomocysteinemia, protein C deficiency, or antithrombin III deficiency were associated with pregnancy loss in this meta-analysis (4). Fetal thrombophilias also have been

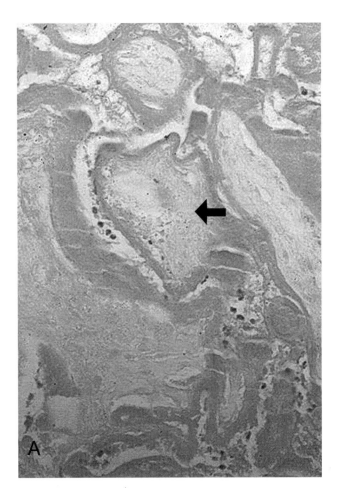
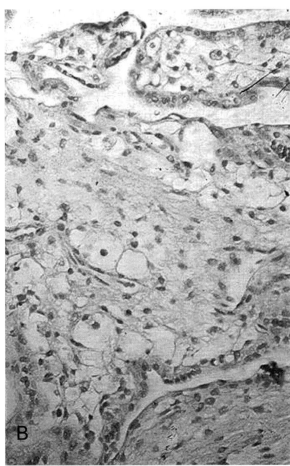

Fig. 11-1. A. Placenta demonstrating villous infarction (arrow) from a case of second-trimester fetal death in a patent with antiphospholipid syndrome (x 40, original magnification). **B.** Normal placenta is shown for comparison (x 100, original magnification). (Silver RM. Fetal death. Obstet Gynecol 2007;109:153–67.)

associated with fetal death but data are inconsistent and should be considered preliminary.

It is important to be careful when attributing fetal death to thrombophilias in women with positive test results. These conditions are extremely common in normal individuals (19), and prospective studies have failed to demonstrate an association between the factor V Leiden mutation and fetal death (or any adverse obstetric outcome) (20). Most pregnancies in women with heritable thrombophilias result in healthy infants, and women with thrombophilias but no prior obstetric complications should be reassured.

As with all potential causes, context is important. Thrombophilia is more likely to contribute to a fetal death if there is objective evidence of placental insufficiency such as intrauterine growth restriction (IUGR), placental infarction, or abnormal laser-Doppler velocimetry findings. It is less plausible as a cause of death in a term fetal demise weighing 8.5 pounds with normal amniotic fluid volume and a normal placenta.

EXPOSURES

Smoking is the most common exposure that has been associated with fetal death. Although most women who smoke give birth to live infants, numerous studies identify smoking as a risk factor for fetal death. The risk is typically 1.5-fold over nonsmokers; the risk decreases to background rate in women who stop smoking after the first trimester. The cause is uncertain but may involve an increase in fetal carboxyhemoglobin and vascular resistance, causing impaired growth and hypoxia. Smoking also increases the risk for potentially catastrophic conditions such as abruption.

Other recreational drugs have been associated with fetal death, although substance abuse is associated with many other risk factors. Cocaine has convincingly been associated with an increased risk for fetal death as well as abruption and IUGR. Although similar pathophysiology should apply to methamphetamines, it has not been linked to fetal death at present. Data regarding alcohol and fetal death are mixed; some studies show an association and some do not (21, 22). Marijuana has not been associated with fetal death. Abrupt narcotic withdrawal (eg, heroin) is another potential cause of fetal death.

Fetal exposure to medications and environmental toxins such as pesticides or radiation has been proposed as a risk for fetal death. This subject is of great interest to communities but is very hard to study. Exposures likely contribute to a very small proportion of fetal deaths.

SYSTEMIC MATERNAL INFECTIONS

Severe maternal infection with any type of organism may result in fetal death. Examples include appendicitis, pneumonia, pyelonephritis, and viruses such as influenza. The pathophysiology of fetal loss may include hypoxia caused by respiratory distress, poor uterine perfusion related to factors such as sepsis and dehydration, the metabolic effects of high fever, and the initiation of a cascade of toxic inflammatory mediators. Systemic infection (as well as intraamniotic infection) also may lead to fetal death by initiating preterm labor, resulting in intrapartum death, especially at previable gestations.

Fetal Conditions

GENETIC CONDITIONS

The best studied genetic cause of fetal death is chromosomal abnormalities (Fig. 11-2). These have been reported in 6–12% of stillbirths. The proportion is higher in first-trimester losses and is likely intermediate for losses

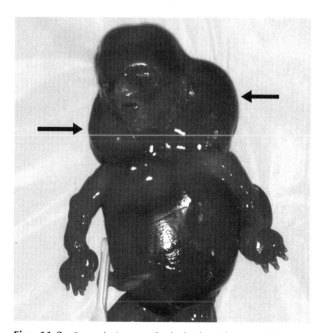

Fig. 11-2. Second-trimester fetal death with cystic hygroma (arrows) and nonimmune hydrops. The fetus had Turner's Syndrome. (Copyright © 1994, J. L. B. Byrne. Used with permission.)

between 10 weeks and 20 weeks of gestation (2). These numbers may underestimate the true percentage because karyotype is not always assessed or successfully obtained in all cases of fetal death. The chances of fetal aneuploidy are increased in the setting of fetal abnormalities noted on the antenatal ultrasonogram or postmortem examination (up to 25%) and if the fetus is small for gestational age (SGA). Conversely, karyotype is more likely to be normal in the absence of these findings. The most common abnormalities are monosomy X (23%), trisomy 21 (23%), trisomy 18 (21%), and trisomy 13 (8%) (23).

Many fetal deaths have genetic abnormalities that are not detected by conventional cytogenetic analysis. Malformations, deformations, syndromes, or dysplasias have been reported in up to 35% of fetal losses undergoing perinatal autopsy (23, 24). Although up to 25% of these fetuses are aneuploid, most will have normal karyotypes. However, it is probable that many of these fetuses have genetic abnormalities that are not identified by traditional cytogenetic analysis.

Genetic abnormalities may contribute to fetal death in cases without obvious malformations. Single gene disorders such as autosomal recessive conditions, including glycogen storage diseases, other metabolic disorders, and hemoglobinopathies, may cause fetal death. X-linked conditions may cause death in male fetuses. There are likely a host of other single gene disorders that contribute to some cases of fetal death, especially early in gestation. Supporting evidence comes from experiments in transgenic mice wherein single gene mutations cause embryonic death. Typically, mice with these mutations suffer abnormal angiogenesis, placental, cardiac, or neurologic development and die at mid gestation.

Other types of genetic abnormalities also contribute to some cases of fetal death. Confined placental mosaicism refers to the presence of abnormal chromosomes in some placental tissue in the setting of normal fetal karyotype. This leads to abnormal placental development and function and has been associated with fetal death and other obstetric abnormalities such as IUGR. Other fetal deaths may have very small deletions or additions of chromosomes that are too small to detect by conventional karyotype. This type of abnormality has been found in some cases of unexplained mental retardation. Newer molecular genetic techniques such as comparative genomic hybridization may allow detection of such "microdeletions."

The identification of genetic causes of fetal death has been somewhat hampered by the fact that there are few syndromes or mutations that account for a large proportion of losses. Instead, many different abnormalities each contribute to a small proportion of cases. Recent developments in molecular genetic technology should greatly facilitate our ability to determine previously unrecognized genetic conditions associated with fetal death.

INFECTION

Infections have been reported to account for 10–25% of fetal deaths in developed countries (25). The proportion is higher in developing countries. In addition to the population studied, the percentage of losses caused by infection is influenced by gestational age and the thoroughness (or lack) of investigation into infectious causes of fetal death. For example, in developed countries, bacterial infections are more common in fetal deaths before 28 weeks of gestation than later in pregnancy.

As with all causes of fetal death, it is important to distinguish causality from association. One may be confident (although not 100% certain) that infection is the cause of death in cases of positive cultures and histologic evidence of inflammation and infection in fetal tissues. It is a different story when there are positive placental or vaginal cultures or maternal serology without histologic evidence of fetal infection.

VIRAL INFECTION

The proportion of fetal deaths caused by viruses is uncertain because of a lack of systematic evaluation. This is especially important for viral infections because they are often hard to culture. Perhaps the most common viral infection associated with pregnancy loss is parvovirus B19 (Fig. 11-3). The virus is thought to cause fetal death through fetal anemia leading to hydrops, direct myocardial toxicity, or other mechanisms. This organism has been reported in 7.5% of fetal deaths in a Swedish study that used polymerase chain reaction to determine infection (26). The proportion of fetal deaths associated with parvovirus has been reported to be as high as 15% when polymerase chain reaction is used to detect parvovirus B19, but is considerably lower (less than 1%) in studies that did not systematically assess for the virus (25). Parvovirus B19 is more likely to cause fetal death in the first or second trimester; deaths late in gestation are rarely caused by the virus.

The most common fetal or neonatal viral infection is cytomegalovirus. Most fetal infections occur after primary maternal infection—which occurs in about 1% of women in the United States. Placental and fetal infection with cytomegalovirus is well documented, as are adverse neonatal sequelae such as IUGR and damage to organ systems, including the brain. Fetal death is rare but has been described.

Coxsackie viruses (A and B) also have been reported to cause fetal death. The organism can cause placental inflammation, myocarditis, and hydrops. Other viruses sporadically linked to fetal death include echoviruses, enteroviruses, chickenpox, measles, rubella, and mumps.

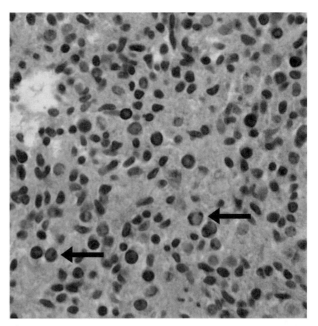

Fig. 11-3. Fetal spleen from a case of parvovirus B19–associated fetal death in the second trimester. Erythroblasts show marginated chromatin and typical amphophilic intra-nuclear inclusions (arrows). Hematoxylin and eosin stain (x 1,000, original magnification). (Copyright © 1994, J. L. B. Byrne. Used with permission.)

For those viruses amenable to vaccine prevention, fetal death is rare in countries with routine vaccination. Human immunodeficiency virus (HIV) may cross the placenta and cause fetal infection. Although fetal death has occasionally been attributed to HIV, HIV-positive women usually have other risk factors for fetal death, making it difficult to document an independent association. Herpes simplex virus rarely causes fetal death because it is rarely transmitted to the fetus in utero.

BACTERIAL INFECTION

Bacterial infections are generally accepted as a cause of some cases of fetal death throughout gestation. In developed countries, a higher proportion of losses in the second trimester are caused by infection compared with term fetal deaths (25). In contrast, fetal deaths caused by bacterial infection persist through term in developing countries. This may be because of increased burden of exposure to infectious agents or a decreased immune response associated with low socioeconomic status in developing nations (25).

Most bacterial infections associated with fetal death are organisms that reach the fetus by ascending from the lower genital tract into the decidua and chorion and occasionally the amniotic fluid. The fetus may then swallow fluid, leading to fetal infection. Examples include Group B Streptococcus, *Escherichia coli, Klebsiella, Ureaplasma urealyticum, Mycoplasma hominis,* and

Bacteroides. Virulent organisms (eg, group B Streptococci) may be associated with clinical evidence of intra-amniotic infection, whereas those responsible for bacterial vaginosis (eg, *Mycoplasma* and *Ureaplasma*) often do not cause clinically apparent disease. Bacteria such as *Listeria monocytogenes* may reach the fetus by hematogenous transmission.

OTHER INFECTIONS

Spirochete, protozoal, and fungal infections may occasionally cause fetal death. *Treponema pallidum*, the organism responsible for syphilis, may cross the placenta in the second and third trimesters and directly infect the fetus. This risk increases with advancing gestation. Fetal death may occur because of direct infection or because of placental vasculopathy associated with placental infection. Syphilis was a common cause of fetal death at the beginning of the twentieth century. Today, syphilis remains a rare cause of fetal death in developed countries and a common one in places with higher prevalence, such as Africa. Other spirochetes that may cause fetal death include *Borrelia burgdorferi*, which causes Lyme disease, Leptospirosis, and African tick-borne relapsing fever.

The parasite *Toxoplasma gondii* may cross the placenta in association with acute maternal infection. The organism may directly infect the fetus and has been linked to sporadic fetal death, which may occur in up to 5% of pregnancies after first trimester infection. However, the rate of primary infection is about 1 per 1,000 in the United States, making it unlikely to cause a substantial proportion of fetal death in the United States (25). Other infectious diseases that have been associated with sporadic fetal death include malaria and Q fever. The relative importance of all of these infections is influenced by the local prevalence of the infectious agent.

Small for Gestational Age Fetus

A major obstetric risk factor for fetal death is the presence of an SGA fetus. This is a complicated subject for several reasons. First, the risk factor of interest is fetal IUGR rather than SGA. However, IUGR implies a downward deflection on a growth curve, requiring several measurements over time, which is unavailable in many populations. In fact, precise knowledge of gestational age is often missing. Second, by definition, many SGA fetuses will be entirely normal, often termed "constitutionally small." Third, the use of population-based tables for weight percentiles does not account for an individual's inherent growth potential. A 6-pound infant may be appropriate for families with constitutionally small children but represent lagging fetal growth in families destined to have larger infants. Recent investigations have focused on developing methods for tracking individual growth potential for fetuses (27). Finally, SGA is not a diagnosis unto itself. Rather it is a sign or a clue for a variety of other conditions that may lead to fetal death.

Despite these concerns, it is increasingly apparent that the presence of an SGA fetus is strongly associated with fetal death. Moreover, there seems to be a "dose–response curve"; the more profound the SGA, the greater the risk for fetal death. This observation strongly supports biologic plausibility. A population-based study from Sweden illustrates the use of customized, rather than population-based growth curves. The odds ratio for stillbirth was 6.1 (95% CI, 5.0–7.5) for SGA fetuses using customized growth charts, compared with 1.2 (95% CI, 0.8–1.9) for SGA fetuses determined by population-based curves (27). Antenatal surveillance, including laser-Doppler velocimetry may be useful in distinguishing which SGA fetuses are at risk for fetal death. Absent end diastolic velocity or reverse flow in the umbilical artery is a particularly worrisome sign and should prompt consideration of delivery.

Obstetric Conditions

FETAL–MATERNAL HEMORRHAGE

Fetal–maternal hemorrhage is one of the most common single disorders responsible for fetal death. The condition has been reported in 5–14% of cases (28). Fetal–maternal hemorrhage may be associated with vaginal bleeding or abdominal pain caused by abruption but also may occur in the absence of symptoms. Because labor and delivery cause fetal–maternal hemorrhage, ideally assessment of fetal blood in the maternal circulation should be done before delivery. However, it is probably useful to assess for the condition after delivery if not done previously. Small amounts of fetal blood routinely enter the maternal circulation. Accordingly, only large amounts of fetal–maternal hemorrhage, ideally in association with autopsy confirmation of fetal anemia and hypoxia, should be considered causal for fetal death. In rare cases of vasa previa, fetal blood passes per vagina rather than entering the maternal circulation. Histologic evaluation of the placenta and cord may confirm the diagnosis.

MULTIPLE GESTATION

The risk of fetal death is substantially increased in multiple gestations. Although they account for about 3% of births in the United States, multiple gestations contribute to 10% of fetal deaths. The proportion is likely higher if second-trimester losses are included. This is of concern given the continued increase in the rate of multiple gestations because of increased use of assisted reproductive technology. The potential causes of fetal death in multiple gestations are numerous and include virtually every obstetric complication, including placental insufficiency, abruption, preeclampsia, and preterm labor. Other problems are unique to multiple gestation, especially in cases of monochorionic placentation, such as twin–twin transfusion syndrome (Fig. 11-4), cord entanglement with monoamniotic gestations, and twin-reverse arterial perfusion sequence.

PLACENTAL ABNORMALITIES

Conditions specific to gestational tissues that may cause fetal death include umbilical cord thrombosis, velamentous cord insertion or vasa previa, and amniotic band syndrome (Fig. 11-5). Placental abnormalities also can provide clues regarding other mechanisms of death, such as infection, thrombosis, inflammation, and vascular abnormalities.

CORD ACCIDENTS

Many cases of fetal death, especially at term, are attributed to umbilical cord accidents. This is thought to occur because of cord occlusion in the presence of nuchal or body cords and true knots in the cord. However, because cord entanglement occurs in up to 30% of uncomplicated pregnancies and because these may be transient findings, caution should be used in attributing fetal death to the presence of these findings. Similarly, true knots are usually associated with live births. Thus, the presence of a true knot or nuchal cord is insufficient evidence that cord accident is the cause of death. Ideally, the demonstration of cord occlusion, fetal hypoxia, and the exclusion of other causes is required to confirm the diagnosis.

OTHER OBSTETRIC DISORDERS

Numerous obstetric disorders may directly or indirectly cause fetal death. Examples include abruption, preeclampsia, cord prolapse, cervical insufficiency, preterm labor, and preterm premature rupture of membranes. These conditions often lead to intrapartum, or early neonatal, rather than antepartum death. Nonetheless, taken together they account for a meaningful proportion of fetal deaths.

Other Conditions

A variety of other disorders such as red blood cell alloimmunization may contribute to some cases of fetal death. Although fetal death from this condition has decreased dramatically because of the use of RhD immune globulin and improved obstetric care, the condition continues to be a cause of fetal death. Uterine malformations have been associated with fetal death and should be considered in cases of recurrent losses and very early preterm labor or preterm premature rupture of membranes. Maternal trauma through motor vehicle accident or violence is a rare but important cause of loss, especially in teenagers.

Unexplained

In most studies of fetal death, the causes are unexplained, even after extensive evaluation. In many cases this is

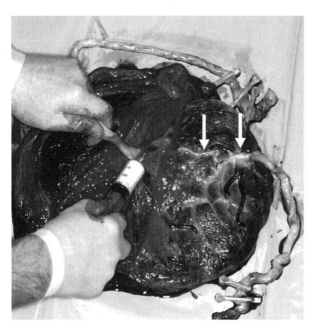

Fig. 11-4. Placenta demonstrating arterial-to-venous anastomoses after injection of milk (arrows) in a pregnancy complicated by twin–twin transfusion syndrome. (Copyright © 1994, J. L. B. Byrne. Used with permission.)

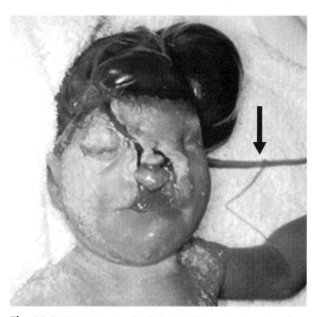

Fig. 11-5. Third-trimester fetal death with acalvarium. On ultrasonography, there was suspicion of possible neural tube defect. However, autopsy demonstrated amniotic band syndrome (arrow points to amniotic band). (Copyright © 1994, J. L. B. Byrne. Used with permission.)

because of inadequate attempts to determine a cause of death. The proportion of unexplained fetal deaths also is influenced by whether conditions that are associated with, but may not be directly causal, are accepted as a cause. Losses later in gestation (third trimester) are more likely to be unexplained than losses earlier in gestation. Such losses are strongly associated with IUGR as well as most of the previously described risk factors for fetal death. Undoubtedly, continued investigation will identify previously unrecognized causes of fetal death so that fewer cases remain unexplained.

Management

The value of an investigation into potential causes of fetal death cannot be overemphasized. First, determining a cause of death helps bring emotional closure to the event. Second, most families at least consider trying to have another child. Invariably, they are quite interested in whether there is a chance for recurrence. Finally, in some cases, medical intervention may reduce the risk of recurrence and improve outcome in subsequent pregnancies. Couples should be counseled regarding these issues in a supportive manner and encouraged to permit an evaluation of their pregnancy loss with sensitivity to their needs and concerns.

The optimal evaluation for potential causes of fetal death is uncertain. It is necessary to balance cost and yield when considering which testing to perform. Thus, it is appropriate to focus on the most common causes of fetal death. It also is desirable to emphasize conditions with recurrence risk, especially those amenable to effective therapies. There is still value, however, in the identification of sporadic conditions. This may allow women to avoid unnecessary tests and interventions in subsequent pregnancies and facilitate emotional healing from the loss.

In most cases, the most valuable test is perinatal autopsy because it provides information that is pertinent to nearly every potential cause of fetal death. Autopsy can identify intrinsic abnormalities such as malformations and metabolic abnormalities, as well as extrinsic problems, including hypoxia and infection. Importantly, perinatal autopsy provides new information that influences counseling and recurrence risk in 26–51% of cases (29, 30). The rate of perinatal autopsy varies widely throughout the United States and the world, but in all but a few centers with dedicated programs is typically less than 50%. If patients are reluctant to proceed with autopsy, it is worthwhile to ask about their reservations. It often is possible to work with individuals so that they are comfortable with the procedure. If families are still uncomfortable with autopsy, partial autopsy, X-rays or postmortem magnetic resonance imaging may provide

valuable information. Other barriers to autopsy are cost (although families are rarely charged), a lack of adequately trained pathologists, and misconceptions on the part of clinicians about its value.

After autopsy, placental evaluation is perhaps the next most valuable test. Gross and histologic examination of gestational tissues is pertinent to a wide variety of conditions, including infection, anemia, hypoxia, and thrombophilias. Patients rarely object to this procedure. Placental examination is considerably more informative in the hands of a trained and interested pathologist.

Karyotype is recommended in all cases of fetal death. However, cost may be an issue, depending upon payor status. In such cases, careful external evaluation by a pathologist or geneticist is invaluable in deciding whether to obtain a karyotype. The risk of chromosomal abnormalities in stillbirths with no dysmorphic features (especially if no abnormalities were noted on antenatal ultrasonography) is probably less than 2%.

In some cases of fetal death it is not possible to successfully culture fetal cells to assess karyotype. This is particularly true if there was a long interval between death and the delivery of the fetus. One strategy to obtain a reliable karyotype is to perform an amniocentesis before delivery. Other approaches are to attempt to culture cells that may survive after demise or under low oxygen tension, such as placenta (especially chorionic plate), fascia lata, tendons, and skin from the nape of the neck. Blood is an excellent cell source if available. In cases of autopsy, tissue should be sent to the cytogenetic laboratory by the pathologist so that the gross examination is not compromised. If autopsy is not obtained, it is important for the clinician to avoid placing the placenta or fetal tissues in formalin so that cells may be grown in culture. If attempts to culture fetal cells are unsuccessful, comparative genomic hybridization has been used to successfully evaluate fetal chromosomes (31). This technique is increasingly available in cytogenetic laboratories.

Autopsy, placental evaluation, and karyotype are worthwhile for most cases of fetal death. Additional testing is controversial and the cost/benefit ratio is uncertain. Screening for fetal–maternal hemorrhage is advised because the test is inexpensive and noninvasive, and the condition is common. This is typically done with a Kleihauer–Betke test, although some laboratories are using alternative methods such as flow cytometry to screen for fetal cells in the maternal circulation.

Testing for infection is probably best accomplished with autopsy and placental histology. Based on histologic findings, the pathologist may choose to culture fetal tissues or to assess for bacterial or viral nucleic acids. Placental cultures should be considered experimental because positive cultures are common in association with live births. Serologic testing for syphilis is advised. In cases of negative first-trimester testing, repeat testing in the third trimester likely can be limited to high-risk populations. It is reasonable to assess parvovirus serology because this organism accounts for a substantial proportion of fetal deaths, and testing is reliable. Although traditionally recommended, the usefulness of "TORCH titers," (serology for toxoplasmosis, rubella, cytomegalovirus, and herpes simplex) remains uncertain.

Routine testing for antiphospholipid syndrome and heritable thrombophilias also is of questionable usefulness. Most authorities advise testing for lupus anticoagulant and anticardiolipin antibodies in all cases of fetal death. However, the condition is rare unless there is clear evidence of placental insufficiency or other features of antiphospholipid syndrome such as thrombosis. Testing for heritable thrombophilias is controversial because positive results in healthy women are common. As with antiphospholipid syndrome, testing cases associated with placental insufficiency or recurrent cases seems most indicated. Testing for antiphospholipid syndrome and heritable thrombophilias is attractive because treatment may improve outcome in subsequent pregnancies.

An antibody screen (indirect Coomb's test) is helpful to exclude red cell alloimmunization. A toxicology screen should always be considered. This is usually accomplished with maternal urine, but measurement of stable metabolites in fetal tissues such as hair or meconium is gaining popularity. Testing for thyroid disease or diabetes in asymptomatic women has been suggested by many authorities, but subclinical thyroid disease and diabetes have not been proved to be associated with fetal death. Uterine imaging studies should be considered in cases of recurrent loss, preterm premature rupture of membranes, and preterm labor.

A summary of recommended tests for the evaluation of fetal death is shown in box 11-1. It seems reasonable to limit testing for rare conditions to cases wherein clinical history or other testing raises suspicion for a particular disorder. Ideally, the clinician should discuss clinical details as well as physical and laboratory findings with the pathologist so that the workup is tailored for each individual loss. Ongoing population-based studies such as that being conducted by the Stillbirth Collaborative Research Network of the National Institute of Child Health and Human Development may clarify the optimal evaluation of fetal death.

Delivery of the Fetus

Most women prefer to proceed with delivery of the fetus after diagnosis of fetal death. It is emotionally stressful to carry a nonviable fetus, especially late in gestation. Nonetheless, there is no medical urgency to effect deliv-

---

BOX 11-1

RECOMMENDED EVALUATION FOR STILLBIRTH

Recommended in most cases
- Perinatal autopsy
- Placental evaluation
- Karyotype
- Antibody screen*
- Serologic test for syphilis†
- Screen for fetal–maternal hemorrhage (Kleihauer–Betke or other)
- Urine toxicology screen
- Parvovirus serology

Recommended if clinical suspicion
- Lupus anticoagulant screen‡
- Anticardiolipin antibodies screen‡
- Factor V Leiden mutation screen‡
- Prothrombin G20210A mutation screen‡
- Protein C, protein S, and antithrombin III deficiency screen§
- Uterine imaging study‖

Not recommended at present
- Thyroid-stimulating hormone screen
- Glycohemoglobin screen
- TORCH titers screen¶
- Placental cultures
- Testing for other thrombophilias

---

*Negative first-trimester screen does not require repeat testing.

†Repeat testing in cases of negative first trimester screen if high-risk population

‡Test in cases of thrombosis, placental insufficiency, and recurrent fetal death

§These thrombophilias are rare in the absence of personal or family history of thrombosis.

‖Test in cases of unexplained recurrent loss, preterm premature rupture of membranes, and preterm labor

¶TORCH titers, serology for toxoplasmosis, rubella, cytomegalovirus, and herpes simplex

---

ery and for some women a delay is emotionally desirable. For example, some women prefer to grieve with their families and do not feel "up to" a medical procedure immediately after diagnosis. Other couples may even prefer prolonged expectant management, usually prompted by a desire to avoid induction of labor. It is important to offer both the options of delivery and expectant management to women experiencing fetal death.

Risks of expectant management include intrauterine infection and maternal coagulopathy. These risks are poorly characterized because of the relative infrequency of expectant management. Older reports state that 80–90% of women will spontaneously go into labor within 2 weeks of fetal death (32). However, this "latency" period may be substantially longer. It seems prudent to perform surveillance for infection and coagulopathy in women undergoing expectant care. Examples include serial assessment of maternal temperature, abdominal pain, bleeding, and labor. Regular office visits (eg, weekly) may be useful for emotional support and medical surveillance. Some authorities advise serial (eg, weekly) determination of complete blood count, platelet count, and fibrinogen level. The usefulness of this is uncertain. A consumptive coagulopathy has been reported in 25% of patients who retain a dead fetus for more than 4 weeks (33), but the condition is rare in clinical practice and is not usually associated with clinical sequelae. A fibrinogen level of less than 100 mg/dL is considered evidence of coagulopathy. Patients should be advised to immediately report symptoms such as fever, pain, bleeding, contractions, leaking fluid, or foul discharge.

Depending on gestational age, evacuation of the uterus may be accomplished medically or surgically. Ideally, the choice of delivery method should be made by the parents based on personal preference. Some women prefer surgical evacuation of the uterus because the procedure is rapid and they may receive a general anesthetic. Others choose induction of labor so that they may experience labor and delivery of an intact fetus.

In experienced hands, dilation and evacuation in the early second trimester is as safe as medical induction of labor. This procedure becomes technically more difficult in the later second and third trimesters. At more advanced gestational ages, labor induction is safer, and dilation and evacuation should be reserved for physicians with more extensive experience and skills in this procedure. Induction of labor has been greatly aided by the availability of prostaglandin preparations. There is considerable experience with the use of prostaglandin E_2 (PGE_2) to induce labor in women with fetal demise. During the past decade, misoprostol has largely replaced PGE_2 for induction of labor in cases of fetal death because of similar efficacy with fewer side effects (34). Adverse effects of prostaglandins include fever, nausea, emesis, and diarrhea, particularly if a PGE_2 preparation is used. Pretreatment with antiemetics, antipyretics, and antidiarrheals may relieve symptoms.

Misoprostol may be administered orally as a lozenge or vaginally in the posterior fornix. The dose of misoprostol is influenced by the size of the uterus, and several approaches have been published. If the uterus is less than 28 weeks size, our approach is to place 200 mg of misoprostol in the posterior fornix every 4 hours until delivery of the fetus and placenta. The dose could be increased to 400 mg every 2 hours, but delivery is not hastened compared with 200 mg every 4 hours. The oral dose (taken as a lozenge) is 200–400 mg every 2–4 hours. The interval to delivery is less when the drug is administered vaginally compared with orally, but some women may prefer to take the drug by mouth. If the uterus is greater than 28 weeks size, we administer an initial dose of 25 mg of misoprostol in the posterior fornix, followed by 25–50 mg every 4 hours. Alternatively, it may be given orally at a dosage of 25 mg every 4 hours. Prostaglandin E_2 should not be used in women with active cardiac, pulmonary or renal disease, and glaucoma. All prostaglandins for medical induction of labor should be avoided in cases of prior cesarean if uterine size is greater than 26 weeks of gestation at the time of induction. In such cases, we use oxytocin (low dose if the cervix is unfavorable). Risks of uterine rupture must be weighed against the desire to avoid hysterotomy in women with fetal death. Although uterine rupture may occur, misoprostol has been used safely for second-trimester induction of labor in women with prior cesarean delivery (35).

In cases of fetal death in the second trimester, especially at less than 20 weeks of gestation, there is an increased risk for retained placenta. Allowing the placenta to deliver spontaneously without "pulling on the umbilical cord" can greatly reduce this risk. Additional doses of misoprostol may be administered (at appropriate intervals) to promote uterine contractility between delivery of the fetus and placenta. In my practice I do not use a "time limit" for the delivery of the placenta in the absence of bleeding or emotional duress. Placental delivery rarely takes more than 2 hours. The use of misoprostol may reduce the incidence of retained placenta to less than 5%, which seems to be lower than seen with oxytocin or PGE_2 (34).

Bereavement

The facilitation of bereavement is an important opportunity for clinicians to help families. Many practitioners, especially obstetric providers, are uncomfortable with death and avoid frank discussions with patients. This is especially true in cases wherein the clinician is worried about being at fault. It is important to overcome these fears and to directly address all of the patient's questions. It is helpful to develop a standard bereavement protocol, particularly in units that rarely encounter stillbirths. Patients should be offered the opportunity to hold their infants and to keep mementos such as pictures, foot and handprints, and plaster casts. Visits with clergy and support groups and psychologic counseling should be offered. Patients should be allowed to make as many choices as possible regarding their experience. Prolonged hospitalizations are unnecessary, and recovery on postpartum wards should be avoided.

Subsequent Pregnancy Management

The risk for virtually all adverse pregnancy outcomes are influenced by prior obstetric history, and fetal death is no exception. The recurrence risk for fetal death is not well studied and reliable numbers for individual patients are often unavailable. A recent population-based study from Missouri noted a stillbirth rate of 22.7 per 1,000 women with prior stillbirth, representing an odds ratio of 4.7 (95% CI, 1.2–5.7) compared with women without prior stillbirth (36). Increased recurrence risks were noted in African Americans (35.9 per 1,000) compared with whites (36). Recurrence risk may be stratified by cause of stillbirth. For example, losses associated with placental insufficiency, prematurity, or some genetic conditions are more likely to recur, whereas those caused by infection or abnormalities of twinning are less likely. Also, fetal death earlier in gestation is more likely to recur than losses at term. Patients with recurrent fetal death are at much higher risk than those with sporadic loss (5).

Strategies to prevent recurrence depend upon the cause of the prior loss(es). Families with identified genetic conditions may be counseled about reproductive options, including antenatal and preimplantation genetic diagnosis. Improved medical care for maternal disorders such as diabetes and hypertension can substantially improve outcome in subsequent pregnancies. The same is true for women with red cell alloimmunization. Although not universally accepted, there is evidence that treatment with thromboprophylaxis can improve the live birth rate in women with antiphospholipid syndrome (37, 38).

Data are less clear for heritable thrombophilias because they are common in healthy women. One well-designed prospective randomized trial compared low molecular weight heparin and low-dose aspirin to low-dose aspirin alone in 160 women with prior fetal death and thrombophilia (39). Pregnancy outcome was dramatically improved in the low molecular weight heparin group with a live birth rate of 71% compared with 14% for low-dose aspirin alone (39). These data are promising but must be interpreted with caution. First, results have not been confirmed in other trials. Second, the rate of pregnancy loss in the control group was extremely high (86%) and much higher than anticipated based on risk factors. Thus, current data are insufficient to recommend routine thromboprophylaxis for women with thrombophilias.

Counseling regarding smoking cessation, weight loss in obese women, and the proper use of seat belts during pregnancy also may reduce the rate of stillbirth. Although of unproved efficacy, these public health measures make good common sense for all women.

Antenatal surveillance is widely recommended in subsequent pregnancies for patients with prior fetal death. Clinical usefulness has been suggested by older studies, and the test is likely to benefit the subset of pregnancies at risk for placental insufficiency. It is noteworthy that in addition to recurrent pregnancy loss, prior fetal death increases the risk for many obstetric complications, including IUGR, abruption, and preterm birth. The most commonly employed surveillance method is the nonstress test. Although some authorities advise testing 2–4 weeks before the gestational age of the fetal death, initiating testing at 32 weeks of gestation likely works as well and may reduce the chance of false-positive results (40). Alternatively, laser-Doppler velocimetry, amniotic fluid indexes, and serial ultrasonography to assess growth may be used to assess placental function. Induction of labor is another common strategy used in women with prior fetal death. As with antenatal surveillance, many clinicians advise delivery at a gestational age 2 weeks before the previous loss. This recommendation should be viewed with caution because of unproved efficacy (with regard to stillbirth prevention) and the potential for clinically relevant prematurity. However, induction has tremendous emotional benefit for many couples with prior fetal death. Accordingly, elective induction in the setting of pulmonary maturity and a favorable cervix may be appropriate in well-selected cases. Indeed, a large component of providing good care in subsequent pregnancies in women with prior fetal death is to attend to the patient's emotional needs. Frequent visits, documentation of fetal heart tones and well-being, and a lot of positive reinforcement are invaluable.

Summary

Fetal death remains a common, traumatic, and in some cases, preventable complication of pregnancy. Delivery may be safely accomplished either medically or surgically, and expectant management is a safe alternative for interested patients. The strongest risk factors for fetal death are African-American race, prior fetal death, obesity, small for gestational age fetus, and advanced maternal age. Common causes and risk factors for fetal death include chromosomal abnormalities, genetic syndromes, infections, placental abnormalities, fetal–maternal hemorrhage, maternal diseases such as diabetes and hypertension, antiphospholipid syndrome, thrombophilias, and abnormalities of multiple gestation. Clinicians should encourage families to allow a thorough investigation of potential causes of fetal death to facilitate emotional closure, to assess recurrence risk, and in some cases to reduce recurrence risk. The optimal "workup" for fetal death is uncertain. Recommended tests include perinatal autopsy, placental evaluation, fetal karyotype, Kleihauer–Betke, antibody screen, and a serologic test for syphilis. Other tests to consider include testing for anticardiolipin anti-bodies, lupus anticoagulant screen, testing for heritable thrombophilias, urine toxicology screen, and parvovirus serology. Subsequent pregnancies may be at increased risk for fetal death and obstetric complications. Treatment of underlying medical or obstetric conditions, antenatal surveillance, and induction of labor with fetal maturity may improve outcome. One hopes that ongoing research will elucidate causes for previously unexplained fetal death and focus efforts on effective prevention.

References

1. Wilcox AJ, Weinberg CR, O'Connor JF, Baird DD, Schlatterer JP, Canfield RE, et al. Incidence of early loss of pregnancy. N Engl J Med 1988;319:189–94.

2. Kline J, Stein Z. Epidemiology of chromosomal abnormalities in spontaneous abortion: prevalence, manifestation and determinants. In: Spontaneous and recurrent abortion. Bennett MJ, Edmonds DK, editors. Oxford (United Kingdom): Blackwell Scientific Publications; 1987. p. 29–50.

3. Oshiro BT, Silver RM, Scott JR, Yu H, Branch DW. Antiphospholipid antibodies and fetal death. Obstet Gynecol 1996;87:489–93.

4. Rey E, Kahn SR, David M, Shrier I. Thrombophilic disorders and fetal loss: a meta-analysis. Lancet 2003;361:901–8.

5. Frias AE Jr, Luikenaar RA, Sullivan AE, Lee RM, Porter TF, Branch DW, et al. Poor obstetric outcome in subsequent pregnancies in women with prior fetal death. Obstet Gynecol 2004;104:521–6.

6. Johansen KS, Hod M. Quality development in perinatal care: the OBSQID project. Obstetrical quality Indicators and Data. Int J Gynaecol Obstet 1999;64:167–72.

7. Cartlidge PH, Stewart JH. Effect of changing the stillbirth definition on evaluation of perinatal mortality rates. Lancet 1995;346:486–8.

8. Baird D, Walker J, Thomson AM. The causes and prevention of stillbirths and first week deaths. III. A classification of deaths by clinical cause; the effect of age, parity and length of gestation on death rates by cause. J Obstet Gynaecol Br Emp 1954;61:433–48.

9. Hey EN, Lloyd DJ, Wigglesworth JS. Classifying perinatal death: fetal and neonatal factors. Br J Obstet Gynaecol 1986;93:1213–23.

10. Gardosi J, Kady SM, McGeown P, Francis A, Tonks A. Classification of stillbirth by relevant condition at death (ReCoDe): population based cohort study. BMJ 2005;331:1113–7.

11. Fretts RC. Etiology and prevention of stillbirth. Am J Obstet Gynecol 2005;193:1923–35.

12. Froen JF, Arnestad M, Frey K, Vege A, Saugstad OD, Stray-Pedersen B. Risk factors for sudden intrauterine unexplained death: epidemiologic characteristics of singleton cases in Oslo, Norway, 1986-1995. Am J Obstet Gynecol 2001;184:694–702.

13. Vintzileos AM, Ananth CV, Smulian JC, Scorza WE, Knuppel RA. Prenatal care and black-white fetal death disparity in the United States: heterogeneity by high-risk conditions. Obstet Gynecol 2002;99:483–9.

14. Fretts RC, Schmittdiel J, McLean FH, Usher RH, Goldman MB. Increased maternal age and the risk of fetal death. N Engl J Med 1995;333:953–7.

15. Bateman BT, Simpson LL. Higher rate of stillbirth at the extremes of reproductive age: a large nationwide sample of deliveries in the United States. Am J Obstet Gynecol 2006;194:840–5.

16. Kristensen J, Vestergaard M, Wisborg K, Kesmodel U, Secher NJ. Pre-pregnancy weight and the risk of stillbirth and neonatal death. BJOG 2005;112:403–8.

17. Cundy T, Gamble G, Townend K, Henley PG, MacPherson P, Roberts AB. Perinatal mortality in Type 2 diabetes mellitus. Diabet Med 2000;17:33–9.

18. Beischer NA, Wein P, Sheedy MT, Steffen B. Identification and treatment of women with hyperglycaemia diagnosed during pregnancy can significantly reduce perinatal mortality rates. Aust N Z J Obstet Gynaecol 1996;36:239–47.

19. Lockwood C, Silver R. Thrombophilias in pregnancy. In: Creasy R, Resnick R, Iams J. Maternal-fetal medicine: principles and practice. 5th ed. Philadelphia (PA): WB Saunders Company; 2003. p. 1005–22.

20. Dizon-Townson D, Miller C, Sibai B, Spong CY, Thom E, Wendel G Jr, et al. The relationship of the factor V Leiden mutation and pregnancy outcomes for mother and fetus. Obstet Gynecol 2005;106:517–24.

21. Kesmodel U, Wisborg K, Olsen SF, Henriksen TB, Secher NJ. Moderate alcohol intake during pregnancy and the risk of stillbirth and death in the first year of life. Am J Epidemiol 2002;155:305–12.

22. Whitehead N, Lipscomb L. Patterns of alcohol use before and during pregnancy and the risk of small-for-gestational-age birth. Am J Epidemiol 2003;158:654–62.

23. Wapner RJ, Lewis D. Genetics and metabolic causes of stillbirth. Semin Perinatol 2002;26:70–4.

24. Pauli RM, Reiser CA. Wisconsin Stillbirth Service Program: II. Analysis of diagnoses and diagnostic categories in the first 1,000 referrals. Am J Med Genet 1994;50:135–53.

25. Goldenberg RL, Thompson C. The infectious origins of stillbirth. Am J Obstet Gynecol 2003;189:861–73.

26. Skjoldebrand-Sparre L, Tolfvenstam T, Papadogiannakis N, Wahren B, Broliden K, Nyman M. Parvovirus B19 infection: association with third-trimester intrauterine fetal death. BJOG 2000;107:476–80.

27. Clausson B, Gardosi J, Francis A, Cnattingius S. Perinatal outcome in SGA births defined by customised versus population-based birthweight standards. BJOG 2001;108:830–4.

28. Laube DW, Schauberger CW. Fetomaternal bleeding as a cause for "unexplained" fetal death. Obstet Gynecol 1982;60:649–51.

29. Faye-Petersen OM, Guinn DA, Wenstrom KD. Value of perinatal autopsy. Obstet Gynecol 1999;94:915–20.

30. Michalski ST, Porter J, Pauli RM. Costs and consequences of comprehensive stillbirth assessment. Am J Obstet Gynecol 2002;186:1027–34.

31. Christiaens GC, Vissers J, Poddighe PJ, de Pater JM. Comparative genomic hybridization for cytogenetic evaluation of stillbirth. Obstet Gynecol 2000;96:281–6.

32. Goldstein DP, Reid DE. Circulating fibrinolytic activity—a precursor of hypofibrinogenemia following fetal death in utero. Obstet Gynecol 1963;22:174–80.

33. Diagnosis and management of fetal death. ACOG Technical Bulletin Number 176—January 1993. Int J Gynaecol Obstet January 1993;42:291–9.

34. Ramsey PS, Savage K, Lincoln T, Owen J. Vaginal misoprostol versus concentrated oxytocin and vaginal PGE2 for secondtrimester labor induction. Obstet Gynecol 2004; 104:138–45.

35. Dickinson JE. Misoprostol for second-trimester pregnancy termination in women with a prior cesarean delivery. Obstet Gynecol 2005;105:352–6.

36. Sharma PP, Salihu HM, Oyelese Y, Ananth CV, Kirby RS. Is race a determinant of stillbirth recurrence? Obstet Gynecol 2006;107:391–7.

37. Kutteh WH. Antiphospholipid antibody-associated recurrent pregnancy loss: treatment with heparin and low-dose aspirin is superior to low-dose aspirin alone. Am J Obstet Gynecol 1996;174:1584–9.

38. Rai R, Cohen H, Dave M, Regan L. Randomised controlled trial of aspirin and aspirin plus heparin in pregnant women with recurrent miscarriage associated with phospholipid antibodies (or antiphospholipid antibodies). BMJ 1997;314:253–7.

39. Gris JC, Mercier E, Quere I, Lavigne-Lissalde G, Cochery-Nouvellon E, Hoffet M, et al. Low-molecular-weight heparin versus low-dose aspirin in women with one fetal loss and a constitutional thrombophilic disorder. Blood 2004;103:3695–9.

40. Weeks JW, Asrat T, Morgan MA, Nageotte M, Thomas SJ, Freeman RK. Antepartum surveillance for a history of stillbirth: when to begin? Am J Obstet Gynecol 1995;172: 486–92.

CHAPTER 12

Preeclampsia; the Syndrome of Hemolysis, Elevated Liver Enzymes, and Low Platelet Count; and Eclampsia

BAHA M. SIBAI

*H*ypertension is the most common medical disorder during pregnancy (1). Approximately 70% of women in whom hypertension is diagnosed during pregnancy will have "gestational hypertension–preeclampsia." The term gestational hypertension–preeclampsia is used to describe a wide spectrum of patients who may have only a mild elevation in blood pressure (BP) or severe hypertension with various organ dysfunctions including acute gestational hypertension; preeclampsia; eclampsia; and hemolysis, elevated liver enzymes, low platelet count (HELLP) syndrome.

Gestational Hypertension and Preeclampsia

Gestational hypertension is defined as a systolic BP of at least 140 mm Hg or a diastolic BP of at least 90 mm Hg or both on at least two occasions at least 6 hours apart after the 20th week of gestation in women known to be normotensive before pregnancy and before 20 weeks of gestation. The BP recordings used to establish the diagnosis should be no more than 7 days apart (1). Gestational hypertension is considered severe if there are sustained elevations in systolic BP to at least 160 mm Hg or in diastolic BP to at least 110 mm Hg or both for at least 6 hours (2).

Gestational hypertension is the most frequent cause of hypertension during pregnancy. The rate is increased in nulliparous women and is further increased in women with previous preeclampsia and in women with multifetal gestation (3). Some women with gestational hypertension will subsequently progress to preeclampsia. The rate of progression depends on gestational age at time of diagnosis; the rate reaches 50% when it develops before 30 weeks of gestation (4).

Preeclampsia is defined as gestational hypertension plus proteinuria (300 mg or more per 24-hour period). If 24-hour urine collection is not available, then proteinuria is defined as a concentration of at least 30 mg/dL (at least 1+ on dipstick) in at least two random urine samples col-lected at least 4 hours apart (should be no more than 7 days apart) (1). The concentration of urinary protein in random urine samples is highly variable. Recent studies have found that urinary dipstick determinations correlate poorly with the amount of proteinuria found in 24-hour urine determinations in women with gestational hypertension (5). Therefore, the definitive test to diagnose proteinuria should be quantitative protein excretion in a 24-hour period. Severe proteinuria is defined as protein excretion of at least 5 g per 24-hour period. Urine dipstick values should not be used to diagnose severe proteinuria (5). In the absence of proteinuria, preeclampsia should be considered when hypertension is associated with persistent cerebral symptoms, epigastric or right upper quadrant pain with nausea or vomiting, or thrombocytopenia and abnormal liver enzymes.

Preeclampsia is considered severe if there is severe gestational hypertension in association with proteinuria or if there is hypertension in association with severe proteinuria (at least 5 g per 24-hour period). In addition, preeclampsia is considered severe in the presence of multiorgan involvement such as pulmonary edema, oliguria (less than 500 mL per 24-hour period), thrombocytopenia (platelet count less than 100,000/mm^3), abnormal liver enzymes in association with persistent epigastric or right upper quadrant pain, or persistent severe central nervous system symptoms.

Etiology and Pathophysiology

The etiology of preeclampsia is unknown. During the past centuries, several etiologies have been suggested, but most of them have not withstood the test of time. The pathophysiologic abnormalities of preeclampsia are numerous. Some of the reported abnormalities include placental ischemia, abnormal hemostasis with activation of the coagulation system, vascular endothelial dysfunction, leukocyte activation, and changes in various cytokines as well as abnormal placental angiogenesis, resulting in reduced placental growth factor and increased levels of soluble fms-like tyrosine kinase 1 (6).

Prediction and Prevention

Prevention of any disease process requires knowledge of its etiology and pathogenesis, as well as the availability of methods to predict or identify those at high risk for this disorder. Numerous clinical, biophysical, and biochemical tests have been proposed for the prediction or early detection of preeclampsia. However, most of these tests have poor sensitivity and poor positive predictive values, and the majority of them are not suitable for routine use in clinical practice (7). At present, there is no single screening test that is considered reliable and cost-effective for predicting preeclampsia or HELLP syndrome (7). As a result, all studies on prevention have included women with various risk factors for preeclampsia (8).

During the past two decades, numerous clinical reports and randomized trials described the use of various methods to reduce the rate and the severity of preeclampsia (8). There are few randomized trials evaluating magnesium, zinc, or fish oil supplementation to prevent preeclampsia. These trials had limited sample size; however, results reveal minimal to no benefit. There are at least eleven placebo-controlled trials evaluating calcium supplementation during pregnancy. Results of these trials conflict (8–10). Most randomized trials for the prevention of preeclampsia have used low-dose aspirin (8). Results of early single-center trials demonstrated an average reduction of 70% with low-dose aspirin. However, results of several large trials that included more than 40,000 women demonstrated minimal to no benefit (11). Moreover, the results of two large multicenter trials using supplementation with vitamins C and E in women identified to be at risk revealed no reduction in rates of preeclampsia (12, 13). Indeed, results of one trial demonstrated adverse maternal and fetal outcome (12), and the other one revealed adverse maternal outcome in those receiving vitamins C and E (13).

Based on the available data, neither calcium supplementation nor low-dose aspirin should be routinely prescribed for preeclampsia prevention in nulliparous women. In addition, zinc, magnesium, fish oil, and vitamins C and E should not be routinely used for this purpose.

Maternal and Perinatal Outcome

GESTATIONAL HYPERTENSION

Most cases of gestational hypertension develop at or beyond 37 weeks of gestation, and thus pregnancy outcome is similar or superior to that seen in normotensive pregnancies (Table 12-1) (4, 14–16). Both gestational age at delivery and birth weight in these pregnancies are higher than those in normotensive pregnancies (4, 14–16). However, women with gestational hypertension are more likely to have higher rates of induction of labor for maternal reasons and higher rates of cesarean delivery

Table 12-1. Pregnancy Outcomes in Women With Mild Gestational Hypertension

	Study			
	Knuist et al (14) (n = 396)	Hauth et al (15) (n = 715)	Barton et al (4) (n = 405)	Sibai et al (16) (n = 186)
Weeks of Gestation at delivery*	Not reported	39.7	37.4†	39.1
Percentage at less than 37 weeks of gestation	5.3	7	17.3	5.9
Percentage at less than 34 weeks of gestation	1.3	1	4.9	1.6
Birth weight (g)*	Not reported	3,303	3,038	3,217
Percentage of small for gestational age infants	1.5‡	6.9	13.8	7
Percentage of newborns less than 2,500 g	7.1	7.7	23.5	Not reported
Percentage of abruptio placentae	0.5	0.3	0.5	0.5
Percentage of perinatal deaths	0.8	0.5	0	0

*Mean values
†Women who developed hypertension at 24–35 weeks
‡Less than one-third percentile

than women with normotensive gestation (1, 14, 15). The increased rate of cesarean delivery in such women is mainly related to failed medical induction or dystocia (1).

Maternal and perinatal morbidities are increased in severe gestational hypertension (15, 17). Indeed, these women have higher morbidities than women with mild preeclampsia (1). In addition, the rates of abruptio placentae, preterm delivery (at less than 37 weeks and 35 weeks of gestation), and small for gestational age infants are similar to those in women with severe preeclampsia. Therefore, these women should be treated as if they had severe preeclampsia (1).

PREECLAMPSIA

Maternal and perinatal outcomes in preeclampsia are dependent on gestational age at onset as well as at time of delivery, the severity of the disease, the presence of multifetal gestation, and the presence of preexisting medical conditions such as pregestational diabetes, renal disease, or thrombophilias (1, 3). In women with mild preeclampsia, the perinatal death rate and rates of preterm delivery, small for gestational age infants, and abruptio placentae are similar to those of normotensive pregnancies (Table 12-2) (15, 17, 18). The rate of eclampsia is less than 1%, but the rate of cesarean delivery is increased because of increased rates of induction of labor (1). In contrast, rates of perinatal mortality and morbidities as well as the rates of abruptio placentae are increased in severe preeclampsia (Table 12-2). The rate of neonatal complications is markedly increased in those who develop severe preeclampsia in the second trimester, whereas it is minimal in those beyond 35 weeks of gestation.

Severe preeclampsia also is associated with increased rates of maternal mortality (0.2%) and morbidity (5%) such as convulsions, pulmonary edema, acute renal or liver failure, liver hemorrhage, disseminated intravascular coagulopathy, and stroke. These complications are usually seen in women who develop preeclampsia before 32 weeks of gestation and in those with preexisting medical conditions (1, 3).

Antepartum Management

HOSPITALIZATION

In the past, treatment of women with mild hypertension–preeclampsia has involved bed rest in the hospital for the duration of pregnancy, with the belief that such treatment diminishes the frequency of progression to severe disease and allows rapid intervention in case of abrupt progression to abruptio placentae, eclampsia, or hypertensive crisis (1). However, these complications are rare among compliant women with mild preeclampsia and absent symptoms. In addition, the results of two randomized trials in women with mild gestational hypertension and several observational studies in women with mild hypertension and mild preeclampsia suggest that most of these women can be safely treated at home or in a daycare facility provided they undergo maternal and fetal evaluation (1).

BED REST

Complete or partial bed rest for the duration of pregnancy is often recommended for women with mild hypertension–preeclampsia. There is no evidence to date that

Table 12-2. Pregnancy Outcomes in Women With Mild and Severe Preeclampsia

	Study					
	Hauth et al (15)		Buchbinder et al (17)		Hnat et al (18)	
	Mild (n = 217)	Severe (n = 109)	Mild* (n = 62)	Severe* (n = 45)	Mild (n = 86)	Severe (n = 70)
Weeks of gestation at delivery*						
Percentage less than 37 weeks	Not reported	Not reported	25.8	66.7	14	33
Percentage less than 35 weeks	1.9†	18.5†	9.7	35.6	2.3	18.6
Percentage of small for gestational age infants*	10.2	18.5	4.8	11.4	NR	NR
Percentage of abruptio placentae	0.5	3.7	3.2	6.7	0	1.4
Percentage of perinatal death	1	1.8	0	8.9	0	1.4

*This study included women with previous preeclampsia. The other studies included only nulliparous women.
†These rates are for delivery at less than 34 weeks of gestation.

suggests that such a recommendation improves pregnancy outcome (19). In addition, there are no published randomized trials comparing complete bed rest and restricted activity in the treatment of women with mild preeclampsia. Prolonged bed rest for the duration of pregnancy increases the risk of thromboembolism.

BLOOD PRESSURE MEDICATIONS

There are several randomized trials describing the use of antihypertensive drugs versus no treatment or a placebo in the treatment of women with mild hypertension or preeclampsia remote from term. Overall, these trials revealed lower rates of progression to severe disease, with no improvement in perinatal outcome (20). Of note, the sample size of these trials was inadequate to evaluate differences in fetal growth restriction, abruptio placentae, perinatal death, or maternal outcome (20).

FETAL AND MATERNAL SURVEILLANCE

There is agreement that fetal testing is indicated during expectant treatment of women with gestational hypertension or preeclampsia (1, 2). However, there is disagreement regarding the test to be used, as well as the frequency of testing. Most authorities in the United States recommend daily fetal movement counts, a nonstress test (NST), or a biophysical profile, to be performed at the time of diagnosis and serially thereafter until delivery (one to two times per week) (1, 2). Ultrasound estimation of fetal weight and amniotic fluid status also are recommended at diagnosis and serially thereafter every 3–4 weeks. Doppler flow velocimetry also is recommended in the presence of fetal growth restriction. The frequency of these tests depends on the severity of hypertension or preeclampsia, gestational age at diagnosis, and fetal growth findings. Most clinical series suggest testing once weekly in women with mild gestational hypertension or preeclampsia, twice weekly if there is suspected fetal growth restriction, and daily during expectant treatment of women with severe preeclampsia at less than 32 weeks of gestation (1). However, there are no large prospective studies assessing the benefits or harms of these monitoring techniques in such women.

Maternal surveillance is indicated in women with gestational hypertension and preeclampsia. The goal of monitoring mild gestational hypertension is to detect progression to severe hypertension or preeclampsia (1, 2). In mild preeclampsia, the goal is early detection of severe preeclampsia. In severe preeclampsia, the goal is to observe patients to detect the development of organ dysfunction. Therefore, all women should be evaluated for symptoms of organ dysfunction such as severe

headaches, visual changes, altered mentation, right upper quadrant or epigastric pain, nausea or vomiting, and shortness of breath (1). In addition, they should undergo laboratory testing for 24-hour urine protein, serum creatinine, platelet count, and liver enzymes. Coagulation function tests are not needed in the presence of a normal platelet count and liver enzymes (21). The frequency of subsequent testing will depend on initial findings, severity of disease, and the ensuing clinical progression. Most authorities recommend evaluation and testing of platelet count, liver enzymes, and serum creatinine once weekly for women with mild gestational hypertension or mild preeclampsia and performing these tests daily during expectant treatment of women with severe preeclampsia remote from term (1).

Expectant Management of Severe Preeclampsia

The clinical course of severe preeclampsia may be characterized by progressive deterioration in both maternal and fetal conditions. Because these pregnancies have been associated with increased rates of maternal morbidity and mortality and with significant risks for the fetus, there is agreement that in such patients prompt delivery is indicated if the disease develops after 34 weeks of gestation. Prompt delivery also is indicated when there is imminent eclampsia (persistent severe symptoms), multiorgan dysfunction, severe fetal growth restriction (fifth percentile), abruptio placentae, or nonreassuring fetal testing before 34 weeks of gestation (22).

There is disagreement about treatment of severe preeclampsia before 34 weeks of gestation in which maternal condition is stable and fetal condition is reassuring. In such patients, some authors consider delivery as the definitive treatment regardless of gestational age, whereas others recommend prolonging pregnancy until development of maternal or fetal indications for delivery or until achievement of fetal lung maturity or 32–34 weeks of gestation (22).

Although delivery is always appropriate for the mother, it may not be optimal for the fetus that is extremely premature. In the past, it was believed that infants born prematurely to severely preeclamptic women had lower rates of neonatal mortality and morbidity than infants of similar gestational age born to nonpreeclamptic women (1). This belief was based on the clinical impression that fetuses of preeclamptic women have accelerated lung and neurologic maturation as a result of stress in utero. However, several recent case–control studies have demonstrated that premature infants born after severe preeclampsia have neonatal complications and mortality similar to those of other premature infants of similar gestational age and have higher rates of admission to neonatal intensive care units (22).

In the past, there was uncertainty regarding the efficacy and safety of corticosteroid use in women with severe preeclampsia before 34 weeks of gestation. A double-blind, randomized trial of 218 women with severe preeclampsia between 26 weeks and 34 weeks of gestation receiving either betamethasone (n = 110) or a placebo (n = 108) reported a significant reduction in the rate of respiratory distress syndrome (relative risk [RR], 0.53; 95% confidence interval [CI], 0.35–0.82) in the steroids group (23). Corticosteroid use also was associated with a reduction in the risks of neonatal intraventricular hemorrhage (RR, 0.35; 95% CI, 0.15–0.86), neonatal infection (RR, 0.39; 95% CI, 0.39–0.97), and neonatal death (RR, 0.5; 95% CI, 0.28–0.89).

Management Strategies

The primary objective of management in gestational hypertension–preeclampsia must always be safety of the mother and then delivery of a newborn who will not require intensive and prolonged neonatal care. This objective can be achieved by formulating a management plan that takes into consideration one or more of the following factors: the severity of the disease process, fetal gestational age, maternal and fetal status at the time of initial evaluation, presence of labor, cervical Bishop score, and the wishes of the mother.

MILD HYPERTENSION OR PREECLAMPSIA

Once mild gestational hypertension or preeclampsia is diagnosed, subsequent therapy will depend on the results of maternal and fetal evaluation (Fig. 12-1). Patients who have a favorable cervix at or near term and patients who are considered noncompliant should undergo induction of labor for delivery. In addition, cervical ripening with prostaglandins and induction of labor can be used in women with mild preeclampsia and an unfavorable cervix at 37 weeks of gestation or more because the mother is at slightly increased risk for development of abruptio placentae and progression to severe disease. Delivery is recommended in patients with a gestational age of greater than or equal to 34 weeks, in the presence of progressive labor or rupture of membranes, abnormal fetal testing, or fetal growth restriction.

For women in whom delivery has not been performed, close maternal and fetal evaluation is essential. These women are instructed to eat a regular diet and to restrict their activity but not to complete bed rest. Diuretics or antihypertensive medication are not used because of the potential to mask the diagnosis of severe

disease. In addition, the current data suggest that antihypertensive therapy in women with mild gestational hypertension or preeclampsia does not improve perinatal outcome (20). Only women considered to have severe disease should be started on antihypertensive medica-

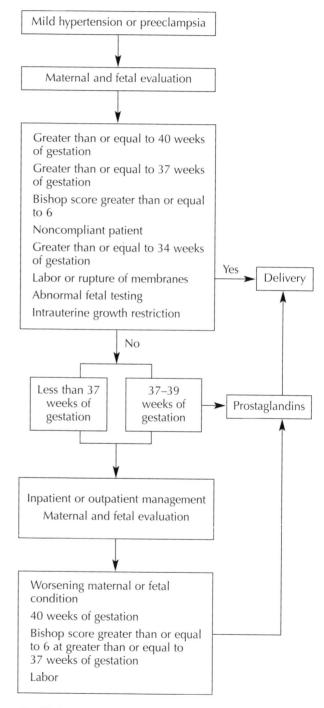

Fig. 12-1. Recommended management of mild gestational hypertension or preeclampsia. (Sibai BM. Diagnosis and management of gestational hypertension and preeclampsia. Obstet Gynecol 2003;102:181–92)

tions, and they require in-hospital management. At the time of initial and subsequent visits, the women are educated and instructed about reporting symptoms of severe preeclampsia. They also are advised to immediately come to the hospital or office if they develop abdominal pain, uterine contractions, vaginal spotting, or decreased fetal movement.

In mild gestational hypertension, fetal evaluation includes an NST and an ultrasound examination of estimated fetal weight and amniotic fluid index. If the results are normal, then there is no need for repeat testing unless there is a change in maternal condition (progression to preeclampsia or severe hypertension) or there is decreased fetal movement or abnormal fundal height growth (1). The development of any of these findings requires prompt fetal testing with a nonstress test or biophysical profile.

Maternal evaluation includes measurements of hematocrit, platelet count, liver function tests, and 24-hour urine protein testing once weekly. The women are usually seen twice a week for evaluation of maternal BP, urine protein by dipstick, and symptoms of impending eclampsia. The onset of maternal symptoms, a sudden increase in BP to severe values, or development of proteinuria (2+ or more on dipstick) may require hospitalization for close evaluation.

For mild preeclampsia at less than 37 weeks of gestation, outpatient management is appropriate in those with a systolic BP of 150 mm Hg or less or a diastolic BP of 100 mm Hg or less and a urine protein count of 1,000 mg or less per 24 hours if they have no symptoms and have normal liver enzyme levels and a normal platelet count (more than 100,000/mm^3). Women who do not satisfy these criteria are managed in the hospital. During ambulatory management, the women are instructed to have relative rest at home, to have BP and urine (dipstick) assessment daily, and to promptly report symptoms of severe disease. These women are then seen twice weekly, during which time they have a laboratory evaluation of platelet count and liver enzymes. Fetal evaluation includes daily fetal movement count, NST twice weekly, and ultrasound evaluation of fetal growth and fluid. If there is evidence of disease progression (significant increase in BP or proteinuria to levels above the threshold mentioned previously), if there is a new onset of symptoms, or if there is evidence of abnormal blood test results or abnormal fetal growth, these women are then hospitalized for the duration of pregnancy. Women managed in the hospital receive similar maternal and fetal evaluations.

SEVERE PREECLAMPSIA

Severe disease mandates immediate hospitalization in labor and delivery. Intravenous (IV) magnesium sulfate to prevent convulsions and antihypertensive medications to lower severe levels of hypertension (systolic BP greater than 160 mm Hg or diastolic BP of at least 110 mm Hg) should be administered. The goal of antihypertensive therapy is to keep systolic BP between 140 mm Hg and 155 mm Hg and diastolic BP between 90 mm Hg and 105 mm Hg (Table 12-3). During the observation period, maternal and fetal conditions are assessed and a decision is made regarding the need for delivery (Fig. 12-2). Those with gestational ages of 24–34 weeks are given corticosteroids to accelerate fetal lung maturity. Maternal evaluation includes monitoring of BP, urine output, cerebral status, and the presence of epigastric pain, tenderness, labor, or vaginal bleeding. Laboratory evaluation includes a platelet count and liver enzyme and serum creatinine testing. Fetal evaluation includes continuous

Table 12-3. Drugs to Treat Severe Hypertension in Preeclampsia–Eclampsia

Drug	Starting Dose	Maximum
Acute treatment*		
Hydralazine	5–10 mg, intravenously every 20 minutes.	30 mg/h
Labetalol	20–40 mg, intravenously every 10–15 minutes	220 mg/h
Nifedipine	10–20 mg, orally every 30 minutes	50 mg/h
Long-term treatment†		
Labetalol	200 mg every 6–8 hours	2,400 mg/d
Nifedipine	10 mg every 6–8 hours	120 mg/d

*Threshold level for women antepartum or intrapartum: systolic blood pressure 160 mm Hg or diastolic blood pressure 110 mm Hg if persistent for 1 hour; threshold level for women with HELLP syndrome and postpartum: systolic blood pressure 155 mm Hg or diastolic blood pressure 105 mm Hg for at least 1 hour.
†Goal during therapy is systolic blood pressure between 140 mm Hg and 155 mm Hg and diastolic blood pressure between 90 mm Hg and 105 mm Hg.

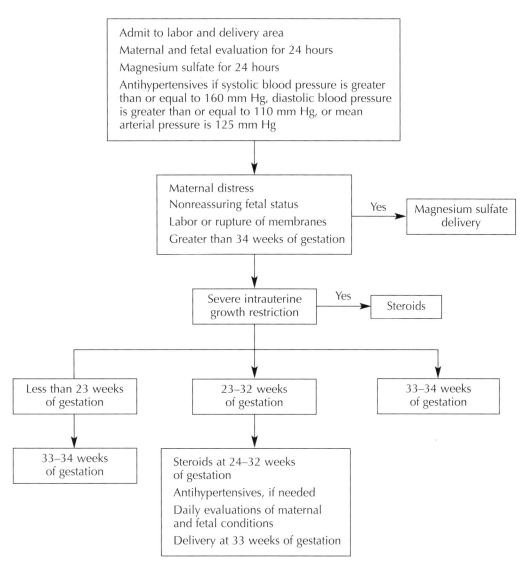

Admit to labor and delivery area
Maternal and fetal evaluation for 24 hours
Magnesium sulfate for 24 hours
Antihypertensives if systolic blood pressure is greater than or equal to 160 mm Hg, diastolic blood pressure is greater than or equal to 110 mm Hg, or mean arterial pressure is 125 mm Hg

Maternal distress
Nonreassuring fetal status
Labor or rupture of membranes
Greater than 34 weeks of gestation

Yes → Magnesium sulfate delivery

Severe intrauterine growth restriction

Yes → Steroids

Less than 23 weeks of gestation

23–32 weeks of gestation

33–34 weeks of gestation

33–34 weeks of gestation

Steroids at 24–32 weeks of gestation
Antihypertensives, if needed
Daily evaluations of maternal and fetal conditions
Delivery at 33 weeks of gestation

Fig. 12-2. Recommended management of severe preeclampsia. Maternal distress: thrombocytopenia, imminent eclampsia, pulmonary edema, and hemolysis plus elevated liver enzyme levels. (Modified from Sibai BM. diagnosis and management of gestational hypertension and preeclampsia. Obstet Gynecol 2003;102:181–92.)

fetal heart monitoring, a biophysical profile, and ultrasound assessment of fetal growth and amniotic fluid. For patients with resistant severe hypertension, despite maximum doses of IV labetalol (220 mg) plus oral nifedipine (50 mg), or persistent cerebral symptoms while taking magnesium sulfate, delivery is performed within 24–48 hours, regardless of fetal gestational age. In addition, patients with either thrombocytopenia or elevated liver enzymes with epigastric pain and tenderness or with serum creatinine of 2 mg/dL or more also undergo delivery within 48 hours (1).

Patients with gestational ages of 33–34 weeks are given corticosteroids and then undergo delivery after 48 hours. Patients with gestational ages below 23 weeks are

offered termination of pregnancy. Patients at 23–32 weeks of gestation receive individualized treatment based on their clinical response during the initial 24-hour observation period. If BP is adequately controlled and fetal test results are reassuring, magnesium sulfate is discontinued and the patients are then observed closely on the antepartum high-risk ward until 32 weeks of gestation or development of a maternal or fetal indication for delivery. During hospitalization, they receive antihypertensive drugs if needed, usually oral nifedipine (40–120 mg/d) plus labetalol (600–2,400 mg/d). The patients also receive daily assessment of maternal and fetal well-being (22). This therapy is appropriate only in a select group of patients and should be practiced only in a tertiary care center with adequate maternal and neonatal intensive care facilities. Once the decision is made for delivery, the patients should receive magnesium sulfate in labor and for at least 24 hours postpartum.

Intrapartum Management

The goals of treatment of women with gestational hypertension–preeclampsia are detection of fetal heart rate abnormalities, detection of progression from mild to severe disease, and prevention of maternal complications. Pregnancies complicated by preeclampsia, particularly those with severe disease or fetal growth restriction, are at risk for reduced fetal reserve and abruptio placentae. Therefore, women with preeclampsia should receive continuous monitoring of fetal heart rate and uterine activity, with special attention to hyperstimulation and development of vaginal bleeding during labor. The presence of uterine irritability or recurrent variable or late decelerations may be the first sign of abruptio placentae.

Some women with mild hypertension–preeclampsia will progress to severe disease as a result of changes in cardiac output and stress hormones during labor. Therefore, women with gestational hypertension–preeclampsia should have BP recordings every hour and need to be questioned about the new onset of symptoms suggesting severe disease. Those who develop severe hypertension or symptoms should be treated as for severe preeclampsia.

Maternal pain relief during labor and delivery can be provided by either systemic opioids or segmental epidural anesthesia. Epidural analgesia is considered the preferred method of pain relief in women with mild gestational hypertension and mild preeclampsia. Although there is no unanimity of opinion regarding the use of epidural anesthesia in women with severe preeclampsia and eclampsia, a significant body of evidence indicates that epidural anesthesia is safe in these women (1, 24). A randomized trial of 116 women with severe preeclampsia receiving either epidural analgesia or patient-controlled analgesia reported no differences in cesarean delivery rates, and the group receiving epidural analgesia had significantly better pain relief during labor (25).

Either epidural, spinal, or combined techniques or regional anesthesia are considered by most obstetric anesthesiologists to be the method of choice during cesarean delivery. In women with severe preeclampsia–eclampsia, general anesthesia increases the risk of aspiration and failed intubation because of airway edema and is associated with marked increases in systemic and cerebral pressures during intubation and extubation (1). Women with airway or laryngeal edema may require awake intubation under fiber optic observation with the availability of immediate tracheostomy. Changes in systemic and cerebral pressures may be attenuated by pretreatment with labetalol or nitroglycerine injections. It is important to emphasize that regional anesthesia is contraindicated in the presence of coagulopathy or severe thrombocytopenia.

Prevention of Convulsions

Magnesium sulfate is the drug of choice to prevent convulsions in women with preeclampsia. Recent randomized trials showed that magnesium sulfate is superior to a placebo for prevention of convulsions in women with severe preeclampsia (26). One of the largest randomized trials to date enrolled 10,141 women with preeclampsia in 33 nations (largely in the third world) (27). Almost all of the enrolled patients had severe disease by U.S. standards; 50% received antihypertensives before randomization, 75% received antihypertensives after randomization, and the remainder had severe preeclampsia or imminent eclampsia. Among all enrolled women, the rate of eclampsia was significantly lower in those assigned to magnesium sulfate (0.8% versus 1.9%; RR, 0.42; 95% CI, 0.29–0.60).

There are two randomized placebo-controlled trials evaluating the efficacy and safety of magnesium sulfate in women with mild preeclampsia. One of these trials included 135 women (28) and the other included only 222 (29). There were no instances of eclampsia in either group in both of these trials. In addition, the findings of both studies revealed that magnesium sulfate does not affect the duration of labor or the rate of cesarean delivery. However, neither of these studies had an adequate sample size to determine the efficacy of magnesium sulfate in preventing convulsions (28, 29). Therefore, the benefit of magnesium sulfate in women with mild preeclampsia remains unclear (21). For women with severe preeclampsia, a loading dose of magnesium sulfate of 6 grams over 15–20 minutes should be given, followed by a maintenance dose of 2 g/h as a continuous IV infusion. In women having elective cesarean delivery, magnesium sulfate is given at least 2 hours before the procedure and continued during delivery and for at least 24 hours postpartum. Serum magnesium levels are not monitored during the infusion because there is no established serum magnesium level that is considered "therapeutic." Serum magnesium levels require monitoring in the presence of renal dysfunction, oliguria (urine output less than 100 mL per 4 hours) or when there are absent reflexes. An occasional patient will have convulsions while receiving the above regimen of magnesium sulfate. In this case, a bolus of 2 grams magnesium sulfate can be given over 3–5 minutes.

Control of Severe Hypertension

The objective of treating acute severe hypertension is to prevent potential cerebrovascular and cardiovascular complications such as encephalopathy, hemorrhage, and congestive heart failure (1). For ethical reasons, there are no randomized trials to determine the level of hypertension to treat to prevent these complications. Antihypertensive therapy is recommended by some for sustained systolic BP values of at least 180 mm Hg and for sustained diastolic values of at least 110 mm Hg. Some experts recommend treating systolic levels of 160 mm Hg or greater, others recommend treating diastolic levels of 105 mm Hg or greater (30, 31), whereas others use a mean arterial BP of 130 mm Hg or greater (1). The definition of sustained hypertension is not clear, ranging from 30 minutes to 2 hours.

The most commonly used and advocated agent for the treatment of severe hypertension in pregnancy is IV hydralazine given as bolus injections of 5–10 mg every 15–20 minutes for a maximum dose of 30 mg. Several drugs were compared with hydralazine in small, randomized trials. The results of these trials were the subject of systematic reviews that suggested that IV labetalol or oral nifedipine is as effective as and has fewer side effects than IV hydralazine (20, 32). The recommended dose of these drugs and levels to treat are summarized in Table 12-3. Blood pressure values of at least 160 mm Hg (systolic) or at least 110 mm Hg (diastolic) are required to initiate therapy intrapartum. For women with thrombocytopenia and those in the postpartum period, use systolic values of at least 155 mm Hg or diastolic values of at least 105 mm Hg. The first-line agent is IV labetalol, and if maximum doses are ineffective, oral nifedipine can be added. Recent studies suggest that nifedipine can be safely used in women receiving magnesium sulfate (20, 33).

Mode of Delivery

There are no randomized trials comparing optimal methods of delivery in women with gestational hypertension–preeclampsia. A plan for vaginal delivery should be attempted for all women with mild disease and for most women with severe disease, particularly those beyond 30 weeks of gestation (1). The decision to perform cesarean delivery should be based on fetal gestational age, fetal condition, presence of labor, and cervical Bishop score. In general, the presence of severe preeclampsia–eclampsia is not an indication for cesarean delivery. It is appropriate to consider cesarean delivery for all women with severe preeclampsia at less than 30 weeks of gestation who are not in labor and whose Bishop score is below 5. Similar consideration for cesarean delivery is given to those with severe preeclampsia plus fetal growth restriction if the gestational age is less than 32 weeks in the presence of an unfavorable Bishop score.

HELLP Syndrome

The HELLP Syndrome—intravascular hemolysis, elevated liver function test results, and thrombocytopenia—has been described in women with severe preeclampsia–eclampsia for many decades (34). In addition, physicians have recognized that the presence of these abnormalities is associated with adverse maternal outcome (35, 36). In 1982, 29 cases of severe preeclampsia–eclampsia complicated by thrombocytopenia, abnormal peripheral blood smear, and abnormal liver function test results were described (37). It was suggested that this collection of laboratory abnormalities constituted an entity separate from traditional severe preeclampsia, and the term HELLP syndrome was coined. Since then, numerous reports claiming to describe this syndrome have appeared in the medical literature. During the past 20 years, numerous retrospective and observational studies as well as a few randomized trials have been published in an attempt to refine the diagnostic criteria for this syndrome, to identify risk factors for adverse pregnancy outcome, and to reduce adverse maternal and perinatal outcomes in women with this syndrome. Despite this recent literature, the diagnosis, management, and pregnancy outcome of HELLP syndrome remain controversial (34).

Diagnosis

LABORATORY CRITERIA

The diagnostic criteria used for HELLP syndrome are variable and inconsistent. Hemolysis, defined as the presence of microangiopathic hemolytic anemia, is the hallmark of the triad of HELLP syndrome (34). The classic findings of microangiopathic hemolysis include abnormal peripheral smear (schistocytes, burr cells, echinocytes), elevated serum bilirubin levels (indirect form), low serum haptoglobin levels, elevated l-lactate dehydrogenase (LDH) levels, and significant decrease in hemoglobin levels (Box 12-1). A significant percentage of published reports included patients who had no evidence of hemolysis; hence, these patients will fit the criteria for "ELLP" (elevated liver enzymes, low platelets) syndrome (38–44). Even in studies in which hemolysis was mentioned, the diagnosis was based on the presence of abnormal peripheral smear (no description of type or degree of abnormalities) (45, 46) or elevated LDH levels (threshold of 180–600 units/L) (47–52).

There is no consensus in the literature regarding which liver function test to use or what degree of elevation in these test results should be used to diagnose elevated liver enzymes (34). In studies in which elevated liver enzymes were mentioned (either aspartate transaminase [AST] or alanine transaminase [ALT]), the values considered abnormal ranged from 17 units/L to 72

BOX 12-1

RECOMMENDED CRITERIA FOR HEMOLYSIS, ELEVATED LIVER ENZYMES, AND LOW PLATELETS SYNDROME

- Hemolysis (at least two)
  —Peripheral smear (schistocytes, burr cells)
  —Serum bilirubin (1.2 mg/dL)
  —Low serum haptoglobin
  —Severe anemia, unrelated to blood loss
- Elevated liver enzymes
  —AST or ALT twice the upper limit of normal
  —LDH twice the upper limit of normal (also elevated in severe hemolysis)
- Low platelets (less than 100,000/mm^3)

Abbreviations: ALT, alanine transaminase; AST, aspartate transaminase; LDH, l-lactate dehydrogenase

units/L (34). In clinical practice, many of these values are considered normal or slightly elevated.

Low platelet count is the third abnormality required to establish the diagnosis of HELLP syndrome. There is no consensus among various published reports regarding the diagnosis of thrombocytopenia. The reported cutoff values range from 75,000/mm^3 to 279,000/mm^3 (39–47). Therefore, some of the patients included in these studies will fit the criteria for "EL" (elevated liver enzymes) syndrome. In essence, these women had severe preeclampsia with mild elevation in liver enzymes (39–41).

Despite well-intentioned efforts at determining a laboratory diagnosis of HELLP syndrome based on elevations in AST, ALT, and LDH levels and the presence of hemolysis, substantial interlaboratory differences remain a major problem. This is partially because of the different number of assays used to measure these tests as well as the cutoff used to establish an abnormal test result. Some studies used the upper limit for a particular test result at their hospital laboratory, some used two standard deviations above the mean for that laboratory, whereas others used more than two times the upper limit in their laboratory. Therefore, clinicians should be familiar with the upper limit value for liver enzyme test results in their own laboratory when diagnosing HELLP syndrome. For example, the upper limit for an LDH level may range from 180 units/L to 618 units/L depending on the assay being used. This is particularly important for patients referred from level I hospitals to tertiary care facilities where different assays are used to measure these tests.

TIME OF ONSET AND MATERNAL CONDITION AT DIAGNOSIS

Some studies included patients who had the abnormalities on admission (35, 36, 53–55), whereas others included

patients who developed the abnormalities during expectant management of preeclampsia (39–41, 56), and others included patients who developed the abnormalities in the postpartum period (49–52, 57–59). Even among the latter group, some had preeclampsia before delivery, some had no clinical evidence of preeclampsia before delivery, some were diagnosed during the first 48 hours postpartum, and others were diagnosed for the first time at or beyond 3 days postpartum (53–57). It is important to recognize that maternal and perinatal outcomes of women who are referred to a tertiary care facility because of HELLP syndrome (usually remote from term or complicated cases) are expected to be different from the respective outcomes of women in whom the diagnosis was based on serial evaluation of liver enzyme levels and platelet counts during management of preeclampsia. In addition, both maternal and perinatal outcomes are expected to be substantially worse in those patients in whom HELLP syndrome develops in the second trimester and who require emergency cesarean deliveries because of nonreassuring fetal test results than in women in whom severe preeclampsia develops at term and have spontaneous vaginal deliveries and subsequently receive the diagnosis of HELLP syndrome because of frequent evaluation of liver enzymes and platelet counts during labor and immediately postpartum.

CLINICAL FINDINGS

One of the major problems with early detection of HELLP syndrome lies in its clinical presentation because patients may present with nonspecific symptoms or subtle signs of preeclampsia. Patients may present with various signs and symptoms, none of which are diagnostic of preeclampsia and all of which may be found in patients with severe preeclampsia–eclampsia without HELLP syndrome (34). Patients frequently will have right upper quadrant or epigastric pain, nausea, or vomiting ranging in frequency from 30% to 90% (Table 12-4) (38, 46, 50, 53, 55). Most patients will give a history of malaise for the past few days before presentation, and some will have nonspecific viral-syndromelike symptoms (34). Headaches are reported by 33–61% of the patients (38, 50, 53) whereas visual changes are reported in approximately 17% of the patients (38). A subset of patients with HELLP syndrome may present with symptoms related to thrombocytopenia such as bleeding from mucosal surfaces, hematuria, petechial hemorrhages, or ecchymosis.

Although most patients will have hypertension (82–88%), it may be only mild in 15–50% of the cases, and absent in 12–18% of the cases. Most patients (86–100%) will have proteinuria by dipstick examination; however, it was reported to be absent in 13% of cases in the two largest series (38, 50, 53).

Table 12-4. Signs and Symptoms of Hemolysis, Elevated Liver Enzymes, and Low Platelets Syndrome

	Study			
	Weinstein (46) (n = 57)	Mercer et al (53) and Audibert et al (38) (n = 509)	Martin et al (50) (n = 501)	Rath et al (55) (n = 50)
Percentage with right upper quadrant or epigastric pain	86	63	40	90
Percentage with nausea or vomiting	84	36	29	52
Percentage with headache	Not reported	33	61	Not reported
Percentage with hypertension	Not reported	85	82	88
Percentage with proteinuria	96	87	86	100

DIFFERENTIAL DIAGNOSIS

The presenting symptoms, clinical findings, and many of the laboratory findings in women with HELLP syndrome overlap with a number of medical syndromes, surgical conditions, and obstetric complications. Therefore, the differential diagnosis of HELLP syndrome should include any of the conditions listed in Box 12-2. Because some patients with HELLP syndrome may present with gastrointestinal, respiratory, or hematologic symptoms in association with elevated liver enzymes or low platelets in the absence of hypertension or proteinuria, many cases of HELLP syndrome will initially be misdiagnosed (34). Conversely, some conditions such as thrombotic thrombocytopenic purpura, hemolytic uremic syndrome, systemic lupus erythematosus, sepsis, or catastrophic antiphospholipid syndrome may be erroneously diagnosed as HELLP syndrome.

Because of the remarkably similar clinical and laboratory findings of these disease processes, even the most experienced physician will face a difficult diagnostic challenge. Therefore, an effort should be made to identify an accurate diagnosis given that management strategies may differ among these conditions.

Maternal and Perinatal Outcome

The presence of HELLP syndrome is associated with an increased risk of maternal death (1%) and morbidities such as pulmonary edema (8%), acute renal failure (3%), disseminated intravascular coagulation (DIC) (15%), abruptio placentae (9%), liver hemorrhage or failure (1%), adult respiratory distress syndrome, sepsis, and stroke (less than 1%). They also are associated with increased rates of wound hematomas and the need for transfusion of blood and blood products (34). The rates of these complications will depend on the population studied, the criteria used to establish the diagnosis, and

the presence of associated preexisting medical conditions (chronic hypertension, lupus) or obstetric complications (abruptio placentae, peripartum hemorrhage, fetal demise, eclampsia). The development of HELLP syndrome in the postpartum period also increases the risk of renal failure and pulmonary edema (60, 61). The presence of abruptio placentae increases the risk of DIC, need for blood transfusions, pulmonary edema, and renal failure (53, 60–62). Patients who have large volume ascites will have a high rate of cardiopulmonary complications (63).

Perinatal mortality and morbidities also are increased in HELLP syndrome. The reported perinatal death rate in recent series ranged from 7.4% to 20.4% (50, 54, 64–66). This high perinatal death rate is mainly experienced at a very early gestational age (less than 28 weeks), in association with severe fetal growth restriction or abruptio placentae (64–66). It is important to

---

BOX 12-2

DIFFERENTIAL DIAGNOSIS IN WOMEN WITH HEMOLYSIS, ELEVATED LIVER ENZYMES, AND LOW PLATELET COUNT SYNDROME

- Acute fatty liver of pregnancy
- Thrombotic thrombocytopenic purpura
- Hemolytic uremic syndrome
- Immune thrombocytopenic purpura
- Systemic lupus erythematosus
- Antiphospholipid syndrome
- Cholecystitis
- Fulminant viral hepatitis
- Acute pancreatitis
- Pulmonary embolism
- Disseminated herpes simplex
- Hemorrhagic or septic shock

emphasize that neonatal morbidities are dependent on gestational age at delivery and similar to those in pre-eclamptic pregnancies without the HELLP syndrome (54, 64–66).

Expectant Management

The clinical course of women with true HELLP syndrome usually is characterized by progressive and sometimes sudden deterioration in the maternal condition (34). Because the presence of this syndrome is associated with increased rates of maternal morbidity and mortality, some authors consider its presence an indication for immediate delivery (37, 55). There also is a consensus that prompt delivery is indicated if the syndrome develops beyond 34 weeks of gestation, or earlier if there is multiorgan dysfunction, DIC, liver infarction or hemorrhage, renal failure, suspected abruptio placentae, or nonreassuring fetal status (34).

However, there is considerable disagreement about the treatment of women with HELLP syndrome at or before 34 weeks of gestation when the maternal condition is stable except for mild to moderate abnormalities in blood test results and a reassuring fetal condition. In such patients, some authors recommend the administration of corticosteroids to accelerate fetal lung maturity followed by delivery after 24 hours (34, 42, 43), whereas others recommend prolonging pregnancy until the development of maternal or fetal indications for delivery or until achievement of fetal lung maturity or 34 weeks of gestation (40, 45, 54, 66). Some of the measures used in these latter cases have included one or more of the following treatments: bed rest, antihypertensive agents, antithrombotic agents, plasma volume expanders, and steroids.

Recently, investigators from the Netherlands reported that expectant management is possible in women with HELLP syndrome before 34 weeks of gestation. In one study, the use of plasma volume expansion, using invasive hemodynamic monitoring and vasodilators, was reported in 128 women with HELLP syndrome before 34 weeks of gestation (54). Magnesium sulfate and steroids were not used in such women. Delivery was performed in 22 of the 128 patients within 48 hours; the remaining 102 patients had pregnancy prolongation for a median of 15 days (range, 3–62 days). Of these 102 women, 55 had antepartum resolution of HELLP syndrome with a median pregnancy prolongation of 21 days (range, 7–62 days). There were no maternal deaths or serious maternal morbidity; however, 11 pregnancies (8.6%) resulted in fetal death at 25–34.4 weeks of gestation, and there were 7 (5.5%) neonatal deaths at 27–32 weeks of gestation (54).

The use of bed rest, antihypertensive medication, and salt restriction was reported in a study of 41 women with HELLP syndrome before 35 weeks of gestation (65). Delivery was performed in 14 women (34%), delivery was performed within 24 hours; in the remaining 27 women, pregnancy was prolonged a median of 3 days (range, 0–59 days). Fifteen of these 27 women showed complete normalization of the laboratory abnormalities. There were no serious maternal morbidities; however, there were 10 fetal deaths at 27–35.7 weeks of gestation.

The results of these studies suggest that expectant management is possible in a very select group of patients with alleged HELLP syndrome before 34 weeks of gestation. However, despite pregnancy prolongation in some of these cases, the overall perinatal outcome was not improved compared with cases at similar gestational age in which delivery was performed within 48 hours after the diagnosis of HELLP syndrome (64). Therefore, such management remains experimental in the absence of randomized trials.

Use of Corticosteroids

Corticosteroids have been suggested as safe and effective drugs for improving maternal and neonatal outcome in women with HELLP or partial HELLP syndrome (48–52). A review of the literature reveals substantial differences in methodology, time of administration, and drug selection among investigators who advocate the use of corticosteroids in women with HELLP syndrome. Different regimens of steroids have been suggested for preventing respiratory distress syndrome as well as accelerating maternal recovery in the postpartum period. The regimens of steroids used included intramuscular betamethasone (12 mg every 12 h or 24 hours apart on two occasions) or IV dexamethasone (various doses at various time intervals) or a combination of the two (42–44, 48–52, 67). Some studies used steroids in the antepartum period only (for 24 hours, 48 hours, repeat regimens, or long-term for weeks until delivery). In other studies, steroids were given for 48 hours before delivery and then continued for 24–48 hours postpartum (43, 44, 51, 52), whereas others recommend their administration in the postpartum period only (58, 59).

In the first randomized, double-blind, placebo-controlled trial of the use of dexamethasone treatment to improve maternal outcome in patients with true HELLP syndrome, a total of 132 women with HELLP syndrome (60 antepartum and 72 postpartum) were studied (68). The primary outcome of the trial was mean days of hospitalization. They found that treatment with high-dose intravenous dexamethasone did not reduce the duration of hospitalizations. In addition, the rates of platelets and fresh frozen plasma transfusions as well as serious maternal complications were not reduced by treatment with dexamethasone (68). Thus, the use of high-dose dexamethasone to improve maternal outcome in women with HELLP syndrome beyond 34 weeks of gestation or postpartum remains experimental (69).

Antepartum Management

Patients in whom HELLP syndrome is suspected should be hospitalized immediately and observed in a labor and delivery unit. Such patients should be treated for severe preeclampsia and should initially receive intravenous magnesium sulfate as prophylaxis against convulsions and antihypertensive medications (34).

The next step in management is to confirm or exclude the diagnosis of HELLP syndrome from other conditions listed in Box 12-2. Blood tests should include a complete blood count with platelet count, a peripheral smear, coagulation studies, serum AST levels, creatinine, glucose, bilirubin, and LDH levels. The diagnosis of HELLP syndrome requires the presence of criteria listed in Box 12-1.

Once the diagnosis of HELLP syndrome is confirmed, a decision is made regarding the need for delivery (Fig. 12-3). Patients with HELLP syndrome who are at less than 35 weeks of gestation should be referred to a tertiary care facility if the maternal and fetal conditions are stable. The first priority is to assess and stabilize the maternal condition, particularly BP and coagulation abnormalities. The next step is to evaluate fetal status with the use of fetal heart rate testing, biophysical profile, or Doppler assessment of fetal vessels. Finally, a decision must be made as to whether delivery should be initiated or delivery could be delayed for 48 hours for corticosteroid benefit. It is recommended to initiate delivery in all patients with true HELLP syndrome except in those with a gestational age between 24 weeks and 34 weeks with stable maternal and fetal conditions. These latter patients are given either betamethasone or dexamethasone, and then delivery is performed within 24 hours

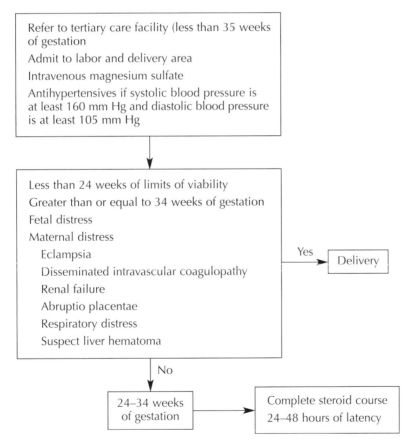

Fig. 12-3. Management of hemolysis, elevated liver enzymes, and low platelet count syndrome. (Modified from Sibai BM. Diagnosis, controversies, and management of the syndrome of hemolysis, elevated liver enzymes, and low platelet count. Obstet Gynecol 2004;103:981–9.)

after the last dose of corticosteroids. Maternal and fetal conditions are assessed continuously during this period. In some of these patients, there may be transient improvement in maternal laboratory test results; however, delivery is still indicated despite such improvement.

Intrapartum Management

The presence of HELLP syndrome is not an indication for immediate cesarean delivery. Such an approach might prove detrimental for both mother and fetus. The decision to perform cesarean delivery should be based on fetal gestational age, fetal conditions, presence of labor, and cervical Bishop score (34). It is recommended to perform elective cesarean delivery for those before 30 weeks of gestation who are not in labor and whose Bishop score is below 5. Patients in labor or with rupture of membranes are allowed to give birth vaginally in the absence of obstetric complications.

Maternal pain relief during labor and delivery can be provided by intermittent use of small doses of systemic opioids. Local infiltration anesthesia can be used for all vaginal deliveries in case of episiotomy or laceration repair. The use of pudendal block is contraindicated in these patients because of the risk of bleeding and hematoma formation into this area (34). Epidural anesthesia also is contraindicated, particularly if the platelet count is less than 75,000/mm³. Therefore, general anesthesia is the method of choice for cesarean delivery in such patients. The impact of corticosteroid administration on the rate of epidural anesthesia use has been assessed in 37 women with partial HELLP syndrome who had a platelet count below 90,000/mm³ before steroid administration (44). The authors found that administration of corticosteroids in these patients increased the rate of epidural anesthesia use, particularly in those who achieved a latency period of 24 hours before delivery (8 of 14 in the steroid group versus 0 of 10 in the no-steroid group, $P = .006$) (44).

Platelet transfusions are indicated either before or after delivery in the presence of significant bleeding (ecchymosis, bleeding from gums, oozing from puncture sites, wound, intraperitoneal), and in those with a platelet count of less than 20,000/mm³. Repeated platelet transfusions are not necessary because of the short half-life of the transfused platelets in such patients. Correction of thrombocytopenia also is important before any surgery. Administer 6 units of platelets in all patients with a platelet count less than 40,000/mm³ before intubation if cesarean delivery is needed. Generalized oozing from the surgical site can occur during surgery or in the immediate postpartum period because of the continued decrease in platelet count in

some of these patients. The risk of hematoma formation at these sites is approximately 20%. It is advisable to use a subfascial drain and to keep the skin incision open for at least 48 hours in patients requiring cesarean delivery (34).

Eclampsia

Eclampsia is defined as the development of convulsions or unexplained coma during pregnancy or postpartum in patients with signs and symptoms of preeclampsia (70). In the Western world, the reported incidence of eclampsia ranges from 1:2,000 pregnancies to 1:3,448 pregnancies (71–73). The reported incidence usually is higher in tertiary referral centers, in multifetal gestation, and in populations with no prenatal care (74, 75).

Diagnosis

The diagnosis of eclampsia is secure in the presence of hypertension, proteinuria, and convulsions. However, women in whom eclampsia develops exhibit a wide spectrum of signs, ranging from severe hypertension, severe proteinuria, and generalized edema to absent or minimal hypertension, no proteinuria, and no edema (75). Hypertension is the hallmark for the diagnosis of eclampsia and can be severe in 20–54% of cases or mild in 30–60% of cases (73, 76). However, in 16% of the cases, hypertension may be absent (76). In addition, severe hypertension is more common in patients who develop antepartum eclampsia (58%) and in those who develop eclampsia at 32 weeks of gestation or earlier (71%) (76).

Eclampsia usually is associated with proteinuria (at least 1+ on dipstick) (75, 76). In a series of 399 women with eclampsia, substantial proteinuria (greater than or equal to 3+ on dipstick) was present in only 48% of the cases, whereas proteinuria was absent in 14% of the cases (76).

Several symptoms are potentially helpful in establishing the diagnosis of eclampsia. These may occur before or after the onset of convulsions, and include persistent occipital or frontal headaches, blurred vision, photophobia, epigastric or right upper-quadrant pain or both, and altered mental status. Patients will have at least one symptom in 59–75% of cases (Table 12-4) (73, 77, 78).

TIME OF ONSET

Eclamptic convulsions can occur during the antepartum, intrapartum, or postpartum periods (Table 12-5) (73, 76–78). Although most cases of postpartum eclampsia occur within the first 48 hours, some develop beyond 48 hours and have been reported as late as 23 days postpartum (76, 78, 79). In the latter cases, an extensive neurologic evaluation is needed to rule out the presence of other cerebral pathologies (78, 79). This evaluation should include neurologic examination, brain imaging, cerebrovascular testing, lumbar puncture, and blood tests, as needed.

Almost all cases (91%) of eclampsia develop at or beyond 28 weeks of gestation (76). The remaining cases occur between 21 weeks and 27 weeks (7.5%) or before 20 weeks of gestation (76). Eclampsia occurring before 20 weeks of gestation usually has been reported with molar or hydropic degeneration of the placenta, with or without a coexistent fetus (80, 81). Eclampsia occurring before 20 weeks of gestation without molar degeneration of the placenta has been described in case reports (76, 80). These women may be misdiagnosed as having hypertensive encephalopathy, seizure disorder, or thrombotic thrombocytopenic purpura. Women in whom convulsions develop in association with hypertension and proteinuria during the first half of pregnancy should be considered to have eclampsia until proved otherwise. These women should have ultrasound examinations of the uterus to rule out molar pregnancy or hydropic or cystic degeneration of the placenta.

Late postpartum eclampsia is defined as eclampsia that occurs more than 48 hours, but less than 4 weeks, after delivery (79). These women will have signs and symptoms consistent with preeclampsia in association with convulsions (78, 79). Some will demonstrate a clinical picture of preeclampsia during labor or immediately postpartum (56%), whereas others will demonstrate these clinical findings for the first time more than 48 hours after delivery (44%) (79). Late postpartum eclampsia can develop despite the use of magnesium during labor and for at least 24 hours postpartum in pre-

viously diagnosed preeclamptic women (78, 79). Therefore, women in whom convulsions develop in association with hypertension or proteinuria or with headaches or blurred vision after 48 hours of delivery should be considered to have eclampsia and initially treated as such (78, 79).

CEREBRAL PATHOLOGY

The pathogenesis of eclamptic convulsions continues to be the subject of extensive investigation and speculation, but the cause is unknown. Several theories and mechanisms have been implicated as possible etiologic factors, but none of these have been conclusively proved. Some of the mechanisms that are implicated in the pathogenesis of eclamptic convulsions have included cerebral vasoconstriction, hypertensive encephalopathy, cerebral edema or infarction.

Cerebral pathology in cortical and subcortical white matter in the form of edema, infarction, and hemorrhage is a common autopsy finding in patients who die from eclampsia (82–84). In patients who died from eclampsia, autopsy information is not necessarily indicative of the central nervous system abnormality present in most patients who survive this condition (85). Focal neurologic signs such as hemiparesis or unconscious state are rare in large eclampsia series reported from developed countries (83, 86, 87). Although eclamptic patients may initially manifest a variety of neurologic abnormalities, including cortical blindness, focal motor deficits, and coma, most of them have no permanent neurologic deficits (85, 87). These neurologic abnormalities are probably caused by a transient insult, such as hypoxia, ischemia, or edema (85).

Several neurodiagnostic tests such as electroencephalography, computed axial tomographic scan, cere-

Table 12-5. Time of Onset of Eclampsia in Relation to Delivery

Symptom	Study			
	Douglas and Redman (73) (n = 383)	Katz et al (77) (n = 53)	Mattar and Sibai (76) (n = 399)	Chames et al (78) (n = 89)
Percentage at antepartum	38	53	53	67*
Percentage at intrapartum	18	36	19	—
Percentage at postpartum	44	11	28	33
less than or equal to 48 h	39	5	11	7
more than 48 h	5	6	17	26

*Includes antepartum and intrapartum cases.

bral laser-Doppler velocimetry, magnetic resonance imaging (MRI), and cerebral angiography (both traditional and MRI angiography) have been studied in women with eclampsia (88). In general, results of electroencephalography (EEG) are acutely abnormal in eclamptic patients, but these abnormalities are not pathognomic of eclampsia. In addition, the abnormal EEG results are not affected by the use of magnesium sulfate (88). Moreover, lumbar puncture is not helpful in the diagnosis and management of eclamptic women. The results of computed tomography scans and MRI reveal the presence of edema and infarction within the subcortical white matter and adjacent gray matter, mostly in the parieto-occipital lobes in approximately 50% of cases (85, 88–90). Cerebral angiography and laser-Doppler velocimetry results suggest the presence of vasospasm (88, 91).

Recently, various forms of brain imaging were used to characterize the relative frequency of vasogenic and cytotoxic edema in two series of eclamptic women (92, 93). Cerebral edema (mostly vasogenic) was present in 93–100% of these women (92, 93). However, concurrent foci of infarction were present in 6 of 27 eclamptic women in one study (92) and in 3 of 17 eclamptic and preeclamptic women in another study (93). In addition, 5 of these 6 women in the former study had persistent abnormalities on repeat MRI testing 6–8 weeks later, suggesting that these lesions might not be reversible (92). Moreover, 4 of the 17 women in the latter study had persistent MRI abnormalities at a follow-up at 8 weeks (median) (93).

Cerebral imaging is not necessary for the diagnosis and management of eclampsia in most women, but is indicated for patients with focal neurologic deficits or prolonged coma. In these patients, hemorrhage and other serious abnormalities requiring specific pharmacologic therapy or surgery must be excluded. Cerebral imaging also may be helpful in patients who have atypical presentation for eclampsia (onset before 20 weeks of gestation or more than 48 hours after delivery, and eclampsia refractory to adequate magnesium sulfate therapy) (70, 88).

DIFFERENTIAL DIAGNOSIS

The presenting symptoms, clinical findings, and many of the laboratory findings overlap with a number of medical and surgical conditions (79, 44–97). The most common cause of convulsions developing in association with hypertension or proteinuria during pregnancy or immediately postpartum is eclampsia. Rarely, other causes producing convulsions in pregnancy or postpartum may mimic eclampsia (Box 12-3).

Maternal and Perinatal Outcome

Although eclampsia is associated with an increased risk of maternal death in developed countries (0 –1.8%) (70, 98), the mortality rate is as high as 14% in developing countries (83, 84, 89). The high rate of maternal mortality reported from the developing countries was noted primarily among patients who had multiple seizures outside the hospital and those without prenatal care (70, 84, 99). In addition, this high mortality rate could be attributed to the lack of resources and intensive care facilities needed to manage maternal complications from eclampsia (75). A review of all reported pregnancy-related deaths in the United States for the years 1979–1992 identified 4,024 pregnancy-related deaths (100). A total of 790 (19.6%) deaths were considered caused by preeclampsia–eclampsia, with 49% of these 790 deaths considered related to eclampsia. The authors found that the risk of death from preeclampsia or eclampsia was higher for women older than 30 years and those with no prenatal care, as well as for African-American women. The greatest risk of death was found among women with pregnancies at or before 28 weeks of gestation (100).

Pregnancies complicated by eclampsia also are associated with increased rates of maternal morbidities, such as abruptio placentae (7–10%) (70), DIC (7–11%) (70), pulmonary edema (3–5%), acute renal failure (5–9%), aspiration pneumonia (2–3%), and cardiopulmonary

---

BOX 12-3

DIFFERENTIAL DIAGNOSIS OF ECLAMPSIA

- Cerebrovascular accidents
  —Hemorrhage
  —Ruptured aneurysm or malformation
  —Arterial embolism or thrombosis
  —Cerebral venous thrombosis
  —Hypoxic ischemic encephalopathy
  —Angiomas
- Hypertensive encephalopathy
- Seizure disorder
- Previously undiagnosed brain tumors
- Metastatic gestational trophoblastic disease
- Metabolic diseases
  —Hypoglycemia
  —Hyponatremia
- Reversible posterior leukoencephalopathy syndrome
- Thrombophilia
- Thrombotic thrombocytopenic purpura
- Postdural puncture syndrome
- Cerebral vasculitis

arrest (2–5%) (70). Adult respiratory distress syndrome and intracerebral hemorrhage are rare complications among eclamptic series reported from the developed world (70). The risks of HELLP syndrome (10–15%) and liver hematoma (1%) are similar in eclamptic and severely preeclamptic patients. Maternal complications are significantly higher among women who develop antepartum eclampsia, particularly among those who develop eclampsia remote from term (73, 76, 84).

Perinatal mortality and morbidities remain high in eclamptic pregnancies. The reported perinatal death rate in recent series ranged from 5.6% to 11.8% (73, 76, 84). This high perinatal death rate is related to prematurity, abruptio placentae, and severe fetal growth restriction (70).

Prevention

The low incidence of eclampsia in developed countries is probably related to prevention of cases of eclampsia in women with a classic presentation and with a classic progression from mild to severe preeclampsia (73, 77). As a result, most cases of eclampsia described in reported series from the United States and Europe were found to have atypical presentation (abrupt onset, development of convulsions while receiving prophylactic magnesium sulfate, or onset of convulsions beyond 48 hours after delivery) (70, 72, 73, 101, 102). Indeed, most eclamptic convulsions in these series developed in hospitalized women, and the onset of convulsions in some of these women was not preceded by warning signs or symptoms (73, 77, 101, 102). Overall, the percentage of eclampsia considered unpreventable in these series ranged from 31% to 87% (72, 73, 101, 102).

There are several randomized trials comparing the efficacy of magnesium sulfate with other anticonvulsive agents for the prevention of recurrent seizures in women with eclampsia (99, 103). In these trials, magnesium sulfate was compared with diazepam, phenytoin, or a lytic cocktail (pethidine, chlorpromazine, and promethazine). Overall, these trials revealed that magnesium sulfate was associated with a significantly lower rate of recurrent seizures (9.4% versus 23.1%; RR, 0.41; 95% CI, 0.32–0.51) and a lower rate of maternal death (3.0% versus 4.8%; RR, 0.62; 95% CI 0.39–0.99) than that observed with other agents (103).

Management

The first priority in the management of eclampsia is to prevent maternal injury and to support respiratory and cardiovascular functions. During or immediately after the acute convulsive episode, supportive care should be given to prevent serious maternal injury and aspiration, assess and establish airway potency, and ensure maternal oxygenation. During this time, the bed's side rails should be elevated and padded, a padded tongue blade should be inserted between the teeth (avoid inducing gag reflex), and physical restraints may be needed (70). To minimize the risk of aspiration, the patient should lie in lateral decubitus position, and vomitus and oral secretion are suctioned as needed.

During the convulsive episode, hypoventilation and respiratory acidosis often occur. Although the initial seizure lasts only a few minutes, it is important to maintain oxygenation by supplemental oxygen administration via a face mask with or without oxygen reservoir at 8–10 L/min (70). After the convulsion has ceased, the patient begins to breathe again and oxygenation is rarely a problem. However, maternal hypoxemia and acidosis may develop in women who have had repetitive convulsions and in those with aspiration pneumonia or pulmonary edema. Transcutaneous pulse oximetry is useful to monitor oxygenation in eclamptic patients. Arterial blood gas analysis is required if the pulse oximetry results are abnormal (oxygen saturation at or below 92%).

The next step is to prevent recurrent convulsions. Magnesium sulfate is the drug of choice to treat and prevent subsequent convulsions in women with eclampsia (99, 103). Give a loading dose of 6 g over 15–20 minutes, followed by a maintenance dose of 2 g/h as a continuous intravenous infusion. Approximately 10% of women with eclampsia will have a second convulsion after receiving magnesium sulfate (99, 103). In these women, another bolus of 2g of magnesium sulfate can be given intravenously over 3–5 minutes. An occasional patient will have recurrent convulsions while receiving adequate doses of magnesium sulfate. In this patient, recurrent seizures can be treated with sodium amobarbital, 250 mg intravenously over 3–5 minutes (70).

The next step is to reduce the blood pressure to a safe range but at the same time avoid significant hypotension. The objective of treating severe hypertension is to avoid loss of cerebral autoregulation and to prevent congestive heart failure without compromising cerebral perfusion or uteroplacental blood flow that is already reduced in many women with eclampsia (88). Keep systolic blood pressure between 140 mm Hg and 160 mm Hg and diastolic blood pressure between 90 mm Hg and 110 mm Hg. The rationale for keeping maternal blood pressure at these levels is to avoid potential reduction in either uteroplacental blood flow or cerebral perfusion pressure. Other potent antihypertensive medications such as sodium nitroprusside or nitroglycerine are rarely needed in eclampsia. Diuretics are not used except in the presence of pulmonary edema.

Maternal hypoxemia and hypercarbia cause fetal heart rate and uterine activity changes during and immediately following a convulsion. Fetal heart rate changes can include bradycardia, transient late decelerations, decreased beat-to-beat variability, and compensatory tachycardia. Changes in uterine activity can include increased frequency and tone (104). These changes usually resolve spontaneously within 3–10 minutes after the termination of convulsions and the correction of maternal hypoxemia. The patient should not be rushed for an emergency cesarean delivery based on these findings, especially if the maternal condition is not stable. It is considered to be advantageous to the fetus to allow in utero recovery from hypoxia and hypercarbia caused by maternal convulsions. However, if the bradycardia or recurrent late decelerations persist beyond 10–15 minutes despite all resuscitation efforts, then a diagnosis of abruptio placentae or nonreassuring fetal status should be considered.

The presence of eclampsia is not an indication for cesarean delivery. The decision to perform cesarean delivery is based on gestational age, fetal condition, presence of labor, and cervical Bishop score (70). Cesarean delivery is recommended for those with eclampsia before 30 weeks of gestation who are not in labor and whose Bishop score is below 5. Patients having labor or rupture of membranes are allowed to give birth vaginally in the absence of obstetric complications. When labor is indicated, it is initiated with either oxytocin infusions or prostaglandins in all patients with a gestational age of 30 weeks or more, regardless of the Bishop score. Maternal pain relief during labor and delivery can be provided by either systemic opioids or epidural anesthesia as recommended for women with severe preeclampsia.

Postpartum Management of Preeclampsia–Eclampsia and HELLP Syndrome

During the immediate postpartum period, women with preeclampsia–eclampsia should receive close monitoring of BP and symptoms and accurate measurements of fluid intake and urinary output. These women usually receive large amounts of IV fluids during labor, as a result of prehydration before the administration of epidural analgesia, and IV fluids given during the administration of oxytocin and magnesium sulfate in labor and postpartum. In addition, during the postpartum period there is mobilization of extracellular fluid leading to increased intravascular volume. As a result, women with severe preeclampsia—particularly those with abnormal renal function, those with capillary leaks, and those with early onset—are at increased risk for pulmonary edema and exacerbation of severe hypertension postpartum. These women should receive frequent evaluation of the

amount of IV fluids, oral intake, blood products, and urine output as well as monitoring by pulse oximetry and pulmonary auscultation.

Patients with HELLP syndrome and those with eclampsia should receive close monitoring of vital signs, fluid intake and output, laboratory values, and pulse oximetry for at least 48 hours. In general, most patients will show evidence of resolution of the disease process within 48 hours after delivery. However, some patients, especially those with abruptio placentae plus DIC, those with severe thrombocytopenia (platelet count less than 20,000/mm^3), and those with severe ascites or significant renal dysfunction may show delayed resolution or even deterioration in their clinical condition. Such patients are at risk of the development of pulmonary edema from transfusion of blood and blood products, fluid mobilization, and compromised renal function. These patients also are at risk of acute tubular necrosis and need for dialysis (34, 70), and may require intensive monitoring for several days.

Severe hypertension or severe preeclampsia, HELLP syndrome, or eclampsia may develop for the first time in the postpartum period (1, 34, 70, 105). Hence, all postpartum women should be educated about the signs and symptoms of severe hypertension or preeclampsia. Therefore, medical care providers as well as personnel who answer phone calls from patients should be educated and instructed about the important information to report to physicians (78, 105). In addition, women who have persistent severe headaches, visual changes, epigastric pain with nausea or vomiting, and severe hypertension require immediate evaluation and potential hospitalization. These women receive magnesium sulfate for at least 24 hours and are given antihypertensive drugs to keep the BP below the severe range. If the patient does not respond to such therapy, then brain imaging should be performed to rule out the presence of other cerebral pathology (78, 94).

In general, most women with gestational hypertension become normotensive during the first week postpartum. In contrast, the hypertension takes a longer time to resolve in women with preeclampsia (106). In addition, there is an initial decrease in BP immediately postpartum in some women with preeclampsia, followed by development of hypertension again between day 3 and day 6 (107). In this case, antihypertensive drugs should be used if the systolic BP is at least 155 mm Hg or if the diastolic BP is at least 105 mm Hg. The drug of choice is oral nifedipine (10 mg every 6 hours) or long-acting nifedipine (30 mg twice daily) to keep BP below that level. Oral nifedipine offers the benefit of diuresis in the postpartum period (108). If BP is well controlled and there are no maternal symptoms, the woman is then discharged with instructions for measurements in one week. Antihypertensive medications are discontinued if the pressure remains below the hypertensive levels.

Subsequent Pregnancy Outcome and Remote Prognosis

Women with a history of preeclampsia–eclampsia are at increased risk of recurrence of all forms of hypertension in subsequent pregnancies. The risk is dependent on body mass index, severity of the disease, gestational age at onset, presence of underlying medical disease, and on the study population. In women with gestational hypertension, the reported recurrence was 29–46.8% (109–111). In women with preeclampsia, the recurrence risk was 7.5–18% (109–112). For those with severe preeclampsia, the risk was 25%. For those with preeclampsia in the second trimester, the risk is 65% (113). The recurrent risk for HELLP syndrome is 2–6% (114–116). The recurrent risk for eclampsia is 1–1.9% (70, 87).

Several studies have suggested that women who develop preeclampsia are at increased risk of cardiovascular complications later in life (117–121). Many risk factors and pathophysiologic abnormalities of preeclampsia are similar to those of coronary artery disease (117–120). Pregnancies complicated by preeclampsia could identify women at risk of cardiovascular disease in later life and provide the opportunity for life-style and risk-factor modification.

Summary

Most adverse pregnancy outcomes occur in women with early onset of preeclampsia and those with severe disease. Expectant management of severe preeclampsia is possible in a select group of patients with stable maternal–fetal conditions at 24–32 weeks of gestation. The use of complete bed rest and antihypertensive medications does not improve perinatal outcome in women with mild hypertension–preeclampsia. Magnesium sulfate is the drug of choice to prevent seizures in severe preeclampsia and to prevent recurrent seizures in eclampsia. The diagnosis of HELLP syndrome requires evidence of hemolysis, elevated liver enzymes, and thrombocytopenia (less than 100,000/mm³). The presence of severe preeclampsia, eclampsia or HELLP syndrome is not an indication for cesarean section. Women with previous history of preeclampsia, HELLP, or eclampsia are at increased risk of recurrence in subsequent pregnancies. Women with a history of preeclampsia–eclampsia are at risk for cardiovascular disease and stroke later in life.

References

1. Sibai BM. Diagnosis and management of gestational hypertension and preeclampsia. Obstet Gynecol 2003; 103:181–92.

2. Diagnosis and management of preeclampsia and eclampsia. ACOG Practice Bulletin No. 33. American College of Obstetricians and Gynecologists. Obstet Gynecol 2002; 99:159–67.

3. Sibai B, Dekker G, Kupferminc M. Preeclampsia. Lancet 2005;365:785–99.

4. Barton JR, O'Brien JM, Bergauer NK, Jacques DL, Sibai BM, Mild gestational hypertension remote from term: progression and outcome. Am J Obstet Gynecol 2001; 184:979–83.

5. Myer NL, Mercer BM, Friedman SA, Sibai BM. Urinary dipstick protein: a poor predictor of absent or severe proteinuria. Am J Obstet Gynecol 1994;170:137–41.

6. Levine RJ, Maynard SE, Qian C, Lim KH, England LJ, Yu KF, et al. Circulating angiogenic factors and the risk of preeclampsia. N Engl J Med 2004;350:672–83.

7. Conde-Aqudelo A, Villar J, Lindheimer M. World Health Organization systemic review of screening tests for preeclampsia. Obstet Gynecol 2004;104:1367–71.

8. Sibai BM. Prevention of preeclampsia: A big disappointment. Am J Obstet Gynecol 1998;179:1275–8.

9. Levine RJ, Hauth JC, Curet LB, Sibai BM, Catalano PM, Morris CD. Trial of calcium to prevent preeclampsia. N Engl J Med 1997;337:69–76.

10. Villar J, Abdel-Aleem H, Merialdi M, Mathai M, Ali MM, Zavaleta N, et al. World Health Organization randomized trial of calcium supplementation among low calcium intake pregnant women. Am J Obstet Gynecol 2006; 194:639–49.

11. Knight M, Duley L, Henderson-Smart DJ, King JF. Antiplatelet agents for preventing and treating preeclampsia. The Cochrane Database or Syst Rev 2000; (2):CD000492. Review.

12. Poston L, Briley AL, Seed PT, Kelly FJ, Shennan AH. Vitamin C and vitamin E in pregnant women at risk for preeclampsia (VIP trial): randomized placebo-controlled trial. Lancet 2006;367:1145–54.

13. Rumbold AR, Crowther CA, Haslam RR, Dekker GA, Robinson JS, for the ACTS Study Group. N Engl J Med 2006;354:1796–806.

14. Knuist M, Bonsel GJ, Zondervan HA, Treffers PE. Intensification of fetal and maternal surveillance in pregnant women with hypertensive disorders. Int J Gynecol. Obstet 1998;61:127.

15. Hauth JC, Ewell MG, Levine RL, Esterlitz JR, Sibai BM, Curet LB. Pregnancy outcomes in healthy nulliparas who subsequently developed hypertension. Obstet Gynecol 2000;95:24–8.

16. Sibai BM, Caritis S, Hauth J, Lindheimer MD, MacPherson C, Klebanoff M, et al. Hypertensive disorders in twin versus singleton gestations. National Institute of Child Health and Human Development Network of Maternal-Fetal Medicine Units. Am J Obstet Gynecol 2000;182:938–42.

17. Buchbinder A, Sibai BM, Caritis S, MacPherson C, Hauth J, Lindheimer MD. Adverse perinatal outcomes

are significantly higher in severe gestational hypertension than in mild preeclampsia. Am J Obstet Gynecol 2002;186: 66–71.

18. Hnat MD, Sibai BM, Caritis S. Hauth J, Lindheimer MD, MacPherson C. Perinatal outcome in women with recurrent preeclampsia compared with women who develop preeclampsia as nulliparas. Am J Obstet Gynecol 2002; 186:422–6.

19. Meher S, Abalos E, Carroli G. Bed rest with or without hospitalization for hypertension during pregnancy. Cochrane Database of Syst Rev 2005;(4):CD003514. Review

20. Von Dadelszen P, Magee LA. Antihypertensive indications in management of gestational hypertension-preeclampsia. Clin Obstet Gynecol 2005;48:441–59.

21. Barron WM, Heckerling P, Hibbard JU, Fisher S. Reducing unnecessary coagulation testing in hypertensive disorders of pregnancy. Obstet Gynecol 1999;94: 364–70.

22. Haddad B, Sibai BM. Expectant management of severe preeclampsia: Proper candidates and pregnancy outcome. Clin Obstet Gynecol 2005;48:430–40.

23. Amorim MMR, Santa LC, Faundes A. Corticosteroid therapy for prevention of respiratory distress syndrome in severe preeclampsia remote from term. Am J Obstet Gynecol 1999;180:1283–8.

24. Hogg B, Hauth JC, Caritis SN, Sibai BM, Lindheimer M, van Dorsten JP, et al. Safety of labor epidural anesthesia for women with severe hypertensive disease. National Institute of Child Health and Human Development Maternal-Fetal Medicine Units Network. Am J Obstet Gynecol 1999;181:1096–101.

25. Head BB, Owen J, Vincent RD Jr, Shih G, Chestnut DH, Hauth JC. A randomized trial of intrapartum analgesia in women with severe preeclampsia. Obstet Gynecol 2002;99:452–7.

26. Sibai BM. Magnesium sulfate prophylaxis in preeclampsia: Lessons learned from recent trials. Am J Obstet Gynecol 2004;190:1520–6.

27. The Magpie Trial Collaborative Group. Do women with preeclampsia, and their babies, benefit from magnesium sulfate? The Magpie trial: A randomized placebo-controlled trial. Lancet 2002;359:1877–90.

28. Witlin AG. Freidman SA, Sibai BM. The effect of magnesium sulfate therapy on the duration of labor in women with mild preeclampsia at term: A randomized, double-blind, placebo-controlled trial. Am J Obstet Gynecol 1997; 176:623–7.

29. Livingston JC, Livingston LW, Ramsey R. Mabie BC, Sibai BM. Magnesium sulfate in women with mild preeclampsia: A randomized, double blinded, placebo-controlled trial. Obstet Gynecol 2003;101:217–20.

30. Martin JN Jr, Thigpen BD, Moore RC, Rose CH, Cushman J, May W. Stroke and severe preeclampsia and eclampsia: A paradigm shift focusing on systolic blood pressure. Obstet Gynecol 2005;105:246–54.

31. Cunningham FG. Severe preeclampsia and eclampsia: systolic hypertension is also important. Obstet Gynecol 2005;105:237–8.

32. Magee LA, Cham C, Waterman EJ, Ohlsson A, von Dadelszen P. Hydralazine for treatment of severe hypertension in pregnancy: meta-analysis. BMJ 2003;327:955–60.

33. Magee LA, Miremadi S, Li J, Cheng C, Ensom MH, Carleton B, et al. Therapy with both magnesium sulfate and nifedipine does not increase the risk of serious magnesium-related maternal side effects in women with preeclampsia. Am J Obstet Gynecol 2005;193:153–63.

34. Sibai BM. Diagnosis, controversies, and management of the syndrome of hemolysis, elevated liver enzymes, and low platelet count. Obstet Gynecol 2004;103:981–91.

35. Pritchard JA, Weisman R. Ratoff OD, Vosburg GJ. Intravascular hemolysis, thrombocytopenia, and other hematologic abnormalities associated with severe toxemia of pregnancy. N Engl J Med 1954;250:89–98.

36. Killam AP, Dillard SH, Patton RC, Pederson PR. Pregnancy-induced hypertension complicated by acute liver disease and disseminated intravascular coagulation. Am J Obstet Gynecol 1975;123:823–8.

37. Weinstein L. Syndrome of hemolysis, elevated liver enzymes, and low platelet count: a severe consequence of hypertension in pregnancy. Am J Obstet Gynecol 1982; 142:159–67.

38. Audibert F, Friedman SA, Frangieh AY, Sibai BM. Clinical utility of strict diagnostic criteria for the HELLP (hemolysis, elevated liver enzymes, and low platelets) syndrome. Am J Obstet Gynecol 1996;183:444–8.

39. Clark SL, Phelan JR, Allen SH, Golde SR. Antepartum reversal of hematologic abnormalities associated with the HELLP syndrome. J Reprod Med 1987;32:781–4.

40. Heyborne KD, Burke MS, Porreca RP. Prolongation of premature gestation in women with hemolysis, elevated liver enzymes and low platelets. J Reprod Med 1990;35: 53–7.

41. Heller CS, Elliott JP. High-order multiple pregnancies complicated by HELLP syndrome: a report of four cases with corticosteroid therapy to prolong gestation. J Reprod Med 1997;42:743–6.

42. Tompkins MJ, Thiagrajah S. HELLP (hemolysis, elevated liver enzymes, and low platelet count) syndrome: the benefit of corticosteroids. Am J Obstet Gynecol 1999;181: 304–9.

43. O'Brien JM, Milligan DA, Barton JR. Impact of high-dose corticosteroid therapy for patients with HELLP (hemolysis, elevated liver enzymes, and low platelet count) syndrome. Am J Obstet Gynecol 2000;183:921–4.

44. O'Brien JM, Shumate SA, Satchwell SL, Milligan DA, Barton JR. Maternal benefit to corticosteroid therapy in patients with HELLP (hemolysis, elevated liver enzymes, and low platelets) syndrome: impact on the rate of regional anesthesia. Am J Obstet Gynecol 202;186:475–9.

45. MacKenna J, Dover NL, Brame RG. Preeclampsia associated with hemolysis, elevated liver enzymes, and low platelets: an obstetric emergency? Obstet Gynecol 1983; 62:751–4.

46. Weinstein L. Preeclampsia/eclampsia with hemolysis, elevated liver enzymes and thrombocytopenia. Obstet Gynecol 1985;66:657–60.

47. Crane JMG, Tabarsi B, Hutchens D. The maternal benefits of corticosteroids with HELLP syndrome. J Obstet Gynaecol Can 2003;25:650–5.

48. Magann EF, Bass D, Chauhan SP, Sullivan DL, Martin JN Jr. Antepartum corticosteroids: disease stabilization in patients with the syndrome of hemolysis, elevated liver enzymes, and low platelets (HELLP). Am J Obstet Gynecol 1994;171:1148–53.

49. Magann EF, Perry KG Jr, Meydrech EF, Harris RL, Chauchan SP, Martin JN Jr. Postpartum corticosteroids: accelerated recovery from the syndrome of hemolysis, elevated liver enzymes, and low platelets (HELLP). Am J Obstet Gynecol 1994;171:1154–8.

50. Martin JN Jr, Rinehart B, May WL, Magann EF, Terrone DA, Blake PG. The spectrum of severe preeclampsia: comparative analysis by HELLP syndrome classification. Am J Obstet Gynecol 1999;180:1373–84.

51. Martin JN Jr, Perry KG, Blake PG, May WA, Moore A, Robinette L. Better maternal outcomes are achieved with dexamethasone therapy for postpartum HELLP (hemolysis, elevated liver enzymes, and thrombocytopenia) syndrome. Am J Obstet Gynecol 1997;177:1011–7.

52. Martin JN Jr, Thigsten BD, Rose CH, Cushman J, Moore A, May WL. Maternal benefit of high-dose intravenous corticosteroid therapy for HELLP. Am J Obstet Gynecol 2003;189:830–4.

53. Mercer BM, Crocker LG, Boe NM, Sibai BM. Induction versus expectant management in premature rupture of the membranes with mature amniotic fluid at 32 to 36 weeks: a randomized trial. Am J Obstet Gynecol 1993; 169(4):775–82.

54. Visser W, Wallenburg HCS. Temporising management of severe preeclampsia with and without the HELLP syndrome. Eur J Obstet Gynecol Reprod Biol 1990;36:43–51.

55. Rath W, Loos W, Kuhn W, Graeff H. The importance of early laboratory screening methods for maternal and fetal outcome in cases of HELLP syndrome. Eur J Obstet Gynecol Reprod Biol 1990;36:43–51.

56. Aarnoudse J, Houthoff HJ, Weits J, Vallenga E, Huisjes JH. A syndrome of liver damage and intravascular coagulation in the last trimester of normotensive pregnancy: a clinical and histopathological study. Br J Obstet Gynaecol 1986;93:145–55.

57. Martin JN Jr, Files JC, Blake PG, Perry KG, Morrison JC, Norman PH. Postpartum plasma exchange for atypical preeclampsia-eclampsia as HELLP syndrome. Am J Obstet Gynecol 1995;172:1107–27.

58. Vigil-DeGracia P, Garcia-Caceres E. Dexamethasone in the postpartum treatment of HELLP syndrome. Int J Gynaecol Obstet 1997;59:217–21.

59. Yalcin OT, Sener T, Hassa H, Ozalp S, Okur A. Effects of postpartum corticosteroids in patients with HELLP syndrome. Int J Gynaecol Obstet 1997;59:217–21.

60. Sibai BM, Ramadan KM. Acute renal failure in pregnancies complicated by hemolysis, elevated live enzymes, and low platelets. Am J Obstet Gyunecol 1993;168:1682–90.

61. Drakeley AJ, LeRoux PA, Anthony J, Penny J. Acute renal failure complicating severe preeclampsia requiring admission to an obstetric intensive care unit. Am J Obstet Gynecol 2002;186:253–6.

62. Haddad B, Barton JR, Livingston JC, Chahine R, Sibai BM. Risk factors for adverse maternal outcomes among women with HELLP syndrome. Am J Obstet Gynecol 2000;183:444–8.

63. Woods JB, Blake PG, Perry KG Jr, Magann EF, Martin RW, Martin JN Jr. Ascites: a portent of cardiopulmonary complications in the preeclamptic patient with the syndrome of hemolysis, elevated liver enzymes, and low platelets. Obstet Gynecol 1992;80:87–91.

64. Abramovici D, Friedman SA, Mercer BM, Audibert F, Kao L, Sibai BM. Neonatal outcome in severe preeclampsia at 24 to 36 weeks' gestation: does HELLP (hemolysis, elevated liver enzymes, and low platelet counts) syndrome matter? Am J Obstet Gynecol 1999;180:221–5.

65. Van Pampus MG, Wolf H, Westenberg SM, van der Post JA, Bonsel GJ, Treffers PE. Maternal and perinatal outcome after expectant management of the HELLP syndrome compared with preeclampsia without HELLP syndrome. Eur J Obstet Gynecol Reprod Biol 1998; 76:31–6.

66. Van Pampus MG, Wolf H, Ilsen A, Treffers PE. Maternal outcome following temporizing management of the (H)ELLP syndrome. Hypertens Pregnancy 2000;19:211-20.

67. Isler CM, Barrilleaux PS, Magann EF, Bass D, Martin JN Jr. A prospective, randomized trial comparing the efficacy of dexamethasone and betamethasone for the treatment of antepartum HELLP syndrome. Am J Obstet Gynecol 2001;184:1332–9.

68. Fonseca JE, Mendez F, Catano C, Arias F. Dexamethasone treatment does not improve the outcome of women with HELLP syndrome: A double-blind, placebo-controlled, randomized clincial trial. Am J Obstet Gynecol 2005;193: 1591–8.

69. Sibai BM, Barton JR. Dexamethasone to improve maternal outcome in women with hemolysis, elevated liver enzymes, and low platelets syndrome. Am J Obstet Gynecol 2005;193:1587–90.

70. Sibai BM. Diagnosis, prevention, and management of eclampsia. Obstet Gynecol 2005;105:402–10.

71. Saftlas AF, Olson DR, Franks AC, Atrash HK, Polaras R. Epidemiology of preeclampsia and eclampsia in the United States: 1979–1986. Am J Obstet Gynecol 1990;163: 460–5.

72. Moller B, Lindmark G. Eclampsia in Sweden. 1976-80. Acta Obstet Gynecol Scand 1986;65:307–14.

73. Douglas KA, Redman CW. Eclampsia in the United Kingdom. BMJ 1994;309:1395–400.

74. Makhseed M, Musimi VM. Eclampsia in Kuwait 1981-1993. Aust NZJ Obstet Gynaecol 1996;36:258–263.

75. Sibai BM. Eclampsia VI. Maternal-perinatal outcome in 254 consecutive cases. Am J Obstet Gynecol 1990;163: 1049–55.

76. Mattar F, Sibai BM. Eclampsia VIII. Risk factors for maternal morbidity. Am J Obstet Gynecol 2000;182: 307–12.

77. Katz VL, Farmer R, Kuller J. Preeclampsia into eclampsia: toward a new paradigm. Am J Obstet Gynecol 2000;182: 1389–96.

78. Chames MC, Livingston JC, Invester TS, Barton JR, Sibai BM. Late postpartum eclampsia: A preventable disease? Am J Obstet Gynecol 2002;186:1174–7.

79. Lubarsky SL, Barton JR, Friedman SA, Nasreddine S, Ramaddan MK, Sibai BM. Late postpartum eclampsia revisited. Obstet Gynecol 1994;83:502–5.

80. Sibai BM, Abdella TH, Taylor HA. Eclampsia in the first half of pregnancy. A report of three cases and review of the literature. J Reprod Med 1982;27:706–08.

81. Newman RB, Eddly GL. Association of eclampsia and hydatidiform mole: case report and review of the literature. Obstet Gynecol Surv 1988;43:185–90.

82. Sheehan JL, Lynch JB. Pathology of toxemia of pregnancy. New York (NY): Churchill Livingstone; 1973.

83. Richards AM, Moodley J, Graham DI, Bullock MRR. Active management of the unconscious eclamptic patient. Br J Obstet Gynaecol 1986;93:554–62.

84. Lopez-Llera M. Main clinical types and subtypes of eclampsia. Am J Obstet Gynecol 1992;166:4–9.

85. Dahmus MA, Barton JR, Sibai BM. Cerebral imaging in eclampsia: Magnetic resonance imaging versus computed tomography. Am J Obstet Gynecol 1992;167:935–41.

86. Pritchard JA, Cunningham FG, Pritchard SA. The Parkland Memorial hospital protocol for treatment of eclampsia: Evaluation of 245 cases. Am J Obstet Gynecol 1984;148:951–63.

87. Sibai BM, Sarinoglu C, Mercer BM. Eclampsia VII. Pregnancy outcome after eclampsia and long-term prognosis. Am J Obstet Gynecol 1992;166:1757–63.

88. Sibai BM. Hypertension. In: Gabbe SG, Niebyl JR, Simpson JL. Obstetrics, normal and problem pregnancies. 4th ed. New York (NY): Churchill Livingstone; 2002.

89. Cunningham FG, Twickler DM. Cerebral edema complicating eclampsia. Am J Obstet Gynecol 2000;182:94–100.

90. Schwartz RB, Feske SK, Polak JF, DeBirolami U, Iaia A, Beckner KM, et al. Preeclampsia-eclampsia: Clinical and neuroradiographic correlates and insights into the pathogenesis of hypertensive encephalopathy. Radiology 2000;217:371–6.

91. Belfort MA, Grunewald C, Saade GR, Varner M, Nisel H. Preeclampsia may cause both overperfusion and underperfusion of the brain. Acta Obstet Gynecol Scand 1999;78:586–1.

92. Zeeman GG, Fleckenstein JL, Twickler DM, Cunningham FG. Cerebral infarction in eclampsia. Am J Obstet Gynecol 2004;190:714–20.

93. Loureiro R, Leite CC, Kahhale S, Freire S, Sousa B, Cardoso EF, et al. Diffusion imaging may predict reversible brain lesions in eclampsia and severe preeclampsia: initial experience. Am J Obstet Gynecol 2003;189:1350–5.

94. Witlin AG, Friedman SA, Egerman RS, Frangieh AY, Sibai BM. Cerebrovascular disorders complicating pregnancy. Beyond eclampsia. Am J Obstet Gynecol 1997;176:139–48.

95. Shearer VE, Harish SJ, Cunningham FG. Puerperal seizures after post-dural puncture headache. Obstet Gynecol 1995;85:255–60.

96. Hinchey J, Chaves C, Appignani B, Breen J, Pao L, Wang A, et al. A reversible posterior leukoencephalopathy syndrome. N Engl J Med 1996;334:494–500.

97. Varner MW. Cerebral vasculopathies masquerading as eclampsia. Obstet Gynecol 2006;107:437–8.

98. Leitch CR, Cameron AD, Walker JJ. The changing pattern of eclampsia over a 60-year period. Br J Obstet Gynaecol 1997;104:917–22.

99. Which anticonvulsant for women with eclampsia? Evidence from the Collaborative Eclampsia Trial [published erratum appears in Lancet 1995;346:258]. Lancet 1995;345:1455–63.

100. MacKay AP, Berg CJ, Atrash HK. Pregnancy-related mortality from preeclampsia and eclampsia. Obstet Gynecol 2001;97:533–8.

101. Sibai BM, Abdella TN, Spinnato JA, Anderson GA. Eclampsia V. The incidence of nonpreventable eclampsia. Am J Obstet Gynecol 1986;154:581–6.

102. Campbell DM, Templeton AA. Is eclampsia preventable? In: Bonnar J, MacGillivray I, Symonds EM, editors. Pregnancy hypertension, proceedings. Baltimore (MD): University Park Press; 1980. p. 483–8.

103. Witlin AG, Sibai BM. Magnesium sulfate in preeclampsia and eclampsia. Obstet Gynecol 1998;92:883–9.

104. Paul RH, Kee SK, Bernstein SG. Changes in fetal heart rate and uterine contraction pattern associated with eclampsia. Am J Obstet Gynecol 1978;130:165–9.

105. Mathys LA, Coppage KH, Lambers DS, Barton JR, Sibai BM. Delayed postpartum preeclampsia: An experience of 151 cases. Am J Obstet Gynecol 2004;190:1464–66.

106. Ferrazani S, DeCarolis S, Pomini F, Testa AC, Mastromarino C, Caruso A. The duration of hypertension in the puerperium of preeclamptic women: Relationship with renal impairment and week of delivery. Am J Obstet Gynecol 1994;17:5060–12.

107. Walters BNJ, Walters T. Hypertension in the puerperium. Lancet 1987;2:330.

108. Barton JR, Hiett AK, Conover WB. The use of nifedipine during the postpartum period in patients with severe preeclampsia. Am J Obstet Gynecol 1990;162:788–92.

109. Campbell DM, MacGillivray I, Carr-Hill R. Preeclampsia in second pregnancy. BJOG 1985;92:131–40.

110. Hjartardottir S, Leifsson BG, Geirsson RT, Steinthorsdottir V. Recurrence of hypertensive disorder in second pregnancy. Am J Obstet Gynecol 2006;194:916–20.

111. Caritis S, Sibai BM, Hauth J. Lindheimer MD, Klebanoff M, Thom E, et al. Low-dose aspirin to prevent preeclampsia in women at high risk. N Engl J Med 1998;338:701–5.

112. Sibai BM, El-Nazer A, Gonzalez-Ruiz A. Severe preeclampsia-eclampsia in young primigravid women: Subsequent pregnancy outcome and remote prognosis. Am J Obstet Gyencol 1986;155:1011–16.

113. Sibai BM, Mercer B. Sarinoglu C. Severe preeclampsia in the second trimester: Recurrence risk and long-term prognosis. Am J Obstet Gynecol 1991;165:1408–12.

114. Sibai BM, Ramadan MK, Chari RS, Friedman SA. Pregnancies complicated by HELLP syndrome: Subsequent pregnancy outcome and long-term prognosis. Am J Obstet Gynecol 1995;172:125–9.

115. Van Pampus MG, Wolf H, Mayruhu G, Treffers PE, Bleker OP. Long-term follow-up in patients with a history of (H)ELLP syndrome. Hypertens. Pregn 2001;20:15–23.

116. Chames MC, Haddad B, Barton JR, Livingston JC, Sibai BM. Subsequent pregnancy outcome in women with a history of HELLP syndrome at 28 weeks of gestation. Am J Obstet Gynecol 2003;188:1504–8.

117. Ramsey JE, Stewart F, Greer IA, Sattar N. Microvascular dysfunction: A link between preeclampsia and maternal coronary heart disease. BJOG 2003;110:2029–31.

118. Wilson BJ, Watson MS, Prescott GJ, Sunderland S, Campbell DM, et al. Hypertensive disease of pregnancy and risk of hypertension and stroke in later life: Results from Cohort study. BMJ 2003;326:1–7.

119. Haukkamaa L, Salminen M, Laivuori H, Leinonen H, Hiilesma V, Kaaja R. Risk for subsequent coronary artery disease after preeclampsia. Am J Cardial 2004;93: 805–8.

120. Wikstrom AK, Haglund B, Olovsson M, Lindberg SN. The risk of ischaemic heart disease after gestational hypertensive disease. BJOG 2005;112:1486–91.

121. Brown DW, Dueker N, Jamieson DJ, Cole JW, Wozniak MA, et al. Preeclampsia and the risk of ischemic stroke among young women: Results from the stroke prevention in young women study. Stoke 2006;37:1055–59.

CHAPTER 13

Prediction and Early Detection of Preterm Labor

JAY D. IAMS

*E*arly detection of pregnant women who will give birth before term has been sought as an avenue to reduce the occurrence of prematurity-related perinatal morbidity and mortality. Preterm birth is associated with 75% of cases of perinatal morbidity and mortality for infants born without congenital anomalies. Sequelae of preterm birth include cerebral palsy, developmental delay, visual and hearing impairment, and chronic lung disease. The rates of preterm and low-birth-weight deliveries have actually increased in recent years despite widespread efforts to address the problem.

The frequency of preterm birth increased from 10.6% to 12.5% of live births in the United States between 1990 and 2004 (1–2). The rise in preterm births has been attributed to increased use of assisted reproductive technologies (3). Between 1996 and 2003, multiple births in the United States increased more than 22%, from 2.7% to 3.3% of live births. The preterm birth rate among multiple deliveries in the United States was 61.2% in 2003 (4). Increased willingness to choose delivery when medical or obstetric complications threaten the health of the mother or fetus after 32–34 weeks of gestation also has contributed to the rise in preterm delivery (5). Approximately 40% of preterm births follow preterm labor and 35% result from preterm premature rupture of membranes. The remaining 25% are caused by medical or obstetric conditions such as hypertension, antenatal hemorrhage, or intrauterine growth restriction (6).

Early detection of preterm labor is difficult because initial symptoms and signs are often mild and may occur in normal pregnancies. Thus, many healthy women will report symptoms during routine prenatal visits, whereas others destined for preterm birth may dismiss the early warning signs as normal in pregnancy. The traditional criteria for preterm labor (persistent contractions accompanied by progressive cervical dilation and effacement) are most accurate when contraction frequency is six or more per hour, cervical dilatation is 3 cm or more, effacement is 80% or more, membranes rupture, or bleeding occurs (7, 8). When lower thresholds for contraction fre-

quency and cervical dilation and effacement (eg, cervical "change" by digital examination) are used, both sensitivity and positive predictive value for true preterm labor decline, and the rate of false-positive diagnosis rises to as much as 40% (9). Consequently, other means have been sought to detect preterm labor early. These include digital and ultrasound examination of the cervix, outpatient monitoring of uterine contractions, and detection of biochemical markers of preterm labor in blood, saliva, and cervicovaginal secretions. These tests have been evaluated as 1) means of identifying women with increased risk of preterm birth before clinical signs or symptoms occur and 2) part of the diagnostic process in women who present with possible preterm labor. The performance of each test varies according to its use to predict preterm birth in women without symptoms, or to detect preterm labor accurately in women with symptoms. This difference, a common source of confusion, occurs because the predictive value of any test result always varies according to the prevalence of the condition or disease in the population. The term "population" refers not only to demographic characteristics or historical risk factors for preterm birth, but also to the presence or absence of symptoms.

Pathophysiology of Preterm Birth

Preterm birth is the ultimate result of several different pathways that culminate in the initiation of labor before 37 weeks of gestation. It is useful to place preterm births in two broad categories—those that are obstetrically indicated (ie, when preterm delivery serves to benefit the mother or fetus) and those that are spontaneous (ie, when preterm delivery occurs in the apparent absence of maternal or fetal jeopardy) (10). Because the clinical presentations may overlap, these categories should be kept in mind during the clinical evaluation of women with signs or symptoms of preterm labor. Sometimes maternal bleeding from a possible abruption accompanies contractions. In other cases, the cause of labor is not evident initially, but may become so when the labor is difficult to stop or fetal status is compromised. This review will focus on spontaneous preterm birth.

Recent studies of the epidemiology and pathophysiology of preterm birth have identified four pathways leading to preterm labor and delivery (11): 1) inflammation, 2) decidual hemorrhage, 3) uterine overdistention, and 4) premature activation of the normal physiologic initiators of labor. Inflammation is more often associated with preterm births before 32 weeks of gestation, whereas decidual hemorrhage may occur at any time. Uterine overdistention may accompany multifetal gestation, polyhydramnios, or a uterine anomaly. Premature activation of the normal maternal–fetal hypothalamic–pituitary–adrenal axis is typical of preterm labor after 32–34 weeks of gestation. Much of the data that underlie these observations have come from studies of markers for preterm delivery, such as cervical ultrasound images (12–14), fetal fibronectin (13–15), the thrombin cascade (16, 17), and maternal salivary estriol (18) measured in asymptomatic women with and without risk factors for preterm birth.

Ultrasound images of the cervix in pregnancy have shown that cervical effacement begins weeks before delivery, approximately 32 weeks of gestation for term births and as early as 16–24 weeks of gestation for preterm births. Effacement begins at the internal cervical os and proceeds caudad through a process called funneling (19). This process is often well established before the external os dilates. The appearance of cervical effacement, as seen by transvaginal ultrasonography has been described, as a progression of the letters T, Y, V, and U to denote the relationship of the cervical canal to the lower uterine segment. This concept is depicted in Figure 13-1.

The length of the cervical canal measured by ultrasonography in the second and early third trimesters ranges from less than 10 mm to 50 mm. The median (50th percentile) length is 35 mm, the 10th percentile is 25 mm, and the 90th is 45 mm (Fig. 13-2) (12). The risk of spontaneous preterm birth increases as the length of the cervix decreases across the entire range of cervical length. A cervical length at 22–24 weeks of gestation that is below 25 mm (the 10th percentile) is associated with a more than sixfold increase in preterm birth before 35 weeks of gestation, relative to women whose cervical length is above the 75th percentile (Fig. 13-2) (12). Some of the range of cervical length is thought to be simply biologic. In other cases, women may experience early effacement or shortening as the result of inflammation caused by hemorrhage or infection or, less commonly, biophysical effects of uterine distention or subclinical contractions (13, 14). This scenario is particularly associated with preterm births before 30–32 weeks of gestation, is more

often followed by long-term morbidity for the infant, and is more likely to recur in subsequent pregnancies (13).

Fibronectin, an extracellular matrix protein, acts as the "glue" that attaches the fetal membranes to the underlying uterine decidua (20). Fibronectin is often found in the cervicovaginal secretions before 16–18 weeks of gestation and again at the end of normal pregnancy as labor approaches. Normally, it is not present in cervicovaginal secretions between 22 weeks and 37 weeks of gestation. Fibronectin found in cervicovaginal secretions after 22 weeks of gestation is a marker of disruption of the decidual–chorionic interface and has been associated with a sixfold increased risk of preterm birth before 35 weeks of gestation and a 14-fold increased risk of preterm birth before 28 weeks of gestation (13, 15). Although fibronectin in the cervicovaginal secretions between 14 weeks and 22 weeks of gestation has been considered to be normal, levels of fibronectin of 50 ng/mL or more in the early second trimester have been associated with an increased risk of preterm birth before 28 weeks of gestation (21). In contrast, preterm births after 32–33 weeks of gestation have been associated with self-reported contractions and a rise in maternal excretion of estriol, an indicator of increasing maturation of the fetal hypothalamic–pituitary–adrenal axis (18).

Although studies of uterine contractions, fibronectin levels, and digital and ultrasound assessment of the cervix have contributed to an expanded understanding of the pathways to preterm birth, use of these tests in clinical practice is still in its infancy. This review addresses the current status of tests for preterm birth in clinical practice. Testing might identify a group of women who could be treated to prevent or reduce the likelihood of preterm birth. No such screening has been found to be consistently effective. Uterine contraction monitoring to identify and treat women with increased contractions (22), cervical ultrasonography to select women for cerclage (23), and fetal fibronectin screening to choose women for antibiotic treatment (24) have failed to reduce the rate of preterm birth in prospective, randomized trials. Recent studies conducted in women with a prior preterm birth have found that prophylactic treatment with 17 α-hydroxyprogesterone caproate can reduce the rate of recurrent preterm birth (25, 26). It does not reduce the rate of preterm birth in women with twin pregnancies, however, based on recent findings by the National Institute of Child Health and Human Development Maternal–Fetal Medicine Units Network. Studies of this intervention in women with other risk factors for preterm birth, such as a short cervix or positive fibronectin test result, are needed. Someday, results from these tests or others yet to be discovered may not only identify a high proportion of women destined for preterm birth (27) but might also be linked to effective interventions to reduce the risk.

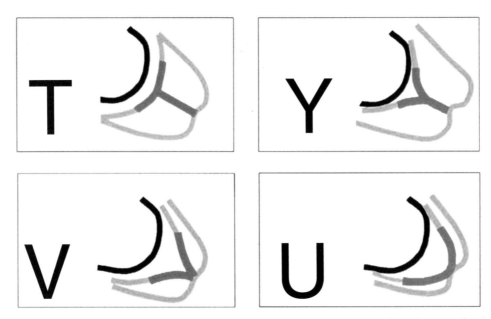

Fig. 13-1. Schematic to display the process of cervical effacement as it proceeds from the internal os, caudad toward the external os, as seen on transvaginal ultrasonography. The letters T, Y, V, and U depict the relationship between the lower uterine segment and the cervical canal. (Modified with permission from Zilianti M, Azuaga A, Calderon F, Pages G, Mendoza G. Monitoring the effacement of the uterine cervix by transperineal sonography: a new perspective. J Ultrasound Med 1995;14:719–24. Copyright © 1995 American Institute of Ultrasound in Medicine.)

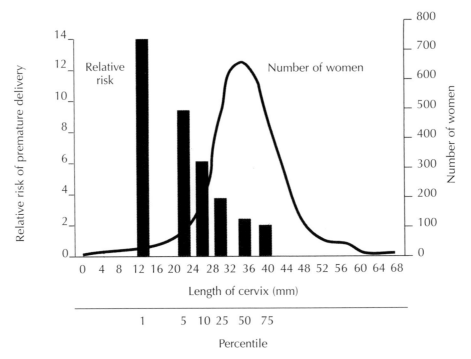

Fig. 13-2. Distribution of subjects among percentiles for cervical length measured by transvaginal ultrasonography at 24 weeks of gestation (solid line) and relative risk of spontaneous preterm delivery before 35 weeks of gestation according to percentiles for cervical length (bars). The risks among women with values at or below the first, fifth, tenth, 25th, 50th, and 75th percentiles for cervical length are compared with the risk among women with values above the 75th percentile. (Modified with permission from Iams JD, Goldenberg RL, Meis PJ, Mercer BM, Moawad A, Das A, et al. The length of the cervix and the risk of spontaneous preterm delivery. N Engl J Med 1996;334:567–72. Copyright © 1996 Massachusetts Medical Society. All rights reserved.)

There are at least two broad areas in which testing might be helpful in clinical practice today. The first is in women with symptoms of preterm labor, in whom early diagnosis is important but notably inaccurate. In some cases, testing these patients with fibronectin screening, cervical ultrasonography, or both can be helpful in improving the accuracy of diagnosis among women with symptoms and the appropriate application of acute interventions such as antenatal steroids or maternal transfer to a tertiary center. The second area is the management of pregnancies with historic risk factors for preterm birth (eg, multiple gestation or a history of preterm birth).

Evaluation of Patients With Symptoms and Signs of Preterm Labor

The goal of early diagnosis of preterm labor in symptomatic women is the appropriate application of three antenatal interventions that are recognized to reduce perinatal morbidity and mortality:

1. Transfer of women with preterm labor to a facility with a neonatal intensive care unit
2. Administration of corticosteroids to the mother
3. Treatment of women in preterm labor with antibiotics effective against the group B streptococci

Tocolytic drugs have been shown to prolong pregnancy for 2–7 days when given to women with symptoms of preterm labor (28), a delay sufficient to allow maternal transfer and treatment with antenatal steroids. Because tocolytic medications can have significant side effects, accurate diagnosis is important to avoid the risks and costs of unnecessary treatment.

The twin hallmarks of preterm labor are persistent uterine contractions accompanied by cervical effacement and dilation. These criteria have suboptimal sensitivity and specificity (29) because of the common occurrence of symptoms and signs of early preterm labor in normal pregnancy and the imprecision of digital examination of the cervix (30). The practice of initiating tocolytic drugs for contraction frequency without any additional diagnostic criteria results in unnecessary treatment of women who do not actually have preterm labor (31). Results of several recent studies have demonstrated that the following indicators are the best clinical predictors of preterm delivery within 24 hours to 7 days in women with preterm labor symptoms (7, 8, 32):

1. Initial cervical dilatation of 3 cm or more
2. Cervical effacement of 80% or more
3. Vaginal bleeding
4. Ruptured membranes

Although specific, these signs often occur too late to allow effective intervention (33). Contraction frequency

is a common initial symptom. The most commonly used clinical threshold for contraction frequency is four or more per hour. The sensitivity of this contraction threshold for delivery within 7–14 days of presentation is approximately 50–60% in women whose cervical dilatation is less than 3 cm (34, 35). Cervical length measurements with ultrasonography and detection of fetal fibronectin in cervical secretions have been studied as methods to improve diagnostic accuracy in this setting.

Cervical Ultrasonography

Studies of transvaginal cervical ultrasonography have reported different thresholds depending on the patients studied (symptoms versus no symptoms) and the goal of the analysis (accurate detection of preterm labor in women with symptoms versus prediction of preterm birth in asymptomatic outpatients). In symptomatic women, the optimal threshold to exclude a diagnosis of preterm labor is a cervical length of 30 mm (36–41). A cervical length of 18–20 mm has optimal positive predictive value in this setting (Fig. 13-3). Because cervical effacement occurs slowly and often precedes clinically evident preterm labor, a cervical length less than 20 mm does not always indicate the presence of preterm labor, but a length of more than 30 mm reliably excludes preterm labor if the examination is done properly (Fig. 13-4). Excessive pressure on the vaginal probe, failure to empty the maternal bladder, and use of transabdominal ultrasonography are all associated with falsely long measurements and should be avoided (42, 43). Multiple dimensions of the cervix have been measured, including the presence and size of a funnel at the internal os, the length of the closed or residual portion of the

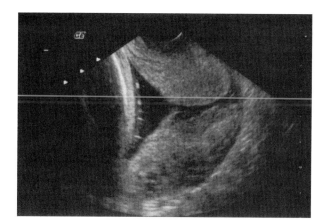

Fig. 13-3. Transvaginal ultrasound image of the cervix obtained from a woman with symptoms of preterm labor. The image supports a diagnosis of preterm labor because of the length (23 mm) and the Y-shaped appearance of the cervix. (Modified from Iams JD. Prediction and early detection of preterm labor. Obstet Gynecol 2003;101:402–12.)

cervix, and the total (funnel length plus length of the closed portion). The residual closed portion is the most reliably measured and is the most consistently correlated with the duration of pregnancy (Fig. 13-5). Funneling, although sometimes a dramatic process when viewed in real time, is a transient process that, to be clinically significant, must be associated with a residual length that is "short" (ie, less than 25 mm). A false or pseudofunnel may occur when the lower uterine segment contracts to form a funnel above a cervix of normal length. This phe-

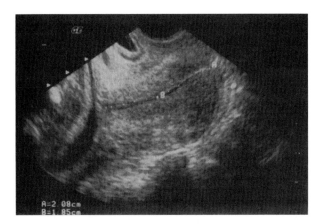

Fig. 13-4. Transvaginal ultrasound image of the cervix obtained from a woman with symptoms of preterm labor. The image excludes a diagnosis of preterm labor because of the length (38 mm) and the T-shaped appearance of the cervix. (Modified from Iams JD. Prediction and early detection of preterm labor. Obstet Gynecol 2003;101:402–12.)

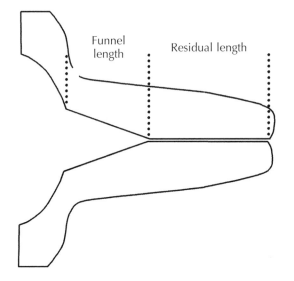

Fig. 13-5. Diagram of a sagittal view of the cervix by transvaginal ultrasonography indicating the appropriate measurement of the cervical length as the residual length. (Modified from Iams JD. Prediction and early detection of preterm labor. Obstet Gynecol 2003;101:402–12.)

nomenon has no clinical significance. Transvaginal images are preferred because transabdominal imaging of the cervix requires at least some urine in the maternal bladder that exerts an unpredictable effect on the measured length of the cervix (42).

Fetal Fibronectin

A positive fibronectin test result (50 ng/mL or more) in a patient with symptoms suggestive of preterm labor has been associated with an increased likelihood of birth before 34 weeks of gestation and birth within 7–14 days of the test (34, 35). However, the positive predictive value for delivery within a week was just 18% in data combined from several studies (6). Given the 40% rate of false-positive diagnosis of preterm labor based on contraction frequency and cervical change by digital examination, the clinical value of the test in symptomatic women is primarily its high negative predictive value. In this respect, the fibronectin test can perform a function similar to cardiac enzymes in the evaluation of chest pain, as a test to avoid overdiagnosis and unnecessary treatment. Several studies have evaluated the performance of fibronectin testing in women with possible preterm labor. In one study, admissions for preterm labor, duration of hospitalization, and use of tocolytic medication all were reduced without affecting neonatal outcome (44). In another study, fibronectin testing was not useful when cervical dilatation was 3 cm or more, but in women with cervical dilatation less than 3 cm, a negative test result was associated with a 90% reduction in maternal transfer to a tertiary care facility (45). A review of multiple studies of fibronectin testing using likelihood ratios found benefits only for a negative test result in women with symptoms before 34 weeks of gestation (46). These reports indicate that to be clinically useful in the diagnosis of preterm labor, the test must be rapidly available and the clinician must be willing to act on a negative test result by not initiating treatment. It is not clear how a positive result should affect clinical management, but there is evidence that a positive fibronectin test result can improve diagnostic sensitivity. Among 235 women with symptoms of preterm labor but no cervical change, the fibronectin assay was positive in 20%. These women were significantly more likely to give birth to preterm infants who experienced morbidity or mortality than women with a negative test result (47).

When fibronectin levels were compared with a contraction frequency of four or more per hour, cervical dilatation of more than 1 cm, vaginal bleeding, and the clinician's diagnosis of preterm labor in symptomatic women with cervical dilatation less than 3 cm to predict birth within 1 week, the addition of the fibronectin assay improved both sensitivity and specificity (34, 35).

Fibronectin tests would appear to be useful in women with symptoms when the following conditions occur:

1. Symptoms occur between 24 weeks and 34 weeks of gestation.
2. Membranes are intact and cervical dilatation is less than 3 cm.
3. Results are available within a few hours (less than 6–8 hours in most settings, perhaps longer in remote sites).
4. The clinician is willing to rely on a negative result by not initiating treatment.

Combined use of fibronectin tests and cervical ultrasonography in the evaluation of symptomatic women has been evaluated in several studies. One found the tests to be complementary in improving the accuracy of (48) diagnosis, and another found that the combination was not superior to either test alone (49). In a third study, both tests were performed in 206 women with possible preterm labor. The fetal fibronectin test improved the performance of ultrasonographic cervical length measurement to predict imminent preterm birth only when the ultrasonographic cervical length measurement was less than 30 mm (Table 13-1) (50).

THE OHIO STATE UNIVERSITY PROTOCOL

At the Ohio State University Medical Center, a swab of cervicovaginal secretions is obtained for fibronectin testing at the time of the initial speculum examination of women with possible preterm labor. Once ruptured membranes have been ruled out, digital examination is performed. When the cervix is effaced 80% or more or dilated 3 cm or more in the presence of regular contractions, the diagnosis of preterm labor is established without any additional testing. Contraction frequency alone is insufficient to establish a diagnosis of preterm labor. The focus of the diagnosis is the evaluation of the cervix. If the cervix is less than 80% effaced, transvaginal ultrasonography is performed after the patient voids. If the cervix is more than 30 mm in length, preterm labor is very unlikely (36–40). A cervical length of less than 20 mm together with regular contractions confirms a diagnosis of preterm labor (41). The fibronectin test is used when the clinical and ultrasound data are equivocal (eg, dilatation of 2 cm and cervical length between 20 mm and 30 mm) or in conflict (eg, the cervix is less than 3 cm dilated, has "changed" by digital examination, but the length measured by ultrasonography is 35 mm). Women who present with mild symptoms and few contractions but whose cervical examination reveals advanced effacement (ie, a length less than 20 mm before 32 weeks of gestation) are observed until a fibronectin test result is returned. Those with a positive fibronectin test result are treated with antenatal corticosteroids but usually do not receive tocolytics unless contraction frequency increases to six or more per hour. The fibronectin swab must be obtained before the digital and ultrasound assessment of the cervix because a pelvic examination within 24 hours invalidates the fibronectin test result, as does coitus within 24 hours. This algorithm is consistent with the current literature in four important respects:

1. It is grounded in the latest information about the pathophysiology of spontaneous preterm birth.
2. Although it is based on the traditional diagnostic criteria of contractions and cervical change, the protocol addresses the importance of accurate diagnosis and the high false-positive rate of these criteria when used alone.
3. It relies on consistent findings from the literature that preterm birth is very unlikely (97–99%) in women with symptoms, intact membranes, and cervical dilatation of less than 3 cm before 34–35 weeks of gestation when transvaginal cervical length exceeds 30 mm (the 25th percentile) and within 14 days when the fetal fibronectin test result is negative.
4. It recognizes the low positive predictive value of both tests and uses them to exclude more than establish the diagnosis of preterm labor. It avoids the use of an algorithm for women with positive tests results because there is no evidence-based guideline for management of these patients.

AN ALTERNATE PROTOCOL FOR DIAGNOSIS OF PRETERM LABOR

The Ohio State University protocol may be easily adopted when the equipment and personnel needed to perform speculum examinations and cervical ultrasonography are continuously available within the hospital. Alternate protocols are appropriate for hospitals without the appropriate personnel or equipment, once ruptured membranes have been excluded by a speculum examination. One such protocol has been studied prospectively in a trial that randomly assigned 179 women with preterm contractions to one of three arms: observation alone, observation plus intravenous hydration, and observation plus a single 0.25-mg dose of subcutaneous terbutaline. The group that received terbutaline spent less time in triage at a lower cost, without any adverse effect on the outcome of pregnancy (51). Women enrolled in the study had intact membranes and cervical dilatation and effacement of less than 1 cm and less than 80%, respectively. The results of this trial suggest that a single dose of subcutaneous terbutaline could be an efficient way to select women with symptoms of preterm labor for fur-

Table 13-1. Frequency of Spontaneous Preterm Delivery According to Cervical Length (Cutoff 30 mm) and Vaginal Fibronectin Results

Cervical Length Less Than 30 mm	Positive Fetal Fibronectin Test Results	Delivery Within 48 Hours	Delivery Within 7 Days	Delivery Within 14 Days	Delivery Less Than or Equal to 32 Weeks of Gestation	Delivery Less Than or Equal to 35 Weeks of Gestation
No	No	2.2% (2 of 93)	2.2% (2 of 93)	3.2% (3 of 93)	0% (0 of 47)	1.1% (1 of 93)
No	Yes	0% (0 of 14)	7.1% (1 of 14)	14.3% (2 of 14)	0% (0 of 5)	21.4% (3 of 14)
Yes	No	7.1% (5 of 70)	11.4% (8 of 70)	12.9% (9 of 70)	6.5% (2 of 31)	17.1% (12 of 70)
Yes	Yes	26.3% (10 of 38)	44.7% (17 of 38)	52.6% (20 of 38)	38.9% (7 of 18)	47.4% (18 of 38)
Prevalence of the outcome		7.9% (17 of 215)	13.0% (28 of 215)	15.8% (34 of 215)	8.9% (9 of 101)	15.8% (34 of 215)

Modified from Gomez R, Romero R, Medina L, Nien J, Chaiworapongsa T, Carstens M et al. Cervicovaginal fibronectin improves the prediction of preterm delivery based on sonographic cervical length in patients with preterm uterine contractions and intact membranes. Am J Obstet Gynecol 2005;192:350–59. Copyright © 2005. Reprinted with permission from Elsevier.

ther evaluation (eg, a cervical ultrasound examination) before a decision about tocolysis is made.

Prediction of Preterm Birth in Women Without Symptoms

Prediction of preterm birth is a logical goal, provided it can meet the criteria required of any screening program:

1. A screening protocol should be efficient—high sensitivity, high negative predictive value, and low cost.
2. An effective prophylactic intervention or treatment for individuals with positive test results should be available.

Protocols to screen for preterm birth do not fulfill either of these prerequisites. Neither an efficient screening protocol nor an effective intervention to prevent or reduce the rate of preterm birth has yet been identified. Screening has been attempted with numerical scoring systems, microbiologic tests, uterine contraction monitoring, digital and ultrasound examinations of the cervix, and fetal fibronectin assays of cervicovaginal secretions. Preterm birth prophylaxis has been attempted with patient education, bed rest, antibiotics, tocolytics, nutritional supplements, cervical cerclage, and social support, all without consistent evidence of benefit. Whether successful reduction of the rate of preterm birth by treatment with 17 α-hydroxyprogesterone caproate in women with a prior preterm birth (25, 26) can be repeated for other groups at risk of preterm labor is to be determined. Interventions could best be applied in women determined to beat high risk of preterm birth, such as multiple

gestation. Quantification of risk in women with singleton pregnancies has been difficult. One recent study evaluated uterine contraction monitoring, digital examination of the cervix (Bishop score), transvaginal ultrasound measurement of cervical length, and fetal fibronectin at 24 weeks, 28 weeks, and 32 weeks of gestation in women with historical risk factors for preterm birth to predict preterm birth before 35 weeks and 37 weeks of gestation (52). In this study, cervical examination, by either ultrasonography (cervical length 25 mm or less) or Bishop score (4 or greater), was the most sensitive; contraction frequency and fibronectin test results were less predictive (Table 13-2) (52). No test had a sensitivity of more than 40%.

Thus, current data do not support routine screening of pregnant women for risks of preterm birth, regardless of the test chosen or the population tested. However, there are instances in which testing can be clinically helpful and others in which testing for preterm birth risk has entered clinical practice, albeit prematurely. For example, selective application of tests to determine preterm birth risk for women with clinical risk factors may have value when the test is used to avoid treatment. Three situations illustrate the potential use of testing:

1. When a negative test result can avert a planned intervention such as the routine recommendation for reduced activity for women with multiple gestation, which is widely practiced despite a lack of supporting data. Studies of cervical ultrasonography in twins show that spontaneous preterm birth is rare when a cervical length of 35 mm or more is present at 24 weeks of gestation (53). Fibronectin test results were less predictive of preterm birth in

Table 13-2. Prediction at 22–24 Weeks of Spontaneous Preterm Birth Before 35 Weeks of Gestation

Test	Sensitivity (%)	Specificity (%)	Predictive Value	
			Positive (%)	Negative (%)
Multiple preterm labor symptoms	50	63.5	21.4	86.4
Uterine contractions greater than or equal to 4 per hour	6.7	92.3	25	84.7
Bishop score greater than or equal to 4	32	91.4	42.1	87.4
Cervical length less than or equal to 25 mm	40.8	89.5	42.6	88.8
Fibronectin greater than or equal to 50 ng/mL	18	95.3	42.9	85.6

Modified from Iams JD. Prediction and early detection of preterm labor. Obstet Gynecol 2003;101:402–12.

twins than in singletons when studied at 24–28 weeks of gestation in asymptomatic women (54). This line of reasoning might someday be appropriate as well to determine the best use of interventions such as 17 α-hydroxyprogesterone caproate. In the study cited (25), 17 α-hydroxyprogesterone caproate was neither uniformly effective (37% of women who received it gave birth preterm) nor necessary (45% of women who did not receive 17 α-hydroxyprogesterone caproate gave birth after 37 weeks of gestation). There are no data to support the use of 17 α-hydroxyprogesterone caproate, but tests such as cervical ultrasonography, fetal fibronectin or others might some day allow accurate selection of women who will benefit from 17 α-hydroxyprogesterone caproate prophylaxis (7).

2. When a test result can be used to help determine the appropriate timing for administration of antenatal corticosteroids or to avoid treatment entirely. A recent study of 189 at-risk pregnancies has highlighted the difficulty in recognizing the "right" time to give steroids based on clinical criteria (55). Only one third of preterm infants received a single course of steroids within 7 days of preterm delivery. In the current climate of concern about timely and repetitive administration of steroids (56), the ability to provide patient-specific risk assessment using cervical length and fibronectin tests could be helpful. The recurrence of risk of preterm birth has been shown to vary considerably according to the length of the cervix and the presence of fibronectin in cervicovaginal secretions (Fig. 13-6) (57). For example, among women with a prior preterm delivery tested at 24 weeks of gestation in a subsequent pregnancy, the chance of another preterm birth was 7% in

women with a negative fibronectin test result and cervical length of more than 35 mm, versus 64% when both fibronectin and cervical length tests were positive (57). Until more definitive information about the benefits and risks of repeated courses of antenatal corticosteroids is available, this information could be helpful in making decisions about antenatal steroid treatment in selected circumstances (eg, a woman at 28 weeks of gestation with a history of preterm birth and symptoms of possible preterm labor).

3. Whether women with a history of early preterm birth may benefit from a cerclage in subsequent pregnancies is an open question. A randomized trial has shown that women with a history of preterm birth before 32 weeks of gestation whose cervical length remained above 25 mm between 18 weeks and 26 weeks of gestation had a rate of preterm birth of 3.4% versus a rate of 10% for women treated with a prophylactic cerclage (58). Once again, a test for preterm birth appears to have clinical value primarily for its ability to identify women who do not need to be treated, rather than to select those who do.

Abdominal Versus Vaginal Ultrasonography of the Cervix

Another application for transvaginal cervical ultrasonography has recently emerged from a recommendation by the American College of Radiology that the cervix and lower uterine segment be imaged as part of every obstetric ultrasound examination in the second trimester (59). The American College of Radiology guidelines specifically mention a search for funneling and a short cervix

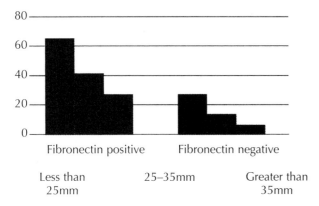

Fig. 13-6. Risk of recurrent preterm birth in women with a prior preterm birth, according to their cervical length and fibronectin test results at 24 weeks of gestation in a subsequent pregnancy. (Modified from Iams JD. Prediction and early detection of preterm labor. Obstet Gynecol 2003;101:402–12.)

(less than 30 mm). This has resulted in an increasing number of apparently normal pregnant women who present to the obstetrician for further evaluation, sometimes with an accompanying report recommending consideration of cervical cerclage. There have even been legal actions brought against obstetricians who have not intervened in response to the report. This has occurred despite the poor reproducibility of transabdominal ultrasonography of the cervix (42, 60) and the absence of any data to support an intervention such as cerclage or bed rest. In this uncertain situation, the American College of Radiology recommends that the obstetrician should obtain a transvaginal ultrasound measurement of the cervix with an empty bladder. A measurement of more than 25 mm in a patient without symptoms and a negative risk history allows the obstetrician to reassure the patient that the risk of preterm birth is not increased. The American College of Radiology uses a cervical length of 30 mm as the threshold of reassurance. When a cervical length of 25 mm or less is obtained, it may be appropriate to obtain a fetal fibronectin test. This opinion is based, paradoxically, on data from a study of cervical length and fibronectin measured in asymptomatic low-risk women that found both tests to have low sensitivity for preterm birth in low-risk pregnancies (61). Despite the poor sensitivity of either test alone, the positive predictive value for preterm birth at less than 35 weeks was 50% when an asymptomatic low-risk patient had both a positive fibronectin test result and a cervical length of less than 25 mm. In the absence of data about how best to manage these pregnancies, education about the signs and symptoms of preterm labor, more frequent visits, and consideration of antenatal corticosteroids seems reasonable.

Summary

New tests for preterm birth have contributed new and important information about the pathways to preterm birth. The use of these tests in clinical practice is currently appropriate in women with symptoms of preterm labor to exclude that diagnosis, with safety for both the mother and the fetus. The use of these tests in asymptomatic women is similarly limited to the selected situations described previously. Use of these tests to screen for risk of preterm birth should be deferred until a successful program of prophylaxis has been reported.

References

1. Hamilton BE, Martin JA, Ventura SJ, Sutton PD, Menacker F. Births: preliminary data for 2004 Natl Vital Stat Rep 2005;54(8):1–17.

2. Martin JA, Hamilton BE, Sutton PD, Ventura SJ, Menacker F, Munson ML. Births: final data for 2003. Natl Vital Stat Rep 2005;54(2): 1–116

3. Wright VC, Schieve LA, Reynolds MA, Jeng G. Assisted reproductive technology surveillance—United States, 2000. MMWR Surveill Summ 2003;52(SS-9):1–16[Erratum in: MMWR 2003;52:942.

4. March of Dimes Peristats. Available at: http://search.marchofdimes.com/cgi-bin/MsmGo.exe?grab_id=13&page_id=262144&query=Peristats&hiword=Peristats+. Retrieved July 26, 2006.

5. Ananth CV, Joseph KS, Oyelese Y, Demissie K, Vintzileos AM. Trends in preterm birth and perinatal mortality among singletons: United States, 1989 Through 2000. Obstet Gynecol 2005;105(5 Pt 1):1084–91.

6. Iams JD. Preterm birth. In: Gabbe SG, Niebyl JR, Simpson JL, editors. Obstetrics: normal and problem pregnancies. 4th ed. Philadelphia (PA): Churchill and Livingstone; 2002. p. 755–826.

7. Hueston WJ. Preterm contractions in community settings: II. Predicting preterm birth in women with preterm contractions. Obstet Gynecol 1998;92:43–6.

8. Macones GA, Segel SY, Stamilio DM, Morgan MA. Predicting delivery within 48 hours in women treated with parenteral tocolysis. Obstet Gynecol 1999;93:432–6.

9. King JF, Grant A, Keirse MJ, Chalmers I. Beta-mimetics in preterm labour: An overview of the randomized clinical trials. Br J Obstet Gynaecol 1988;95:211–22.

10. Meis PJ, Ernest JM, Moore ML. Causes of low birthweight births in public and private patients. Am J Obstet Gynecol 1987;156:1165–8.

11. American College of Obstetricians and Gynecologists. Preterm labor and delivery. Precis: Obstetrics. 2nd ed. Washington, DC: ACOG; 1999.

12. Iams JD, Goldenberg RL, Meis PJ, Mercer BM, Moawad A, Das A, et al. The length of the cervix and the risk of spontaneous preterm delivery. N Engl J Med 1996;334:567–72.

13. Goldenberg RL, Iams JD, Mercer BM, Meis PJ, Moawad AH, Copper RL, et al. The preterm prediction study: the value of new vs standard risk factors in predicting early and all spontaneous preterm births. Am J Public Health 1998;88:233–8.

14. Goldenberg RL, Iams JD, Das A, Mercer BM, Meis PJ, Moawad AH, et al. The preterm prediction study: sequential cervical length and fibronectin testing for the prediction of spontaneous preterm birth. Am J Obstet Gynecol 2000;182:636–43.

15. Goldenberg RL, Mercer BM, Meis PJ, Copper RL, Das A, McNellis D. The preterm prediction study: fetal fibronectin testing and spontaneous preterm birth. Obstet Gynecol 1996;87:643–8.

16. Lockwood CJ, Kuczynski E. Risk stratification and pathological mechanisms in preterm delivery. Paediatr Perinat Epidemiol 2001;15 Suppl 2:78–89.

17. Elovitz MA, Baron J, Phillippe M. The role of thrombin in preterm parturition. Am J Obstet Gynecol 2001;185: 1059–63.

18. Heine RP, McGregor JA, Goodwin TM, Artal R, Hayashi RH, Robertson PA, et al. Serial salivary estriol to detect an increased risk of preterm birth. Obstet Gynecol 2000;96: 490–7.

19. Zilianti M, Azuaga A, Calderon F, Pages G, Mendoza G. Monitoring the effacement of the uterine cervix by transperineal sonography: a new perspective. J Ultrasound Med 1995;14:719–24.

20. Feinberg RF, Kleiman HJ, Lockwood CJ. Is oncofetal fibronectin a trophoblast glue for human implantation? Am J Pathol 1991;138:537–43.

21. Goldenberg RL, Klebanoff M, Carey JC, Macpherson C, Leveno KJ, Moawad AH, et al. Vaginal fetal fibronectin measurements from 8 to 22 weeks' gestation and subsequent spontaneous preterm birth. Am J Obstet Gynecol 2000;183:469–75.

22. Dyson DC, Danbe KH, Bamber JA, Crites YM, Field DR, Maier JA, et al. Monitoring women at risk for preterm labor. N Engl J Med 1998;338:15–9.

23. Rust OA, Atlas RO, Jones KJ, Benham BN, Balducci J. A randomized trial of cerclage versus no cerclage among patients with ultrasonographically detected second-trimester preterm dilatation of the internal os. Am J Obstet Gynecol 2000;183:830–5.

24. Andrews WW. Randomized clinical trial of metronidazole plus erythromycin to prevent spontaneous preterm delivery in fetal fibronectin positive women. J Soc Gynecol Investig 2001;8 Suppl:47A.

25. Meis PJ, Klebanoff M, Thom E, Dombrowski MP, Sibai B, Moawad A et al. Prevention of recurrent preterm delivery by 17 alpha-hydroxyprogesterone caproate. N Engl J Med 2003;348:2379–85

26. Meis PJ for the Society for Maternal Fetal Medicine. 17 Hydroxyprogesterone for the prevention of preterm delivery. Obstet Gynecol 2005;105:1128–35

27. Goldenberg RL, Iams JD, Mercer BM, Meis PJ, Moawad A, Das A, et al. The preterm prediction study: Toward a multiple-marker test for spontaneous preterm birth. Am J Obstet Gynecol 2001;185:643–51.

28. Berkman ND, Thorp JM Jr, Hartmann KE, Lohr KN, Idicula AE, McPheeters M, et al. Management of preterm labor. Evidence report/technology assessment no. 18. AHRQ publication no. 01-E021. Rockville, Maryland: U.S. Department of Health and Human Services, Agency for Healthcare Research and Quality. 2000. Available at: http://www.gov/clinic/epcix.htm. Retrieved October 8, 2002.

29. Pircon RA, Strassner HT, Kirz DS, Towers CV. Controlled trial of bed rest and hydration vs. rest alone in the evaluation of preterm uterine contractions. Am J Obstet Gynecol 1989;161:775–9.

30. Jackson GM, Ludmir J, Bader TJ. The accuracy of digital examination and ultrasound in the evaluation of cervical length. Obstet Gynecol 1992;79:214–8.

31. Hueston WJ. Preterm contractions in community settings: I. Treatment of preterm contractions. Obstet Gynecol 1998;92:38–42.

32. Macones GA, Segel SY, Stamilio DM, Morgan MA. Prediction of delivery among women with early preterm labor by means of clinical characteristics alone. Am J Obstet Gynecol 1999;181:1414–8.

33. Utter GO, Dooley SL, Tamura RK, Socol ML. Awaiting cervical change for the diagnosis of preterm labor does not compromise the efficacy of ritodrine tocolysis. Am J Obstet Gynecol 1990;163:882–6.

34. Iams JD, Casal D, McGregor JA, Goodwin TM, Kreaden US, Lowensohn R, et al. Fetal fibronectin improves the accuracy of diagnosis of preterm labor. Am J Obstet Gynecol 1995;173:141–5.

35. Peaceman AM, Andrews WW, Thorp JM, Cliver SP, Lukes A, Iams JD, et al. Fetal fibronectin as a predictor of preterm birth in patients with symptoms: a multicenter trial. Am J Obstet Gynecol 1997;177:13–8.

36. Murakawa H, Utumi T, Hasagawa I, Tanaka K, Fuzimori R. Evaluation of threatened preterm delivery by transvaginal ultrasonographic measurement of cervical length. Obstet Gynecol 1993;82:829–32.

37. Iams JD, Paraskos J, Landon MB, Teteris JN, Johnson FF. Cervical sonography in preterm labor. Obstet Gynecol 1994;84:40–6.

38. Gomez R, Galasso M, Romero R, Mazor M, Sorokin Y, Goncalves L, et al. Ultrasonographic examination of the uterine cervix is better than cervical digital examinations a predictor of the likelihood of preterm delivery in patients with preterm labor and intact membranes. Am J Obstet Gynecol 1994;171:956–64.

39. Timor-Tritsch I, Boozarjomehri F, Masakowski Y, Monteagudo A, Chao CR. Can a snapshot sagittal view of the cervix by transvaginal ultrasonography predict active preterm labor? Am J Obstet Gynecol 1996;174:990–5.

40. Crane JMG, Van den Hof F, Armson BA, Liston R. Transvaginal ultrasound in the prediction of preterm delivery: Singleton and twin gestations. Obstet Gynecol 1997;90:357–63.

41. Leitich H, Brumbauer M, Kaider A, Egarter C, Husslein P. Cervical length and dilation of the internal os detected by vaginal ultrasonography as markers for preterm delivery: a systematic review. Am J Obstet Gynecol 1999;181:1465–72.

42. Mason GC, Maresh MJA. Alterations in bladder volume and the ultrasound appearance of the cervix. Br J Obstet Gynaecol 1990;97:547–8.

43. Yost NP, Bloom SL, Twickler DM, Leveno KJ. Pitfalls in ultrasonic cervical length measurement for predicting preterm birth. Obstet Gynecol 1999;93:510–6.

44. Joffe GM, Jacques D, Bemis-Hayes R, Burton R, Skram B, Shelburne P. Impact of the fetal fibronectin assay on admissions for preterm labor. Am J Obstet Gynecol 1999; 180:581–6.

45. Giles W, Bisits A, Knox M, Madsen G, Smith R. The effect of fetal fibronectin testing on admissions to a tertiary maternal fetal medicine unit and cost savings. Am J Obstet Gynecol 2000;182:439–42.

46. Chien PF, Khan KS, Ogston S, Owen P. The diagnostic accuracy of cervico-vaginal fetal fibronectin in predicting preterm delivery: an overview. Br J Obstet Gynaecol 1997; 104:436–44.

47. Rinehart BK, Terrone DA, Isler CM, Barrilleaux PS, Bufkin L, Morrison JC. Pregnancy outcome in women with preterm labor symptoms without cervical change. Am J Obstet Gynecol 2001;184:1004–7.

48. Rizzo G, Capponi A, Arduini A, Lorido C, Romanini C. The value of fetal fibronectin in cervical and vaginal secretions and of ultrasonographic examination of the uterine cervix in predicting premature delivery in patients with preterm labor and intact membranes. Am J Obstet Gynecol 1996;175:1146–51.

49. Rozenberg P, Goffinet A, Malagrida L, Giudicelli Y, Perdu M, Houssin I, et al. Evaluating the risk of preterm delivery: a comparison of fetal fibronectin and transvaginal ultrasonographic measurement of cervical length. Am J Obstet Gynecol 1997;176:196–9.

50. Gomez R, Romero R, Medina L, Nien J, Chaiworapongsa T, Carstens M et al. Cervicovaginal fibronectin improves the prediction of preterm delivery based on sonographic cervical length in patients with preterm uterine contractions and intact membranes. Am J Obstet Gynecol 2005; 192:350–59.

51. Guinn DA, Goepfert AR, Owen J, Brumfield C, Hauth JC. Management options in women with preterm contractions: a randomized clinical trial. Am J Obstet Gynecol 1997;177:814–8.

52. Iams JD, Newman RB, Thom EA, Goldenberg RL, Mueller-Heubach E, Moawad A, et al. Frequency of uterine contractions and the risk of spontaneous preterm birth. N Engl J Med 2002;346:250–5.

53. Imseis HM, Albert TA, Iams JD. Identifying twin gestations at low risk for preterm birth with transvaginal ultrasonographic cervical measurement at 24-26 weeks. Am J Obstet Gynecol 1997;177:1149–55.

54. Goldenberg RL, Iams JD, Miodovnik M, Van Dorsten JP, Thurnau G, Bottoms SF, et al. The preterm prediction study: risk factors in twin gestations. Am J Obstet Gynecol 1996;175:1047–53.

55. Mercer B, Egerman R, Beazley D, Sibai B, Carr T, Sepesi J. Weekly antenatal steroids in women at risk for preterm birth: a randomized trial [abstract]. Am J Obstet Gynecol 2001;184:S6

56. National Institutes of Health Consensus Development Panel. Antenatal corticosteroids revisited: Repeat courses— National Institutes of Health Consensus Development Conference statement, August 17–18, 2000. Obstet Gynecol 2001;98:144–50.

57. Iams JD, Goldenberg RL, Mercer BM, Moawad A, Thom E, Meis PJ, et al. The preterm prediction study: recurrence risk of spontaneous preterm birth. Am J Obstet Gynecol 1998;178:1035–40.

58. Althuisius SM, Dekker GA, van Geijn HP, Bekedam DJ, Hummel P. Cervical incompetence prevention randomized cerclage trial (CIPRACT): study design and preliminary results. Am J Obstet Gynecol 2000;183:823–9.

59. Expert Panel on Women's Imaging. Premature cervical dilatation. Reston, Virginia: American College of Radiology, 1999 Available at: http://www.acr.org/dyna/?id appropriateness_criteria. Retrieved October 8, 2002.

60. Andersen HF. Transvaginal and transabdominal ultrasonography of the uterine cervix during pregnancy. J Clin Ultrasound 1991;19:77–83.

61. Iams JD, Goldenberg RL, Mercer BM, Moawad AH, Meis PJ, Das A, et al. The preterm prediction study: can low risk women destined for spontaneous preterm birth be identified? Am J Obstet Gynecol 2001;184:652–5.

CHAPTER 14

Cerclage and Cervical Insufficiency

John Owen and James H. Harger[†]

Preterm birth remains the most important problem in obstetrics, resisting solution and yielding its secrets slowly and reluctantly. Our continued inability to effectively predict and prevent preterm birth has caused many clinicians to adopt empiric methods to determine the risk of the problem, detect its precursors and early stages, and treat various degrees of early labor and cervical dilatation (1, 2). At the beginning of a new millennium dominated by the promise of understanding disease processes through molecular biology and genetics, physicians look forward to providing improved care for many old afflictions. We now emphasize the importance of evidence-based medicine, and routinely advocate the assessment of new treatments through randomized clinical trials with sufficient statistical power and thorough statistical analysis. At present, however, we remain polarized about the value of cervical cerclage (3).

Incidence and Clinical Importance

The incidence of preterm birth varies widely among different populations but is now approximately 13% in the United States. Most (80%) of these are from spontaneous causes and not effected for maternal or fetal indications. Risk factors include low maternal prepregnancy weight and socioeconomic status, racial and ethnic factors, physical effort during pregnancy, tobacco use, shorter intervals between pregnancies, altered vaginal flora, uterine abnormalities, and multiple gestations. The incidence of cervical insufficiency is very difficult to determine because there are no objective criteria for the diagnosis. Rather, the clinical diagnosis is determined by history, physical examination, and exclusion of other causes of midtrimester birth. Nevertheless, many retrospective series of cerclage suggest that the frequency of cerclage operations in some large delivery cohorts around the world ranges from 1:54 to 1:2000 pregnancies (4–8).

The major clinical importance of cervical insufficiency is the difficulty that confronts physicians in differentiating this condition from other causes of early preterm delivery and pregnancy loss. Presuming the diagnosis of cervical insufficiency based on historical criteria alone may divert the attention of the physician from first excluding other causes of preterm birth.

Pathophysiology

Although the pathophysiology of cervical insufficiency is still poorly understood, as early as 1962, it was suggested that cervical competence was not an all-or-none phenomenon as traditionally taught (9). Rather, it comprised degrees of insufficiency, and combinations of factors could cause "cervical failure." In their proposed classification, one group of patients had ostensibly normal cervical tissue, whose integrity as a fibrous ring had been previously damaged as the result of antecedent obstetric trauma. These defects might even be concealed by a normal-appearing external os and ectocervix. The second group possessed an abnormally low collagen/muscle ratio that would compromise its mechanical function and lead to premature dilation. The third group comprised women who had no history of antecedent trauma and who also had normal collagen/muscle ratios but whose obstetric histories mimicked those of groups 1 and 2, presumably from premature triggering of other factors (ie, cervical ripening).

Although tradition has viewed the cervix as either competent or incompetent, recent evidence, including clinical data (10–13) and interpretative reviews (14–16), suggest that, as with most other biologic processes, cervical competence is rarely an all-or-none phenomenon, as it likely functions along a continuum of reproductive performance. Although some women have tangible anatomic evidence of poor cervical integrity, most women with a clinical diagnosis of cervical insufficiency have ostensibly normal cervical anatomy. In a concept of cervical competence as a continuum, a poor obstetric history results from a process of premature cervical ripening induced by infection, inflammation, local or systemic hormonal effects, or even genetic predisposition.

In broader terms, spontaneous preterm birth may be best characterized as a syndrome comprising several

[†]Deceased February 5, 2004

anatomic and related functional components (17). These components include the uterus and its myometrial contractile function (eg, preterm labor), decidual activation and loss of chorioamnionic integrity (eg, preterm rupture of membranes), and diminished cervical competence, either from a primary anatomic defect or from early pathologic cervical ripening (eg, cervical insufficiency). In a particular pregnancy, a single anatomic feature may appear to predominate, even though it is more likely that most cases of spontaneous preterm birth result from the interaction of multiple stimuli and pathways, which culminate in the overt clinical syndrome. Nevertheless, the relative significance of these components varies, not only among different women, but also in successive pregnancies of the same patient. This model supports the variable, and often unpredictable, clinical course of women with a history of cervical insufficiency (18). Thus, correcting just one factor may have such a small, incremental effect that it appears to be insignificant or does not account for most cases of preterm birth. To significantly diminish the incidence of preterm birth, several pathways must be treated simultaneously during the pregnancy. For example, a woman may have an appreciable component of cervical insufficiency but not respond to mechanical support offered by cerclage unless the underlying cause(s) of the midtrimester cervical changes, which may also cause early membrane rupture, also are identified and modified. Although this concept remains largely unproved, it represents an attractive and useful hypothesis for further testing.

Diagnosis

Clinically, the important distinction between cervical insufficiency and preterm labor is usually made through the presence or absence of "painless cervical dilatation." Physicians have been taught that women with perceived, painful uterine contractions or vaginal bleeding underwent delivery because of preterm labor or abruption. Cervical insufficiency was a diagnosis by exclusion. The clinical presentation of cervical insufficiency was often preceded by a history of cervical trauma caused by cone biopsy, intrapartum cervical lacerations, or excessive, forced dilatation in the course of induced abortion. This clinical diagnosis, supported by antecedent pelvic pressure, increased mucoid vaginal discharge, and presenting advanced cervical dilatation without appreciable discomfort or painful uterine contractions, was considered to be sufficient to warrant a trial of prophylactic cerclage in a subsequent pregnancy.

The clinical diagnosis of cervical insufficiency was classically given to women with a history of spontaneous pregnancy loss in the second or rarely the early third trimester; each successive pregnancy loss caused by cervical insufficiency occurred at an earlier gestational age than the previous one. In another variation, a woman could silently dilate, letting the amnionic sac prolapse through a minimally dilated cervix, after which the membranes could rupture spontaneously. Contrary to optimal scientific methods, many of these symptoms and signs were not evaluated by determining the sensitivity, specificity, and predictive values of the various clinical features. Rather, they were assumed to be correct because they appeared plausible and theoretically likely. Confounding these analyses was the lack of an objective "gold" standard for the diagnosis, against which these clinical criteria could be tested.

Previous authors have suggested a variety of diagnostic studies to confirm the presence of cervical insufficiency, but none of these tests has been validated in rigorous scientific studies. Widening of the cervical canal demonstrated by hysterosalpingography, ease of insertion of cervical dilators, force required to withdraw an inflated Foley catheter bulb through the internal os, and several different methods to measure the force required to stretch the cervix using an intracervical balloon have been reported. These tests had significant flaws, including a requirement that they be performed when the subject is not pregnant, use of ionizing radiation, ignoring the known effects of pregnancy on the dynamic response of the cervix, and failing to account for the effect of estrogens and progesterone during the menstrual cycle. At present, there is no valid preoperative test for confirming or refuting the clinical diagnosis of cervical insufficiency in women with historical risk factors.

With the advent of endovaginal ultrasound assessment of the cervix in the past 20 years came new criteria for establishing the diagnosis of some degree of cervical insufficiency. In this new paradigm, the diagnosis is not a dichotomy in which the cervix is proclaimed either "incompetent" or competent (19). Rather, the cervix may be viewed as having a continuum of competency, varying in its ability to remain closed and uneffaced throughout gestation, in spite of the presence of mechanical forces and uterine activity as well as various hormonal, biochemical, bacteriological, and immunological stimuli. Numerous investigators have asserted that cervical incompetence can be diagnosed by midtrimester ultrasound evaluation of the cervix. Various ultrasound findings, including shortened cervical length, funneling at the internal os, and dynamic responses to provocative maneuvers, such as fundal pressure, have been used to select women for treatment, generally cerclage. In most of these earlier reports, the ultrasound evaluations were not blinded, leading to uncontrolled interventions and difficulty determining their effectiveness. In many instances the ultrasound criteria for cervical incompetence were only qualitatively described and, thus, were not reproducible.

More recently large, blinded observational studies using reproducible methods have been published (11, 20, 21). These investigators studied the relationship between midtrimester cervical ultrasound findings and the risk of preterm birth. Members of the National Institute of Child Health and Human Development Maternal–Fetal Medicine Units Network (11) completed a study of 2,915 unselected women with a singleton pregnancy who underwent a blinded cervical ultrasound evaluation at 24 weeks of gestation. The relative risk (RR) of spontaneous preterm birth increased proportional to shortened cervical length. In spite of this highly significant relationship, as a test for predicting spontaneous preterm birth at less than 35 weeks of gestation, a cervical length cutoff of less than 26 mm (the population 10th percentile) had low sensitivity (37%) and poor positive predictive value (18%). Although shortened cervical length less than 25 mm has been suggested as a diagnostic criterion for cervical insufficiency, the extremely low predictive value observed in an unselected population and the realization that approximately 10% of a given population would be given this diagnosis makes this a clinically untenable indication.

In a subsequent study, members of the National Institute of Child Health and Human Development Maternal–Fetal Medicine Units Network (21) examined the utility of cervical ultrasonography as a predictor of spontaneous preterm birth at less than 35 weeks of gestation in high-risk women, defined as at least one prior spontaneous preterm birth at less than 32 weeks of gestation. Women believed to have cervical insufficiency (based on a typical clinical history) and who underwent cerclage were not eligible. Beginning at 16–18 weeks of gestation, 183 pregnant women underwent serial, biweekly ultrasound evaluations until the 23rd week of gestation. The study design permitted an analysis of the shortest observed cervical length over time, which also included any fundal pressure-induced (or spontaneously occurring) cervical length shortening. As in the previous study (11), there was a highly significant inverse relationship between cervical length and spontaneous preterm birth. However, in this high-risk population at a cervical length cutoff of less than 25 mm (the population 10th percentile at the initial evaluation), the sensitivity increased to 69% and the positive predictive value to 55%. Importantly, a secondary analysis of the data suggested that these high-risk women with shortened cervical length may have a clinically significant component of cervical insufficiency because there was a preponderance of midtrimester births at less than 27 weeks of gestation in this cohort (22).

These reports (21, 22) and others support the concept that cervical length, as a surrogate function for cervical competence, operates along a continuum of reproductive performance and provides prospective confirmation of an earlier published retrospective analysis (10). Nevertheless, in spite of the consistent relationship between shortened cervical length and spontaneous preterm birth, the identification of an appropriate cervical length action cutoff and confirmation of the potential contribution of related cervical ultrasound findings (eg, funneling at the internal os) remains problematic. Cervical ultrasonography performs poorly as a screening test in low-risk women (11), but it appears to have significant utility in high-risk women, defined as women with a prior early spontaneous preterm birth (20, 21). Whether cervical ultrasonography has similar predictive values in other populations of at risk women (eg, exposure to diethylstilbestrol, prior cervical surgery, multiple induced abortions) remains speculative because it has not been well studied. Whereas some investigators have included women with these risk factors in their study populations composed primarily of women with prior spontaneous preterm birth, the results could not been subcategorized because of small sample sizes (20). However, in a recent series of 64 women with various uterine anomalies, the authors observed an overall preterm delivery rate at less than 35 weeks of gestation of 11% and a significant relationship between cervical length less than 25 mm and preterm birth (23), with summary predictive values similar to other high-risk populations (21). A recent systematic review (24) summarized the predictive value of vaginal ultrasonography for preterm birth in 46 published series of both asymptomatic and symptomatic gravida women carrying singleton or twin gestations.

Management

Patient Selection for Prophylactic Cerclage

Over the past 40 years, women have been selected for cervical cerclage for a variety of indications. Initial reports suggested cerclage for women with a visible defect in the exocervix, a scar or laceration that could be repaired as if it were a hernia (25). In contemporary practice, overt cervical trauma has become increasingly uncommon and such palpable cervical defects rare in the United States. Cervical damage from surgery also is diminishing as indications for cone biopsy and more radical surgical procedures are diminishing. More common is the patient who has undergone a loop electrosurgical excision procedure (LEEP), usually for cervical dysplasia. This procedure is plausibly a risk factor for cervical insufficiency.

A study of 574 women who had undergone LEEP examined the reproductive performance of 55 women who conceived after the surgery (26). Their goal had been to obtain a nominal 7 mm thick specimen, and they cited a maximum excisional depth of 1.5 cm. In this series, no spontaneous preterm birth at less than 37 weeks was observed. A similar series of 52 women reported an incidence of spontaneous preterm birth of less than 10% and no midtrimester losses that might suggest a clinical diagnosis of cervical incompetence (27). A more recent and much larger retrospective cohort study (28) examined 652 women treated with laser conization, laser ablation, or LEEP, and compared these women to a cohort of 426 untreated patients. The overall adjusted rates of preterm birth before 37 weeks of gestation were similar; however, the group with the highest tertile of specimen height (greater than or equal to 1.7 cm) had more than a three-fold increased risk of preterm chorioamnionic rupture compared with untreated women. Even considering the effect on preterm membrane rupture, the overall effect on preterm birth was not statistically significant because the 95% confidence interval included 1.

Nevertheless, the most accepted indication for prophylactic cerclage was a typical history consistent with the clinical diagnosis (ie, recurrent painless dilation and midtrimester birth) and no satisfactory alternate explanation for the preterm birth (29). More than 100 non-controlled studies have employed this indication to various degrees, but none has proved the efficacy of cerclage in such cases. Interestingly, a German randomized trial published in 1986 compared prophylactic cerclage with the use of a vaginal pessary and found no difference in perinatal outcome (30).

Branch in 1986 (31) and Cousins in 1980 (32) collectively tabulated over 25 case series of cerclage efficacy published between 1959 and 1981. Branch estimated a precerclage survival range of 10–32% versus a perinatal survival range of 75–83% in the same cohorts of women managed with Shirodkar cerclage. Similarly, case series that used McDonald cerclage reported a cohort perinatal survival range of 7–50% before, and 63–89% with cerclage. Cousins estimated a "mean" survival before Shirodkar of 22% versus 82% after therapy and 27% and 74%, respectively, for investigators who used the McDonald technique. In total, experience with over 2,000 patients has been reported in these historic cohort comparisons. Interpretation of these series is limited by several important observations: 1) diagnostic criteria were not consistent or always reported, 2) definitions of treatment success were inconsistent (but generally recorded as perinatal survival, as opposed to a gestational age-based end point) 3) treatment approaches were not always detailed and might involve multiple combinations of surgery, medication, bed rest and other uncontrolled therapies, and 4) cases were not subcategorized according to etiology (ie, anatomic defects versus a presumed functional cause) (32). Nevertheless, based on compelling, but potentially biased efficacy data, the surgical management of women with clinically defined cervical insufficiency has become common (29).

As a consequence of largely uncontrolled studies suggesting a benefit from cerclage in women with a typical history, firm, evidence-based guidelines for the management of women with a history of at least two (ie, recurrent) pregnancy losses associated with painless cervical dilatation in the second (or early third) trimester are lacking but may include prophylactic cerclage (Fig. 14-1). The cerclage should be performed at 13–16 weeks of gestation after ultrasound evaluation shows a live fetus with no apparent anomalies. Although there are no rigorous scientific data to guide the management of women with a previous successful pregnancy treated with prophylactic cerclage for appropriate indications, another prophylactic cerclage is probably warranted; most women with a successful previous cerclage are understandably reluctant to attempt future pregnancies without another cerclage. In the absence of data from a randomized trial, this decision should be made by consensus between physician and patient. Women with a history of only one second-trimester pregnancy loss can be monitored with serial endovaginal ultrasonography beginning at 16–20 weeks of gestation, depending on the gestational timing of the previous pregnancy loss. These are continued to around 23 weeks of gestation, the threshold of fetal viability, after which the risks of cerclage may outweigh any potential benefit. At present, there is no scientific evidence supporting cervical cerclage for any indication in the first trimester.

A small proportion of patients has the obstetric history appropriate for the diagnosis of cervical insufficiency but, in addition, displays cervical hypoplasia. Such women may have had an extensive cold cone biopsy or a severe, deep obstetric laceration of the cervix, whereas a few suffer such lacerations as a consequence of uterine rupture or displaced cerclage. Some cases appear to result from congenital anomalies of the cervix and are sometimes associated with exposure in utero to nonsteroidal estrogens such as diethylstilbestrol. Other cases are associated with sporadic müllerian anomalies. The literature on cerclage in women exposed in utero to diethylstilbestrol is unclear (33, 34) and lacks randomized trials. Regardless, the last systematic diethylstilbestrol administration to pregnant women ended more than 35 years ago, so this appears to be a moot point.

Because transvaginal insertion of a cerclage band in these women with a hypoplastic cervix by any technique

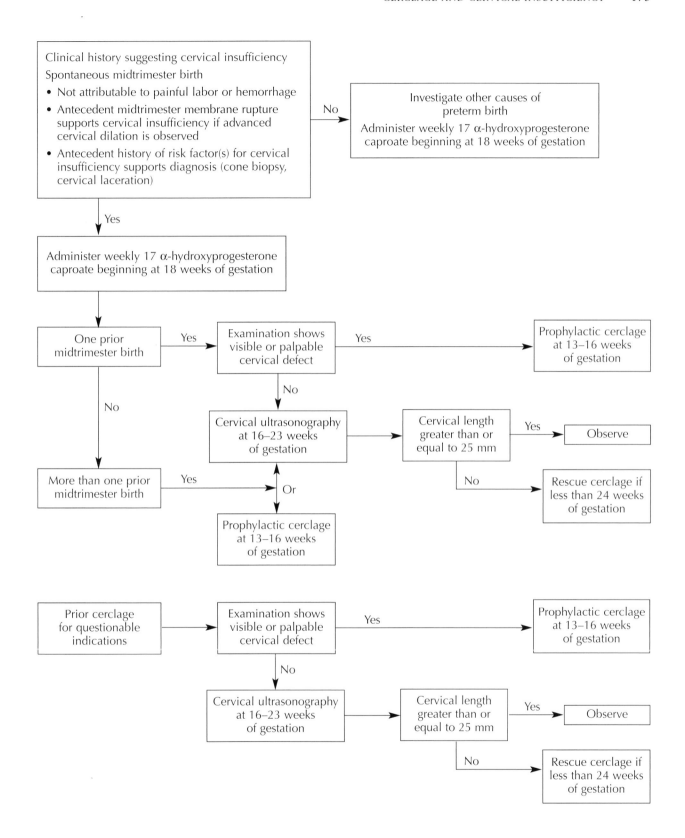

Fig. 14-1. Indicated cerclage: obstetric history and physical findings. (Modified from Harger JH. Cerclage and cervical insufficiency: An evidence-based analysis. Obstet Gynecol 2002;100:1313–27.)

would be technically difficult or impossible, some authors have advocated a transabdominal approach (35–38). Indications for this laparotomy-based cerclage method include technical failure in previous transvaginal attempts to place the cerclage band, failure of the transvaginal cerclage with or without displacement of the band, and occasional instances in which there is either a deep cervical laceration or absence of sufficient cervical tissue to anchor the transvaginal cerclage. The morbidity of transabdominal cerclage can be formidable. There are significant risks from surgical hemorrhage and the required laparotomy during early pregnancy. To the usual serious operative risks of cerclage placement, postoperative intestinal obstruction and thrombophlebitis must be added. The physician and patient also must consider the requirement for cesarean delivery not only for the index pregnancy but also for subsequent pregnancies if the band is left in place; this is usually done if future fertility is desired. Because of the rarity of indications for transabdominal cerclage, the available published series on transabdominal cerclage are too small to establish sound, evidence-based scientific proof for this approach (39).

Regardless of the clinical history or original cerclage indication, once a woman had a successful pregnancy with a cerclage, few obstetricians would refrain from using a cerclage in subsequent pregnancies. Because few, if any, controlled data support the utility of prophylactic cerclage, this practice will likely lead to overuse of the procedure. Although a placebo-controlled trial of cerclage in women with a typical clinical history might be difficult to perform, trials with other therapeutic options, such as vaginal pessary, ultrasound cervical assessment, or pharmacologic interventions should define the role of cerclage in contemporary obstetric practice.

Other indications for cerclage (in women lacking a typical or classic history) have included: 1) the presence of various "risk factors" (eg, prior cervical surgery such as LEEP or induced abortion), 2) shortened cervical length or funneling on a midtrimester ultrasonogram and 3) the observation of cervical dilation with membrane prolapse in the midtrimester. The evidence for cerclage in these clinical settings will be reviewed.

Cerclage for Risk Factors

To date, four randomized clinical trials of prophylactic cerclage (40–43) for risk factors have failed to show any benefit except the largest, multinational study of 1,292 women who lacked a typical clinical history, but whose managing physicians were unsure whether cerclage was indicated based on any of six historical risk factors (41). In the entire study population, the frequency of delivery before 33 weeks of gestation was significantly lower (RR, 0.75; 95% confidence interval [CI], 0.57–0.98) in cerclage-treated women (83 of 647, 13%) than in the controls (110 of 645, 17%). Because most untreated women delivered near term regardless, this benefit only amounts to the saving of one preterm birth at less than 33 weeks of gestation in every 25 treated with prophylactic cerclage for risk factors. Moreover, women assigned to cerclage received more tocolytic medications and spent more time in the hospital. Puerperal fever was significantly more common in the cerclage group.

In subgroup analyses, the authors divided their study subjects into six mutually exclusive cohorts: 1) 554 singleton pregnancies with exactly one second-trimester abortion or preterm delivery but no cone biopsy or cervical amputation, 2) 196 singleton pregnancies with exactly two second-trimester abortions or preterm deliveries but no cone biopsy or cervical amputation, 3) 107 singleton pregnancies with three or more second-trimester abortions or preterm deliveries but no cone biopsy or cervical amputation, 4) 138 singleton pregnancies with a history of cone biopsy or cervical amputation, 5) 269 singleton pregnancies with other indications, and 6) 28 twin pregnancies. Only in the subgroup of 107 women with at least three previous second-trimester pregnancy losses or premature births was there a significant reduction in the frequency of delivery before 33 weeks of gestation, 8 of 54 (15%) in the cerclage group compared with 17 of 53 (32%) in the control group (P = .02). In the other five subgroups, there was no significant improvement in neonatal outcome or rate of preterm birth. The authors concluded that this latter subgroup should undergo further study. This failure to find a clear benefit for elective cerclage based on risk factors known to be associated with cervical insufficiency perplexed many obstetricians.

Cerclage for Ultrasound Indications

Asymptomatic women who are found to have shortened cervical length or cervical funneling in the midtrimester comprise a group with suspected cervical insufficiency. Many retrospective studies in the past decade have attempted to address this group of "urgent" or "rescue" cerclages with contradictory findings (Table 14-1) (38, 44–47).

More recently, the publication of four randomized trials of cerclage for shortened cervical length has increased our awareness of the limitations of cerclage for this theoretical indication (Table 14-1) (48–52). In the Netherlands (48–49) a two-tiered randomized clinical trial of high-risk patients, most of whom were believed to have cervical incompetence based on their obstetric history, was performed. In the first tier, eligible patients

Table 14-1. Cohort Series and Randomized Trials of Cerclage for Ultrasonographically Suspected Cervical Insufficiency in Singleton Gestations

Author, Year	Population	N	Selection Criteria	Gestational Age	Outcome	Benefit
Retrospective Cohort Series						
Heath, 1998 (46)	Unselected	43	Cervical length, less than or equal to l5 mm	23 weeks	Preterm birth at less than 32 weeks of gestation Cerclage (5%) versus no cerclage (50%)	Yes
Berghella, 1999 (45)	Risk factors	63	Cervical length less than 25 mm or more than 25% funneling	14–24 weeks	Adjusted odds ratio for preterm birth at less than 35 weeks of gestation with cerclage: 1.1; 95% confidence interval, 0.3–4.6	No
Novy, 2001 (47)	Symptomatic and asymptomatic women with certain physical findings	35	Cervical length less than 30 mm plus funneling and softening or less than 60% effaced and external os less than 2 cm dilated	18–27 weeks	Mean 4 wk increase in delivery gestational age with cerclage: 29 versus 25 weeks	Yes
Hassan, 2001 (44)	Unselected	70	Cervical length less than or equal to 15 mm	14–24 weeks	Preterm birth at less than 34 weeks of gestation Cerclage (68%) versus no cerclage (53%)	No
Randomized Clinical Trials						
Althuisius, 2001 (48, 49)	High-risk history consistent with cervical insufficiency	35	Cervical length less than 25 mm	Less than 27 weeks	Preterm birth at less than 34 weeks of gestation Cerclage (0%) versus no cerclage (44%)	Yes
Rust, 2001 (50)	Unselected, but many had risk factors	113	Cervical length less than 25 mm or more than 25% funneling	16–24 weeks	Preterm birth at less than 34 weeks of gestation Cerclage (35%) versus no cerclage (36%)	No
To, 2004 (51)	Unselected, low risk	253	Cervical length less than or equal to 15 mm	22–24 weeks	Preterm birth at less than 33 weeks of gestation Cerclage (22%) versus no cerclage (26%)	No
Berghella, 2004 (52)	Unselected, but most had risk factors	61	Cervical length less than 25 mm or more than 25% funneling	14–23 weeks	Preterm birth at less than 35 weeks of gestation Cerclage (45%) versus no cerclage (47%)	No

were randomly assigned to receive either prophylactic cerclage or to begin ultrasound surveillance. Thirty-five of the patients assigned to the cervical ultrasound group were found to have a shortened cervical length less than 25 mm and underwent a second randomization to either cerclage or no cerclage. Both cerclage and no cerclage groups were instructed to use modified home rest. Of the 19 assigned to cerclage, there was no preterm birth at less than 34 weeks of gestation versus a 44% preterm birth rate in the no cerclage, home rest group (*P* = .002). None

of the women who maintained a cervical length of at least 25 mm experienced a preterm birth. The women who received cerclage for shortened cervical length had outcomes almost identical to women who received the earlier prophylactic cerclage. In one study, 138 women who had various risk factors for preterm birth (including 12% with multiple gestations) were randomly assigned to receive McDonald cerclage or no cerclage after their cervical length shortened to less than 25 mm or they developed funneling greater than 25% (50). Preterm birth at less than 34 weeks of gestation was observed in 35% of the cerclage group versus 36% of the control group.

In a multinational trial comprising 12 hospitals in 6 countries, 47,123 unselected women were screened at 22–24 weeks of gestation with vaginal ultrasonography to identify 470 with a shortened cervical length of 15 mm or less (51). Of these 470 women, 253 participated in a randomized trial in which the primary outcome was the rate of delivery prior to 33 weeks of gestation. Women assigned to the (Shirodkar) cerclage group (n = 127) had a similar rate of preterm birth as the control population (n = 126), 22% versus 26%; $P = .44$. The authors did not specifically comment on the proportion of women in the control group who underwent deliveries in the midtrimester after a presentation consistent with clinically defined cervical incompetence; however, they observed four stillbirths attributed to birth at 23–24 weeks of gestation and five neonatal deaths in deliveries at 23–26 weeks of gestation. In the cerclage group, the respective counts were three and four. Finally, women with various risk factors for spontaneous preterm birth (prior preterm birth, curettages, cone biopsy, and diethylstilbestrol exposure) were screened with vaginal scans every 2 weeks from 14–23 weeks of gestation, and 61 women with a cervical length less than 25 mm or funneling greater than 25% were randomly assigned to McDonald cerclage or to a no-cerclage control group (52). Preterm birth at less than 35 weeks of gestation was observed in 45% of the cerclage group and 47% of the control group.

Of the four published randomized trials, the findings of two (50, 52) seem most applicable to obstetric practice in the United States, and these reports did not support the use of cerclage for ultrasound findings commonly cited as "abnormal" in women with various types of risk factors. The multinational trial (51) confirmed that shortened cervical length less than or equal to 15 mm identified a very high-risk group; however, approximately 100 women in a general obstetric population would have to be screened to find one with this risk factor. None of these studies demonstrated a clinical benefit from ultrasound-indicated cerclage.

One trial (48, 49) included women who the authors believed had a clinical diagnosis of cervical incompetence based on past obstetric history and who would have likely been candidates for prophylactic cerclage in the United States. Nevertheless, their study does suggest a potential role for cervical ultrasonography in women with a clinical diagnosis of cervical incompetence, if the intent is to avoid cerclage when the cervical length is maintained at greater than or equal to 25 mm. This also has been the conclusion of other investigators (53). In one case series of 35 women in whom cerclage had been placed in prior pregnancies for questionable indications, it was found that, collectively, these women had been managed through 58 pregnancies with cerclage (54). These investigators followed the cohort through an additional 52 pregnancies managed with clinical examinations and ultrasonography up to 28 weeks of gestation without elective, prophylactic cerclage. Compared with the pregnancies managed with elective cerclage, fewer perinatal losses were observed in the group managed with serial examinations (0% versus 16% in the elective cerclage group; $P = .01$). Thus, it may be reasonable to suggest that women with a prior cerclage for questionable indications be followed in a similar manner to that for women with one prior midtrimester loss consistent with cervical insufficiency (Fig. 14-1).

A meta-analysis (55) of the previously described four randomized trials analyzed patient-level data to determine if certain subgroups of women with midtrimester cervical shortening might benefit from cerclage, defined as a reduction in the RR of preterm birth at less than 35 weeks of gestation. Paradoxically, they demonstrated a significant detriment in women with multiple gestations (RR, 2.15; 95% CI, 1.15–4.01), although this has not been confirmed in other retrospective series (56, 57). They did observe a marginal benefit from cerclage in women with singleton gestations, and particularly those who also had experienced a prior spontaneous preterm birth (RR, 0.61; 95% CI, 0.4–0.9). However, some of this apparent beneficial effect may have been because of the inclusion of women with a prior spontaneous birth attributed to a clinical diagnosis of cervical insufficiency (48, 49). Whether patients with a prior preterm birth attributed to other components of the spontaneous preterm birth syndrome would benefit from ultrasound-indicated cerclage remains speculative. A large, multicenter randomized trial in high-risk women, defined as women who had one or more early spontaneous preterm births but who lack a clinical history of cervical incompetence, is needed to further define the potential utility of cervical ultrasound screening to select patients for interventions such as cerclage. Such a trial is currently in progress (2, 58).

Emergent Cerclage

Women who present with incompetence in evolution have been considered for an emergent cerclage. Advanced, painless cervical dilatation was a key diagnostic criterion, but obstetric history was not necessary for this diagnosis. Any woman, even a primigravida, could be considered for this diagnosis if her cervix were found to be dilated more than 2 cm with no perceived uterine contractions and no bleeding to suggest abruption. Cervical effacement of greater than 50% and 1) the presence of pelvic pressure,

2) the symptom of a heavy, mucoid vaginal discharge, and 3) bulging membranes prolapsed through the cervical os would support the immediate diagnosis of cervical insufficiency. If electronic contraction monitoring revealed no evidence of labor and the fetus was normal without evidence of chorioamnionitis, then an emergent cerclage would be inserted at once.

Similar to case series describing the presumed benefit of prophylactic cerclage, reports describing the outcome of women who present with incompetence in evolution generally have not always included a contemporary control group managed with bed rest or other therapy. In one review of eight series published between 1980 and 1992 comprising 249 patients who received an emergent midtrimester cerclage, a mean neonatal survival rate of 64% (reported range, 22–100%) was estimated (59). In a series of 35 cases of incompetence in evolution (cervical dilation, 2–5 cm), the two cohorts included 19 women who received emergent cerclage and 16 who were managed with bed rest (47). The neonatal survival rate was 80% in the cerclage cohort versus 75% in the bed rest group.

In a prospective, though uncontrolled evaluation of cerclage versus bed rest (cerclage was used at the discretion of the attending physician), women presenting with more advanced cervical dilation greater than 4 cm (Fig. 14-2) were studied (60). The cerclage group comprised 22 women versus 15 in the bed-rest group. Although neonatal survival was not significantly different (17:22 with cerclage versus 9:15 with bed rest, P = .3), gestational age at birth was a mean 4 weeks greater in the cerclage group (33 weeks versus 29 weeks, P = .001). Rates of chorioamnionitis were similar between the two groups. In spite of obvious flaws in study design and size, the authors claim that their series showed that "the superiority of emergency cervical cerclage to bed rest was clearly demonstrated." They also stated that ethical restrictions precluded randomizing the enrollment process but simultaneously called for a larger randomized clinical trial of emergency cerclage (60).

In a randomized clinical trial, emergency cerclage plus bed rest versus bed rest alone was evaluated in 23 women who presented with cervical dilation and membranes prolapsing to or beyond the external os prior to 27 weeks of gestation (61). Both singleton and twin gestations were eligible; however, no information on the amount of cervical dilation was reported, and so it is not known whether the groups were comparable in this important aspect. They observed a longer mean interval from presentation to delivery (54 days versus 20 days, P = .046) in the cerclage group. The neonatal survival rate was 9:16 with cerclage and 4:14 in the bed-rest group. Although the survival differences were not statistically significant, there were significantly lower rates of neonatal composite morbidity (which included death) in the cerclage group (10:16 versus 14:14, P = .02).

Although, these reports are not of sufficient scientific quality on which to base firm management recommendations, collectively they demonstrate several important concepts. The earlier the gestational age at presentation and the more advanced the cervical dilation, the greater the risk of poor neonatal outcome. Other reports show that women who present with incompetence in evolution have an appreciable (nominal 50%) incidence of bacterial colonization of their amniotic fluid or other markers of subclinical chorioamnionitis (16, 62, 63) or proteomic markers of inflammation or bleeding (64). Women with abnormal amniotic fluid markers have a much shorter presentation-to-delivery interval, regardless of whether they receive cerclage or are managed expectantly with bed rest.

In a study in which amniocentesis was performed in 18 women who presented with incompetence in evolution and the amniotic fluid analyzed for glucose, l-lactate dehydrogenase, Gram stain, and culture, abnormal results suggested subclinical infection (62). Of 11 women who underwent cerclage with no evidence of subclinical infection, the neonatal survival was 100%, and the mean latent phase duration from presentation to delivery was 93 days. Of the 7 women with abnormal biochemistry profiles in whom cerclage was withheld, no neonatal survivors were observed, and the mean latent phase was 4 days. Recognizing that at least a portion of the 7 women who declined amniocentesis but who received emergent cerclage also had subclinical infection, it was predictable that the mean latent phase in this cohort was intermediate (17 days) as compared with the groups with disparate amniotic fluid analyses. These investigators suggested

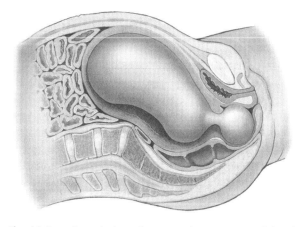

Fig. 14-2. Prolapsed ("hourglass") membranes in a candidate for "emergency" cerclage. Illustration: Thomas Sims. (Harger JH. Cerclage and cervical insufficiency: an evidence-based analysis. Obstet Gynecol 2002;100:1313–27.)

that amniocentesis could aid in selecting candidates for emergent therapeutic cerclage.

The optimal management of women who present with incompetence in evolution remains indefinite. Although emergent cerclage may benefit some, patient selection remains largely empiric. Although it is not standard care, the evaluation of amniotic fluid makers of infection and inflammation appear to have important prognostic value, but it is still unclear whether and to what extent the results should direct patient management. Further clinical investigation is clearly warranted.

Selection of Cerclage Technique

Many variations on the technique of cerclage have been published. The current standard techniques employed for transvaginal cerclage were first described by Shirodkar (65) and McDonald (66); since then, both have been modified in minor ways without any real change in the basic approach. The original Shirodkar band was composed of a fascia lata autograft inserted at the level of the internal cervical os by dissecting the bladder cephalad. Currently, most surgeons employ a 5-mm wide Mersilene band anchored with silk sutures to cervical stroma (65). Transabdominal cerclages employ the same Mersilene band applied through a laparotomy with several minor alterations in approach to reduce the disruption of uterine vessels and consequent hemorrhage. The McDonald purse-string suture with large silk sutures or, in some authors' hands, a 5-mm Mersilene band or no.1 nonabsorbable suture is easier and faster to insert, but neither technique has ever been shown to be superior to the other in a randomized trial. The same surgeons who favor one cerclage technique over the other are likely to select different women for the cerclage than the surgeons who favor the other technique, leading to the inevitable selection biases that render comparisons invalid (4, 67). Efforts to bolster the marginal efficacy of cerclage have led to other methods, such as the Wurm procedure, using large, U-shaped horizontal mattress silk sutures through the cervix. Some authors even advocate suturing the cervix entirely shut, but none of these procedures has gained many adherents. The McDonald procedure remains the most often employed because of its simplicity, speed, lack of need for dissection of the urinary bladder, and ease in later removal.

Complications

The sheer simplicity of most cerclage operations, especially the most commonly used McDonald purse-string suture, may obscure the hazards of cerclage procedures. This perceived simplicity and safety could lead the physician to employ cerclage as a therapeutic trial in a woman with a marginal diagnosis. Faced with uncertain reasons for a history of pregnancy losses, a physician could reason that, if a pregnancy treated empirically with cerclage results in a satisfactory perinatal outcome, the diagnosis must have been cervical insufficiency. Such reasoning leads the physician to overlook other indicated diagnostic studies, such as hysterosalpingography and parental karyotyping. Further, the physician could overlook other treatable factors in the development of preterm birth, such as progesterone. Recently the National Institute of Child Health and Human Development Maternal–Fetal Medicine Units Network reported the results of a clinical trial comparing weekly injections of 17 α-hydroxyprogesterone caproate for the prevention of preterm birth in women with a history of spontaneous preterm delivery. Patients receiving 17 α-hydroxyprogesterone caproate had a 33% reduction in preterm birth compared with those receiving placebo (68). At this time, it is less clear how this information may be applied to patients with a clinical history of cervical insufficiency because this population has not been specifically investigated. Nevertheless its use should be considered because these patients, by definition, have all experienced at least one prior spontaneous preterm birth.

The complications associated with nonemergent cerclage have been reported in many publications (Table 14-2). Of these complications, membrane rupture and pelvic infection are the most serious because they generally lead to pregnancy loss. The series in Table 14-2 tend to be from older publications and most comprise relatively small patient populations; the point estimates necessarily involve wide confidence limits. Many are from centers outside of the United States and, in some cases, the distinction between acute and later complications is difficult to ascertain. Recent data on cerclage-associated complications are lacking. Of the eight series using cerclage for ultrasound indications, only two reported procedure-associated complications (46, 51). In each of these series there was one occurrence of membrane rupture at less than 12 hours after cerclage. There appears to be no clear explanation for the dearth of data about cerclage complications in reports published in the past two decades. If, however, cerclage complications were actually less frequent at present, authors supporting the use of cerclage should be likely to emphasize that point and assert the increased safety of the operations.

Other complications associated with cerclage include displacement of the suture and cervical scarring leading to significant lacerations in labor. Suture displacement requiring cerclage revision or removal is uncommon; if cervical lacerations result, their long-term consequences have not been well-characterized. Another complication of cerclage, regardless of its indications,

Table 14-2. Acute Complications of Nonemergent Cerclage

Author	Year	N	Chorioamnionic rupture (%)	Chorioamnionitis (%)
Cushner) (69)	1963	25		3
Harger (3)	1980	202	1.1	1
Jennings (70)	1972	61	1.6	
Lipshitz (71)	1975	71	1.4	
Nishijima (72)	1969	46		2.2
Peters et al (73)	1979	32	9	6.2
Taylor et al (74)	1959	40	5	
Toaff et al (7)	1977	381		1

Modified from Harger JH. Cerclage and cervical insufficiency: an evidence-based analysis. Obstet Gynecol 2002;100:1313–27.

includes the ill-defined problem called "cervical dystocia" in 1.4–5% of later pregnancies (4, 5, 71). Papers published in the past decade have not mentioned this problem, which is attributed to scarring of the cervix caused by the presence of the suture itself. Although plausible, this complication has been difficult to distinguish from other causes of slow progress in labor and can be minimized in the counseling of cerclage candidates.

Increased uterine contractile activity may follow surgical manipulation of the cervix itself or insertion of a foreign body such as a McDonald or Shirodkar suture. Prevention of this postoperative problem has been addressed in many ways by different authors. Some authors employ preoperative contraction monitoring to differentiate women with appreciable uterine activity from those with none, and they generally refrain from performing a cerclage in those women with evidence of frequent contractions. Most authors suggest bed rest after cerclage for widely varying lengths of time ranging from 24 hours to 5 days. Some reasonably require reduced maternal activity and pelvic rest for the remainder of the pregnancy, considering this relatively benign proscription as part of the multifactorial approach to reducing the risk of preterm delivery. Nevertheless, the insistence on prolonged bed rest could cause deep vein thrombosis and pulmonary embolism. In general, the recommendation of bed rest has not been associated with improved perinatal outcomes (75). Many authors augment postoperative rest with administration of tocolytic drugs such as terbutaline and indomethacin.

These drugs are administered orally and, sometimes, intravenously for hours to days after placement of cerclage. Although such adjunctive treatments may be appealing intuitively, they have never been evaluated in an appropriately designed randomized study of women after cerclage placement.

Overt chorioamnionitis has been reported in association with nonemergent cerclages in 1.0–7.7% of older reports (4, 5, 7, 76). Such reports have led some authors to advocate the use of perioperative prophylactic antibiotic therapy and precerclage screening and treatment of presumed cervical pathogens. As with tocolytic therapy around the time of cerclage, however, no randomized trials have presented controlled data supporting the efficacy of this practice and excluding the effect of confounding treatments. Future study analysis should include multivariable regression to account for these confounding variables.

Elective cesarean delivery also was reported in the older literature as a consequence of the decision to leave successful Shirodkar sutures in place. Previous papers calculated that elective cesarean delivery was performed for this indication in 3–18% of all cerclage-treated pregnancies (4, 7, 77). Since the McDonald technique has largely supplanted the Shirodkar procedure, there are no data supporting the superiority of the Shirodkar technique, and this issue also has disappeared from the literature of the past decade.

Future Problems for Study

Given the present limited state of our knowledge about the pathophysiology of cervical insufficiency, more research must be conducted. Clarifying the molecular biology of the cervix is essential if we are to improve our diagnosis of this elusive condition and if we are to design effective interventions that minimize complications. Accurate patient selection for the correct preventive therapy is paramount. Seminal work (78, 79) has provided some provocative early information about this crucial area, but the difficulty of obtaining human cervical biopsy specimens just before, during, and after labor has led investigators to employ a rat model as a surrogate. The hypothesis that disorganization and rearrangement of collagen fibrils by a decorin-collagen interaction, rather than collagen degradation through an enzymatic activity, are a primary mechanism in the weakening of the tensile strength of the cervix has been studied in rat models (73).

At present, randomized clinical trials are essential to determine which patients actually benefit from cerclage, the optimal surgical technique in various clinical settings, and the efficacy of adjunctive tocolytic agents and antibiotics in the perioperative period. These trials must be large enough and diverse enough for subgroup analysis and for external validity. Although some authorities have questioned the ethics of performing clinical trials of cerclage because randomized trials have shown no clear benefit from cerclage for most indications, an evidence-based approach suggests that the recommendation for cerclage itself may be unethical. Forty-five years of retrospective reports supporting cerclage have failed to provide contemporary, evidence-based support for the procedure.

Summary

Spontaneous preterm birth is best characterized as a syndrome comprised of uterine, chorioamnionic–decidual and cervical components. Multiple stimuli and poorly defined interactive pathways result in preterm birth. In some patients one component may appear to dominate the clinical presentation.

Cervical insufficiency is primarily a clinical diagnosis characterized by recurrent painless dilation and midtrimester birth. As a component of the preterm birth syndrome, cervical competence usually functions along a continuum of reproductive performance. The efficacy of prophylactic cerclage for a clinical diagnosis of cervical insufficiency has never been confirmed in properly designed randomized clinical trials but may improve perinatal outcome in carefully selected patients. In the absence of a clinical history of cervical insufficiency, prophylactic cerclage for women with various "risk factors" and "rescue" cerclage for ultrasound evidence of cervical length shortening has been proved ineffective in large randomized trials.

Additional research is needed to define the optimal candidate for cerclage, especially women who present with advanced midtrimester dilation and women with prior early spontaneous preterm birth and cervical length shortening.

References

1. Goldenberg RL, Rouse DJ. Prevention of premature birth. NEJM 1998;339:313–20.

2. Romero R, Espinoza J, Erez O, Hassan S. The role of cerclage in obstetric practice: can the patient who could benefit from this procedure be identified? Am J Obstet Gynecol 2006;194:1–9.

3. Alfirevic Z. Cerclage: We all know how to do it but can't agree when to do it. Obstet Gynecol 2006;107:219–20.

4. Harger JH. Comparison of success and morbidity in cervical cerclage procedures. Obstet Gynecol 1980;56:543–9.

5. Kuhn RJP, Pepperell RJ. Cervical ligation: A review of 242 pregnancies. Aust N Z J Obstet Gynaecol 1977;17:79–83.

6. Barter RH, Dusbabek JA, Riva HL, Parks J. Surgical closure of the incompetent cervix during pregnancy. Am J Obstet Gynecol 1958;75:511–24.

7. Toaff R, Toaff ME. Cervical incompetence: Diagnostic and therapeutic aspects. Isr J Med Sci 1977;13:39–49.

8. Lidegaard O. Cervical incompetence and cerclage in Denmark 1980–1990. A register-based epidemiological survey. Acta Obstet Gynecol Scand 1994;73:35–8.

9. Danforth DN, Buckingham JC. Cervical incompetence: A re-evaluation. Postgrad Med 1962;32:345–51.

10. Iams JD, Johnson FF, Sonek J, Sachs L, Gebauer C, Samuels P. Cervical competence as a continuum: A study of ultrasonographic cervical length and obstetric performance. Am J Obstet Gynecol 1995;172:1097–106. (G)

11. Iams JD, Goldenberg RL, Meis PJ, Mercer BM, Moawad A, Das A, et al. The length of the cervix and the risk of spontaneous premature delivery. National Institute of Child Health and Human Development Maternal Fetal Medicine Unit Network. N Engl J Med 1996;334:567–72.

12. Buckingham JC, Buethe RA Jr, Danforth DN. Collagen-muscle ratio in clinically normal and clinically incompetent cervices. Am J Obstet Gynecol 1965;91:232–7.

13. Ayers JWR, DeGrood RM, Compton AA, Barclay M, Ansbacher R. Sonographic evaluation of cervical length in pregnancy; diagnosis and management of preterm cervical effacement in patients at risk for premature delivery. Obstet Gynecol 1988;71:939–44.

14. Craigo SD. Cervical incompetence and preterm delivery. (Editorial) N Engl J Med 1996;334:595–6.

15. Olah KS, Gee H. The prevention of preterm delivery-can we afford to continue to ignore the cervix? Br J Obstet Gynaecol 1992;99:278–80.

16. Romero R, Gomez R, Sepulveda W. The uterine cervix, ultrasound and prematurity. Editor Comments. Ultrasound Obstet Gynecol 1992;2:385–8.

17. Romero R, Mazor M, Munoz H, Gomez R, Galasso M. Sherer DM. The preterm labor syndrome. Ann HY Acad Sci 1994;734:414–29.

18. Dunn LJ, Dans P. Subsequent obstetrical performance of patients meeting the historical criteria for cervical incompetence. Bull Sloan Hosp Women 1962;7:43–5.

19. Iams JD. Cervical ultrasonography. Ultrasound Obstet Gynecol 1997;10:156–60.

20. Berghella V, Tolosa JE, Kuhlman K, Weiner S, Bolognese RJ, Wapner RJ. Cervical ultrasonography compared with manual examination as a predictor of preterm delivery. Am J Obstet Gynecol 1997;177:723–30.

21. Owen J, Yost N, Berghella V, Thom E, Swain M, Dildy GA, Mirodovnik M, Langer O, Sibai B, McNellis D. Mid-trimester endovaginal sonography in women at high risk for spontaneous preterm birth. JAMA 2001;286:1340–8.

22. Owen J, Yost N, Berghella V, et al. Can shortened midtrimester cervical length predict very early spontaneous preterm birth? Am J Obstet Gynecol 2004;191:298–303.

23. Airoldi J, Berghella V, Sehdev H, Ludmir J. Transvaginal Ultrasonography of the cervix to predict preterm birth in women with uterine anomalies. Obstet Gynecol 2005; 106(3):553–6.

24. Honest H, Bachman LM, Coomarasamy A, Gupta JK, Kleijnen J, Khan KS. Accuracy of cervical transvaginal sonography in predicting preterm birth; a systematic review. Ultrasound Obstet Gynecol 2003;22:305–22.

25. Lash AF, Lash A. Incompetent internal os of the cervix—diagnosis and treatment. Am J Obstet Gynecol 1957;79:346.

26. Ferenczy A, Choukroun D, Falcone T, Franco E. The effect of cervical loop electrosurgical excision on subsequent pregnancy outcome: North American experience. Am J Obstet Gynecol 1995;172:1246–50.

27. Althuisius SM, Shornagel Ga, Dekker GA, van Geijn HP, Hummel P. Loop electrosurgical excision procedure of the cervix and time of delivery in subsequent pregnancy. Int J Gynecol Obstet 2001;72:31–4.

28. Sadler L, Saftkas A, Wang W, Exeter M, Whittaker J, McCowan L. Treatment for cervical intraepithelial neoplasia and risk of preterm delivery. JAMA 2004;291:2100–6.

29. Cervical Insufficiency. ACOG Practice bulletin No. 48, American College of Obstetricians and Gynecologists. Obstet Gynecol 2003;102:1091–9.

30. Forster VF, During R, Schwartzlos G. Treatment of cervical incompetence: Cerclage or pessary? Zentralbl Gynakol 1986;168:230–6.

31. Branch DW. Operations for cervical incompetence. Clin Obstet Gynecol 1986;29:240–54.

32. Cousins LM. Cervical incompetence 1980: A time for re¬appraisal. Clin Obstet Gynecol 1980;23:467–79.

33. Ludmir J, Landon MB, Gabbe SG, Samiels P, Mennuti MT. Management of the diethylstilbestrol-exposed pregnant patient: A prospective study. Am J Obstet Gynecol 1987; 157:665–9.

34. Mangan CE, Borow L, Burnett-Rubin MM, Egan V, Giuntoli RL, Mikuta JJ. Pregnancy outcome in 98 women exposed to diethylstilbestrol in utero, their mothers, and unexposed siblings. Obstet Gynecol 1982;59:315–9.

35. Anthony GS, Walker RG, Cameron AD, Price JL, Walker JJ, Calder AA. Transabdominal cervico-isthmic cerclage in the management of cervical incompetence. Eur J Obstet Gynecol Reprod Biol 1997;72:127–30.

36. Benson RG, Durfee RD. Transabdominal cervicouterine cerclage during pregnancy for the treatment of cervical incompetence. Obstet Gynecol 1965;25:145–55.

37. Gibb DMF, Salaria DA. Transabdominal cervicoisthmic cerclage in the management of recurrent second trimester miscarriage and preterm delivery. Br J Obstet Gynaecol 1995;102:802–6.

38. Novy MJ. Transabdominal cervicoisthmic cerclage: A reappraisal 25 years after its introduction. Am J Obstet Gynecol 1991;164:1635–42.

39. Lotgering FK, Gaughler-Senden IPM, Lotgering SF, Wallenburg HCS. Outcome after Transabdominal cervicoisthmic cerclage. Obstet Gynecol 2006;107:779–84.

40. Dor J, Shalev J, Mashiach G, Blankstein J, Serr DM. Elective cervical suture of twin pregnancies diagnosed ultrasonically in the first trimester following induced ovulation. Gynecol Obstet Invest 1982;13:55–60.

41. Medical Research Council/Royal College of Obstetricians and Gynecologists Working Party on Cervical Cerclage. Final report of the Medical Research Council/Royal College of Obstetricians and Gynecologists multicentre randomised trial of cervical cerclage. Br J Obstet Gynaecol 1993;100:516–23.

42. Lazar P, Gueguen S, Dreyfus J, Renaud R, Pontinnier G, Papiernik E. Multicentred controlled trial of cervical cerclage in women at moderate risk of preterm delivery. Br J Obstet Gynaecol 1984;91:731–5.

43. Rush RW, Isaacs S, McPherson K, Jones L, Chalmers I, Grant A. A randomized controlled trial of cervical cerclage in women at high risk of spontaneous preterm delivery. Br J Obstet Gynaecol 1984;91:724–30.

44. Hassan SS, Romero R, Maymon E, Berry SM, Blackwell SC, Treadwell MC, et al. Does cervical cerclage prevent preterm delivery in patients with a short cervix? Am J Obstet Gynecol 2001;184:1325–31.

45. Berghella V, Daly SF, Tolosa JE, DiVito MM, Chalmers R, Garg N, et al. Prediction of preterm delivery with intravaginal ultrasonography of the cervix in patients with high-risk pregnancies: Does cerclage prevent prematurity? Am J Obstet Gynecol 1999;181:809–15.

46. Heath VC, Souka AP, Erasmus I, Gibb DM, Nicolaides KH. Cervical length at 23 weeks of gestation: The value of Shirodkar suture for the short cervix. Ultrasound Obstet Gynecol 1998;12:318–22.

47. Novy J, Gupta A, Wothe DD, Gupta S, Kennedy KA, Gravett MG. Cervical cerclage in the second trimester of pregnancy: A historical cohort study. Am J Obstet Gynecol 2001;184:1447–56.

48. Althuisius SM, Dekker GA, van Geijn HP, Bekedam DJ, Hummel P. Cervical Incompetence Prevention Randomized Cerclage Trial (CIPRACT): Study design and preliminary results. Am J Obstet Gynecol 2000;183:823–9.

49. Althuisius SM, Dekker GA, Hummel P, Bekedam DJ, van Geijn HP. Final results of the Cervical Incompetence Prevention Randomized Cerclage Trial (CIPRACT): therapeutic cerclage with bed rest versus bed rest alone. Am J Obstet Gynecol. 2001 Nov;185(5):1106–12.

50. Rust OA, Atlas RO, Jones KJ, Benham BN, Balducci J. A randomized trial of cerclage versus no cerclage among patients with ultrasonographically detected second-trimester preterm dilatation of the internal os. Am J Obstet Gynecol 2000;183:830–5.

51. To MS, Alfirevic Z, Heath VCF, Cicero S, Cacho AM, Williams PR, Nicolaides KH on behalf of the Fetal Medicine Foundation Second Trimester Screening Group. Cervical Cerclage for prevention of preterm delivery in women with short cervix: randomized controlled trial. Lancet 2004;363:1849–53.

52. Berghella V, Odibo AO, Tolosa JE. Cerclage for prevention of preterm birth in women with a short cervix found on transvaginal ultrasound: A randomized trial. Am J Obstet Gynecol 2004;191:1311–7.

53. Berghella V, Haas S, Chervoneva I, Hyslop T. Patients with prior second-trimester loss: prophylactic cerclage or serial transvaginal sonograms. Am J Obstet Gynecol 2002;187: 747–51.

54. Fejgin MD, Gabai B, Golberger S, Ben-Nun I, Beyth Y. Once a cerclage, not always a cerclage. J Reprod Med 1994; 39:880–2.

55. Berghella V, Odibo AO, To MS, Rust OA, Althuisius SM. Cerclage for short cervix on ultrasonography, meta-analysis of trials using individual patient-level data. Obstet Gynecol 2005;106:181–9.

56. Newman RB, Krombach SR, Myers MC, McGee DL. Effect of cerclage on obstetrical outcome in twin gestations with a shortened cervical length. Am J Obstet Gynecol 2002;186:634–40.

57. Roman AS, Rebarber A, Pereria L, Sfakianski AK, Mulholland J, Berghella V. The Efficacy of sonographically indicated cerclage in multiple gestations. J Ultrasound Med 2005;24:763–8.

58. Owen J, Iams JD, Hauth JC. Vaginal sonography and cervical incompetence. Am J Obstet Gynecol 2003;188: 586–96.

59. Aarts JM, Brons JTJ, Bruinse HW. Emergency cerclage: A review. Obstet Gynecol Surv 1995;50:459–69.

60. Olatunbosun OA, Nuaim LA, Turnwell RW. Emergency cerclage compared with bed rest for advanced cervical dilatation in pregnancy. Int Surg 1995;80:170–4.

61. Althuisius SM, Dekker GA, Hummel P, van Geijn HP. Cervical incompetence prevention randomized cerclage trial: emergency cerclage with bed rest versus bed rest alone. Am J Obstet Gynecol 2003;189:907–10.

62. Mays JK, Figuerioa R, Shah J, Khakoo H, Kaminsky S, Tejani N. Amniocentesis for selection before rescue cerclage. Obstet Gynecol 2000;95:652–5.

63. Treadwell MC, Bronsteen RA, Bottoms SF. Prognostic factors and complication rates for cervical cerclage: A review of 482 cases. Am J Obstet Gynecol 1991;165:555–8.

64. Weiner CP, Lee KY, Buhimschi CS, Christner R, Buhimschi IA. Proteomic biomarkers that predict the clinical success of rescue cerclage. Am J Obstet Gynecol 2005;192:710–8.

65. Shirodkar VN. A new method of treatment for habitual abortions in the second trimester of pregnancy. Antiseptic 1955;52:299–300.

66. McDonald IA. Suture of the cervix for inevitable miscarriage. J Obstet Gynecol Br Emp 1957;64:346–50.

67. Harger JH. Cervical cerclage: Patient selection, morbidity and success rates. Clin Perinatol 1983;10:321–41.

68. Meis PJ, Klebanoff M, Thom E, Dombrowski MP, Sibai B, Moawad AH et al. Prevention of recurrent preterm birth by 17 alpha-hydroxyprogesterone caproate. NEJM 2003;348:2379–85.

69. Cushner IM. The management of cervical incompetence by purse-string suture. Am J Obstet Gynecol 1963;87: 882–91.

70. Jennings CL. Temporary submucosal cerclage. Report of 48 cases. Am J Obstet Gynecol 1972;113:1097–102.

71. Lipshitz J. Cerclage in the treatment of cervical incompetence. S Afr Med J 1975;49:2013–5.

72. Nishijima S. Antepartum cervical cerclage operations. Am J Obstet Gynecol 1969;104:273–8.

73. Peters MA, Thiagarajah S, Harbert GM. Cervical cerclage: Twenty years' experience. South Med J 1979;72:933–7.

74. Taylor ES, Hansen RR. Incompetent os of the cervix as a cause for fetal loss. JAMA 1959;171:1312–4.

75. Goldenberg RL, Cliver SP, Bronstein J, Cutter GR, Andrews WW. Bed rest in pregnancy. Obstet Gynecol 1994;84:131–6.

76. Aarnoudse JG, Huisjes HJ. Complications of cerclage. Acta Obstet Gynecol Scand 1979;58:255–7.

77. Seppala M, Vara P. Cervical cerclage in the treatment of incompetent cervix. Acta Obstet Gynecol Scand 1970;49: 343–6.

78. Leppert PC, Kokenyesi R, Klemenich CA, Fisher J. Further evidence of a decorin-collagen interaction in the disruption of cervical collagen fibers during rat gestation. Am J Obstet Gynecol 2000;182:805–11.

79. Leppert PC. Proliferation and apoptosis of fibroblasts and smooth muscle cells in rat uterine cervix throughout gestation and the effect of the antiprogesterone onapristone. Am J Obstet Gynecol 1998;178:713–25.

CHAPTER 15

Preterm Premature Rupture of Membranes

Brian M. Mercer

Incidence and Clinical Importance

Preterm premature rupture of membranes (PROM) occurs in 3% of pregnancies and is responsible for approximately one third of all preterm births. Preterm PROM is an important cause of perinatal morbidity and mortality, particularly because it is associated with brief latency from membrane rupture to delivery, perinatal infection, and umbilical cord compression caused by oligohydramnios. Even with conservative management, 50–60% of women with preterm PROM remote from term will deliver within 1 week of membrane rupture. Amnionitis (13–60%) and clinical abruptio placentae (4–12%) are commonly associated with preterm PROM. The risk of these complications increases with decreasing gestational age at membrane rupture.

The frequency and severity of neonatal complications after preterm PROM vary with the gestational age at which rupture and delivery occur and are increased with perinatal infection, abruptio placentae, and umbilical cord compression. Respiratory distress syndrome (RDS) is the most common serious complication after preterm PROM at any gestational age. Other serious acute morbidities, including necrotizing enterocolitis, intraventricular hemorrhage, and sepsis are common with early preterm birth but relatively uncommon near term. Remote from term, serious perinatal morbidities that may lead to long-term sequelae or death are common. Figures 15-1, 15-2, and 15-3 present recent gestational age-dependent morbidity and mortality curves from a prospective community-based evaluation of 8,523 women giving birth consecutively at six hospitals in Shelby County, Tennessee, between July 1997 and March 1998. In this evaluation, 33% of live-born and resuscitated infants delivered at 23 weeks of gestation survived to discharge from the hospital (Fig. 15-1). One-week increments in gestational age were associated with improvements in survival when delivery occurred between 23 weeks and 32 weeks of gestation. Among infants surviving to discharge, RDS (more than 24 hours

of oxygen requirement or ventilation in the absence of other evident causes of respiratory compromise) was the most common acute morbidity at any gestational age (Fig. 15-2). Among surviving infants, intraventricular hemorrhage and necrotizing enterocolitis were rare when delivery occurred after 32 weeks of gestation. Blood- or cerebrospinal culture-proved sepsis decreased rapidly among those women giving birth between 27 weeks and 30 weeks of gestation, with a modest decrease in sepsis for each week gained thereafter. Although this evaluation did not measure long-term morbidity, retinopathy of prematurity and bronchopulmonary dysplasia occurred commonly among survivors born at 23 weeks of gestation and were almost never seen with delivery at or after 32 weeks of gestation (Fig. 15-3). These findings were similar to a recent multicenter observational study of women who gave birth to infants who weighed less than 1,000 g (1). In that study, 15 of 40 liveborn singletons delivered at 23 weeks of gestation survived (37.5%). However, two thirds of survivors experienced major morbidities potentially associated with long-term morbidity (any of the following: grades 3–4 intraventricular hemorrhage, grades 3–4 retinopathy of prematurity, necrotizing enterocolitis requiring surgery, oxygen dependence at 120 days or at discharge, or seizures). Current data specific to infants delivered after preterm PROM are not available. However, it has been found that perinatal sepsis is twofold more common in the setting of preterm PROM than preterm birth after preterm labor with intact membranes (2).

Definitions

Premature rupture of the membranes is defined as spontaneous membrane rupture that occurs before the onset of labor. When spontaneous membrane rupture occurs before 37 weeks of gestation, it is referred to as preterm PROM. The term "latency" refers to the time from membrane rupture to delivery. The term "conservative management" is defined as treatment directed at continuing the pregnancy. Preterm PROM that occurs at or before 26 weeks of gestation complicates 0.6–0.7% of pregnancies, and has been defined as "midtrimester PROM." Although the delineation of midtrimester PROM was clinically relevant in the 1970s and 1980s, the gestational age of fetal viability has progressively declined over the past 3 decades. As such, it is currently more clinically relevant to differentiate preterm PROM into "previable PROM," which occurs before the limit of viability (less than 23 weeks of gestation), "preterm PROM remote from term" (from viability to about 32 weeks of gestation), and "preterm PROM near term" (approximately 31–36 weeks of gestation). When previable PROM occurs, immediate delivery will lead to neonatal death. Conservative management may lead to previable or periviable birth, but also may lead to extended latency and delivery of a potentially viable infant. Immediate delivery after preterm PROM remote from term is associated with a high risk of significant perinatal morbidity and mortality that decreases with advancing gestational age at delivery. Alternatively, with preterm PROM near term, expeditious delivery of a noninfected and nonasphyxiated infant is associated with a high likelihood of survival and a low risk of severe morbidity.

Pathophysiology

Premature rupture of membranes is multifactorial in nature. In any given patient, one or more pathophysiologic processes may be evident. Choriodecidual infection or inflammation appears to play an important role in the cause of preterm PROM, especially at early gestational ages (3). Decreased membrane collagen content has been demonstrated in the setting of preterm PROM and with increasing gestational age (4). In support of this, increases in amniotic fluid matrix metalloproteases (1, 8, and 9) as well as decreases in tissue inhibitors of matrix metalloproteases (1 and 2) have been identified among women with preterm PROM (5–6). Supporting these findings, recent studies have implicated a potential genetic link to preterm birth and PROM through polymorphisms for inflammatory cytokines (7–10). Other factors associated with preterm PROM include lower socioeconomic status, cigarette smoking, sexually transmitted infections, prior cervical conization, prior preterm delivery, prior preterm labor in the current pregnancy, uterine distention (eg, twins, hydramnios), cervical cerclage, amniocentesis, and vaginal bleeding in pregnancy. Each of these factors may be associated with

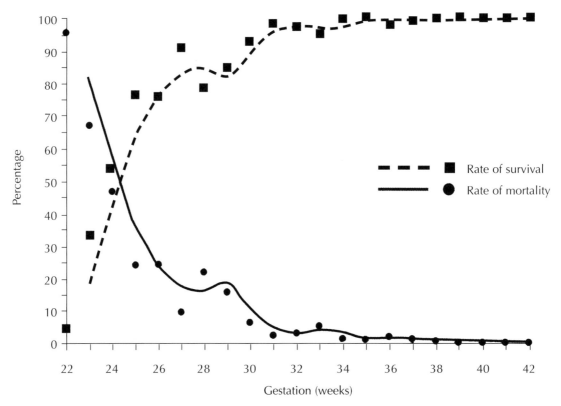

Fig. 15-1. Survival by gestational age among live-born resuscitated infants. (Mercer BM. Preterm premature rupture of the membranes. Obstet Gynecol 2003;101:178–193.)

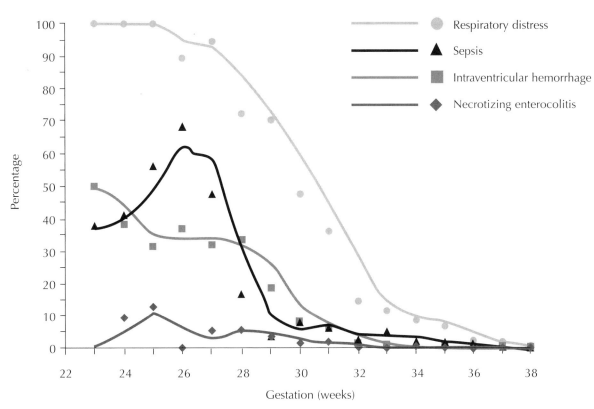

Fig. 15-2. Acute morbidity by gestational age among surviving infants. (Mercer BM. Preterm premature rupture of the membranes. Obstet Gynecol 2003;101:178–193.)

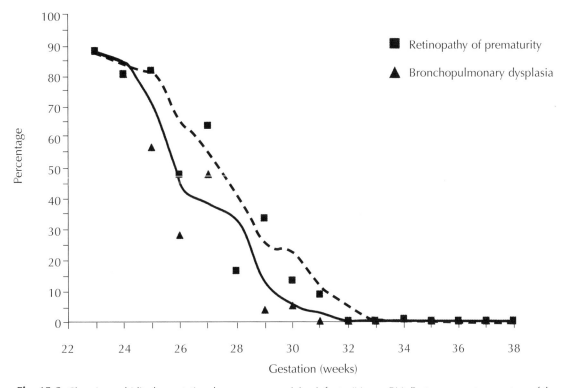

Fig. 15-3. Chronic morbidity by gestational age among surviving infants. (Mercer BM. Preterm premature rupture of the membranes. Obstet Gynecol 2003;101:178–193.)

preterm PROM through membrane stretch or degradation, local inflammation, or a weakening of maternal resistance to ascending bacterial colonization. However, in many cases, the ultimate cause of premature membrane rupture is unknown.

Prediction of Preterm Premature Rupture of Membranes

Because the clinical course of preterm PROM is often one of brief latency and increased infectious risk, it would be preferable to prevent it from occurring. In a large prospective study, the National Institute of Child Health and Human Development (NICHD) Maternal–Fetal Medicine Units Network found prior preterm birth and preterm birth caused by preterm PROM to be associated with subsequent preterm birth caused by preterm PROM (11). Those with a prior preterm birth at 23–27 weeks of gestation had a 27.1% risk of preterm birth subsequently (P <.001). Those with a history of preterm PROM had a 13.5% risk of preterm birth caused by preterm PROM in a subsequent gestation (versus 4.1%, relative risk 3.3, P <.01) and a 13.5-fold higher risk of preterm PROM at less than 28 weeks of gestation in the subsequent gestation (1.8% versus 0.13%, P <.01). In a separate publication from this study, the investigators found medical complications, work in pregnancy, symptomatic contractions, bacterial vaginosis, and low body mass index to be associated with preterm birth caused by preterm PROM in nulliparas. Preterm PROM in multiparas was associated with prior preterm PROM, prior preterm birth caused by preterm labor, and low body mass index. The presence of a short cervix (less than 25 mm by transvaginal ultrasonography) was associated with preterm PROM in both nulliparas and multiparas. A positive fetal fibronectin screen also was associated with preterm PROM in multiparas. Nulliparas with a positive cervicovaginal fetal fibronectin and a short cervix had a 16.7% risk of preterm birth caused by preterm PROM, whereas multiparas with a prior history, a short cervix, and a positive fetal fibronectin had a 25% risk of preterm PROM. Multiparas with all three risk factors had a 31-fold increased risk of PROM with delivery before 35 weeks of gestation relative to those without risk factors (25% versus 0.8%, P = .001) (12). Despite our developing ability to identify women at increased risk for preterm PROM, such testing is expensive and inconvenient to the patient and will identify only a small fraction of those ultimately giving birth preterm. Although recent studies regarding the prevention of spontaneous preterm birth or PROM with progesterone or vitamin C supplementation have been encouraging, the majority of preterm PROM will not be prevented with these interventions (13–15). Thus, our clinical efforts remain focused on management of preterm PROM once it has occurred, rather than its prevention.

Diagnostic Approach

The approach to the diagnosis of membrane rupture is clinical, with over 90% of cases confirmed based on the presence of a suspicious history or ultrasound finding followed by documentation of fluid passing from the cervix or the presence of a phenaphthazine ferning positive vaginal pool of fluid. Other plausible causes of vaginal discharge (eg, urinary incontinence, vaginitis, cervicitis, mucous "show" with cervical effacement and dilatation, semen, vaginal douches) should be excluded if the diagnosis is unclear. The Nitrazine test result can be "falsely positive" if the vaginal pH level is increased by blood or semen contamination or alkaline antiseptics, or if bacterial vaginosis is present. The ferning test should be performed on a sample collected from the posterior fornix or lateral vaginal sidewall to avoid cervical mucus, which may also yield a false-positive result. Prolonged leakage with minimal residual fluid can lead to a false-negative Nitrazine or ferning test result. Should initial test results be negative but a clinical suspicion of membrane rupture remains, the patient can be retested after prolonged recumbency or alternate measures can be considered. Ultrasound evaluation may prove useful if the diagnosis remains in doubt after speculum examination. The diagnosis of membrane rupture can be confirmed unequivocally with ultrasound-guided amnioinfusion of indigo carmine (1 mL in 9 mL of sterile normal saline), followed by observation for passage of blue fluid per vaginum. Although oligohydramnios without evident fetal urinary tract malformations or fetal growth restriction may be suggestive of membrane rupture, ultrasonography alone cannot diagnose or exclude membrane rupture with certainty. Cervicovaginal screening for fetal fibronectin has been suggested as a marker for preterm PROM when the diagnosis remains in doubt after initial speculum examination. However, the impact of prolonged membrane rupture on the fibronectin result has not been elucidated. Further, a positive test result may reflect disruption of the decidua rather than membrane rupture. As such, fetal fibronectin testing for the diagnosis of preterm PROM is not recommended for routine practice.

Until such time as the diagnosis of membrane rupture is excluded, it is prudent to avoid digital cervical examinations, which have been shown to decrease latency and increase infectious morbidity without adding substantial information to that obtained by careful visualization during a sterile speculum examination

(16, 17). The speculum examination also offers the opportunity to perform appropriate cultures (eg, endocervical chlamydia and gonorrhea) if these have not been recently performed or clinical suspicion of new infection is present. Anovaginal cultures for group B streptococcus should be obtained if these tests have not been performed within 5 weeks.

Therapeutic Approach

General Considerations

Because the risk of perinatal complications changes dramatically with gestational age at membrane rupture and delivery, a gestational age-based approach to the management of preterm PROM is appropriate. Although there is no apparent neonatal benefit to conservative management after membrane rupture at term, there is a potential for neonatal benefit when conservative management of preterm PROM is undertaken for the immature fetus. This benefit may only be accrued if conservative measures lead to pregnancy prolongation resulting in a reduction of gestational age-dependent morbidity, or through prevention of perinatal infection. Management should be based on individual assessment of the estimated risk for maternal, fetal, and neonatal complications should conservative management or expeditious delivery be pursued (Fig. 15-4).

Although practice varies and there is considerable controversy regarding the optimal management of preterm PROM, there is general consensus regarding some issues. First, gestational age should be established based on clinical history and prior ultrasound assessment where available. Ultrasonography should be performed, if feasible, to estimate gestational age (if no prior ultrasonography has been performed) as well as fetal growth, position, and residual amniotic fluid volume and to evaluate for gross fetal abnormalities that may cause polyhydramnios. The woman with preterm PROM should be evaluated clinically for evidence of advanced labor, chorioamnionitis, abruptio placentae, and fetal distress. Fetuses of women with advanced labor, intrauterine infection, significant vaginal bleeding, or nonreassuring fetal test results are best delivered regardless of gestational age. If fetal malpresentation coexists with significant cervical dilation, there is an increased risk of umbilical cord prolapse, which may increase the risk of fetal loss. This circumstance may justify early delivery given the increased fetal risk. Cases of women with genital herpes simplex virus (HSV) infection or human immunodeficiency virus (HIV) infection generally should not be managed conservatively. In certain cases (eg, recurrent HSV infection or HIV infection near the limit of viability), conservative management of preterm

PROM may be justified because of the extremely high risk of mortality and chronic morbidity when immediate delivery is undertaken. These cases should be managed individually. Although there are published case series supporting conservative management in the setting of recurrent HSV infection, there are no data in this regard for women infected with HIV (18). Intrapartum prophylaxis against group B streptococcus is recommended for gravida women giving birth preterm, unless recent anovaginal group B streptococcus cultures are negative (19). If conservative management of preterm PROM is to be pursued, the patient should be admitted to a facility capable of providing emergent delivery for abruptio placentae, fetal malpresentation in labor, and fetal distress caused by umbilical cord compression or in utero infection. The facility should also be capable of providing 24-hour neonatal resuscitation and intensive care because conservative management generally should be performed only in pregnancies in which there is a significant risk of neonatal morbidity and mortality should delivery occur. If adequate facilities for maternal and neonatal care do not exist, patient transfer should be undertaken early in the course of management to avoid emergent transfer once complications arise.

Preterm Premature Rupture of Membranes Near Term

When preterm PROM occurs at 34–36 weeks of gestation, the risk of severe acute morbidity and mortality occurring is low when expeditious delivery is pursued. Corticosteroids are generally not given to accelerate fetal pulmonary maturity. Conversely, conservative management at 34–36 weeks of gestation is associated with an increased risk of amnionitis (16% versus 2%, $P = .001$), prolonged maternal hospitalization (5.2 versus 2.6 days, $P = .006$), and a lower mean umbilical cord pH at delivery (7.25 versus 7.35, $P = .009$) without the benefit of a significant reduction of perinatal complications related to prematurity (20). A "mature" phosphatidyl glycerol, fluorescence polarization assay, lecithin–sphingomyelin ratio, or a lamellar body count result from fluid collected from either the vaginal pool or amniocentesis is associated with a low risk of significant pulmonary complications after preterm PROM near term, regardless of the presence of blood or meconium contamination. The presence of blood or meconium in the setting of preterm PROM should raise the level of suspicion for abruptio placentae or fetal compromise and lead to reconsideration of the benefits of conservative management. Should pulmonary maturity be evident based on vaginal pool amniotic fluid or from amniocentesis at 32–36 weeks of gestation, it is evident that the risk of major nonpulmonary perinatal complications are low and that conser-

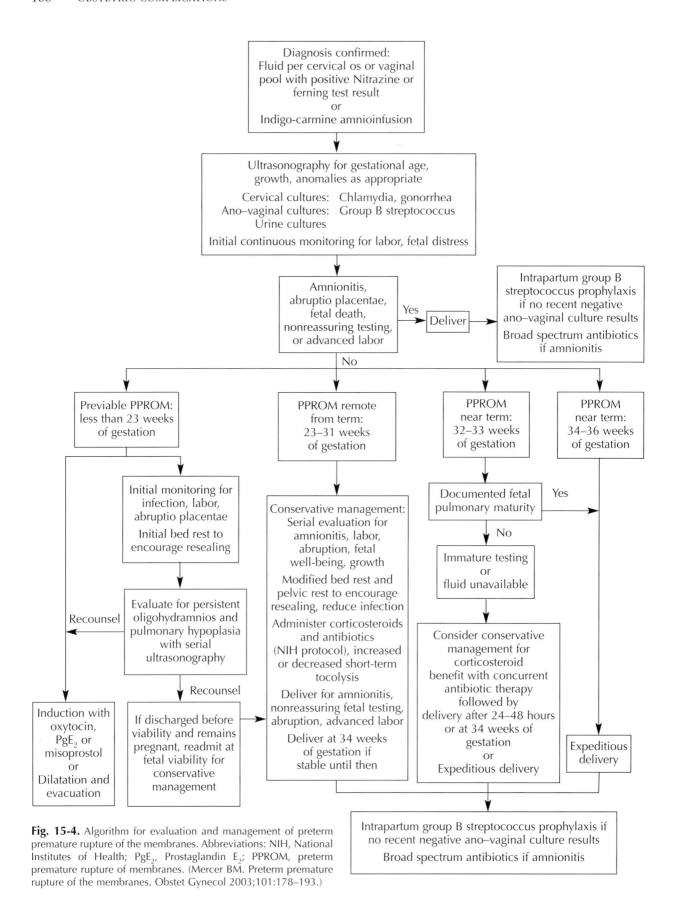

Fig. 15-4. Algorithm for evaluation and management of preterm premature rupture of the membranes. Abbreviations: NIH, National Institutes of Health; PgE₂, Prostaglandin E₂; PPROM, preterm premature rupture of membranes. (Mercer BM. Preterm premature rupture of the membranes. Obstet Gynecol 2003;101:178–193.)

vative management will prolong pregnancy only briefly (36 versus 14 hours, $P < .001$), increase the risk of amnionitis (27.7% versus 10.9%, $P = .06$), and place the fetus at risk for occult cord compression while unmonitored, without offering a significant reduction in neonatal morbidity (21). Thus, the woman who suffers preterm PROM at 34–36 weeks of gestation generally is best served by expeditious delivery. When preterm PROM occurs at 32–33 weeks of gestation, it is recommended that fetal pulmonary maturity be assessed by vaginal pool specimen if available, and that amniocentesis by a skilled clinician be considered should there be inadequate vaginal fluid for pulmonary maturity evaluation. When fetal pulmonary maturity is evident after preterm PROM at 32–33 weeks, there is little to be gained by continued pregnancy, and expeditious delivery is recommended (21–22).

There are no studies on which to guide practice for women in which pulmonary maturity testing is not performed or unavailable after preterm PROM at 32–33 weeks of gestation. At this gestation, the likelihood of survival with delivery is high, but there remains significant risk of pulmonary immaturity and other gestational age-dependent morbidity should the fetus be immature. The practice of immediate delivery versus conservative management was evaluated in 129 unselected women with preterm PROM at 30–33½ weeks of gestation (23). Tocolytics and antenatal steroids were not administered, and group B streptococcus prophylaxis was not given. Conservative management of preterm PROM was associated with only a brief increase in latency to delivery (59% versus 100% delivered within 48 hours, $P < .001$), but a significant increase in amnionitis (15% versus 2%, $P = .009$), and no evident reduction in gestational age-dependent morbidity. There was a significant risk of RDS in this population (35%). In addition, there was one stillbirth caused by suspected occult umbilical cord compression in the conservatively managed group, and three neonatal deaths in the immediately delivered group (two from sepsis and one from pulmonary hypoplasia). Although this study does suggest that immediate delivery might reduce fetal exposure to intrauterine infection and avoid fetal loss caused by cord compression, it confirms that infants delivered at 30–33 weeks of gestation remain at risk for neonatal sepsis and other significant gestational age-dependent morbidity in the absence of documented pulmonary maturity. As such, should fetal pulmonary immaturity be suspected at 32–33 weeks of gestation or should fluid for testing be unavailable, an option would be to treat the patient conservatively with close fetal monitoring, adjunctive antibiotic therapy, and antenatal corticosteroid administration for fetal maturation. At 32 weeks of gestation, if all is stable after antenatal corticosteroid

benefit has been achieved, generally conservative management can be continued to 34 weeks of gestation. With PROM at 33 weeks of gestation, one can proceed to delivery after corticosteroid benefit has been achieved because there is little additional benefit achieved by prolonging the pregnancy less than one week. If there is no plan to either induce fetal maturation with corticosteroids (eg, previously administered) or to suppress infection with antibiotics in an attempt to prolong the pregnancy more than 1 week, women with PROM at 32–33 weeks of gestation are likely better served by expeditious delivery.

Preterm Premature Rupture of Membranes Remote From Term

Delivery before 32 weeks of gestation is associated with a significant risk of neonatal complications, including severe acute morbidity and mortality. Because of this, the stable patient with preterm PROM remote from term is generally best served by conservative management in an attempt to prolong pregnancy and reduce the risk of gestational age-dependent morbidity in the newborn. Despite conservative efforts, many women ultimately will deliver after a brief latency. However, a subset of these women will remain pregnant for an extended period, allowing the fetus to mature in utero. A low initial amniotic fluid index has been shown to be associated with shorter latency and an increased risk of amnionitis (24–25). However, amniotic fluid volume assessment does not accurately predict who ultimately will deliver quickly despite conservative measures and, thus, should not be used in isolation to make decisions regarding conservative management (26).

During conservative management, care should be directed toward the early detection of labor, abruptio placentae, amnionitis, and umbilical cord compression or occult fetal distress. This generally is best accomplished by inpatient observation unless the membranes reseal. Conservative management consists of initial prolonged continuous fetal and maternal monitoring combined with subsequent modified bed rest to increase the opportunity for amniotic fluid reaccumulation and spontaneous membrane sealing. The fetus with preterm PROM remote from term is at significant risk (32–76%) for umbilical cord compression and fetal distress (27–28). Because abnormal fetal heart rate patterns and contractions can occur in otherwise asymptomatic women, fetal assessment should be performed at least daily on those with initially reassuring testing. Although both the nonstress test and the biophysical profile have the ability to confirm fetal well-being or identify fetal compromise in the setting of preterm PROM, fetal heart rate monitoring offers the opportunity to identify periodic heart rate changes, such as variable and late decelerations, in addition to allowing concurrent assessment of uterine activity. Biophysical profile test results may be confounded by the presence of oligohydramnios but can be helpful should the nonstress test result be equivocal, particularly remote from term when the fetal heart rate pattern is less likely to be "reactive." Those with intermittent umbilical cord compression but otherwise reassuring test results should undergo continuous fetal heart rate monitoring, pending reassessment on successful attainment of antenatal corticosteroid benefit (24–48 hours after initial dose). During conservative management, complete pelvic rest and avoidance of digital pelvic examinations should be undertaken to reduce the risk of intrauterine infection and enhance latency.

The combination of fever (temperature exceeding 38°C [100.4°F]) with uterine tenderness or maternal or fetal tachycardia, or both in the absence of another source of infection, are suggestive of intrauterine infection and should lead to expeditious delivery. Maternal white blood cell counts may be artificially elevated if antenatal corticosteroids have been administered within 5–7 days. Alternatively, a rising white blood cell count in the presence of suspicious clinical findings may be useful in identifying those who require closer observation, continuous fetal monitoring, or delivery. Maternal fever is not always present early in the course of amnionitis. Should maternal symptoms, physical findings, and hematologic findings be equivocal, amniocentesis may provide further suggestive information regarding the presence of intrauterine infection, including a glucose concentration of less than 16–20 mg/dL, a positive Gram stain, or a positive amniotic fluid culture. Although positive amniotic fluid cultures and elevated interleukin levels have been clearly associated with an increased risk of early delivery and perinatal infectious morbidity, these test results are not rapidly available in most clinical laboratories, limiting their utility in clinical practice. If amnionitis is suspected but the diagnosis is equivocal, amniocentesis should be considered with Gram stain, differential count, and glucose level used for acute management. Should a positive amniotic fluid culture become evident later, this information should be considered by the obstetrician, if the patient has not given birth, and provided to the neonatologist if the patient delivers subsequent to the amniocentesis.

Optimal treatment of the woman reaching an advanced gestational age after conservative management of preterm PROM remote from term has not been studied. In the absence of labor, abruption, nonreassuring fetal testing, or intrauterine infection, it is reasonable to consider labor induction when the pregnancy reaches 34 weeks of gestation. It also may be reasonable to assess fetal pulmonary maturity at any time from 32–34 weeks and consider delivery once maturity has been documented.

ADJUNCTIVE TREATMENT WITH ANTIBIOTICS

The benefits of narrow-spectrum intrapartum prophylaxis with intravenous penicillin or ampicillin to prevent vertical transmission and early-onset neonatal sepsis by group B streptococcus (Streptococcus agalactiae) have been well established. Intrapartum group B streptococcus prophylaxis with intravenous penicillin as a 5,000,000-unit initial bolus followed by 2,500,000 units every 4 hours or ampicillin (2 g) followed by 1 g intravenous (IV) every 4 hours (erythromycin, 500 mg IV every 6 hours, or clindamycin, 900 mg IV every 8 hours, or vancomycin, 1 g IV every 12 hours if the patient is allergic to penicillin) should be administered during labor or before cesarean delivery after preterm PROM, unless there is inadequate time or a negative anovaginal culture obtained within 5 weeks of delivery (19). Because of increasing resistance of group B streptococcus to erythromycin and clindamycin, some investigators have suggested careful confirmation of penicillin allergy before alternate treatment, and intravenous cefazolin for those with documented penicillin allergy (29, 30). Should the latter approach be taken, the caregiver should closely observe the patient for allergy to cephalosporins. It may be prudent to restrict such alternative treatment to women with minor allergic reactions to penicillin therapy.

The goal of adjunctive antibiotic therapy during the conservative management of preterm PROM remote from term is to treat or prevent ascending decidual infection in order to prolong pregnancy and offer the opportunity for reduced neonatal infectious and gestational age-dependent morbidity. More than two dozen randomized, prospective, controlled trials have been undertaken to determine if there is value in the adjunctive administration of antibiotics during conservative management of preterm PROM remote from term (31–34). The broad range of antibiotics administered, differing routes and duration of administration, inclusion of pregnancies at low risk for neonatal morbidity, and the variability of concurrent tocolytic and corticosteroid administration make interpretation of the findings difficult. However, two large multicenter clinical trials with different approaches to this issue have adequate power to evaluate the utility of adjunctive antibiotics after preterm PROM in reducing infant morbidity. The combination of these studies, as well as specific details from individual smaller trials, offer valuable insights regarding the potential role of adjunctive antibiotics in this setting.

The NICHD Maternal–Fetal Medicine Units Network elected to study women with preterm PROM from the limit of 24–32 % weeks of gestation (35). The primary goal was to see if adjunctive antibiotic therapy during conservative management of preterm PROM would reduce the number of infants who were acutely ill after birth. A secondary goal was to see if such treatment reduced individual infectious or gestational age-dependent morbidities. The NICHD Maternal–Fetal Medicine Units Network elected to use initial aggressive IV therapy (48 hours) with ampicillin (2 g IV every 6 hours) and erythromycin (250 mg IV every 6 hours) followed by limited duration oral therapy (5 days) with amoxicillin (250 mg orally every 8 hours) and enteric-coated erythromycin base (333 mg orally every 8 hours). These agents were chosen because of their broad-spectrum antimicrobial coverage and their demonstrated safety when used in pregnancy. The duration of therapy was limited because of concerns that prolonged therapy might lead to selective survival of resistant bacteria that might be more difficult to treat should neonatal infection occur. Once group B streptococcus carriage was identified based on initial cultures, carriers were treated with ampicillin for 1 week and then again in labor, regardless of whether they were assigned to study antibiotics or placebo therapy. Similar to other studies, this trial found that antibiotic treatment prolonged pregnancy, increasing twofold the likelihood that patients would not have delivered after 7 days of treatment. Despite discontinuation of antibiotics at 7 days, treated women continued to be more likely to remain pregnant up to 3 weeks after randomization, suggesting that the therapy successfully treated subclinical infection rather than just suppressing it. Regarding infant morbidity, the NICHD Maternal–Fetal Medicine Units Network trial found that antibiotics improved neonatal health by reducing the number of infants with one or more major infant morbidities (composite morbidity: death, RDS, early sepsis, severe intraventricular hemorrhage, severe necrotizing enterocolitis) from 53% to 44% (P <.05). Additionally, aggressive antibiotic therapy was associated with significant reductions in individual gestational age-dependent morbidity including RDS (40.5% versus 48.7%), stages 3 to 4 necrotizing enterocolitis (2.3% versus 5.8%), patent ductus arteriosus (11.7% versus 20.2%), and chronic lung disease (bronchopulmonary dysplasia: 13.0% versus 20.5%) (P<.05 for each). Regarding infectious morbidity, the antibiotic study group had a lower incidence of neonatal group B streptococcus sepsis (0% versus 1.5%, P = .03). Amnionitis was also reduced with study antibiotics (23% versus 32.5%, P = .01). Neonatal sepsis (8.4% versus 15.6%, P = .009) and pneumonia (2.9% versus 7.0%, P = .04) were less frequent in those who were not group B streptococcus carriers. In support of this study's findings, Mantel-Haenszel χ^2 tests of prospective randomized clinical trials with initial broad-spectrum parenteral therapy for women with preterm PROM at less than 34 weeks of gestation shows that antibiotics increase the likelihood of women remaining pregnant for longer than 1 week (odds ratio [OR], 2.52;

and 95% confidence interval [CI], 1.92–3.30), reduce amnionitis (OR, 0.60; CI, 0.47–0.78), reduce neonatal sepsis (OR, 0.47; CI, 0.33–0.67), reduce RDS (OR, 0.76; CI, 0.60–0.96), and reduce intraventricular hemorrhage (OR, 0.70; CI, 0.52–0.95), without an increase in the risk of cesarean delivery (OR, 1.00; CI, 0.78–1.28) or necrotizing enterocolitis (OR, 1.28; CI, 0.84–1.98) (33–42). Because of these findings, limited-duration aggressive antibiotic therapy is recommended during conservative management of preterm PROM remote from term.

A large multiarm, multicenter placebo-controlled trial of oral antibiotic therapy of women with preterm PROM at less than 37 weeks of gestation was performed (43). Women were randomized to receive oral erythromycin, amoxicillin–clavulonic acid, both, or a placebo for up to 10 days. More than 400 presented and nonpresented statistical analyses were performed. In summary, oral erythromycin was associated with brief pregnancy prolongation (not significant at 7 days), reduced need for supplemental oxygen (31.1% versus 35.6%, P = .02), reduced positive blood cultures (5.7% versus 8.2%, P = .02), but no significant reduction in the composite primary outcome (an infant suffering one or more of the following: death, chronic lung disease, major cerebral abnormality on ultrasonography) (12.7% versus 15.2%, P = .08). Subanalysis of singleton gestations revealed a reduction in oxygen dependence at 28 days (6.9% versus 8.9%, P = .03), positive blood cultures (5.3% versus 7.4%, P = .04), abnormal cerebral ultrasonography (3% versus 4.6%, P = .04), and composite morbidity (11.2% versus 14.4%, P = .02) with erythromycin. Oral amoxicillin–clavulonic acid prolonged pregnancy (43.3% versus 36.7% undelivered after 7 days, P = .005) and reduced the need for supplemental oxygen (30.1% versus 35.6%, P = .05), but was associated with an increased risk of necrotizing enterocolitis (1.9% versus 0.5%, P = .001) without reducing other neonatal morbidity or composite morbidity. The combination of oral amoxicillin–clavulonic acid and erythromycin yielded similar findings. Subanalysis of women with preterm PROM remote from term was not presented but was reported to reveal the same pattern of findings. There was no analysis of the benefits of oral antibiotics during conservative management at 32–36 weeks of gestation. The study concluded that oral "erythromycin, when given to women with preterm PROM, has effects on the occurrence of major neonatal disease, and might therefore have a substantial health benefit on the long-term respiratory and neurologic function of many children." They raised concern regarding the potential negative effects of oral amoxicillin–clavulonic acid because of the increased incidence of necrotizing enterocolitis. An alternate conclusion would be that oral antibiotic therapy with erythromycin reduces perinatal morbidity when given to women with preterm PROM before 37 weeks of gestation but, given the small differences in the actual incidences of morbidity in the study groups, many women would need to be treated to prevent one adverse outcome. Although the finding regarding increased necrotizing enterocolitis with oral amoxicillin–clavulonic acid is concerning, it is at odds with the NICHD Maternal–Fetal Medicine Units Network trial finding of reduced stages 2–3 necrotizing enterocolitis with aggressive antibiotic therapy in a higher risk population. Further, there is no consistent trend toward a positive or negative effect of antibiotics for necrotizing enterocolitis in the literature.

There appears to be a role for adjunctive aggressive antibiotic therapy with erythromycin and amoxicillin or ampicillin during conservative management of preterm PROM remote from term. If aggressive therapy is not given, oral erythromycin may offer some benefit. The combination of erythromycin and extended-spectrum ampicillin–clavulonic acid in a lower risk population near term does not appear to be beneficial and may be harmful. This latter regimen is not recommended. Although two recent randomized trials have attempted to evaluate the value of limiting the duration of antibiotic treatment to less than 7 days, they were not adequately powered to confirm that infant morbidities would not increase with treatments of shorter duration (44, 45). Thus 7 days of therapy, according the NICHD protocol, is recommended. Intrapartum group B streptococcus prophylaxis should be given to carriers, regardless of prior therapy.

ADJUNCTIVE TREATMENT WITH CORTICOSTEROIDS

It is well established that administration of antenatal corticosteroids to women at high risk of delivering an immature preterm infant is one of the most effective obstetric interventions directed to reduce perinatal morbidity and mortality. Antenatal corticosteroids reduce the risk of RDS, intraventricular hemorrhage, and perinatal death and have been shown to have long-term neurologic benefits when given in a timely fashion before preterm birth. The current National Institutes of Health consensus conference recommendations regarding corticosteroid administration in the setting of preterm PROM are that a single course of betamethasone (12 mg intramuscular [IM], two doses every 24 hours) or dexamethasone (6 mg IM, four doses every 12 hours) be given during conservative management of preterm PROM before 30–32 weeks of gestation because of the potential for reduction of intraventricular hemorrhage (46). There continues to be discussion regarding the efficacy of corticosteroids in the setting of preterm PROM in the prevention of RDS. It has been suggested that antenatal corticosteroids may be inappropriate in this setting

because 1) women with preterm PROM will deliver too quickly to accrue the potential benefits; 2) preterm PROM itself might induce fetal pulmonary maturation, thereby making corticosteroids unnecessary; and 3) antenatal corticosteroids might delay the diagnosis or increase the risk of perinatal infection through their immunosuppressive effects. It is now clear that most women with preterm PROM remote from term who undergo conservative management will remain pregnant for at least 24–48 hours, particularly if adjunctive antibiotics are administered. Although there have been conflicting reports regarding the relative risk of RDS with preterm birth after preterm PROM, it is clear that RDS remains the most common acute morbidity after preterm birth caused by preterm PROM. In the NICHD Maternal–Fetal Medicine Units trial, the incidence of RDS after conservatively managed preterm PROM was 41% when corticosteroids were not administered, despite adjunctive antibiotic administration. Regarding perinatal infection, studies performed before the era of adjunctive antibiotic administration revealed conflicting results as to the risk of neonatal infection when antenatal corticosteroids were administered. There are two recent randomized clinical trials that have assessed the utility of antenatal corticosteroid administration concurrent to adjunctive antibiotic administration. In the first, a reduced incidence of RDS (18.4% versus 43.6%, $P = .03$) with no obvious increase in perinatal infection (3% versus 5%, $P = NS$) was found when antenatal corticosteroids were administered after initiation of ampicillin-sulbactam for preterm PROM at 24–34 weeks of gestation (47). In a multicenter trial, women with preterm PROM were evaluated after being allocated to either a single course of dexamethasone (12 mg IM, two doses every 24 hours) or placebo at 28–34 weeks of gestation (48). All patients received amoxicillin and metronidazole for 5 days. Although there was no significant reduction in morbidity in the overall population, no increase in maternal or neonatal morbidity was evident in the corticosteroid group. Among those remaining pregnant at least 24 hours after study entry, newborns exposed to antenatal steroids had a lower incidence of perinatal death (1.3% versus 8.3%, $P = .05$). The most recent meta-analysis regarding this issue includes data from the original trial of corticosteroid administration published in 1972 (49). Corticosteroid administration in the setting of preterm PROM was found to substantially reduce the risks of RDS (20% versus 35.4%; OR, 0.56; CI, 0.46–0.70), intraventricular hemorrhage (7.5% versus 15.9%; OR, 0.47; CI, 0.31–0.70), and necrotizing enterocolitis (0.8% versus 4.6%; OR, 0.21; CI, 0.05–0.82) without significantly increasing the risks of maternal infection (9.2% versus 5.1%; OR, 1.95; CI, 0.83–4.59) or neonatal infection

(7.0% versus 6.6%; OR, 1.05; CI, 0.66–1.68). The analysis suggested that there was no need for additional study of this specific issue. Maternal–fetal medicine providers appear to agree. A recent survey found that 99.4% would administer antenatal corticosteroids in this setting (50).

Thus, based on current information, it is recommended that a single course of antenatal corticosteroids be administered concurrently to initial adjunctive antibiotic therapy during conservative management of preterm PROM before 32 weeks of gestation. Similar treatment also should be considered if conservative management is pursued for suspected fetal pulmonary immaturity at 32–34 weeks of gestation. The risks and benefits of repeated corticosteroid administration after an initial course of antenatal corticosteroids near the limit of viability remain to be determined. Currently routine repeated administration of antenatal corticosteroid is not recommended.

ADJUNCTIVE TREATMENT WITH TOCOLYSIS

There are inadequate data from which to make firm recommendations regarding tocolytic therapy in the setting of preterm PROM. Two small studies of prophylactic intravenous or oral betamimetic therapy and a study of prophylactic betamimetic or magnesium sulfate tocolysis after preterm PROM have suggested brief pregnancy prolongation in this setting (51–53). Alternatively, a practice of expectant management with therapeutic tocolysis initiated only after the onset of contractions did not show that tocolysis prolonged latency (54). Similarly, improved neonatal outcome has not been conferred with a practice of tocolysis and serial assessment of fetal pulmonary maturity followed by delivery (55).

Although no study has demonstrated that tocolytics improve or worsen neonatal outcome, studies of conservative management have not evaluated tocolysis when corticosteroids and antibiotics are given concurrently. It is plausible that short-term pregnancy prolongation with prophylactic tocolysis could enhance the potential for corticosteroid effect and allow more time for antibiotics to act against subclinical decidual infection. Given evidence of short-term pregnancy prolongation without evident risk in some studies, it is not unreasonable to initiate tocolysis in women at high risk for infant morbidity should there be concurrent attempts to prevent infection, prolong pregnancy, and induce fetal pulmonary maturity. However, this approach should not be considered an expected practice because further research is needed.

Previable Preterm Premature Rupture of Membranes

Approximately one half of women with second-trimester PROM will deliver within 1 week of membrane rupture.

Alternatively, up to 22% will remain pregnant for at least 1 month. In addition to the high risk of chorioamnionitis (39%), maternal morbidities associated with conservative management of second-trimester PROM include endometritis (14%), abruptio placentae (3%), retained placenta, and postpartum hemorrhage necessitating dilation and curettage (12%). Maternal sepsis is a rare but serious complication, complicating 0.8% of cases. One maternal death from sepsis has been reported in 731 pregnancies complicated by second-trimester PROM (0.14%) (56). The incidence of stillbirth subsequent to second-trimester PROM (15%) is higher than that seen with preterm PROM later in pregnancy (1%). This may reflect increased fetal susceptibility to umbilical cord compression, hypoxia, and intrauterine infection but also may reflect a practice of nonintervention for fetal distress in the previable or periviable fetus.

Previable delivery is immediately lethal. Periviable delivery after preterm PROM may be associated with more frequent morbidity and mortality than that seen with delivery from other causes because previable and periviable PROM are associated with perinatal infection and pulmonary hypoplasia. Women with early previable PROM, before 20 weeks of gestation, and those with persistent oligohydramnios are at particular risk for pulmonary hypoplasia. Lethal pulmonary hypoplasia rarely occurs with membrane rupture subsequent to 24 weeks of gestation, presumably because alveolar growth adequate to support postnatal development has occurred. Ultrasound estimates of interval fetal lung growth including lung length, chest circumference, chest to abdomen circumference ratio, or chest circumference to femur length ratio carry a high-positive predictive value for lethal pulmonary hypoplasia (57–60). The pattern of fetal restriction deformities occurring after prolonged intrauterine crowding is similar to that seen with Potter's syndrome. The nonpulmonary features include abnormal facies and limb positioning abnormalities. The ears may be low set, and epicanthal folds may be present. The extremities may be flattened and malpositioned.

It is estimated that 56–84% of survivors will be "neurologically intact" after midtrimester PROM (56, 61–65). However, developmental delay (24%), delayed motor development (23%), and other less frequent complications, including cerebral palsy, chronic lung disease, hydrocephalus, and mental retardation, are serious reported sequelae. The frequency of these outcomes may be biased because of the lack of follow-up in more than 40% of cases. There are no available recent data regarding the outcomes of survivors delivering after conservatively managed previable preterm PROM.

Women presenting with PROM before viability should be counseled regarding the impact of immediate delivery and the potential risks and benefits of conservative management. Counseling should include a realistic appraisal of neonatal outcomes, including the availability of obstetric monitoring and neonatal intensive care facilities. Because of the significant risk of adverse maternal and neonatal sequelae after previable PROM, some women will desire expeditious delivery. Depending on the experience of the healthcare provider and the patient's wishes, this can be accomplished by dilation and evacuation, or by labor induction with high-dose oxytocin or vaginal prostaglandin therapy in the absence of contraindications. There currently are no data on which to make recommendations regarding initial conservative management of the woman with previable PROM. The benefits of an initial period of inpatient observation may include strict bed and pelvic rest to enhance the opportunity for resealing, and for early identification of infection and abruption. Ultrasonography should be performed to exclude the presence of associated fetal anomalies. Serial ultrasonography should be offered every 1–2 weeks initially to evaluate for reaccumulation of amniotic fluid and to evaluate interval pulmonary growth. Some women will elect not to continue the pregnancy if interval ultrasonography results suggest a high likelihood of lethal pulmonary hypoplasia based on the presence of persistent severe oligohydramnios or lagging pulmonary growth. A number of novel treatments, including amnioinfusion and fibrin–platelet–cryoprecipitate or gel foam sealing of the membranes, have been investigated preliminarily (66–68). In some approaches, cervical cerclage placement concurrent to attempted membrane sealing is used. The maternal risks and fetal benefits of these aggressive interventions have not been adequately demonstrated, so currently they should not be incorporated into routine clinical practice. Many clinicians will discharge the patient to bed rest at home after an initial observation period, with readmission to hospital bed rest once the patient reaches a gestation at which they would intervene for fetal benefit should labor, amnionitis, nonreassuring test results, or abruption occur. There are no published data evaluating the risks and benefits of this strategy versus continued hospitalization with PROM before viability.

Cervical Cerclage

Cervical cerclage is a widely described risk factor for PROM and other adverse pregnancy outcomes. Preterm PROM complicates about one in four pregnancies with a cerclage and approximately half of pregnancies after emergent cerclage. Although women undergoing cerclage placement, whether elective or emergent, are at high risk for preterm birth, a thorough discussion of the

potential adverse sequelae despite cerclage placement should be undertaken before the procedure. There are no prospective studies regarding the treatment of preterm PROM subsequent to cervical cerclage in situ. A number of retrospective studies have suggested that when cerclage is removed on admission the risk of adverse perinatal outcomes is not higher than those seen after preterm PROM without a cerclage (69–70). Alternatively, studies comparing pregnancies in which the cerclage was retained or removed have been small and have yielded conflicting results (71–73). Each study found a statistically insignificant trend toward increased maternal infection with retained cerclage. One study found increased infant mortality and death from sepsis with retained cerclage, with the only evident benefit being a decreased likelihood of delivery within 24 hours (71). One study, which largely reflected differing practices at two institutions, found significant pregnancy prolongation with cerclage retention (72). Among those with preterm PROM before 28 weeks of gestation, cerclage retention was associated with improved birth weight (942 g versus 758 g, $P = .04$). However, no controlled study has found a significant reduction in infant morbidity with cerclage retention after preterm PROM. Given the potential risk without evident neonatal benefit, the general approach to management should include early cerclage removal after preterm PROM. The role for short-term cerclage retention while attempting to enhance fetal maturation with antenatal corticosteroids in the periviable gestation has not been determined.

Cerebral Palsy and Adverse Neurologic Outcome

It is established that preterm birth is a significant risk factor for long-term sequelae such as chronic lung disease, neurosensory impairment, cerebral palsy, and developmental delay. There are accumulating data linking perinatal infection to neurologic complications. Because preterm PROM is associated with early delivery and perinatal infection, it is a potential risk factor for long-term neurologic morbidity. Cerebral palsy and cystic periventricular leukomalacia have been linked to the presence of amnionitis, which is commonly seen after preterm PROM (74). Similarly, elevated amniotic fluid cytokines and fetal systemic inflammation, which may accompany or reflect maternal or fetal infection, have been associated with preterm PROM as well as brain lesions such as periventricular leukomalacia, the subsequent development of cerebral palsy, or both (75–77). Currently, there are no data to suggest that immediate delivery of the candidate for conservative management after preterm PROM will prevent these sequelae. Therefore, conservative management, with adjunctive antibiotics to reduce the risk of intrapartum infection, is recommended. However, at more advanced gestational ages, particularly if pulmonary maturity can be documented, expeditious delivery may reduce the risk of exposure to intrauterine infection and subsequent morbidity.

Summary

Premature rupture of the membranes affects more than 120,000 pregnancies annually in the United States and is associated with significant maternal, fetal, and neonatal risk. Management of PROM requires an accurate diagnosis and evaluation of the risks and benefits of continued pregnancy or expeditious delivery. An understanding of gestational age-dependent neonatal morbidity and mortality is important in determining the potential benefits of conservative management of preterm PROM at any gestation. When possible, the treatment of pregnancies complicated by PROM remote from term should be directed toward conserving the pregnancy and reducing perinatal morbidity caused by prematurity while monitoring closely for evidence of infection, abruptio placentae, labor, or fetal compromise caused by umbilical cord compression. Alternatively, when preterm PROM occurs near term, the patient generally is best served by expeditious delivery, particularly if fetal pulmonary maturity is evident. It is important that the patient be well informed regarding the potential for subsequent maternal, fetal, and neonatal complications regardless of the management approach.

References

1. Bottoms SF, Paul RH, Mercer BM, MacPherson CA, Caritis SN, Moawad AH, et al. Obstetric determinants of neonatal survival: Antenatal predictors of neonatal survival and morbidity in extremely low birth weight infants. Am J Obstet Gynecol 1999;180:665–9.

2. Seo K, McGregor JA, French JI. Preterm birth is associated with increased risk of maternal and neonatal infection. Obstet Gynecol 1992;79:75–80.

3. Bendon RW, Faye-Petersen O, Pavlova Z, Qureshi F, Mercer B, Miodovnik M, et al. Fetal membrane histology in preterm premature rupture of membranes: Comparison to controls, and between antibiotic and placebo treatment. The National Institute of Child Health and Human Development Maternal Fetal Medicine Units Network. Pediatr Dev Pathol 1999;2:552–8.

4. Skinner SJ, Campos GA, Liggins GC. Collagen content of human amniotic membranes: Effect of gestation length and premature rupture. Obstet Gynecol 1981;5:487–9.

5. Vadillo-Ortega F, Hernandez A, Gonzalez-Avila G, Bermejo L, Iwata K, Strauss JF 3rd. Increased matrix metalloproteinase activity and reduced tissue inhibitor of metalloproteinases-1 levels in amniotic fluids from pregnancies complicated by premature rupture of membranes. Am J Obstet Gynecol 1996;174:1371–6.

6. Maymon E, Romero R, Pacora P, Gomez R, Athayde N, Edwin S, et al. Human neutrophil collagenase (matrix metalloproteinase 8) in parturition, premature rupture of the membranes, and intrauterine infection. Am J Obstet Gynecol 2000;183:94–9.

7. Fuks A, Parton LA, Polavarapu S, Netta D, Strassberg S, Godi I, Hsu CD. Polymorphism of Fas and Fas ligand in preterm premature rupture of membranes in singleton pregnancies. Am J Obstet Gynecol 2005;193:1132–6.

8. Kalish RB, Vardhana S, Gupta M, Perni SC, Chasen ST, Witkin SS. Polymorphisms in the tumor necrosis factor-alpha gene at position -308 and the inducible 70 kd heat shock protein gene at position +1267 in multifetal pregnancies and preterm premature rupture of fetal membranes. Am J Obstet Gynecol 2004;191:1368–74.

9. Wang H, Parry S, Macones G, Sammel MD, Ferrand PE, Kuivaniemi H, Tromp G, Halder I, Shriver MD, Romero R, Strauss JF 3rd. Functionally significant SNP MMP8 promoter haplotypes and preterm premature rupture of membranes (PPROM). Hum Mol Genet 2004;13:2659–69.

10. Macones GA, Parry S, Elkousy M, Clothier B, Ural SH, Strauss JF 3rd. A polymorphism in the promoter region of TNF and bacterial vaginosis: preliminary evidence of gene-environment interaction in the etiology of spontaneous preterm birth. Am J Obstet Gynecol 2004;190:1504–8.

11. Mercer BM, Goldenberg RL, Moawad AH, Meis PJ, Iams JD, Das AF, et al. The preterm prediction study: Effect of gestational age and cause of preterm birth on subsequent obstetric outcome. Am J Obstet Gynecol 1999;181:1216–21.

12. Mercer BM, Goldenberg RL, Meis PJ, Moawad AH, Shellhaas C, Das A, et al. The preterm prediction study: Prediction of preterm premature rupture of the membranes using clinical findings and ancillary testing. Am J Obstet Gynecol 2000;183:738–45.

13. Meis PJ, Klebanoff M, Thom E, Dombrowski MP, Sibai B, Moawad AH, et al. Prevention of recurrent preterm delivery by 17 alpha-hydroxyprogesterone caproate. N Engl J Med 2003;348:2379–85.

14. da Fonseca EB, Bittar RE, Carvalho MH, Zugaib M. Prophylactic administration of progesterone by vaginal suppository to reduce the incidence of spontaneous preterm birth in women at increased risk: a randomized placebo-controlled double-blind study. Am J Obstet Gynecol 2003;188:419–24.

15. Casanueva E, Ripoll C, Tolentino M, Morales RM, Pfeffer F, Vilchis P, et al. Vitamin C supplementation to prevent premature rupture of the chorioamniotic membranes: a randomized trial. Am J Clin Nutr 2005;81:859–63.

16. Lewis DF, Major CA, Towers CV, Asrat T, Harding JA, Garite TJ. Effects of digital vaginal examinations on latency period in preterm premature rupture of membranes. Obstet Gynecol 1992;80:630–4.

17. Alexander JM, Mercer BM, Miodovnik M, Thurnau GR, Goldenberg RL, Das AF, et al. The impact of digital cervical examination on expectantly managed preterm rupture of membranes. Am J Obstet Gynecol 2000;183:1003–7.

18. Major CA, Towers CV, Lewis DF, Garite TJ. Expectant management of preterm premature rupture of membranes

complicated by active recurrent genital herpes. Am J Obstet Gynecol 2003;188:1551–4.

19. Prevention of early-onset group B streptococcal disease in newborns. ACOG Committee Opinion No. 279. American College of Obstetricians and Gynecologists. Obstet Gynecol 2002;100:1405–12.

20. Naef RW 3rd, Allbert JR, Ross EL, Weber BM, Martin RW, Morrison JC. Premature rupture of membranes at 34 to 37 weeks' gestation: Aggressive versus conservative management. Am J Obstet Gynecol 1998;178:126–30.

21. Mercer BM, Crocker L, Boe N, Sibai B. Induction versus expectant management in PROM with mature amniotic fluid at 32-36 weeks: A randomized trial. Am J Obstet Gynecol 1993;82:775–82.

22. Edwards R, Stickler L, Johnson I, Duff P. Outcomes with premature rupture of membranes at 32 or 33 weeks when management is based on evaluation of fetal lung maturity. J Matern Fetal Neonatal Med. 2004;16:281-5.

23. Cox SM, Leveno KJ. Intentional delivery versus expectant management with preterm ruptured membranes at 30-34 weeks' gestation. Obstet Gynecol 1995;86:875–9.

24. Park JS, Yoon BH, Romero R, Moon JB, Oh SY, Kim JC, et al. The relationship between oligohydramnios and the onset of preterm labor in preterm premature rupture of membranes. Am J Obstet Gynecol 2001;184:459–62.

25. Vermillion ST, Kooba AM, Soper DE. Amniotic fluid index values after preterm premature rupture of the membranes and subsequent perinatal infection. Am J Obstet Gynecol 2000;183:271–6.

26. Mercer BM, Rabello YA, Thurnau GR, Miodovnik M, Goldenberg RL, Das AF, et al. The NICHD-MFMU antibiotic treatment of preterm PROM study: impact of initial amniotic fluid volume on pregnancy outcome. Am J Obstet Gynecol 2006;194:438–45.

27. Smith CV, Greenspoon J, Phelan JP, Platt LD. Clinical utility of the nonstress test in the conservative management of women with preterm spontaneous premature rupture of the membranes. J Reprod Med 1987;32:1–4.

28. Moberg LJ, Garite TJ, Freeman RK. Fetal heart rate patterns and fetal distress in patients with preterm premature rupture of membranes. Obstet Gynecol 1984;64:60–4.

29. Fiore Mitchell T, Pearlman MD, Chapman RL, Bhatt-Mehta V, Faix RG. Maternal and transplacental pharmacokinetics of cefazolin. Obstet Gynecol 2001;98:1075–9.

30. Silverman NS, Morgan M, Nichols WS. Antibiotic resistance patterns of group B streptococcus in antenatal genital cultures. J Reprod Med 2000;45:979–82.

31. Mercer B. Antibiotic therapy for preterm premature rupture of membranes. Clin Obstet Gynecol 1998;41:461–8.

32. Egarter C, Leitich H, Karas H, Wieser F, Husslein P, Kaider A, et al. Antibiotic treatment in premature rupture of membranes and neonatal morbidity: A meta-analysis. Am J Obstet Gynecol 1996;174:589–97.

33. Cox SM, Leveno KJ, Sherman ML, Travis L, DePalma R. Ruptured membranes at 24 to 29 weeks: A randomized double blind trial of antimicrobials versus placebo. Am J Obstet Gynecol 1995;172:412.

34. Ovalle-Salas A, Gomez R, Martinez MA, Rubio R, Fuentes A, Valderrama O, et al. Antibiotic therapy in patients with preterm premature rupture of membranes: A prospective, randomized, placebo-controlled study with microbiologi-

cal assessment of the amniotic cavity and lower genital tract. Prenat Neonat Med 1997;2:213–22.

35. Mercer B, Miodovnik M, Thurnau G, Goldenberg R, Das A, Merenstein G, et al. Antibiotic therapy for reduction of infant morbidity after preterm premature rupture of the membranes: A randomized controlled trial. JAMA 1997; 278:989–95.

36. Amon E, Lewis SV, Sibai BM, Villar MA, Arheart KL. Ampicillin prophylaxis in preterm premature rupture of the membranes: A prospective randomized study. Am J Obstet Gynecol 1988;159:539–43.

37. Johnston MM, Sanchez-Ramos L, Vaughn AJ, Todd MW, Benrubi GI. Antibiotic therapy in preterm premature rupture of membranes: A randomized, prospective, double-blind trial. Am J Obstet Gynecol 1990;163:743–7.

38. Christmas JT, Cox SM, Andrews W, Dax J, Leveno KJ, Gilstrap LC. Expectant management of preterm ruptured membranes: Effects of antimicrobial therapy. Obstet Gynecol 1992;80:759–62.

39. McCaul JF, Perry KG Jr, Moore JL Jr, Martin RW, Bucovaz ET, Morrison JC. Adjunctive antibiotic treatment of women with preterm rupture of membranes or preterm labor. Int J Gynaecol Obstet 1992;38:19–24.

40. Lockwood CJ, Costigan K, Ghidini A, Wein R, Chien D, Brown BL, et al. Double-blind; placebo-controlled trial of piperacillin prophylaxis in preterm membrane rupture. Am J Obstet Gynecol 1993;169:970–6.

41. Morales WJ, Angel JL, O'Brien WF, Knuppel RA. Use of ampicillin and corticosteroids in premature rupture of membranes: A randomized study. Obstet Gynecol 1989; 73:721–6.

42. Owen J, Groome LJ, Hauth JC. Randomized trial of prophylactic antibiotic therapy after preterm amnion rupture. Am J Obstet Gynecol 1993;169:976–81.

43. Kenyon SL, Taylor DJ, Tarnow-Mordi W, Oracle Collaborative Group. Broad spectrum antibiotics for preterm, prelabor rupture of fetal membranes: The ORACLE I randomized trial. Lancet 2001;357:979–88.

44. Lewis DF, Adair CD, Robichaux AG, Jaekle RK, Moore JA, Evans AT, et al. Antibiotic therapy in preterm premature rupture of membranes: Are seven days necessary? A preliminary, randomized clinical trial. Am J Obstet Gynecol 2003;188:1413–6.

45. Segel SY, Miles AM, Clothier B, Parry S, Macones GA. Duration of antibiotic therapy after preterm premature rupture of fetal membranes. Am J Obstet Gynecol 2003; 189:799–802.

46. National Institutes of Health. NIH Consensus Development Conference Statement: Effect of corticosteroids for fetal maturation on perinatal outcomes, February 28–March 2, 1994. Am J Obstet Gynecol 1995;173:246–52.

47. Lewis DF, Fontenot MT, Brooks GG, Wise R, Perkins MB, Heymann AR. Latency period after preterm premature rupture of membranes: A comparison of ampicillin with and without sulbactam. Obstet Gynecol 1995;86:392–5.

48. Pattinson RC, Makin JD, Funk M, Delport SD, Macdonald AP, Norman K, et al. The use of dexamethasone in women with preterm premature rupture of membranes—a multicentre, double-blind, placebo-controlled, randomised trial. Dexiprom Study Group. S Afr Med J 1999;89:865–70.

49. Harding JE, Pang J, Knight DB, Liggins GC. Do antenatal corticosteroids help in the setting of preterm rupture of membranes? Am J Obstet Gynecol 2001;184:131–9.

50. Ramsey PS, Nuthalapaty FS, Lu G, Ramin S, Nuthalapaty ES, Ramin KD. Contemporary management of preterm premature rupture of membranes (PPROM): a survey of maternal-fetal medicine providers. Am J Obstet Gynecol 2004;191:1497–502.

51. Christensen KK, Ingemarsson I, Leideman T, Solum T, Svenningsen N. Effect of ritodrine on labor after premature rupture of the membranes. Obstet Gynecol 1980;55:187–90.

52. Levy DL, Warsof SL. Oral ritodrine and preterm premature rupture of membranes. Obstet Gynecol 1985;66:621–3.

53. Weiner CP, Renk K, Klugman M. The therapeutic efficacy and cost-effectiveness of aggressive tocolysis for premature labor associated with premature rupture of the membranes. Am J Obstet Gynecol 1988;159:216–22.

54. Garite TJ, Keegan KA, Freeman RK, Nageotte MP. A randomized trial of ritodrine tocolysis versus expectant management in patients with premature rupture of membranes at 25 to 30 weeks of gestation. Am J Obstet Gynecol 1987;157:388–93.

55. How HY, Cook CR, Cook VD, Miles DE, Spinnato JA. Preterm premature rupture of membranes: Aggressive tocolysis versus expectant management. J Matern Fetal Med 1998;7:8–12.

56. Moretti M, Sibai B. Maternal and perinatal outcome of expectant management of premature rupture of the membranes in midtrimester. Am J Obstet Gynecol 1988;159:390–6.

57. Yoshimura S, Masuzaki H, Gotoh H, Fukuda H, Ishimaru T. Ultrasonographic prediction of lethal pulmonary hypoplasia: Comparison of eight different ultrasonographic parameters. Am J Obstet Gynecol 1996;175:477–83.

58. Lauria MR, Gonik B, Romero R. Pulmonary hypoplasia: Pathogenesis, diagnosis, and antenatal prediction. Obstet Gynecol 1995;86:466–75.

59. D'Alton M, Mercer B, Riddick E, Dudley D. Serial thoracic versus abdominal circumference ratios for the prediction of pulmonary hypoplasia in premature rupture of the membranes remote from term. Am J Obstet Gynecol 1992;166:658–63.

60. Vintzileos AM, Campbell WA, Rodis JF, Nochimson DJ, Pinette MG, Petrikovsky BM. Comparison of six different ultrasonographic methods for predicting lethal fetal pulmonary hypoplasia. Am J Obstet Gynecol 1989;161:606–12.

61. Taylor J, Garite TJ. Premature rupture of membranes before fetal viability. Obstet Gynecol 1984;64:615–20.

62. Bengtson JM, VanMarter LJ, Barss VA, Greene MF, Tuomala RE, Epstein MF. Pregnancy outcome after premature rupture of the membranes at or before 26 weeks' gestation. Obstet Gynecol 1989;73:921–7.

63. Major CA, Kitzmiller JL. Perinatal survival with expectant management of midtrimester rupture of membranes. Am J Obstet Gynecol 1990;163:838–44.

64. Morales WJ, Talley T. Premature rupture of membranes at 25 weeks: A management dilemma. Am J Obstet Gynecol 1993;168:503–7.

65. Rib DM, Sherer DM, Woods JR Jr. Maternal and neonatal outcome associated with prolonged premature rupture of membranes below 26 weeks' gestation. Am J Perinatol 1993;10:369–73.

66. Quintero RA. New horizons in the treatment of preterm premature rupture of membranes. Clin Perinatol 2001;28:861–75.

67. Sciscione AC, Manley JS, Pollock M, Maas B, Shlossman PA, Mulla W, et al. Intracervical fibrin sealants: A potential treatment for early preterm premature rupture of the membranes. Am J Obstet Gynecol 2001;184:368–73.

68. O'Brien JM, Milligan DA, Barton JR. Gelatin sponge embolization: A method for the management of iatrogenic preterm premature rupture of the membranes. Fetal Diagn Ther 2002;17:8–10.

69. Blickstein J, Katz Z, Lancet M, Molgilner BM. The outcome of pregnancies complicated by preterm rupture of the membranes with and without cerclage. Int J Obstet Gynecol 1989;28:237–42.

70. Yeast JD, Garite TR. The role of cervical cerclage in the management of preterm premature rupture of the membranes. Am J Obstet Gynecol 1988;158:106–10.

71. Ludmir J, Bader T, Chen L, Lindenbaum C, Wong G. Poor perinatal outcome associated with retained cerclage in patients with premature rupture of membranes. Obstet Gynecol 1994;84:823–6.

72. Jenkins TM, Berghella V, Shlossman PA, McIntyre CJ, Maas BD, Pollock MA, et al. Timing of cerclage removal after preterm premature rupture of membranes: Maternal and neonatal outcomes. Am J Obstet Gynecol 2000;183:847–52.

73. McElrath TF, Norwitz ER, Lieberman ES, Heffner LJ. Management of cervical cerclage and preterm premature rupture of the membranes: Should the stitch be removed? Am J Obstet Gynecol 2000;183:840–6.

74. Wu YW, Colford JM Jr. Chorioamnionitis as a risk factor for cerebral palsy: A meta-analysis. JAMA 2000;20;284:1417–24.

75. Yoon BH, Jun JK, Romero R, Park KH, Gomez R, Choi JH, et al. Amniotic fluid inflammatory cytokines (interleukin-6, interleukin-1beta, and tumor necrosis factor-alpha), neonatal brain white matter lesions, and cerebral palsy. Am J Obstet Gynecol 1997;177:19–26.

76. Yoon BH, Romero R, Kim CJ, Koo JN, Choe G, Syn HC, et al. High expression of tumor necrosis factor-alpha and interleukin-6 in periventricular leukomalacia. Am J Obstet Gynecol 1997;177:406–11.

77. Yoon BH, Romero R, Yang SH, Jun JK, Kim IO, Choi JH, et al. Interleukin-6 concentrations in umbilical cord plasma are elevated in neonates with white matter lesions associated with periventricular leukomalacia. Am J Obstet Gynecol 1996;174:1433–40.

CHAPTER 16

Management of Preterm Labor

Robert L. Goldenberg

Preterm birth is the leading cause of neonatal mortality and constitutes a substantial portion of all birth-related short- and long-term morbidity. Spontaneous preterm labor is responsible for more than one half of preterm births. Its management is the topic of this review. Although there are many maternal characteristics associated with preterm birth, the etiology in most cases is not clear, although, for the earliest cases, the role of intrauterine infection is assuming greater importance. Most efforts to prevent preterm labor have not proved to be effective, and equally frustrating, most efforts at arresting preterm labor once started have failed. The most important components of management, therefore, are aimed at preventing neonatal complications through the use of corticosteroids and antibiotics to prevent group B streptococcal neonatal sepsis and avoiding traumatic deliveries. Delivery in a medical center with an experienced resuscitation team and the availability of a newborn intensive care unit will ensure the best possible neonatal outcomes. Obstetric practices for which there is little evidence of effectiveness in preventing or treating preterm labor include: bed rest, hydration, sedation, home uterine activity monitoring, oral terbutaline after successful intravenous tocolysis, and tocolysis without the concomitant use of corticosteroids.

Prematurity

A preterm delivery, as defined by the World Health Organization, is one that occurs at less than 37 weeks of gestation and more than 20 weeks of gestation. In the United States, the preterm delivery rate is approximately 12%, whereas in Europe it varies between 5% and 7%. In spite of advances in obstetric care, the rate of prematurity has not decreased over the past 40 years. In fact, in most industrialized countries it has increased slightly (Fig. 16-1). Prematurity remains a leading cause of neonatal morbidity and mortality in developed countries, accounting for 60–80% of deaths of infants without congenital anomalies. Because the risk of neonatal morbidity and mortality near term is low, greater attention is

now being focused on early preterm birth (less than 32 weeks of gestation). Although births in this gestational age group represent 1–2% of all deliveries, they account for nearly 50% of all long-term neurologic morbidity and approximately 60% of perinatal mortality.

Neonatal mortality rates have decreased in recent years largely because of improved neonatal intensive care and better access to these services. With appropriate medical care, neonatal survival dramatically improves as gestational age progresses, with more than 50% of neonates surviving at 25 weeks of gestation, and more than 90% surviving by 28–29 weeks of gestation (Table 16-1). In the United States, survival rates of 20–30% have been reported in neonates delivered at 22–23 weeks of gestation; however, these premature infants are often left with long-term neurologic impairment (1). Because of the rapid improvement in both survival and freedom from major handicap as delivery gestational age increases from 22 weeks to 28 weeks, the major benefits from delaying delivery are seen in this time. Short-term morbidities associated with preterm delivery include respiratory distress syndrome, intraventricular hemorrhage, periventricular leukomalacia, necrotizing enterocolitis, bronchopulmonary dysplasia, sepsis, and patent ductus arteriosus. Long-term morbidities include cerebral palsy, mental retardation, and retinopathy of prematurity. The risk of these morbidities is directly related to the gestational age and birth weight. For example, cerebral palsy, defined as a nonprogressive motor dysfunction with origin around the time of birth, complicates approximately 2 per 1,000 of all live births. The relative risk for a preterm infant developing cerebral palsy is nearly 40 times that for term infants. Approximately 8–10% of surviving newborns weighing less than 1,000 g at birth will develop cerebral palsy. These infants also have substantially higher rates of mental retardation and visual disabilities, as well as neurobehavioral dysfunction and poor school performance (2).

Preterm Labor

Preterm labor is usually defined as regular contractions accompanied by cervical change occurring at less than 37

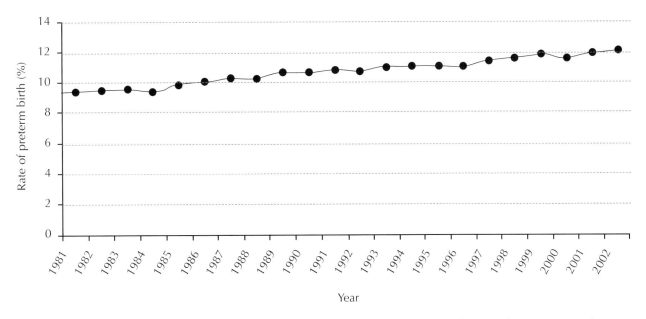

Fig. 16-1. Incidence of preterm birth in the United States, 1981–2002. (Modified from Goldenberg RL. The management of preterm labor. Obstet Gynecol 2002;100:1020–37.)

weeks of gestation. Spontaneous preterm labor accounts for 40–50% of all preterm deliveries, with the remainder resulting from preterm premature rupture of membranes (PROM) (25–40%) and obstetrically indicated preterm delivery (20–25%) (3).

The pathogenesis of preterm labor is not well understood, and it is often not clear whether preterm labor represents early idiopathic activation of the normal labor process or results from a pathologic mechanism. Several theories exist regarding the initiation of labor, including 1) progesterone withdrawal, 2) oxytocin initiation, and 3) premature decidual activation. The progesterone withdrawal theory stems from the large body of work previously done with sheep. As parturition nears, the fetal–adrenal axis becomes more sensitive to adrenocorticotropic hormone, increasing the secretion of cortisol. Fetal cortisol then stimulates trophoblast 17 α-hydroxylase activity, which decreases progesterone secretion and leads to a subsequent increase in estrogen production. This reversal in the estrogen/progesterone ratio results in increased prostaglandin formation, initiating a cascade of events that culminate in labor and subsequent delivery. Although this mechanism is well established in sheep, its role in humans has not been confirmed.

The second parturition theory involves oxytocin as an initiator of labor. Because intravenously administered oxytocin increases the frequency and intensity of uterine contractions, it is natural to assume that oxytocin plays an important role in the initiation of labor. Accepting oxytocin as the initiating agent for the onset of labor, however, is difficult for two reasons: 1) blood levels of

oxytocin do not increase before labor, and 2) the clearance of oxytocin remains constant during pregnancy. Thus, although oxytocin likely plays a role in the support of labor, its role in the initiation of labor, either at term or preterm, is not established. The most likely pathway to the initiation of preterm labor probably involves prema-

Table 16-1. Neonatal Survival by Gestational Age and Improvement in Survival by Week

Gestational Age (wk)	Approximate Survival Rate (%)	Approximate Improvement in Survival Rate (%)
21	0	—
22	Rare	—
23	25	25
24	50	25
25	70	20
26	80	10
27	86	6
28	91	5
29	94	3
30	95	1
31	96	1
32	97	1
33	98	1
34	99	1
35	more than 99	less than 1
36	more than 99	less than 1

Goldenberg RL. The management of preterm labor. Obstet Gynecol 2002;100:1020–37.

ture decidual activation. Although decidual activation may be mediated in part by the fetal–decidual paracrine system, and potentially by intrauterine bleeding, in many cases, especially those involving early preterm labor, it appears that this activation occurs in the context of an occult upper genital tract infection (Fig. 16-2).

Infection and Preterm Birth

A growing body of evidence suggests that infection of the decidua, fetal membranes, and amniotic fluid is associated with preterm delivery (4). Clinical chorioamnionitis complicates 1–5% of term pregnancies, but nearly 25% of preterm deliveries. In one study (5), histologic

chorioamnionitis was more common in preterm deliveries than in term deliveries (32.8% versus 10%). An investigation of patients in preterm labor demonstrated that positive amniotic fluid culture results were present in 19% of women with intact membranes with no clinical evidence of intrauterine infection (6). In women with spontaneous preterm labor, an inverse relationship exists between colonization of the chorioamnion and amniotic fluid and gestational age at delivery. In one study, chorioamnion colonization was associated with 83% of the very early spontaneous preterm births, but played a much less important role in the initiation of parturition at or near term (4). Organisms that have been associated with histologic chorioamnionitis include *Ureaplasma*

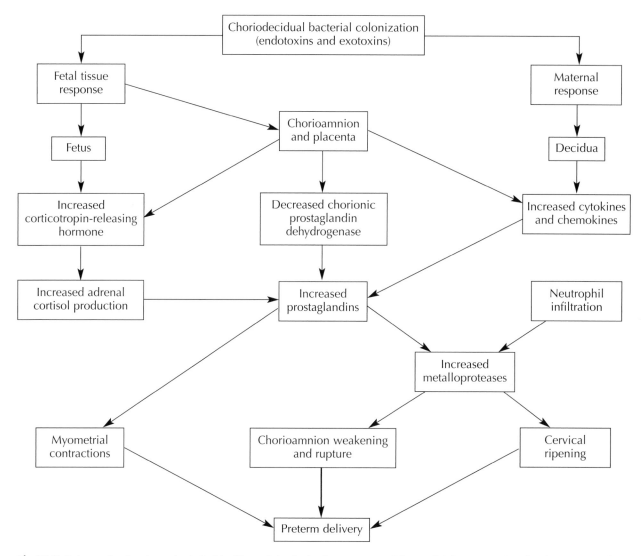

Fig 16-2. Pathways leading from choriodecidual bacterial colonization to preterm labor and delivery. (Reprinted with permission from Goldenberg RL, Hauth JC, Andrews WW. Intrauterine infection and preterm birth. N Engl J Med 2000;342:1500–7. Copyright © 2000 Massachusetts Medical Society. All rights reserved.)

urealyticum, Mycoplasma hominis, Gardnerella vaginalis, Peptostreptococcus, and *Bacteroides* species (4).

Risk Factors

In the United States, race is a significant risk factor for preterm delivery. African-American women have a prematurity rate of approximately 16–18%, compared with 7–9% for white women. Women younger than 17 years and older than 35 years have a higher risk of preterm delivery. Less education and lower socioeconomic status also are risk factors, although they probably are not independent of one other. The relative contribution of various causes of preterm birth differs by ethnic group. For example, preterm labor more commonly leads to preterm birth in white women, whereas preterm PROM is more common in African-American women (7). Various behavioral factors also increase the risk for preterm delivery. Both poor and excessive weight gain are associated with an increase in preterm birth, whereas women with a low body mass index (less than 19.8) are at higher risk for preterm delivery (8). Smoking plays a more significant role in fetal growth restriction than it does in preterm delivery. However, women who smoke still have an approximate 20–30% increase in preterm birth (9). In the United States approximately 20% of pregnant women smoke, and 10–15% of all preterm births can be attributed to maternal smoking. A history of a preterm delivery is one of the most significant risk factors. The recurrence risk of preterm birth in women with a history of preterm delivery ranges from 17% to 40%, and appears to depend on the number of prior preterm deliveries. Women who have had a prior preterm delivery have been reported to have a 2.5-fold increased risk of spontaneous preterm delivery with their next pregnancy (10). The earlier the gestational age of the prior preterm delivery, the greater the risk for a subsequent early spontaneous preterm delivery.

Multiple gestations carry one of the highest risks of preterm delivery. Approximately 50% of twin and nearly all higher multiple gestations end before 37 completed weeks of gestation. The average length of gestation is significantly shorter for twins (36 weeks), triplets (33 weeks), and quadruplets (31 weeks) than it is for singletons (39 weeks) (11). Vaginal bleeding caused by placenta previa or marginal placental separation is associated with almost as high a risk of preterm delivery as multiple gestations. Additionally, second-trimester bleeding not associated with either placenta previa or separation also has been significantly associated with preterm birth.

In addition to the risk factors discussed previously, a variety of other factors have been associated with an increased risk of preterm labor. Extremes in the volume of amniotic fluid, such as hydramnios or oligohydramnios, have been associated with an increased risk of preterm labor. Maternal abdominal surgery in the late second and third trimesters can cause an increase in uterine activity that may culminate in preterm delivery. Maternal medical conditions, such as gestational or preexisting diabetes and hypertension (essential or pregnancy induced), are associated with a higher rate of preterm delivery; however, these preterm births are often indicated preterm deliveries because of maternal complications rather than the result of spontaneous preterm labor. Asymptomatic bacteriuria is associated with an increased rate of prematurity (12). Systemic infections, such as bacterial pneumonia, pyelonephritis, and acute appendicitis, often lead to increased uterine activity, potentially leading to premature delivery.

Another potentially important clinical risk factor is the presence of uterine contractions. In a study involving approximately 2,500 patients, in which multiple gestations, vaginal bleeding, preterm PROM, and hydramnios were excluded, uterine activity was evaluated in patients with preterm, term, and postterm deliveries (13). The authors demonstrated an increase in uterine activity beginning 6 weeks before delivery, regardless of gestational age at birth. A surge in uterine activity occurred within 72 hours of delivery in all three groups. Unfortunately, these patients depended on tocodynamometry to determine this increase in frequency. When patients are instructed to self-detect an increase in uterine activity, they can identify only 15% of the contractions noted by tocodynamometry. The use of tocodynamometry and cervical examination at 28 weeks of gestation was evaluated in 589 nulliparous women to determine whether patients at risk for preterm delivery could be identified (14). The investigators noted that the best predictor of spontaneous preterm birth was the presence of a soft or medium consistency cervix. In this study, the risk of spontaneous preterm delivery increased from 4.2% for those women with no contractions detected to 18.2% for those patients having four or more contractions in 30 minutes. A study from the National Institute of Child Health and Human Development Maternal–Fetal Medicine Units Network (15) again found an association between the presence of contractions and preterm delivery. However, because of the large overlap in contraction frequency between those women who gave birth at term and those who gave birth preterm, monitoring contraction frequency was not found to be useful in defining a population at especially high risk for spontaneous preterm birth. Similar results were reported in a study confined to twins (16). For this reason, among others, the use of home uterine activity monitoring has not generally resulted in a reduction of preterm births.

Biochemical and Ultrasound Predictors

The biochemical processes leading to the initiation of either term or preterm labor have not been well established in humans. Recently, however, important insights into the pathophysiology of spontaneous preterm labor have helped to identify various biochemical markers that may predict preterm delivery. The most powerful biochemical marker identified to date is fetal fibronectin. Fetal fibronectin is a glycoprotein found in the extracellular matrix and, when found in the vagina or cervix, appears to be a marker of choriodecidual disruption. Typically, fetal fibronectin is absent from cervicovaginal secretions from around the 20th week of gestation until near term. In women undergoing routine screening during prenatal care or when tested with a diagnosis of potential preterm labor, detection of elevated cervicovaginal levels of fetal fibronectin has been shown to be strongly associated with an increased risk for preterm delivery (17, 18). For clinical care, the most important characteristic of the fetal fibronectin test is its negative predictive value. In women in questionable preterm labor, if the test result is negative, less than 1% of women will give birth within 1–2 weeks. If the test result is positive, the risk of subsequent preterm delivery within 1–2 weeks is higher—approximately 20%.

As labor approaches, the cervix tends to shorten, soften, rotate anteriorly, and then dilate. These changes tend to begin weeks before delivery, regardless of gestational age. Digital examination is the traditional method used to detect cervical maturation, but quantifying these changes is often difficult. For example, if the external portion of the cervix is closed, it is impossible to evaluate the internal os by digital examination. Vaginal ultrasonography allows a more objective approach to the examination of the cervix. In asymptomatic women, cervical changes determined by ultrasonography, including shortening and funneling, appear to have high predictive value for subsequent preterm birth. Alterations in length begin to occur approximately 10 weeks before delivery (19). Digital examination changes, however, tend to occur only 3–4 weeks before delivery.

One of the most difficult decisions an obstetrician has to make is determining whether a woman presenting with symptoms of preterm labor, such as contractions and a small amount of cervical effacement or dilation, is in preterm labor. Numerous studies confirm that between 50% and 75% of women who fit this description will, without treatment, go on to give birth at term. For this reason, traditionally, patients are observed for several hours or more to await additional cervical change before a decision is made to initiate tocolytic treatment, give corticosteroids, or discharge the patient. In many cases, a decision regarding true or false labor cannot be made with assurance even then. In recent years, it has become apparent that, in some women, the presence of cervical or vaginal fetal fibronectin, and perhaps a short cervix, as determined by ultrasonography, can separate those women not in labor from those who have a more significant risk for early delivery. Therefore, for women in whom the diagnosis of preterm labor is uncertain, obtaining one of these tests is a reasonable strategy. For those women whose fetal fibronectin test result is negative and perhaps for those with a cervical length greater than 30 mm, the likelihood of delivery within 1 week is less than 1%. Thus, most women with a negative test result can safely be sent home without treatment.

Prevention

Conceptually, prevention of preterm labor may be divided into two major areas. The first involves a reduction in the presence of one or more of the specific risk factors or, in a more general approach, an improvement in quality of life, including income and nutritional enhancement, and a reduction in physical and emotional stress. Although space does not permit a thorough review of these attempts, suffice it to say that in developed countries these approaches have not consistently been found to reduce the incidence of preterm labor. Other programs attempting to decrease the rate of preterm delivery have focused on screening for detection of preterm contractions or cervical change before the onset of true labor. These approaches include: 1) patient education to recognize preterm contractions, 2) health care provider surveillance for cervical changes, and 3) home uterine activity monitoring. Educational programs generally train women to recognize symptoms of preterm labor, including contractions, pelvic pressure, and vaginal discharge. In addition, weekly vaginal examinations have been used in an attempt to detect early cervical changes before the onset of labor. Several explanations have been advanced as to why these interventions have generally failed to demonstrate significant reductions in the preterm birth rate. For example, the level of education and supervision may have been inadequate for the patient population under evaluation. One of the more important reasons, however, may be that early symptoms of premature labor are often subtle and varied, and women often do not perceive contractions until labor is relatively advanced. In a study of women who had been trained in self-palpation of uterine activity, they identified only 15% of the contractions detected by a monitor, and as few as 11% could identify 50% of their contractions (20). Home uterine activity monitoring was proposed as a potential solution to this problem. Although some of the early, small trials with home uterine activity monitoring demonstrated a significant decrease in preterm births among enrolled participants, subsequent larger studies have not (21). Hence, it appears that home uterine activity monitoring is of little or no benefit in reducing the frequency of preterm birth. One potential reason for this failure is that the interventions available to treat early preterm labor once detected are, for the most part, not effective. Thus, overall, attempts at prevention and treatment of preterm labor through risk reduction and early detection, although conceptually appealing, have not generally led to reductions in preterm birth.

Treatment

The therapeutic interventions considered in the setting of preterm labor generally have the following goals: 1) to inhibit or reduce the strength and frequency of contractions, thus delaying the time to delivery; and 2) to optimize fetal status before preterm delivery. In this section, many of the contemporary obstetric therapeutic strategies proposed to achieve these goals are reviewed.

Bed Rest

Bed rest represents one of the most common interventions used for the prevention and treatment of threatened preterm labor. In fact, it is recommended for a wide range of pregnancy-related conditions. One survey found that bed rest was prescribed for at least 1 week for 20% of pregnant women in the United States (22). Unfortunately, there are no prospective randomized studies that have independently evaluated the effectiveness of bed rest for the prevention of preterm labor or its treatment in singleton pregnancies. In four randomized trials of hospitalization and bed rest for the prevention or treatment of preterm delivery in twin pregnancies, two studies found no benefit, and two showed an increase in preterm birth. Therefore, although a reduction of physical activity may seem appropriate for some women at risk for preterm birth, there is no evidence that this intervention, especially when extended to full bed rest, will result in a reduction in preterm birth. In fact, in twins this intervention may be harmful. Therefore, no evidence exists that bed rest should be a standard component of prevention or treatment for preterm labor.

Hydration and Sedation

Another common practice used for the initial treatment of preterm labor is oral or intravenous hydration. Some physicians attempt to differentiate true preterm labor from false labor using this strategy. Several theories are offered as to why hydration may be effective in treating preterm labor. First, at least in animals, hydration inhibits the release of antidiuretic hormone through the Henry–Gauer reflex. Second, women in preterm labor may have plasma volumes below normal. Few studies have evaluated the use of hydration in a prospective manner. In a prospective randomized study of 48 women with preterm contractions, no benefit from hydration was found (23). In a prospective randomized study of 179 women with preterm contractions, similar findings were reported (24). Patients in this investigation were randomized to observation alone, intravenous hydration, or a single dose of subcutaneous terbutaline. No significant differences were noted between the three groups in the mean days to delivery or the incidence of preterm delivery. Hence, intravenous hydration does not appear to reduce preterm birth, and the routine use of hydration to treat preterm labor or to differentiate true from false labor cannot be recommended.

Sedation also is a commonly used strategy to differentiate true preterm labor from preterm contractions. Similar to hydration, there are limited data documenting the efficacy of sedation in this clinical setting. In a prospective comparative study, 119 women with preterm labor were randomly assigned to treatment with hydration and sedation or to treatment with bed rest alone (25). Women randomized to the hydration group, sedation group, or both received 500 mL of lactated Ringer's solution intravenously over 30 minutes and 8–12 mg of intramuscular morphine sulfate. There was no significant difference between hydration and sedation and bed rest alone with regard to contraction cessation and rates of preterm delivery. Therefore, the literature does not support the use of hydration, sedation, or both in the initial treatment of preterm labor. In many cases, initial hydration with intravenous infusion of fluid occurs before the start of intravenous infusion of a tocolytic agent. A large fluid bolus may increase the risk of fluid overload and subsequent development of pulmonary edema.

Progesterone

Based on the progesterone withdrawal hypothesis of labor initiation, over the years there has been interest in the use of progesterone and other progestins for the treatment and prevention of preterm labor. A meta-analysis of six randomized controlled trials of 17 α-hydroxyprogesterone caproate used prophylactically to prevent preterm labor revealed a significant decrease in preterm birth (odds ratio, 0.5; 95% confidence interval, 0.3–0.85) (26). More recently, two studies in high-risk women with a history of preterm birth, one using weekly intramuscular injections of 17 α-hydroxyprogesterone caproate and the other using daily administration of a progesterone vaginal suppository, have both shown significant reductions in preterm birth rates (27, 28). At present, however, no evidence exists for the use of 17 α-hydroxyprogesterone caproate in women with a multiple pregnancy, a short cervix, or other high-risk conditions (29). Furthermore, the use of progestins, including large doses of intramuscular progesterone or 6-methyl-17-acetoxyprogesterone, has not successfully inhibited active preterm labor (30, 31).

Tocolytics

BETA-SYMPATHOMIMETIC AGENTS

There are three known types of β-adrenergic receptors in humans: 1) β_1 receptors occur primarily in the heart, small intestine, and adipose tissue; 2) β_2 receptors are found in the uterus, blood vessels, bronchioles, and liver; and 3) β_3 receptors are found predominantly on white and brown adipocytes. Beta-sympathomimetic agents are structurally related to catecholamines and, when administered in vivo, stimulate all β-receptors throughout the body. Stimulation of the β_2 receptors results in uterine smooth muscle relaxation. Although some β-sympathomimetic agents have been proposed as β_2-selective agents, at the dosages used pharmacologically, stimulation of all receptor types often occurs. Such stimulation results in many of the side effects associated with the β-sympathomimetic agents. Of the β-sympathomimetic agents, the β_2-selective agents (eg, ritodrine, terbutaline)

(Table 16-2) have been the primary drugs used for the treatment of preterm labor.

Ritodrine is the only medication approved by the U.S. Food and Drug Administration for the treatment of preterm labor. This approval resulted largely from studies demonstrating efficacy similar to that of other tocolytic agents but with fewer side effects (32, 33). The initial reports also suggested an increase in pregnancy duration with a reduction in neonatal morbidity and mortality rates. Subsequent reports have not been as positive. The Canadian Preterm Labor Investigators Group (34) conducted a large multicenter clinical trial comparing ritodrine with a placebo. They concluded that ritodrine treatment significantly delayed delivery for 24 hours, but that it did not significantly improve other perinatal outcomes. In a meta-analysis involving 16 clinical trials with a total of 890 women, it was demonstrated that women treated with ritodrine had significantly fewer deliveries within 24–48 hours of the start of therapy (35). However, no statistically significant decrease in the incidence of respiratory distress syndrome, birth weight less than 2,500 g, or perinatal death was demonstrated. These studies were completed before the use of antenatal steroid therapy became widespread.

Although ritodrine can be administered either intravenously or orally, treatment usually begins with intravenous infusion. The initial recommended infusion rate was 100 mcg/min. However, more recently, an initial

Table 16-2. Some Currently Used Tocolytic Agents

Generic Name	Brand Name	Mechanism of Action	Usual Dosages	Major Side Effects	Comments
Magnesium sulfate	—	Calcium antagonist	4-g loading dose IV, then 1–3 g/h	Respiratory arrest; cardiac arrest	Monitor deep tendon reflexes and serum magnesium levels
Ritodrine	Utopar	β_2 activator	Start at 50 mcg/min IV, increasing to a maximum of 350 mcg/min	Cardiac arrhythmias, pulmonary edema, myocardial ischemia	Monitor cardiac rhythm and fluid and electrolyte status
Terbutaline	Brethine	β_2 activator	5–10 mcg/min IV, increasing to a maximum of 80 mcg/min	Cardiac arrhythmias, pulmonary edema, myocardial ischemia	Monitor cardiac rhythm and fluid and electrolyte status
Nifedipine	Procardia	Calcium channel blocker	20 mg orally followed by 10–20 mg orally every 6–8 h	Maternal hypotension	Monitor blood pressure
Indomethacin	Indocin	Prostaglandin synthetase inhibitor	50-mg loading dose PO, PV, or PR, followed by 25–50 mg every 6 h	Maternal gastrointestinal disturbance, oligohydramnios, ductal constriction	Not usually used after 32 weeks of gestation, careful monitoring required for more than 48 h

Abbreviations: IV, intravenously; PO, orally; PV, per vagina; PR per rectum.
Goldenberg RL. The management of preterm labor. Obstet Gynecol 2002;100:1020–37.

infusion of 50 mcg/min with a maximal rate of 350 mcg/min has been suggested (36). With cessation of uterine activity the infusion rate should be reduced. The patient should be closely monitored for fluid balance, cardiac status, and electrolyte levels, including potassium and glucose. Relative contraindications to any type of β-mimetic therapy include diabetes mellitus, underlying cardiac disease, use of digitalis, hyperthyroidism, severe anemia, and hypertension.

Many of the maternal side effects are caused by stimulation of β-receptors throughout the body. Serious maternal cardiopulmonary side effects include pulmonary edema, myocardial ischemia, arrhythmia, and even maternal death. Pulmonary edema may occur in approximately 4% of patients receiving parenteral ritodrine. Predisposing factors associated with this complication include multiple gestation, positive fluid balance, blood transfusion, anemia, infection, polyhydramnios, and underlying cardiac disease. The associated use of corticosteroids also has been implicated in the development of pulmonary edema. However, because the two most commonly used antepartum steroids, betamethasone and dexamethasone, have minimal mineralocorticoid activity, it is unlikely that these drugs contribute significantly to this complication. The maternal mortality that has been reported with intravenous ritodrine therapy is generally associated with pulmonary edema or cardiac arrhythmia. For those reasons pulse, blood pressure, and respiratory status should be closely monitored and discontinuation of therapy strongly considered with any respiratory distress or a heart rate greater than 130 beats per minute. Metabolic effects of ritodrine include hypokalemia, resulting from an increase in insulin and glucose concentrations, which drives potassium intracellularly. This condition generally resolves within 6–12 hours of discontinuing therapy.

A wide range of fetal cardiac complications has been described, including rhythm disturbances such as supraventricular tachycardia and atrial flutter. These usually resolve within a few days to 2 weeks after cessation of therapy. Fetal cardiac septal hypertrophy has been described with maternal ritodrine treatment. The degree of hypertrophy correlates with the duration of therapy and usually resolves within 3 months of age. Other, more serious fetal complications have included hydrops, pulmonary edema, and cardiac failure. Fetal and neonatal death, with histologic evidence of myocardial ischemia, also have been reported. Neonatal hypoglycemia is another potential complication with β-sympathomimetics and usually develops when delivery occurs within 2 days of treatment. The hypoglycemia is transient and results in medication-induced hyperinsulinemia. Neonatal periventricular–intraventricular hemorrhage

may be increased with β-sympathomimetic therapy. In a retrospective study of 2,827 women who gave birth preterm, there was a twofold increase in intraventricular hemorrhage in neonates whose mothers received β-mimetics, but this finding has not been consistently demonstrated in other studies (37). Studies evaluating long-term exposure to β-sympathomimetics demonstrate no differences in Apgar scores, head circumference, or neurologic status. Largely as a result of potential complications, as well as the limited evidence for improvements in important perinatal outcomes associated with its use and perhaps because of its cost relative to magnesium sulfate, ritodrine has fallen out of favor as a tocolytic agent in the United States.

Terbutaline is now the most commonly used β$_2$-selective β-mimetic agent in pregnancy and can be administered via oral, subcutaneous, or intravenous routes. In its itinial study, 30 patients with preterm labor were randomly assigned to intravenous terbutaline therapy and demonstrated an 80% success rate, in comparison with 20% for the placebo (38). Unfortunately, as with other tocolytic agents, subsequent studies have not reported similar success rates. Similar to ritodrine, terbutaline has been effective in temporarily arresting premature labor, but not reducing the rate of preterm birth. The initial infusion is 5–10 mcg/min, with the rate increased when necessary every 10–15 minutes to a maximum of 80 mcg/min. Terbutaline may be administered subcutaneously in 0.25-mg doses every 20–30 minutes (four to six doses) as the first-line tocolytic agent for preterm labor. In one study, the use of the terbutaline pump was compared with oral terbutaline therapy (39) and, in another study, a prospective double-blind randomized clinical trial comparing terbutaline pump maintenance therapy with a placebo was conducted (40). These investigators demonstrated no significant decreases in the preterm delivery rate or improvement in neonatal outcomes with use of the terbutaline pump. Orally administered terbutaline has mostly been used to prevent recurrence of already inhibited contractions. The usual oral dosages range from 2.5 mg to 5 mg every 4–6 hours, titrated by patient response and maternal pulse. Most studies of oral terbutaline have not shown a reduction in preterm birth. Maternal and neonatal side effects and complications are generally similar to those stated for ritodrine.

MAGNESIUM SULFATE

The use of magnesium sulfate as a tocolytic agent was first described in a randomized study of 71 women with preterm labor (41). Patients were allocated to intravenous infusion of magnesium, ethanol, or dextrose in water. The magnesium group received a 4-g bolus followed by a maintenance infusion of 2 g/h. The success rate, defined by the absence of contractions for 24 hours, was 77% for the magnesium group versus 45% for the ethanol group and 44% for the placebo group. In a randomized comparison of magnesium and terbutaline, it was demonstrated that magnesium had efficacy similar to terbutaline, with fewer side effects (42). Orally administered magnesium has not been shown to be effective in reversing preterm labor or preventing its recurrence (43–45). Overall, the evidence that magnesium sulfate, regardless of how it is administered, is an effective tocolytic is weak, and a Cochrane systematic review concluded that magnesium sulfate is ineffective as a tocolytic agent (46).

Magnesium sulfate is usually administered intravenously as an initial bolus of 4–6 g over 30 minutes, followed by a maintenance infusion of 1–3 g/h. Serum magnesium levels of 5–8 mg/dL are considered therapeutic for inhibiting myometrial activity. Once cessation of uterine activity is achieved, the patient is generally maintained at the lowest effective infusion rate for 12–24 hours and then weaned. Maternal side effects secondary to magnesium sulfate are typically dose related. Common side effects noted with the use of magnesium sulfate include flushing, nausea, headache, drowsiness, and blurry vision. Diminishment of deep tendon reflexes occurs when serum magnesium levels exceed 12 mg/dL (10 mEq/L). Significant respiratory depression can occur as serum levels reach 14–18 mg/dL (12–14 mEq/L), and cardiac arrest may occur with levels greater than 18 mg/dL (15 mEq/L). In general, respiratory depression does not occur before loss of deep tendon reflexes. The toxic effects of high magnesium levels can be rapidly reversed with the infusion of 1 g of calcium gluconate.

Absolute contraindications to the use of magnesium sulfate include myasthenia gravis and heart block. Relative contraindications include underlying renal disease and recent myocardial infarction. Concurrent use of calcium channel blockers and magnesium sulfate can theoretically result in profound hypotension and probably should be avoided, especially because there is no evidence of greater efficacy for combination treatment relative to either treatment used alone (47). Pulmonary edema has been reported in approximately 1% of women treated with magnesium sulfate, and the risk is increased in patients with multifetal gestations and those receiving combined tocolytic therapy. Because of the potential risk of fluid overload and the subsequent development of pulmonary edema, periodic assessment of fluid intake and output is essential.

Magnesium readily crosses the placenta, achieving fetal steady-state levels within hours of the start of treatment. No significant alterations in neurologic states or Apgar scores have been reported with umbilical cord concentrations of 4 mg/dL or less. At cord concentrations between 4 mg/dL and 11 mg/dL, respiratory depression and motor depression have been seen. Serum calcium levels in the fetus and newborn are unchanged or minimally reduced. Several observational reports have suggested that antenatal magnesium sulfate treatment for preterm labor or preeclampsia is associated with a decreased risk for cerebral palsy in very low birth weight infants (48). A large prospective multicenter trial is now ongoing to further explore the neonatal benefits of antenatal magnesium sulfate therapy.

In summary, although both maternal and neonatal side effects occur with magnesium use, they appear to be less common as well as generally less severe when compared with those seen with β-sympathomimetic therapy. If tocolytic drugs, none of which work particularly well in reducing preterm birth or improving important neonatal outcomes, are to be used, the one with the least side effects should be considered. For now, this seems to be magnesium sulfate, and it is possible that, for this reason, most U.S. practitioners now use magnesium sulfate as the primary tocolytic agent.

PROSTAGLANDIN SYNTHETASE INHIBITORS

Prostaglandins are 20-carbon cyclopentane carboxylic acids derived from membrane phospholipids (primarily arachidonic acid) via the enzymatic action of phospholipase A and cyclooxygenase (prostaglandin synthetase). Therefore, this pathway represents a key target for pharmacologic intervention. A number of drugs that inhibit the action of prostaglandin synthetase (eg, aspirin, ibuprofen, indomethacin, sulindac) are available. Of these drugs, indomethacin has been the most extensively studied.

Indomethacin was first used as a tocolytic agent in a study in which it was administered to 50 patients with preterm labor (49). Tocolysis was achieved in 40 of the 50 patients for at least 48 hours. In the first prospective, randomized, double-blind, placebo control study of 30 women with preterm labor, only one of 15 women in the indomethacin group failed therapy after 24 hours, in comparison with 9 of 15 women in the placebo group (50). In a comparison of indomethacin with ritodrine in a randomized trial, similar efficacy in delaying deliveries 48 hours and 7 days was found (51). Maternal side effects causing discontinuation of treatment were much more common in the ritodrine group (24% versus 0%). Similar efficacy was noted by the same authors in a comparative trial of indomethacin and magnesium sulfate (52).

Indomethacin is usually administered orally or rectally. A loading dose of 50–100 mg is followed by a total 24-hour dose not greater than 200 mg. Indomethacin blood concentrations usually peak 1–2 hours after oral administration, whereas rectal administration is associated with levels that peak slightly sooner. Most studies have limited the use of indomethacin to 24–48 hours because of concerns regarding the development of oligohydramnios and constriction of the ductus arteriosus. Maternal side effects are infrequent. Gastrointestinal upset may occur but usually can be relieved by taking the medication with meals or using an antacid. Maternal contraindications to indomethacin use include peptic ulcer disease; allergies to indomethacin or related compounds; hematologic, hepatic, or renal dysfunction; or drug-induced asthma. Fetal contraindications include preexisting oligohydramnios and congenital fetal heart disease in which the fetal circulation is dependent on the ductus arteriosus.

Indomethacin readily crosses the placenta, with fetal levels equilibrating with maternal concentrations about 5 hours after administration. Several fetal side effects have been reported with the use of indomethacin. Fetal urine output has been shown to decrease after administration of indomethacin. Long-term therapy may result in the development of oligohydramnios, although the timing of the onset is unpredictable. Therefore, the amniotic fluid index should be followed while the patient is receiving long-term therapy, and if the amniotic fluid index falls below 5 cm, therapy is usually discontinued. Resolution of oligohydramnios usually occurs within 48 hours of discontinuation of treatment. However, persistent anuria, renal microcystic lesions, and neonatal death have been reported with prenatal indomethacin exposure. Most of these infants were exposed to doses greater than 200 mg per day for more than 48 hours without adequate amniotic fluid assessment. Another important potential complication related to indomethacin use is the development of ductal constriction or closure, which leads to the diversion of right ventricular blood flow into the pulmonary vasculature. With time, this causes pulmonary arterial hypertrophy. After birth, relative pulmonary hypertension can cause shunting of blood through the foramen ovale and away from the lungs, resulting in persistent fetal circulation. This complication has been described with long-term indomethacin therapy but not in fetuses exposed to the drug for less than 48 hours. For this reason, it has been recommended that, for long-term treatment, patency of the ductus arteriosus be monitored and, if the pulsatility index is less than 2 cm per second, discontinuation of therapy be considered. The effects on ductal constriction have been shown to increase with advancing gestational age. At 32 weeks of gestation, it is estimated that 50% of fetuses will demonstrate ductal constriction. On the basis of these data, indomethacin therapy should be discontinued by 32 weeks of gestation at the latest.

Another reported complication in fetuses exposed to indomethacin prenatally and delivered at less than 30 weeks of gestation is an increased risk of necrotizing enterocolitis. In a retrospective case–control study, 57 fetuses delivered at less than 30 weeks of gestation after recent exposure to indomethacin were compared with 57 matched control fetuses (53). The incidence of necrotizing enterocolitis was 29% in the indomethacin group, versus 8% in the control group. Additionally, higher incidences of intraventricular hemorrhage and patent ductus arteriosus were noted in the indomethacin treatment group. The effect of the duration of treatment and the timing of the exposure in relation to delivery were not reported. Although these results are of concern, when used with appropriate caution (less than 48 hours of therapy, less than 30–32 weeks of gestation), indomethacin appears to be a relatively safe and effective tocolytic agent.

Sulindac is another prostaglandin synthetase inhibitor, closely related to indomethacin in structure, which likely has similar efficacy in inhibiting preterm labor. Initially, sulindac was reported to have fewer side effects than indomethacin when used for tocolysis. However, in a randomized double-blind study to evaluate the comparative effects of sulindac and terbutaline on fetal urine production and amniotic fluid volume, the authors concluded that sulindac administration resulted in a significant decrease in fetal urine flow and amniotic fluid volume (54). Additionally, two fetuses developed severe ductal constriction. Thus, sulindac shares many of the fetal side effects associated with indomethacin, and its safety, relative to indomethacin, is unknown.

CALCIUM CHANNEL BLOCKERS

Calcium channel blockers are agents that reduce transmembrane calcium influx, thus controlling muscle contractility and pacemaker activity in cardiac, vascular, and uterine tissue. To date, most clinical investigations evaluating the use of calcium channel blockers for the treatment of preterm labor have used nifedipine. The first reported use of nifedipine for the treatment of preterm labor was in a study involving 10 patients, with resultant cessation of uterine activity for 3 days in all patients undergoing treatment (55). In a subsequent randomized study, the nifedipine group had a significantly longer interval from presentation to delivery than either a ritodrine or placebo control group (56). Nifedipine has been shown to be as effective as ritodrine in prolonging pregnancy, but has far fewer side effects leading to discontinuation of therapy (57). The results of several subsequent studies and meta-analyses also suggest that nifedipine has a better safety profile than ritodrine and is at least equally effective in delaying delivery (58–60). Nifedipine is reported to be as effective in delaying delivery as magnesium sulfate (61, 62). In women with a diagnosis of successfully treated preterm labor, maintenance oral nifedipine did not prolong pregnancy relative to a no-treatment or control group (63).

Nifedipine can be administered orally or in sublingual form. It is rapidly absorbed by the gastrointestinal tract, with detectable blood levels attained within 5 minutes of sublingual administration. Nifedipine readily crosses the placenta, and serum concentrations of the fetus and the mother are comparable. An initial loading dose of 20 mg orally is typically given, followed by 10–20 mg every 6–8 hours. The sublingual form is not recommended for treatment of preterm labor because it acts more rapidly than the oral form and can cause acute hypotension. Contraindications to the use of nifedipine, or any of the calcium channel blockers include hypotension, congestive heart failure, and aortic stenosis. Concurrent use of calcium channel blockers and magnesium sulfate can theoretically result in profound hypotension and probably should be avoided (47). Maternal side effects of orally administered nifedipine result from the vasodilatory effects and include dizziness, lightheadedness, flushing, headache, and peripheral edema. The incidence of these side effects is approximately 17%, with severe effects resulting in the discontinuation of therapy in 2–5% of patients.

Studies evaluating the fetal effects of calcium channel blocker therapy have been limited to date. One concern is the potential adverse effect calcium channel blockers may have on uteroplacental blood flow, as has been reported in animal studies. However, several reports have examined uteroplacental blood flow in patients receiving nifedipine and have demonstrated no significant adverse effects on fetal or uteroplacental blood flow during treatment (64). As with many of the other tocolytic agents, additional studies are needed to more completely evaluate the potential fetal effects of calcium channel blocker therapy and the overall role of calcium channel blockers as a tocolytic agent for the treatment of preterm labor (65).

OXYTOCIN ANTAGONISTS

Although oxytocin antagonists are not available for use in the United States, their use to inhibit preterm labor will be discussed because they are available elsewhere. Oxytocin antagonists have been shown to effectively inhibit oxytocin-induced uterine contractions in both in vitro and in vivo animal models. The initial human studies were performed in the late 1980s. In one study, it was reported that a short-term infusion of an oxytocin antagonist in 13 patients resulted in inhibition of premature labor in all patients; however, 10 of these patients sub-

sequently required treatment with β-agonists (66). Similarly, in a report of 12 patients who were treated with an oxytocin receptor antagonist, nine had arrest of contractions (67). The most studied oxytocin antagonist is atosiban, which is a nonapeptide oxytocin analogue that competitively binds with the oxytocin–vasopressin receptor and is capable of inhibiting oxytocin-induced uterine contractions. Atosiban is typically administered intravenously, beginning with a single bolus of 6.75 mg, followed by an infusion at 300 mcg/min for 3 hours, and then 100 mcg/min for up to 18 hours.

Several prospective randomized, blinded clinical trials have demonstrated that atosiban is effective in diminishing uterine contractions in women with threatened preterm birth without causing significant maternal fetal or neonatal adverse effects. In one study, a 2-hour infusion of atosiban significantly decreased contraction frequency relative to placebo (68). In a prospective randomized, double-blind investigation of 501 women with preterm labor, atosiban was significantly more effective than a placebo in delaying delivery 24 hours, 48 hours, and 7 days (69). However, there was no improvement in perinatal outcomes. In a comparison of atosiban with ritodrine for the treatment of preterm labor in a randomized controlled trial involving 212 women, it was demonstrated that atosiban's tocolytic efficacy was comparable to that of ritodrine therapy (70). However, atosiban use was associated with fewer adverse side effects. No differences were noted between the groups with respect to neonatal outcomes. In a recent international study of atosiban versus β-mimetic agents (71), the efficacy of atosiban was similar to that of β-mimetic therapy, but the maternal cardiovascular side effects were considerably fewer in those women receiving atosiban. The potential use of atosiban for maintenance therapy in patients with arrested preterm labor also has recently been evaluated in a multicenter double-blind, placebo-controlled trial of 513 women with arrested preterm labor (72). Median time from start of maintenance therapy to first recurrence of labor was significantly longer for women treated with atosiban (32.6 days) than for the placebo-treated women (27.6 days). These data suggest that atosiban may be useful in delaying delivery 24–48 hours in the setting of preterm labor. However, this delay appears to have minimal impact on neonatal outcomes. Further studies are needed to more clearly elucidate the role of the oxytocin antagonists for the treatment of preterm labor.

NITRIC OXIDE DONORS

Nitric oxide is a potent endogenous hormone that facilitates smooth muscle relaxation in the vasculature, the gut, and the uterus. The use of nitric oxide donors (eg, nitroglycerin, glycerol trinitrate) for tocolytic therapy has been investigated. In a comparison of transdermal glycerol trinitrate with ritodrine for tocolysis in 245 women with documented preterm labor between 24 weeks and 36 weeks of gestation, there were no differences with respect to tocolytic effect and neonatal outcomes (73). However, in a comparison of intravenous nitroglycerin with magnesium sulfate in 31 women studied before 35 weeks of gestation, tocolytic failures (tocolysis 12 hours or longer) were significantly more common in patients treated with nitroglycerin than in the women treated with magnesium sulfate (74). Importantly, 25% of the patients treated with nitroglycerin experienced significant hypotension that required discontinuation of treatment. Given the potential profound hemodynamic effects of these nitric oxide donors on the central and peripheral circulation, these agents should be used with caution in the pregnant patient. Clinical use of these agents for the treatment of preterm labor remains experimental.

SUMMARY OF TOCOLYTICS

More than 20 years ago, in an editorial (75), the *British Medical Journal* indicated that, "in women in preterm labor, the use of tocolytics was frequently unnecessary, often ineffective, and occasionally harmful." Not much is different today. In many women, tocolytics seem to stop contractions temporarily, but rarely prevent preterm birth. Most importantly, used alone, they appear to convey little or no benefit for any fetal or neonatal outcome. For example, a meta-analysis of tocolytic therapy (76) concluded that although tocolytics may prolong pregnancy, they have not been shown to improve perinatal outcomes but do have adverse health effects on women. However, in some women they do appear to delay delivery long enough for successful administration of corticosteroids, one of the few interventions of clear benefit. Therefore, as a general rule, if tocolytics are given, they should be given concomitantly with corticosteroids. The gestational age range in which tocolytics should be used is open to debate, but because corticosteroids are not generally used at or after 34 weeks of gestation and because the perinatal outcomes in later-gestational-aged preterm infants are generally good, most authorities do not recommend the use of tocolytics at or after 34 weeks of gestation. There is no consensus on a lower gestational age limit for the use of tocolytic agents.

Antibiotics

Preterm labor, especially at less than 30 weeks of gestation, has been associated with occult upper genital tract infection (Fig. 16-2). Many, if not all, of the bacterial species involved in this occult infection are capable of inciting an inflammatory response, which ultimately may culminate in preterm labor and delivery. Antibiotics, therefore, have the potential to prevent or treat spontaneous preterm labor or both. Initial investigations of the use of antibiotics to prevent preterm birth showed that treatment of nonbacteriuric asymptomatic pregnant patients with daily tetracycline therapy resulted in fewer preterm births (77). However, although the data are mixed, many subsequent prospective trials of prenatal administration of antibiotics in women colonized with *Chlamydia trachomatis, Ureaplasma urealyticum*, and group B streptococcus have not shown a significant decrease in preterm birth. Recently, however, the association of bacterial vaginosis with preterm birth has prompted renewed interest in the use of antibiotics to prevent preterm birth in asymptomatic women. The results of these trials have been mixed as well, although two trials of clindamycin use, one orally and one vaginally, with the drugs started early in pregnancy, both found benefit in reducing preterm birth (78, 79). Similarly, the use of antibiotics for the treatment of documented preterm labor also has produced mixed results (Table 16-3) (80–97). A Cochrane meta-analysis (80) summarizing eight of the randomized controlled clinical trials comparing antibiotic therapy (mostly penicillin derivatives) with a placebo for the treatment of documented preterm labor demonstrated no difference between the placebo and antibiotic treatment in pregnancy prolongation, preterm delivery, respiratory distress syndrome, or neonatal sepsis. One potential reason for the failure of antibiotics to prevent preterm birth may be related to the fact that they do not seem to prevent or treat the histologic chorioamnionitis associated with preterm birth (97, 98). Antibiotics were, however, associated with a significantly decreased risk for maternal infection and neonatal necrotizing enterocolitis. Two randomized studies in women in early preterm labor, one performed in South Africa and one in Denmark, suggest that a combination of metronidazole and ampicillin, given to women with preterm labor for 6–8 days, may significantly delay delivery, increase birth weight, and improve neonatal outcomes such as sepsis and necrotizing enterocolitis (90, 94). As a profession, we adopt many clinical practices without such randomized trial evidence and, in specific cases, this intervention might be considered. Clearly, further studies are needed to evaluate various antibiotic regimens for the treatment of women with preterm labor with intact membranes. However, in the interim period, treatment of women in preterm labor with antibiotics for the sole purpose of preventing preterm delivery is not generally recommended.

Table 16-3. Randomized Controlled Trials of Antibiotics in Women in Preterm Labor With Intact Membranes

					Outcomes		
Author	Year	Weeks of Gestation	N	Antibiotics (Type)	Delay in Delivery	Decrease in Preterm Delivery	Decrease in Perinatal Mortality and Morbidity
McGregor et al	1986	Less than 34	17	Erythromycin	Yes	No	No
Morales et al	1988	21–34	150	Erythromycin, ampicillin	Yes	Yes	Not stated
Newton et al	1989	24–34	95	Ampicillin, erythromycin	No	No	No
McGregor et al	1991	Less than or equal to 34	103	Clindamycin	Yes	No	No
Newton et al	1991	24–33	86	Ampicillin, sulbactam	No	No	No
McCaul et al	1992	19–33	40	Ampicillin	No	No	No
Romero et al	1993	24–34	277	Ampicillin, erythromycin, amoxicillin	No	No	No
Norman et al	1994	26–34	81	Ampicillin, amoxicillin, metronidazole	Yes	No	Yes
Watts et al	1994	Less than 34	56	Mezlocillin, erythromycin	No	No	No
Gordon et al	1995	24–35	95	Ceftizoxine	No	No	No
Cox et al	1996	24–34	78	Ampicillin, sulbactam, Augmentin	No	No	No
Svare et al	1997	26–34	110	Ampicillin, metronidazole	Yes	Yes	No
Oyarzun et al	1998	22–36	170	Amoxicillin, erythromycin	No	No	No
Kenyon et al	2001	24–33	6,295	Erythromycin, amoxicillin, clavulonic acid	No	No	No

Goldenberg RL. The management of preterm labor. Obstet Gynecol 2002;100:1020–37.

Group B Streptococcus Prophylaxis

Group B streptococcus is an important cause of neonatal morbidity and death, especially in premature infants, but its role in the initiation of preterm labor is uncertain. Approximately 10–20% of U.S. women are group B streptococcus positive during pregnancy. The risk of preterm birth appears to be greatest in women with group B streptococcus in the urine, perhaps indicating a greater degree of colonization; thus, treatment of the urinary tract infection may result in a reduction in preterm birth. As an example, in a randomized trial of women who had a urine culture positive for group B streptococcus treated with antibiotics, the treated group had a lower incidence of premature delivery than the nontreated group (37.5% versus 5.4%) (99). These studies may be interpreted as showing that asymptomatic bacteriuria

with group B streptococcus (or in fact with any organism) is a risk factor for preterm delivery and that eradication with antibiotics decreases the risk. From a labor management perspective, these and other data suggest that women in preterm labor should be evaluated for bacteriuria and, if the results are positive, treated. However, whether this strategy applied to patients in labor will result in a significant reduction in preterm birth is unknown.

Group B streptococcus can cause significant neonatal morbidity and mortality. Usually acquired from the maternal genital tract after membrane rupture, the port of entry is generally the fetal lung. Sepsis often follows. In 1996, the Centers for Disease Control and Prevention in conjunction with the American College of Obstetricians and Gynecologists and the American Academy of Pediatrics set forth recommendations regarding two different approaches to the prevention of early-onset neonatal group B streptococcus disease (100). In the first strategy, intrapartum antibiotic prophylaxis was offered to women identified as being at high risk for having infants who develop early-onset group B streptococcus sepsis. Unless recently shown to be group B streptococcus negative, all women in preterm labor were in this category. In the second strategy, prenatal screening cultures were to be collected at 35–37 weeks of gestation, and women who were positive or of unknown status and preterm were considered to be high risk and treated. More recently, most authorities have settled on some variation of the second strategy, which includes vaginal–rectal screening of all women at 35–37 weeks of gestation, with the exception of those women with a previous infant infected with group B streptococcus or those with group B streptococcus bacteriuria (101, 102). Within this strategy, all women in preterm labor or with preterm PROM with 1) a history of an infected infant, 2) with a history of group B streptococcus bacteriuria, 3) with no recent culture results, or 4) with a positive recent culture should receive intrapartum antibiotic prophylaxis. For intrapartum chemoprophylaxis, intravenous penicillin G (5 million units initially and then 2.5 million units every 4 hours) until delivery is recommended. Intravenous ampicillin (2 g initially and then 1 g every 4 hours until delivery) is an acceptable alternative to penicillin G. Clindamycin or erythromycin may be used for women allergic to penicillin, although the efficacy of these drugs for group B streptococcus disease prevention has not been measured in controlled trials. It should be emphasized that the goal of this strategy is to prevent transmission of the group B streptococcus from the mother to the fetus and subsequent neonatal sepsis, and not to prevent preterm birth. Therefore, unless proved to be group B streptococcus negative, all women in preterm labor should receive group B streptococcus prophylaxis. A number of studies have shown a reduction in group B streptococcal neonatal sepsis with the adoption of one of the two strategies described previously (103, 104).

Corticosteroids

The use of antenatal corticosteroids for the prevention of neonatal respiratory distress syndrome stems from animal work in the late 1960s (105). Researchers observed that gravid sheep, which had received corticosteroids to induce preterm labor, gave birth to lambs that had accelerated fetal lung maturity and decreased respiratory problems at birth. After this observation, these investigators conducted the first trial of antenatal cocorticosteroid therapy in humans and found that 12 mg of betamethasone given on two occasions, 24 hours apart, resulted in a significant decrease in the incidence of respiratory distress syndrome, which was associated with a decrease in rates of perinatal mortality in newborns born before 34 weeks of gestation. The beneficial effect was noted only if delivery occurred after more than 24 hours had elapsed from the first dose and before 7 days.

Since then, 15 additional prospective randomized controlled trials have been performed. A meta-analysis of these trials confirmed that antenatal corticosteroid therapy significantly decreased the incidence and severity of neonatal respiratory distress syndrome (106). Neonatal mortality also was significantly reduced, as was the incidence of intraventricular hemorrhage and necrotizing enterocolitis. These benefits appeared to be maximal if delivery occurred more than 24 hours after start of the treatment but within 7 days.

Despite these data, antenatal corticosteroids remained underused throughout the 1980s and early 1990s. For this reason, the National Institutes of Health convened a Consensus Development Conference on Antenatal Steroids in 1994 to review the potential risks and benefits of antenatal corticosteroid therapy (107). The panel concluded that antenatally administered corticosteroids (betamethasone or dexamethasone) significantly reduce the risk of respiratory distress syndrome, intraventricular hemorrhage, and neonatal death. The panel recommended that all women between 24 weeks and 34 weeks of gestation at risk for preterm delivery should be considered candidates for antenatal corticosteroid treatment. Additionally, given that treatment for less than 24 hours was associated with a significantly decreased risk for respiratory distress syndrome, intraventricular hemorrhage, and mortality, the panel concluded that steroids should be administered unless delivery is imminent. For patients with preterm PROM, treatment was recommended for patients at less than 30–32 weeks of gestation because of the high risk of intraventricular hemorrhage. Recent studies suggesting worse outcomes in newborns whose mothers received multiple courses of corticosteroids and one randomized trial showing no benefit strongly suggest that the practice of giving repetitive weekly-dose courses until 34 weeks of gestation be discontinued unless data from ongoing randomized clinical trials demonstrate benefit for this practice. Long-term follow-up of infants exposed in utero to a single course of antenatal corticosteroid therapy has not demonstrated any adverse effect on growth, physical development, motor or cognitive skills, or school progress at 3 years and 6 years. Hence, the use of a single course of corticosteroids appears to be an efficacious and safe treatment for improving neonatal outcomes in patients with preterm labor.

The commonly used steroids for the enhancement of fetal maturity are betamethasone (12 mg intramuscularly every 24 hours, two doses) and dexamethasone (6 mg intravenously every 6 hours, four doses). These two corticosteroids have been identified because the most appropriate for antenatal use as they readily cross the placenta and have long half-lives and limited mineralocorticoid activity. One study (108), however, suggests that betamethasone is more effective in reducing intraventricular hemorrhage and periventricular leukomalacia than dexamethasone. Therefore, in the absence of other data, betamethasone given as a single course appears to be the better choice.

Delivery

The remarkable reduction in neonatal mortality rates that has occurred in the past several decades is mostly because of the widespread use of newborn intensive care for preterm newborns. Birth in proximity to a newborn intensive care unit with an experienced resuscitation team in attendance is one of the best predictors of neonatal survival. Obstetricians and other delivery attendants should do all in their power to ensure that each preterm newborn can benefit from this technology.

Women in preterm labor are more likely to have fetuses in the breech presentation than those at term, and the earlier the preterm labor, the more likely the breech fetus is to have a nonfrank presentation. Fetuses in the breech position, especially those less than 32 weeks of gestation, when delivered vaginally are prone to cord prolapse, muscle trauma, and head entrapment. They appear less likely to have traumatic and asphyxial injuries when delivered by cesarean delivery. Vaginally delivered preterm breech fetuses near term appear to have outcomes nearly comparable to those of vertex infants of the same gestational age, but few randomized trials exist to guide our choice of delivery method. Nevertheless, in most institutions virtually all preterm breech infants are delivered by cesarean delivery. Given the limited experience of most obstetricians in conducting breech deliveries and the reported increases in rates of morbidity and mortality with vaginal delivery, this practice seems appropriate, and is consistent with the American College of Obstetricians and Gynecologists' position on breech delivery at term (109). There is little or no evidence that routinely delivering preterm vertex infants by cesarean delivery improves outcome. Therefore, in preterm vertex infants, cesarean delivery should generally be performed for the same indications as in term infants. How to select the earliest gestational age for which cesarean delivery should be offered is a complicated issue. However, factors considered should include the gestational age-specific survival and short- and long-term neonatal morbidity rates at the delivering institution. In specific cases, after appropriate counseling, the parents' wishes should be strongly considered as a guide to management. It is the practice in many institutions with a good newborn intensive care unit to offer cesarean deliveries when indicated at about 24 weeks of gestation and to strongly recommend them when indicated beginning at 26 weeks of gestation.

Preterm infants, and especially very early preterm infants, are more vulnerable to trauma during delivery than fetuses at term. They are far more likely to have soft tissue damage, neurological injury, and traumatic intracranial hemorrhage than term infants. For this reason, special care should be taken not to traumatize these infants, especially during cesarean delivery or when using forceps. Vacuum extraction in preterm births may add extra risk and is considered to be contraindicated by some authorities. Although there are no randomized trials to confirm it, there appears to be less labor and delivery trauma when preterm labor is conducted with intact membranes. For this reason, especially for early preterm deliveries, artificial membrane rupture should be performed only for a clear indication. For the very early preterm breech fetus of borderline viability for which a cesarean delivery will not be performed, an en caul delivery appears to result in the least trauma (110). The choice of anesthesia should be based on similar considerations for both term and preterm labor.

Summary

The epidemiology, pathophysiology, and current therapeutic strategies used in the setting of preterm labor have been reviewed. Despite our best efforts, preterm delivery remains a significant clinical problem, accounting for a substantial component of all neonatal morbidity and mortality. Although we have gained important insights into the pathophysiology of preterm labor over the past several decades, effective therapeutic interventions to decrease spontaneous preterm delivery have not been discovered (111). Therefore, the successful management of preterm labor includes preventing neonatal disease when possible, including the use of corticosteroids and, when appropriate, group B streptococcus prophylaxis and reducing trauma and asphyxia during delivery. Preterm newborns should be delivered at a site that can perform expert resuscitation and provide intensive care when necessary. Clearly, additional research is needed to further explore the pathophysiology of spontaneous preterm labor and potential therapeutic approaches to deal with this important clinical problem. In the meantime, it seems important to practice evidence-based medicine, doing the things that work, and to eliminate from practice those things for which there is no evidence of efficacy. The latter practices include hydration, sedation, bed rest, home uterine activity monitoring, tocolysis without the concomitant use of corticosteroids, and oral terbutaline after successful intravenous tocolysis.

References

1. Hack M, Fanaroff AA. Outcomes of children of extremely low birthweight and gestational age in the 1990s. Early Hum Dev 1999;53:193–218.

2. Hack M, Taylor HG, Klein N, Eiben R, Schatschneider C, Mercuri-Minich N. School-age outcomes in children with birth weights under 750 g. N Engl J Med 1994;331:753–9.

3. Tucker JM, Goldenberg RL, Davis RO, Copper RL, Winkler CL, Hauth JC. Etiologies of preterm birth in an indigent population: Is prevention a logical expectation? Obstet Gynecol 1991;77:343–7.

4. Goldenberg RL, Hauth JC, Andrews WW. Intrauterine infection and preterm birth. N Engl J Med 2000;342:1500–7.

5. Guzick DS, Winn K. The association of chorioamnionitis with preterm delivery. Obstet Gynecol 1985;65:11–6.

6. Watts DH, Krohn MA, Hillier SL, Eschenbach DA. The association of occult amniotic fluid infection with gestational age and neonatal outcome among women in preterm labor. Obstet Gynecol 1992;79:351–7.

7. Meis PJ, Ernest JM, Moore ML. Causes of low birthweight births in public and private patients. Am J Obstet Gynecol 1987;156:1165–8.

8. Wen SW, Goldenberg RL, Cutter G, Hoffman HJ, Cliver SP. Intrauterine growth retardation and preterm delivery: Prenatal risk factors in an indigent population. Am J Obstet Gynecol 1990;162:213–8.

9. Shiono PH, Klebanoff MA, Rhoads GG. Smoking and drinking during pregnancy. JAMA 1986;255:82–4.

10. Mercer BM, Goldenberg RL, Moawad AH, Meis PJ, Iams JD, Das AF, et al. The preterm prediction study: Effect of gestational age and cause of preterm birth on subsequent obstetric outcome. National Institute of Child Health and Human Development Maternal-Fetal Medicine Units Network. Am J Obstet Gynecol 1999;181:1216–21.

11. Cunningham FG, Gant NF, Leveno KJ, Gilstrap LC III, Hauth JC, Wenstrom KD, editors. Williams Obstetrics. 21st ed. New York (NY): McGraw Hill; 2001. p. 780.

12. Romero R, Oyarzun E, Mazor M, Sirtori M, Hobbins JC, Bracken M. Meta-analysis of the relationship between asymptomatic bacteriuria and preterm delivery/birth weight. Obstet Gynecol 1989;73:576–82.

13. Nageotte MP, Dorchester W, Porto M, Keegan KA Jr, Freeman RK. Quantitation of uterine activity preceding preterm, term, and postterm labor. Am J Obstet Gynecol 1988;158:1254–9.

14. Copper RL, Goldenberg RL, Dubard MB, Hauth JC, Cutter GR. Cervical examination and tocodynamometry at 28 weeks' gestation: Prediction of spontaneous preterm birth. Am J Obstet Gynecol 1995;172:666–71.

15. Iams JD, Newman RB, Thom EA, Goldenberg RL, Mueller-Heubach E, Moawad A, et al. Frequency of uterine contractions and the risk of spontaneous preterm delivery. N Engl J Med 2002;346:250–5.

16. Newman RB, Iams JD, Das A, Goldenberg RL, Meis P, Moawad A, et al for the National Institute of Child Health and Human Development Network of Maternal-Fetal Medicine Units. A prospective masked observational study of uterine contraction frequency in twins. Am J Obstet Gynecol 2006;195:1564–70.

17. Peaceman AM, Andrews WW, Thorp JM, Cliver SP, Lukes A, Iams JD, et al. Fetal fibronectin as a predictor of preterm birth in patients with symptoms: A multicenter trial. Am J Obstet Gynecol 1997;177:13–8.

18. Goldenberg RL, Iams JD, Das A, Mercer BM, Meis PJ, Moawad AH, et al. The preterm prediction study: Fetal fibronectin testing and spontaneous preterm birth. Obstet Gynecol 1996;87:636–43.

19. Okitsu O, Mimura T, Nakayama T, Aono T. Early prediction of preterm delivery by transvaginal ultrasonography. Ultrasound Obstet Gynecol 1992;2:402.

20. Newman RB, Gill PJ, Wittreich P, Katz M. Maternal perception of prelabor uterine activity. Obstet Gynecol 1986;68:765–9.

21. Dyson DC, Danbe KH, Bamber JA, Crites YM, Field DR, Maier JA, et al. Monitoring women at risk for preterm labor. N Engl J Med 1998;338:15.

22. Goldenberg RL, Cliver SP, Bronstein J, Cutter GR, Andrews WW, Mennemeyer ST. Bed rest in pregnancy. Obstet Gynecol 1994;84:131–6.

23. Pircon RA, Strassner HT, Kirz DS, Towers CV. Controlled trial of hydration and bed rest versus bed rest alone in the evaluation of preterm uterine contractions. Am J Obstet Gynecol 1989;161:775–9.

24. Guinn DA, Goepfert AR, Owen J, Brumfield C, Hauth JC. Management options in women with preterm uterine contractions: A randomized clinical trial. AmJ Obstet Gynecol 1997;177:814–8.

25. Helfgott AW, Willis D, Blanco J. Is sedation beneficial in the treatment of threatened preterm labor? A preliminary report. J Matern Fetal Med 1994;3:37–42.

26. Keirse MJ. Progestogen administration in pregnancy may prevent preterm delivery. Br J Obstet Gynaecol 1990;97:149–54.

27. Meis PJ, Klebanoff M, Thom E, Dombrowski MP, Sibai B, Moawad AH, et al. Prevention of recurrent preterm delivery by 17 alpha-hydroxyprogesterone caproate [published erratum appears in N Engl J Med 2003;349:1299]. N Engl J Med 2003;348:2379–85.

28. da Fonseca EB, Bittar RE, Carvalho MHB, Zugaib M. Prophylactic administration of progesterone by vaginal suppository to reduce the incidence of spontaneous preterm birth in women at increased risk: a randomized placebo-controlled double-blind study. Am J Obstet Gynecol 2003;188:419–24.

29. Meis PJ. 17 hydroxyprogesterone for the prevention of preterm delivery. Obstet Gynecol 2005;105(5 Pt 1):1128–35.

30. Fuchs AR, Stakemann G. Treatment of threatened premature labor with large doses of progesterone. Am J Obstet Gynecol 1960;79:172–6.

31. Ovlisen B, Iversen J. Treatment of threatened premature labor with 6-methyl-17-acetoxyprogesterone. Am J Obstet Gynecol 1963;86:291–5.

32. Barden TP, Peter JB, Merkatz IR. Ritodrine hydrochloride: A beta-mimetic agent for use in preterm labor. I. Pharmacology, clinical history, administration, side effects, and safety. Obstet Gynecol 1980;56:1–6.

33. Merkatz JR, Peter JB, Barden TP. Ritodrine hydrochloride: A beta-mimetic agent for use in preterm labor. II. Evidence of efficacy. Obstet Gynecol 1980;56:7–12.

34. Canadian Preterm Labor Investigators Group. The treatment of preterm labor with beta-adrenergic agonist ritodrine. N Engl J Med 1992;327:308–12.

35. King JF, Grant A, Keirse MJ, Chalmers I. Beta-mimetics in preterm labour: An overview of randomized, controlled trials. Br J Obstet Gynaecol 1998;95:211–22.

36. Caritis SN, Venkataramanan R, Darby MJ, Chiao JP, Krew M. Pharmacokinetics of ritodrine administered intravenously: Recommendations for changes in the current regimen. Am J Obstet Gynecol 1990;162:429–37.

37. Groome LJ, Goldenberg RL, Cliver SP, Davis RO, Copper RL. Neonatal periventricular-intraventricular hemorrhage after maternal β-sympathomimetic tocolysis. Am J Obstet Gynecol 1992;167:873–9.

38. Ingemarsson I. Effect of terbutaline on premature labor. Am J Obstet Gynecol 1976;125:520–4.

39. Lam F, Gill P, Smith M, Kitzmiller JL, Katz M. Use of the subcutaneous terbutaline pump for long-term tocolysis. Obstet Gynecol 1988;72:810–3.

40. Guinn DA, Goepfert AR, Owen J, Wenstrom KD, Hauth JC. Terbutaline pump maintenance therapy for prevention of preterm delivery: A double-blind trial. Am J Obstet Gynecol 1998;179:874–8.

41. Steer CM, Petrie RH. A comparison of magnesium sulfate and alcohol for the prevention of premature labor. Am J Obstet Gynecol 1977;129:1–4.

42. Miller JM, Keane MW, Horger EO 3rd. A comparison of magnesium sulfate and terbutaline for the arrest of premature labor. J Reprod Med 1982;27:348–51.

43. Martin RW, Perry KG Jr, Hess LW, Martin JN Jr, Morrison JC. Oral magnesium and the prevention of preterm labor in a high-risk group of patients. Am J Obstet Gynecol 1992;166:144–7.

44. Ricci JM, Hariharan S, Helfgott A, Reed K, O'Sullivan MJ. Oral tocolysis with magnesium chloride: A randomized controlled prospective clinical trial. Am J Obstet Gynecol 1991;165:603–10.

45. Ridgeway LE 3rd, Muise K, Wright JW, Patterson RM, Newton ER. A prospective randomized comparison of oral terbutaline and magnesium oxide for the maintenance of tocolysis. Am J Obstet Gynecol 1990;163:879–82.

46. Crowther CA, Hiller JE, Doyle LW. Magnesium sulphate for preventing preterm birth in threatened preterm labour. Cochrane Database Syst Rev 2002;CD001060.

47. Ben-Ami M, Giladi Y, Shalev E. The combination of magnesium sulfate and nifedipine: A cause of neuromuscular blockade. Br J Obstet Gynaecol 1994;101:262–3.

48. Grether JK, Hoogstrate J, Walsh-Greene E, Nelson KB. Magnesium sulfate for tocolysis and risk of spastic cerebral palsy in premature children born to women without preeclampsia. Am J Obstet Gynecol 2000;183:717–25. 44. Zuckerman H, Reiss U, Rubinstein I. Inhibition of human premature labor by indomethacin. Obstet Gynecol 1974;44:787–92.

49. Zuckerman, H et al. Inhibition of human premature labor by indomethacin. Obstet Gynecol 1974;44:787.

50. Niebyl JR, Blake DA, White RD, Kumor KM, Dubin NH, Robinson JC, et al. The inhibition of premature labor with indomethacin. Am J Obstet Gynecol 1980;136:1014–9.

51. Morales WJ, Smith SG, Angel JL, O'Brien WF, Knuppel RA. Efficacy and safety of indomethacin versus ritodrine in the management of preterm labor: A randomized study. Obstet Gynecol 1989;74:567–72.

52. Morales WJ, Madhav H. Efficacy and safety of indomethacin compared with magnesium sulfate in the management of preterm labor: A randomized study. Am J Obstet Gynecol 1993;169:97–102.

53. Norton ME, Merrill J, Cooper BA, Kuller JA, Clyman RI. Neonatal complications after the administration of indomethacin for preterm labor. N Engl J Med 1993;329:1602–7.

54. Kramer WB, Saade GR, Belfort M, Dorman K, Mayes M, Moise KJ Jr. A randomized, double-blind study comparing the fetal effects of sulindac to terbutaline during the management of preterm labor. Am J Obstet Gynecol 1999;180:396–401.

55. Ulmsten U, Andersson KE, Wingerup L. Treatment of premature labor with the calcium antagonist nifedipine. Arch Gynecol 1980;229:1–5.

56. Read MD, Wellby DE. The use of a calcium antagonist (nifedipine) to suppress preterm labour. Br J Obstet Gynaecol 1986;93:933–7.

57. Ferguson JE II, Dyson DC, Schutz T, Stevenson DK. A comparison of tocolysis with nifedipine or ritodrine: Analysis of efficacy and maternal, fetal, and neonatal outcome. Am J Obstet Gynecol 1990;163:105–11.

58. Koks CA, Brolmann HA, de Kleine MJ, Manger PA. A randomized comparison of nifedipine and ritodrine for suppression of preterm labor. Eur J Obstet Gynecol Reprod Biol 1998;77:171–6.

59. Papatsonis DN, Kok JH, van Geijn HP, Bleker OP, Ader HJ, Dekker GA. Neonatal effects of nifedipine and ritodrine for preterm labor. Obstet Gynecol 2000;95:477–81.

60. Tsatsaris V, Papatsonis D, Goffinet F, Dekker G, Carbonne B. Tocolysis with nifedipine or beta-adrenergic agonists: A meta-analysis. Obstet Gynecol 2001;97:840–7.

61. Haghighi L. Prevention of preterm delivery: Nifedipine or magnesium sulfate. Int J Gynaecol Obstet 1999;66:297–8.

62. Glock JL, Morales WJ. Efficacy and safety of nifedipine versus magnesium sulfate in the management of preterm labor: A randomized study. Am J Obstet Gynecol 1993;169:960–4.

63. Carr DB, Clark AL, Kernek K, Spinnato JA. Maintenance oral nifedipine for preterm labor: A randomized clinical trial. Am J Obstet Gynecol 1999;181:822–7.

64. Mari G, Kirshon B, Moise KJ Jr, Lee W, Cotton DB. Doppler assessment of the fetal and uteroplacental circulation during nifedipine therapy for preterm labor. Am J Obstet Gynecol 1989;161:1514.

65. van Geijn HP, Lenglet JE, Bolte AC. Nifedipine trials: effectiveness and safety aspects. BJOG: An International Journal of Obstetrics & Gynaecology. 2005;112(Suppl 1): 79–83.

66. Akerlund M, Stromberg P, Hauksson A, Andersen LF, Lyndrup J, Trojnar J, et al. Inhibition of uterine contractions of premature labour with an oxytocin analogue. Results from a pilot study. Br J Obstet Gynaecol 1987;94: 1040–4.

67. Andersen LF, Lyndrup J, Akerlund M, Melin P. Oxytocin receptor blockade: A new principle in the treatment of preterm labor? Am J Perinatol 1989;6:196–9.

68. Goodwin TM, Paul R, Silver H, Spellacy W, Parsons M, Chez R, et al. The effect of the oxytocin antagonist atosiban on preterm uterine activity in the human. Am J Obstet Gynecol 1994;170:474.

69. Romero R, Sibai BM, Sanchez-Ramos L, Valenzuela GJ, Veille JC, Tabor B, et al. An oxytocin receptor antagonist (atosiban) in the treatment of preterm labor: A randomized, double-blind, placebo-controlled trial with tocolytic rescue. Am J Obstet Gynecol 2000;182:1173–83.

70. Moutquin JM, Sherman D, Cohen H, Mohide PT, Hochner-Celnikier D, Fejgin M, et al. Double-blind, randomized, controlled trial of atosiban and ritodrine in the treatment of preterm labor: A multicenter effectiveness and safety study. Am J Obstet Gynecol 2000;182:1191–9.

71. The Worldwide Atosiban Versus Beta-agonists Study Group. Effectiveness and safety of the oxytocin antagonist atosiban versus beta-adrenergic agonists in the treatment of preterm labour. Br J Obstet Gynaecol 2001;108: 133–42.

72. Valenzuela GJ, Sanchez-Ramos L, Romero R, Silver HM, Koltun WD, Millar L, et al. Maintenance treatment of preterm labor with the oxytocin antagonist atosiban. The Atosiban PTL-098 Study Group. Am J Obstet Gynecol 2000;182:1184–90.

73 Lees CC, Lojacono A, Thompson C, Danti L, Black RS, Tanzi P, et al. Glyceryl trinitrate and ritodrine in tocolysis: An international multicenter randomized study. GTN Preterm Labour Investigation Group. Obstet Gynecol 1999;94:403–8.

74. El-Sayed YY, Riley ET, Holbrook RH Jr, Cohen SE, Chitkara U, Druzin ML. Randomized comparison of intravenous nitroglycerin and magnesium sulfate for treatment of preterm labor. Obstet Gynecol 1999;93:79–83.

75. Drugs in threatened preterm labour [editorial]. Br Med J 1979;I:71.

76. Gyetvai K, Hannah ME, Hodnett ED, Ohlsson A. Tocolytics for preterm labor: A systematic review. Obstet Gynecol 1999;94:869–77.

77. Elder HA, Santamarina BA, Smith S, Kass EH. The natural history of asymptomatic bacteriuria during pregnancy: The effect of tetracycline on the clinical course and outcome of pregnancy. Am J Obstet Gynecol 1971;111: 441–62.

78. Lamont RF, Jones BM, Mandal D, Hay PE, Sheehan M. The efficacy of vaginal clindamycin for the treatment of abnormal genital tract flora in pregnancy. Infect Dis Obstet Gynecol. 2003;11(4):181–9.

79. Ugwumadu A, Manyonda I, Reid F, Hay P. Effect of early oral clindamycin on late miscarriage and preterm delivery in asymptomatic women with abnormal vaginal flora and bacterial vaginosis: a randomised controlled trial. Lancet. 2003;361(9362):983–8.

80. King J, Flenady V. Antibiotics for preterm labour with intact membranes. Cochrane Database Syst Rev 2000; 2:CD000246.

81. Mazor M, Chaim W, Maymon E, Hershkowitz R, Romero R. The role of antibiotic therapy in the prevention of prematurity. Clin Perinatol 1998;25:659–85.

82. Thorp JM, Hartmann KE, Berkman ND, Carey TS, Lohr KN, Gavin NI, et al. Antibiotic therapy for the treatment of preterm labor: A review of the evidence. Am J Obstet Gynecol 2002;186:587–92.

83. McGregor JA, French JI, Reller LB, Todd JK, Makowski EL. Adjunctive erythromycin treatment for idiopathic preterm labor: Results of a randomized, double-blinded, placebo-controlled trial. Am J Obstet Gynecol 1986;154: 98–103.

84. Morales WJ, Angel JL, O'Brien WF, Knuppel RA, Finazzo M. A randomized study of antibiotic therapy in idiopathic preterm labor. Obstet Gynecol 1988;72:829–33.

85. Newton ER, Dinsmoor MJ, Gibbs RS. A randomized blinded, placebo-controlled trial of antibiotics in idiopathic preterm labor. Obstet Gynecol 1989;74:562–6.

86. McGregor JA, French JI, Seo K. Adjunctive clindamycin therapy for preterm labor: Results of a double-blind, placebo-controlled trial. Am J Obstet Gynecol 1991; 165:867–75.

87. Newton ER, Shields L, Ridgway LE 3rd, Berkus MD, Elliott BD. Combination antibiotics and indomethacin in idiopathic preterm labor: A randomized double-blind clinical trial. Am J Obstet Gynecol 1991;165:1753–9.

88. McCaul JF, Perry KG Jr, Moore JL Jr, Martin RW, Bucovaz ET, Morrison JC. Adjunctive antibiotic treatment of women with preterm rupture of membranes or preterm labor. Int J Gynaecol Obstet 1992;38:19–24.

89. Romero R, Sibai B, Caritis S, Paul R, Depp R, Rosen M, et al. Antibiotic treatment of preterm labor with intact membranes: A multicenter, randomized, double-blinded, placebo-controlled trial. Am J Obstet Gynecol 1993;169: 764–74.

90. Norman K, Pattinson RC, de Souza J, de Jong P, Moller G, Kirsten G. Ampicillin and metronidazole treatment in preterm labour: A multicentre, ramdomised controlled trial. Br J Obstet Gynaecol 1994;101:404–8.

91. Watts DH, Krohn MA, Hillier SL, Eschenbach DA. Randomized trial of antibiotics in addition to tocolytic therapy to treat preterm labor. Infect Dis Obstet Gynecol 1994;1:220–7.

92. Gordon M, Samuels P, Shubert P, Johnson F, Gebauer C, Iams J. A randomized, prospective study of adjunctive ceftizoxime in preterm labor. Am J Obstet Gynecol 1995;172:1546–52.

93. Cox SM, Bohman VR, Sherman L, Leveno KJ. Randomized investigation of antimicrobials for the prevention of preterm birth. Am J Obstet Gynecol 1996;174: 206–10.

94. Svare J, Langhoff-Roos J, Anderson LF, Kryger-Baggesen N, Borch-Christensen H, Heisterberg L, et al. Ampicillin/ metronidazole treatment in idiopathic preterm labour: A randomised controlled multicentre trial. Br J Obstet Gynaecol 1997;104:892–7.

95. Oyarzun E, Gomez R, Rioseco A, Gonazalez P, Gutierrez P, Donoso E, et al. Antibiotic treatment in preterm labor and intact membranes: A randomized, double-blinded, placebo-controlled trial. J Matern Fetal Med 1998;7: 105–10.

96. Kenyon SL, Taylor DJ, Tarnow-Mordi W. Broad-spectrum antibiotics for spontaneous preterm labour: The ORACLE II randomised trial. Lancet 2001;357:989;94.

97. Goldenberg RL, Mwatha A, Read JS, Adeniyi-Jones S, Sinkala M, Msmanga G, et al. The HPTN 024 study: the efficacy of antibiotics to prevent chorioamnionitis and preterm birth. Am J Obstet Gynecol. 2006;194(3): 650-61.

98. Ugwumadu A, Reid F, Hay P, Manyonda I, Jeffrey I. Oral clindamycin and histologic chorioamnionitis in women with abnormal vaginal flora. Obstet Gynecol 2006;107(4): 863–8.

99. Thomsen AC, Morup L, Hansen KB. Antibiotic elimination of group B streptococci in urine in prevention of preterm labour. Lancet 1987;1:591–3.

100. Centers for Disease Control and Prevention. Prevention of perinatal group B streptococcal disease: A public health perspective. MMWR Morb Mortal Wkly Rep 1996;45 (RR-7):1.

101. Gibbs RS, Schrags S, Schuchat A. Perinatal infections due to Group B Streptococci. Obstet Gynecol 2004;104 (5 Pt 1):1062-76. Review.

102. Centers for Disease Control and Prevention. Prevention of Perinatal Group B Streptococcal Disease. MMWR 2002; 51(RR-11):4.

103. Schrag S, Schuchat A. Prevention of neonatal sepsis. Clinics in Perinatology 2005;32(3):601–15.

104. Sutkin G, Krohn MA, Heine RP, Sweet RL. Antibiotic prophylaxis and non-group B streptococcal neonatal sepsis. Obstet Gynecol 2005;105(3):581–6.

105. Liggins GC, Howie RN. A controlled trial of antepartum glucocorticoid treatment for prevention of the respiratory distress syndrome in premature infants. Pediatrics 1972; 50:515–25.

106. Crowley P. Prophylactic corticosteroids for preterm birth. Cochrane Database Syst Rev 2000;2:CD000065.

107. National Institutes of Health (NIH) Consensus Development Conference. Effect of corticosteroids for fetal maturation on perinatal outcomes. Am J Obstet Gynecol 1995;173:246.

108. Baud O, Foix-L'Helias L, Kaminski M, Audibert F, Jarreau PH, Papiernik E, et al. Antenatal glucocorticoid treatment and cystic periventricular leukomalacia in very premature infants. N Engl J Med 1999;341:1190–6.

109. American College of Obstetricians and Gynecologists. ACOG committee opinion no. 265. Mode of term single breech delivery. Obstet Gynecol 2001;98:1189–90.

110. Goldenberg RL, Davis RO. In caul delivery of the very premature infant. Am J Obstet Gynecol 1983;145:645–6.

111. Goldenberg RL, Rouse DJ. The prevention of premature birth. N Engl J Med 1998;339:313–20.

CHAPTER 17

17 α-Hydroxyprogesterone Caproate for the Prevention of Preterm Delivery

PAUL J. MEIS

The concept that progesterone therapy may improve pregnancy outcome has been under consideration for more than 50 years. Early studies of this therapy examined the use of progesterone in women with threatened abortion or as a treatment for women with a history of repeated early pregnancy loss. The results of randomized controlled trials of progesterone for these indications have failed to show efficacy, and progesterone treatment is not currently recommended for the treatment of threatened abortion. However, other studies of progesterone examined whether this treatment might be effective in preventing preterm birth (1). Since that time, a number of trials of progesterone for prevention of preterm delivery have been reported. In this review, we will discuss historically important trials of progesterone for the prevention of preterm delivery, including two meta-analyses and more recent trials of progesterone, 17 α-hydroxyprogesterone caproate, and medroxyprogesterone. In preparation for this review, we performed a search of all literature in English from 1966 to February 2005 in MEDLINE for the terms "progesterone" and "preterm birth," which yielded 150 citations.

The most successful of these early trials employed 17 α-hydroxyprogesterone caproate. Although most of these trials reported efficacy for progesterone therapy in reducing the rate of preterm delivery, the trials had relatively small numbers of subjects, and the treatment never achieved wide acceptance. Recently, the publication of two large randomized trials, one of 17 α-hydroxyprogesterone caproate (2) and the other of progesterone vaginal suppositories (3), have stimulated renewed interest in the use of this treatment modality and have also stimulated basic research about the mechanisms of progesterone function.

Preterm birth, that is, delivery before 37 completed weeks of gestation, is the major determinant of infant mortality in developed countries (4). The rate of preterm birth is greater in the United States than in most developed countries and is the factor most responsible for the relatively high rate of infant mortality in the United States (4). In addition, the rate of preterm birth in the United

States has increased progressively over the past two decades, from 9% to 12% of all births (Fig. 17-1) (5). The rate of preterm delivery is particularly high for African-American women, who experience rates of low birth weight and preterm delivery twice as high as those for white women in the United States (4). Preterm birth is hazardous to the surviving children. Preterm birth increases the risk for developmental problems, and preterm birth is the largest single cause of cerebral palsy (4). In addition, the financial costs of preterm birth are high. In 2001, the total national bill for premature babies was estimated at $13.6 billion (6). For these reasons, preterm birth is a very significant public health problem in the United States.

Many attempts have been made to find ways to reduce the incidence of preterm birth. Beginning in the 1970s, drug therapy for the prevention of preterm delivery became widely used and focused mainly on the use of tocolytic drugs to halt preterm labor after it had begun. Although trials of various tocolytic drugs have shown effectiveness in halting labor for up to several days, the use of these drugs has not reduced the incidence of preterm delivery and has not resulted in any improvement

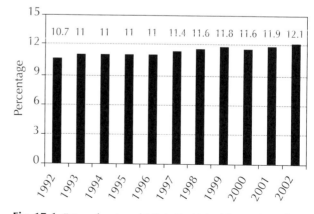

Fig. 17-1. Rates of preterm birth in the United States. (Data from National Center for Health Statistics. Final natality data. Available at: www.marchofdimes.com/peristats. Retrieved February 10, 2005.)

in perinatal outcome (7). Cervical cerclage has long been employed for women thought to have a weakness of cervical integrity, but randomized trials of cervical cerclage have generally not shown effectiveness (8). Although vaginal infections are known to be associated with an increased risk of preterm delivery, the largest and best controlled trials in low-risk women have found no improvement in rates of preterm birth as a result of screening for and treating vaginal infections (9, 10). Despite many trials of reduced physical activity, the use of tocolytic drugs to halt labor, antibiotic therapy, and other strategies for prevention, no effective and reproducible method of preventing preterm birth has been discovered (11). Thus, the enigma of preterm birth is widely considered to be the greatest problem in obstetrics in the developed world.

Actions of Progesterone

Progesterone, produced by secretion from the corpus luteum and the placenta, is known to be essential for the maintenance of pregnancy early in gestation (12, 13). In addition, progesterone is known to have actions that maintain pregnancy later in gestation. Progesterone acts to relax smooth muscle in many organs, including the pregnant uterus. Progesterone has immunosuppressive activity against the activation of T lymphocytes and blocks the effects of oxytocin on the myometrium (13, 14). Perhaps most importantly, progesterone is a potent inhibitor of the formation of gap junctions between myometrial cells (15). These intercellular communications are essential for the propagation of coordinated uterine muscle activity leading to labor.

In addition to actions of progesterone for general maintenance of pregnancy, evidence exists, from data obtained from both animals and humans, that changes in local or systemic concentrations of progesterone may play a role in the initiation of labor. The importance of progesterone in regulating the onset of labor is supported by the observation that, in sheep, goats, and many other mammalian species, a decrease in plasma progesterone and an increase in estrogen precede the onset of labor (16). These findings of changes in the progesterone/estrogen ratio are consistent with the concept of "progesterone block," which was advanced and championed by Csapo in the 1950s (17), based on his extensive and pioneering experiments in pregnant rabbits.

The role of progesterone or of changes in the progesterone/estrogen ratio in human beings and other primates is less well known. Although investigators have described low progesterone concentrations or low progesterone/estrogen ratios in the plasma of women destined to give birth prematurely (18, 19), no consistent evidence exists of changes in plasma progesterone or the progesterone/estrogen ratio before the onset of labor at term or before term. Nonetheless, some evidence exists that local changes in progesterone or the progesterone/estrogen ratio in the placenta, decidua, or fetal membranes may be important in the initiation of labor in human beings (20, 21). Several investigators have reported the effects of administering progesterone antagonists to women at term. The results were an increased rate of spontaneous onset of labor and, in the women whose labor was induced with oxytocin, an increased sensitivity to oxytocin compared with placebo-treated controls (22–24). Although these data support the concept that progesterone plays a role in maintaining gestation in human beings, the actual mechanisms by which progesterone therapy may avert preterm labor and delivery are not known.

Early Trials

One of the earliest prophylactic trials of 17 α-hydroxyprogesterone caproate for the prevention of preterm delivery enrolled women identified as being at risk of preterm delivery by using a risk-scoring system (1). Ninety-nine women were randomly assigned to receive 17 α-hydroxyprogesterone caproate or placebo injections. Preterm delivery occurred less frequently in the treated group (4%) than in the placebo group (18%). A subsequent trial evaluated 17 α-hydroxyprogesterone caproate for women who had a history of two spontaneous abortions, two preterm deliveries, or a combination of these outcomes in the pregnancies immediately preceding the index pregnancy (25). Of the 43 women in the trial, 18 were randomized to weekly injections of 250 mg of 17 α-hydroxyprogesterone caproate, and 22 were randomized to placebo injections. The treatment was started as soon as the patients registered for care and was continued to 37 weeks of gestation. Three patients in the placebo group and four patients in the treatment group also received a cervical cerclage. The primary outcome was delivery at less than 36 weeks of gestation. The rate of preterm delivery in the placebo group was 41% (nine women), whereas none of the treatment group gave birth before 36 weeks of gestation. The treatment group showed significant differences from the control group in mean duration of pregnancy, mean birth weight, and perinatal mortality rate. The publication of this trial in a major medical journal stimulated considerable interest in the use of this drug to prevent preterm birth. The conclusion was that large-scale trials were needed to demonstrate the efficacy of this treatment. No support for a larger trial was available, however, and the funding agency for this trial indicated that, in view of the positive results of the trial, a further placebo-controlled trial could not be supported ethically (19).

The results of these early reported trials of progesterone for prevention of preterm labor and delivery were evaluated by two different meta-analyses. A meta-analysis of randomized controlled trials involved the use of progesterone or other progestational agents for the maintenance of pregnancy (26). Fifteen trials of variously defined high-risk subjects were felt to be suitable for analysis. The trials employed six different progestational drugs. The pooled odds ratios (OR) for these trials showed no statistically significant effect on rates of miscarriage, stillbirth, neonatal death, or preterm birth. The authors concluded that "progestogens should not be used outside of randomized trials at present" (26).

In response to this publication, the results of an analysis of a more focused selection of trials were presented (27). This meta-analysis was restricted to trials that employed 17 α-hydroxyprogesterone caproate, the most fully studied progestational agent, and included all placebo-controlled trials that used this drug. Pooled ORs found no significant effect on rates of miscarriage, perinatal death, or neonatal complications. However, in contrast to the previously mentioned review, the OR for reduction of preterm birth was significant, 0.5 (95% confidence interval [CI], 0.30–0.85), as was the OR for birth weight less than 2,500 g, 0.46 (95% CI, 0.27–0.80). The results demonstrated by these trials contrasted markedly with the poor effectiveness of other efforts to reduce the occurrence of preterm birth, but that since no effect was demonstrated to result in lower perinatal mortality or morbidity, "further well-controlled research would be necessary before it is recommended for clinical practice" (27).

Although most of these trials employing 17 α-hydroxyprogesterone caproate showed positive results for the prevention of preterm birth, two trials did not show efficacy. In a trial in twin pregnancies (28), 77 women were identified as having twin gestations at 28–33 weeks of gestation and were then randomly assigned to receive weekly injections of either 250 mg of 17 α-hydroxyprogesterone caproate or a placebo injection until 37 weeks of gestation. No significant differences were seen for rates of preterm delivery (30.8% in the treatment group versus 23.7% in the placebo group), mean duration of pregnancy, mean birth weight, or rates of perinatal mortality. To date, this remains the only reported trial of 17 α-hydroxyprogesterone caproate or other progestogen in multiple gestation. A trial of 17 α-hydroxyprogesterone caproate in a relatively low-risk group of pregnant women included women on active duty in the military (29). The women were randomly assigned at 16–20 weeks of gestation to receive weekly injections of 1,000 mg of 17 α-hydroxyprogesterone caproate (80 subjects) or placebo injections (88 subjects), continuing until 36 weeks of gestation. No difference was seen for any pregnancy outcome studied. The rate of low birth weight birth for the treatment group was 7.5%, compared with 9% for the placebo infants. The results of this trial are notable for the low rate of preterm and low birth weight delivery in the population studied. Because of the low prevalence of the outcome studied in this population, the trial did not have sufficient power to detect a difference in rates of low birth weight birth. To show a 40% reduction in the treatment group compared with placebo in the rate of the outcome measured (ie, low birth weight) would have required a total sample of 1,540 subjects. The results of this trial suggest that progesterone therapy is not useful in women at low risk for preterm delivery.

Recent Trials

In a randomized, placebo-controlled trial of progesterone vaginal suppositories in 142 women (3), the subjects were selected as being at high risk for preterm birth. The risk factor in more than 90% of the subjects was that of a previous preterm delivery. The patients were randomly assigned to daily insertion of either a 100-mg progesterone suppository or a placebo suppository. The treatment period was 24–34 weeks of gestation. All patients were monitored for uterine contractions once weekly for 1 hour with an external tocodynamometer. Although 81 progesterone and 76 placebo patients were entered into the study, several patients were excluded from analysis because of premature rupture of the fetal membranes or were lost to follow-up, leaving 72 progesterone and 70 placebo subjects. The rate of preterm delivery at less than 37 weeks of gestation in the progesterone patients was 13.8%, significantly less than the rate in the placebo patients of 28.5%. The rate of preterm delivery at less than 34 weeks of gestation in the treatment group was 2.8%, compared with 18.6% in the placebo group. These differences were statistically significant. The rate of uterine contractions measured by the weekly hour-long recording was significantly less between 28 weeks and 34 weeks in the progesterone patients compared with the placebo patients. Analysis of the results by intent to treat showed smaller differences between the groups, but these differences remained statistically significant.

A large multicenter trial of 17 α-hydroxyprogesterone caproate conducted by the Maternal–Fetal Medicine Units Network of the National Institute of Child Health and Human Development enrolled women with a documented history of a previous spontaneous preterm delivery, which occurred as a consequence of either spontaneous preterm labor or preterm premature rupture of the fetal membranes (2). After receiving an ultrasound examination to rule out major fetal anomalies and to determine gestational age, the subjects were offered the study and given a test dose of the placebo injection to assess compliance. If they chose to continue, they were randomly assigned, using a 2:1 ratio, to weekly injections of 250 mg of 17 α-hydroxyprogesterone caproate or a placebo injection. Treatment was begun between 16 weeks and 20 weeks of gestation and was continued until delivery or 37 weeks of gestation, whichever came first. The study planned to enroll 500 subjects, a sample size estimated to be sufficient to detect a 37% reduction in the rate of preterm birth. However, enrollment was halted at 463 subjects, 310 in the treatment group and 153 in the placebo group, following a scheduled evaluation by the Data Safety and Monitoring Committee, which found that the evidence of efficacy for the primary outcome was such that further entry of patients would not be ethical. In this study, delivery at less than 37 weeks of gestation was reduced from 54.9% in the placebo group to 36.3% in the treatment group. Similar reductions were seen in delivery at less than 35 weeks of gestation, from 30.7% to 20.6%, and delivery at less than 32 weeks of gestation, from 19.6% to 11.4% (Fig. 17-2A). Rates of birth weight less than 2,500 g were reduced. All of these differences were statistically significant. Although the sample size of the study was not powered to examine effects on neonatal morbidity and mortality, a strong trend was found for reduction in rates of neonatal death, transient tachypnea, respiratory distress syndrome, bronchopulmonary dysplasia, need for ventilatory support, supplementary oxygen, intraventricular hemorrhage, necrotizing enterocolitis, patent ductus arteriosis, and

retinopathy. These differences were statistically significant for rates of intraventricular hemorrhage (but not for grades III–IV), necrotizing enterocolitis, and need for supplemental oxygen and ventilatory support (Fig. 17-2B). Further analysis of the results of one trial found that treatment with 17 α-hydroxyprogesterone caproate was especially efficacious in preventing recurrent preterm delivery for women whose prior preterm delivery occurred very early in gestation at 20–27 weeks (30).

The women enrolled in this study had unusually high rates of preterm birth. This could be explained in part by the fact that the mean gestational age of their previous preterm delivery was quite early, at 31 weeks of gestation. In addition, one third of the women had more than one previous spontaneous preterm delivery. Despite random allocation, more women in the placebo group had more than one preterm delivery. Adjustment of the analysis controlling for the imbalance found that the treatment effect remained significantly different from that of the placebo. A majority of the women were African American, and the treatment with 17 α-hydroxyprogesterone caproate showed equal efficacy in the African-American women and the non–African-American subjects.

Recently, two systematic reviews have evaluated the results of progesterone trials to prevent preterm birth (31, 32). The meta-analyses of these reviews included the Maternal–Fetal Medicine Units Network trial and the da Fonseca trial (3) as well as some earlier trials. Although the reviews differed as to which of the earlier trials were included, the results of the meta-analyses were similar in showing efficacy for progesterone treatment to prevent preterm delivery at less than 37 weeks of gestation, with odds ratios of approximately 0.5.

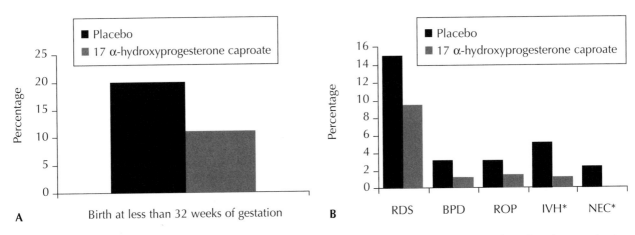

Fig. 17-2. Rates of births at less than 32 weeks of gestation (A) and rates of respiratory distress syndrome, bronchopulmonary dysplasia, retinopathy of prematurity, intraventricular hemorrhage, and necrotizing enterocolitis (B) in treatment (17 α-hydroxyprogesterone caproate) and placebo groups. *P <.05. Abbreviations: BPD, bronchopulmonary dysplasia; IVH, intraventricular hemorrhage; NEC, necrotizing enterocolitis; RDS, respiratory distress syndrome; ROP, retinopathy of prematurity. (Meis PJ, for the Society for Maternal–Fetal Medicine. 17 Hydroxyprogesterone for the Prevention of Preterm Delivery. Obstet Gynecol 2005;105:1128–1135.)

Safety Issues

The evidence for the safety of the use of 17 α-hydroxyprogesterone caproate in pregnancy consists of theoretical considerations, animal studies, and clinical studies. The substance 17 α-hydroxyprogesterone is a naturally occurring metabolite of progesterone. Progesterone and 17 α-hydroxyprogesterone are produced in large amounts in human pregnancy (33). The quantities produced in pregnancy, mainly by the placenta, exceed pharmacologic doses in clinical use. Additionally, 17 α-hydroxyprogesterone has no androgenic activity (34). It is not reasonable to expect ill effects of a nonandrogenic progestin, naturally found in large quantities, upon human gestation.

The effects of 17 α-hydroxyprogesterone caproate on pregnancy in experimental animals have been studied in rats, rabbits, mice, and monkeys (Macaca mulatta) (35–38). Results of these studies have shown no evidence of androgenic or glucocorticoid activity, no virilizing effects upon female fetuses, and no teratogenic effects.

Well-controlled clinical studies have been done to examine the safety of 17 α-hydroxyprogesterone caproate in human pregnancy. The outcome of 150 pregnancies in patients treated with 17 α-hydroxyprogesterone caproate because of threatened abortion was examined and compared with 150 patients who experienced early pregnancy bleeding but were not treated with the drug (39). No evidence was found that the drug had any adverse effect on the fetus or the outcome of the pregnancy. In a cohort study of 13,643 pregnancies in Germany, no increase was found in malformations in infants exposed in utero to 17 α-hydroxyprogesterone caproate, compared with controls (40). In 24,000 pregnancies delivered in Olmstead County, Minnesota, 1936–1974, the 649 offspring exposed to 17 α-hydroxyprogesterone caproate showed no increase in congenital anomalies or other ill effects compared with controls (41). In a follow-up study by questionnaire of 382 women treated with progestins during pregnancy, no increase in anomalies was found (42). In a comparison of 1,608 infants exposed to progestins in utero with 1,146 control infants, no difference was found in rates of all malformations (120/1,000 and 123.9/1,000, respectively) or in rates of major malformations (63.4/1,000 and 71.5/1,000, respectively) (43). In a comparison of 502 cases of hypospadias with 1,286 randomly selected male control children, a higher rate of exposure to progestogens in utero between 4 weeks and 14 weeks of gestation in the cases was found (OR, 3.7) (44). The type of progestational agent was not known for most of the exposed cases. In a study of a group of adolescent males who were exposed in utero to 17 α-hydroxyprogesterone caproate, a battery of psychologic tests performed on the subjects and on matched control subjects disclosed no significant differences between the groups in psychologic testing (45). Longer-term evaluations of any possible effects of in utero exposure to 17 α-hydroxyprogesterone caproate are in progress.

Several extensive reviews of the safety of the use of progestins in pregnancy have been published. In one review, it was found that "no justification (exists) for undue concern over the induction of nongenital malformations through hormone use in pregnancy" (46). The author found that, although some androgenic compounds have the potential for masculinization of the female fetus, progesterone and 17 α-hydroxyprogesterone caproate have no such potential. In a meta-analysis of 186 published articles, no association between first-trimester exposure to sex hormones and external genital malformations was shown (47). In the current REPROTOX17 computer database, supported by Micomedex, the review of 17 α-hydroxyprogesterone caproate concludes that "There is no available evidence that the administration of this agent (17 α-hydroxyprogesterone caproate) during pregnancy is harmful" (48). The safety of 17 α-hydroxyprogesterone caproate administration in pregnancy is well documented by animal and clinical studies. Knowledgeable authors have uniformly concluded that no evidence exists that administration of 17 α-hydroxyprogesterone caproate in pregnancy represents a significant risk to mother, fetus, or newborn. Although evidence of possible teratogenic effects of 17 α-hydroxyprogesterone caproate is slight, it would be prudent to withhold 17 α-hydroxyprogesterone caproate treatment for the prevention of preterm delivery until 16 weeks of gestation.

Choice of Drug

At present, the greatest body of evidence for efficacy in preventing preterm delivery in women at high risk exists for 17 α-hydroxyprogesterone caproate, with five reported successful trials of this compound (1, 2, 25, 49, 50). One trial of progesterone suppositories has found efficacy for this preparation (3). No other progestational drugs have been shown to have efficacy in randomized trials, but insufficient data are available for these other compounds. The dose of 17 α-hydroxyprogesterone caproate used in most of the reported trials has been 250 mg/wk. Little data exist from pharmacokinetic or pharmacotherapeutic studies to argue for or against this dosage. The rate of adverse effects from this drug or from the inert oil vehicle (castor oil) appears to be small, even with higher doses. One author (29) used 1,000 mg/wk of the drug and comparable volumes of the placebo oil, and another (51) used up to 2,000 mg of 17 α-hydroxyprogesterone caproate with no reported maternal or fetal adverse effects. Without doubt, new studies of the pharmacokinetic and pharmacotherapeutic characteristics of 17 α-hydroxyprogesterone caproate would be of significant value. At the time of this writing, 17 α-hydroxyprogesterone caproate is available in the United States only from compounding pharmacies. We anticipate that the U.S. Food and Drug Administration will approve its manufacture by pharmaceutical companies for the indication of preventing recurrent preterm birth.

Little information exists for the potential efficacy of oral progestational agents. The only drug submitted to a large prophylactic trial to prevent preterm delivery is medroxyprogesterone. This drug has been shown to have effective antiinflammatory and pregnancy-preserving properties in a rat model of uterine infection in pregnancy (52). However, in one clinical trial, no evidence of efficacy was found by intent-to-treat analysis (53). The possible reasons for the failure of prevention of preterm delivery in this trial include the fact that the subjects were at fairly low risk for preterm delivery, and the rate of compliance was very low.

Indications for Treatment

Currently, the patients who have been found to benefit from prophylactic treatment with progesterone to prevent preterm delivery are women at high risk for preterm delivery because of a history of a prior spontaneous preterm delivery caused by spontaneous preterm labor or preterm premature rupture of the fetal membranes. Treatment with progesterone for other high-risk conditions, such as multiple gestation or short uterine cervix, should not be encouraged outside of randomized trials. Several such trials are in progress or in development at the time of this writing. The only published trial of progesterone therapy for twin pregnancy failed to show efficacy, although this failure may have been related to the fact that therapy was started at 29 weeks of gestation or later (28).

Although 17 α-hydroxyprogesterone caproate treatment is effective in preventing recurrent preterm delivery in women at risk, this treatment can have only a modest impact on the rate of preterm birth in the general population (54). More trials are urgently needed to determine whether 17 α-hydroxyprogesterone caproate treatment is effective for women with other high-risk pregnancy conditions. In addition, improved methods of screening for risk and subsequent prophylactic treatment are needed for women in their first pregnancy.

The timing of initiation of progesterone therapy is likely to be important for its effectiveness. Successful trials have started treatment at no later than 24 weeks of gestation. It is reasonable to wait until 16 weeks of gestation to start treatment, and we recommend beginning as soon after this time as possible.

Four published trials have used a progestational drug for patients in preterm labor, and one trial, in an attempt to prolong pregnancy in patients close to term, used a progestational drug (55–59). Although the design of these trials and the drugs they used varied, none of these studies have demonstrated any efficacy in prolonging pregnancy. Thus, the use of progesterone as a tocolytic drug, or as an adjunct to tocolytic agents for patients in preterm labor, is to be discouraged outside of randomized trials. It is likely that, once the physiologic or pathologic processes that precede labor (such as the formation of gap junctions or activation of the inflammatory cascade) have occurred, treatment with progesterone is not effective in halting this process.

Summary

Evidence is sufficient for clinicians to choose to use progesterone therapy to prevent recurrent preterm delivery in women at risk. The greater body of evidence of efficacy at this time is for treatment of 17 α-hydroxyprogesterone caproate at 250 mg/wk beginning as soon as possible after 16 weeks of gestation and continuing to 36 weeks of gestation. The safety of the use of this drug has been clearly documented. Some evidence exists to support the use of daily progesterone suppositories. Further research will be necessary to support the use of progesterone for other high-risk conditions. In addition, further research is needed to elucidate the mechanism of action of 17 α-hydroxyprogesterone caproate and progesterone in preventing preterm labor and delivery.

References

1. Papiernik E. Double blind study of an agent to prevent pre-term delivery among women at increased risk. In: Edition Schering, Serie IV, fiche 3. 1970;65–8.

2. Meis PJ, Klebanoff M, Thom E, Dombrowski MP, Sibai B, Moawad AH, et al. Prevention of recurrent preterm delivery by 17 alpha-hydroxyprogesterone caproate [published erratum appears in N Engl J Med. 2003;349:1299]. N Engl J Med 2003;348:2379–85.

3. da Fonseca EB, Bittar RE, Carvalho MHB, Zugaib M. Prophylactic administration of progesterone by vaginal suppository to reduce the incidence of spontaneous preterm birth in women at increased risk: a randomized placebo-controlled double-blind study. Am J Obstet Gynecol 2003;188:419–24.

4. Paneth NS. The Problem of Low Birth Weight. Future Child 1995;5:19–34.

5. Mattison DR, Damus K, Fiore E, Petrini J, Alter C. Preterm delivery: a public health perspective. Paediatr Perinat Epidemiol 2001;15(suppl 2):7–16.

6. Agency of Heathcare Research and Quality. Overview of the HCUP Nationwide Inpatient Sample 2001. Available at: http://www.hcup-us.ahrq.gov/nisoverview.jsp. Retrieved March 2, 2005.

7. Gyetvai D, Hannah ME, Hodnett ED, Ohlsson A. Tocolytics for preterm labor: a systematic review. Obstet Gynecol 1999;94:869–77.

8. Harger JH. Cerclage and cervical insufficiency: an evidence-based analysis. Obstet Gynecol 2002;100:1313–27.

9. Carey JC, Klebanoff MA, Hauth JC, Hillier SL, Thom EA, Ernest JM, et al. Metronidazole to prevent preterm delivery in pregnant women with asymptomatic bacterial vaginosis. N Engl J Med 2000;342:534–40.

10. Klebanoff MA, Carey JC, Hauth JC, Hillier SL, Nugent RP, Thom EA, et al. Failure of metronidazole to prevent preterm delivery among pregnant women with asymptomatic *Trichomonas vaginalis* infection. N Engl J Med 2001;345:487–93.

11. Creasy RK. Preterm birth prevention: where are we? Am J Obstet Gynecol 1993;168:1223–30.

12. Rebar RW, Cedars MI. Hypergonadotropic forms of amenorrhea in young women. Endocrinol Metab Clin North Am 1992;21:173–91.

13. Stites DP, Siiteri PK. Steroids as immunosuppressants in pregnancy. Immunol Rev 1983;75:117–38.

14. Siiteri PK, Seron-Ferre M. Some new thoughts on the feto-placental unit and parturition in primates. In: Novy MJ, Reskko JA, editors. Fetal endocrinology. New York (NY): Academic Press; 1981. p. 1–34.

15. Garfield RE, Dannan MS, Daniel EE. Gap junction formation in myometrium: control by estrogens, progesterone, and prostaglandins. Am J Physiol 1980;238:C81–9.

16. Challis JRG. Sharp increase in free circulating oestrogens immediately before parturition in sheep. Nature 1971; 229:208.

17. Csapo AI. Progesterone block. Am J Anat 1956;98:273–91.

18. Cousins LM, Hobel CJ, Chang RJ, Okada DM, Marshall JR. Serum progesterone and estradiol-17b levels in premature and term labor. Am J Obstet Gynecol 1977;127: 612–5.

19. Johnson JWC, Lee PA, Zachary AS, Calhoun S, Migeon CJ. High-risk prematurity–progestin treatment and steroid studies. Obstet Gynecol 1979;54:412–8.

20. Mitchell B, Cruickshank B, McLain, Challis J. Local modulation of progesterone production in human fetal membranes. J Clin Endocrinol Metab 1982;55:1237–9.

21. Romero R, Scoccia B, Mazor M, Wu YK, Benveniste R. Evidence for a local change in the progesterone/estrogen ratio in human parturition at term. Am J Obstet Gynecol 1988;159:657–60.

22. Frydman R, LeLaidier C, Baton-Saint-Mleux C, Fernandez H, Vial M, Bourget P. Labor induction in women at term with mifepristone (RU 486): a double-blind, randomized, placebo-controlled study. Obstet Gynecol 1992;80:972–5.

23. LeLaidier C, Baton C, Benifla JL, Fernandez H, Bourget P, Frydman R. Mifepristone for labour induction after previ-

ous caesarean section. Br J Obstet Gynaecol 1994;101: 501–3.

24. Chwalisz K, Fahrenholz F, Hackenbery M, Hackenberg M, Garfield R, Elger W. The progesterone antagonist onapristone increases the effectiveness of oxytocin to produce delivery without changing the myometrial oxytocin receptor concentrations. Am J Obstet Gynecol 1991;165:1760–70.

25. Johnson JWC, Austin KL, Jones GS, Davis GH, King TM. Efficacy of 17alpha-hydroxyprogesterone caproate in the prevention of premature labor. N Engl J Med 1975;293: 675–80.

26. Goldstein P, Berrier J, Rosen S, Sacks HS, Chalmers TC. A meta-analysis of randomized control trials of progestational agents in pregnancy. Br J Obstet Gynaecol 1989; 96:265–74.

27. Keirse MJNC. Progesterone administration in pregnancy may prevent preterm delivery. Br J Obstet Gynaecol 1990;97:149–54.

28. Hartikainen-Sorri AL, Kauppila A, Tuimala R. Inefficacy of 17 alpha hydroxyprogesterone caproate in the prevention of prematurity in twin pregnancy. Obstet Gynecol 1980;56:692–5.

29. Hauth JC, Gilstrap LC 3rd, Brekken AL, Hauth JM. The effect of 17 alpha-hydroxyprogesterone caproate on pregnancy outcome in an active-duty military population. Am J Obstet Gynecol 1983;146:187–90.

30. Spong CY, Meis PJ, Thom EA et al. Progesterone for the prevention of recurrent preterm birth: impact of gestational age at previous delivery. Am J Obstet Gynecol 2005;193:1127–31.

31. Dodd J, Flenady V, Cincotta R, and Crowther C. Prenatal administration of progesterone for preventing preterm birth. Cochrane Database Syst Rev. 2006 Jan 25;(1) CD004947

32. Sanchez-Ramos L, Kaunitz AM, and Delke I. Progestational agents to prevent preterm birth: A meta-analysis of randomized controlled trials. Obstet Gynecol 2005;105: 273–9

33. Tulchinsky D, Simmer H. Sources of plasma 17alpha-hydroxyprogesterone in human pregnancy. J Clin Endocrinol Metab 1972;35:799–808.

34. Kessler W, Borman A. Some biological activities of certain progestogens.I. 17 alpha-hydroxyprogesterone 17-n-caproate. Ann N Y Acad Sci 1958;71:486–93.

35. Johnstone EE, Franklin RR. Assay of progestins for fetal virilizing properties using the mouse. Obstet Gynecol 1964;23:359–62.

36. Courtney KD, Valerio DA. Teratology in the Macaca mulatta. Teratology 1968;1:163–72.

37. Carbone JP, Brent RL. Genital and nongenital teratogenesis of prenatal progesterone therapy: the effects of 17 alpha-hydroxyprogesterone caproate on embryonic and fetal development and endochondral ossification in the C57B1/6L mouse. Am J Obstet Gynecol 1993;169:1292–8.

38. See miller RE, Nelson GW, Johnson CK. Evaluation of teratogenic potential of Delalutin, (17 alpha-hydroxyprogesterone caproate) in mice. Teratology 1983;28:201–8.

39. Varma T, Morsman J. Evaluation of the use of Proluton-Depot (hydroxyprogesterone hexonate) in early pregnancy. Int J Gnyaecol Obstet 1982;20:13–7.

40. Michaelis J, Michaelis H, Gluck E, Keller S. Prospective studies of suspected association between certain drugs administered in early pregnancy and congenital malformations. Teratology 1983;27:57–64.

41. Resseguie LJ, Hick JF, Bruen JA, Noller KL, O'Fallon WM, Kurland LT. Congenital malformations among offspring exposed in utero to progestins, Olmstead County, Minnesota 1936-1974. Fertil Steril 1985;43:514–9.

42. Check JH, Rankin A, Teichman M. The risk of fetal anomalies as a result of progesterone therapy during pregnancy. Fertil Steril 1986;45:575–7.

43. Katz Z, Lancet M, Skornik J, Chemke J, Mogilner BM, Klinberg M. Teratogenicity of progestogens given during the first trimester of pregnancy. Obstet Gynecol 1985;65: 775–80.

44. Carmichael SL, Shaw GM, Laurent C et al. Maternal progestin intake and risk of hypospadias. Arch Pediatr Adolesc Med 2005;159:957–962.

45. Kester PA. Effects of prenatally administered 17 alpha-hydroxyprogesterone caproate in adolescent males. Arch Sex Behav 1984;13:441–55.

46. Schardein JL. Congenital abnormalities and hormones during pregnancy: a clinical review. Teratology 1980;22: 251–70.

47. Raman-Wilms L, Tseng AL, Wighardt S, Einarson TR, Koren G. Fetal genital effects of first-trimester sex hormone exposure: a meta-analysis. Obstet Gynecol 1995;85:141–9.

48. REPROTOX 1997 Healthcare Series. Vol 92. Greenwood Village (CO): Micromedex Inc; 1997.

49. LeVine L. Habitual abortion: a controlled clinical study of pregestational therapy. West J Surg Obstet Gynecol 1964; 72:30–6.

50. Yemini M, Borenstein R, Dreazen E, Apelman Z, Mogilner BM, Kessler I, et al. Prevention of premature labor by 17 alpha-hydroxyprogesterone caproate. Am J Obstet Gynecol 1985;151:574–7.

51. Sherman AI. Hormonal therapy for control of the incompetent os of pregnancy. Obstet Gynecol 1966;28:198–205.

52. Elovitz M, Wang Z. Medroxyprogesterone acetate, but not progesterone, protects against inflammation-induced parturition and intrauterine fetal demise. Am J Obstet Gynecol 2004;190:693–701.

53. Hobel CJ, Ross MG, Bemis RL, Bragonier JR, Nessim S, Sandhu M, et al. The West Los Angeles Preterm Birth Prevention Project. I. Program impact on high-risk women. Am J Obstet Gynecol 1994;170:54–62.

54. Petrini JR, Callaghan WM, Klebanoff M, Green NS, Lackritz EM, Howse JL, et al. Estimated effect of 17 alpha-hydroxyprogesterone caproate on preterm birth in the United States. Obstet Gynecol 2005;105:267–72.

55. Fuchs F, Stakemann G. Treatment of threatened premature labor with large doses of progesterone. Am J Obstet Gynecol 1960;79:172–6.

56. Kauppila A, Hartikainen-Sorri AL, Janne O, Tuimala R, Jarvinen PA. Suppression of threatened premature labor by administration of cortisol and 17 alpha-hydroxyprogesterone caproate: a comparison with ritodrine. Am J Obstet Gynecol 1980;138:404–8.

57. Erny R, Pigne A, Prouvost C, Gamerre M, Malet C, Serment H, et al. The effects of oral administration of progesterone for premature labor. Am J Obstet Gynecol 1986;154:525–9.

58. Noblot G, Audra P, Dargent D, Faguer B, Mellier G, et al. The use of micronized progesterone in the treatment of menace of preterm delivery. Eur J Obstet Gynecol Reprod Biol 1991;40:203–9.

59. Brenner WE, Hendricks CH. Effect of medroxyprogesterone acetate upon the duration and characteristics of human gestation and labor. Am J Obstet Gynecol 1962;83: 1094–8.

CHAPTER 18

Management of Rh Alloimmunization in Pregnancy

Kenneth J. Moise Jr

With the dawn of the new millennium, medical science has made little impact on the major complications of pregnancy. The one notable exception is rhesus alloimmunization and its associated fetal–neonatal consequence—hemolytic disease of the fetus/newborn. In the early 1960s, the first successful in utero therapy was described. Later that decade, an effective method of prevention, rhesus immunoglobulin, was studied and introduced into clinical practice. By the end of the second millennium, new refinements in genetics and ultrasonography had further advanced the care of what was once a major perinatal disease.

Incidence

Although effective prophylaxis has been available since 1968, the now Centers for Disease Control and Prevention noted in 1991 that one in every 1,000 live-born infants exhibited some effect from rhesus hemolytic disease (1). Although not considered as reliable a source of data, a 2003 review of U.S. birth certificates indicated that 6.8 pregnancies per 1,000 live births were complicated by rhesus sensitization (2).

Pathophysiology

Several investigators have reported that spontaneous fetomaternal hemorrhages occur with increasing frequency and volume with advancing gestational age. Using a sensitive Kleihauer–Betke test, 0.01 mL of fetal cells have been noted in 3%, 12%, and 46% of women in each of the three successive trimesters (3). In most cases, the antigenic load of RhD antigen on the fetal erythrocytes and erythrocytic precursors is insufficient to stimulate the maternal immune system. However, in the case of a large antenatal fetomaternal hemorrhage or a fetomaternal hemorrhage at delivery, maternal B lymphocyte clones that recognize the RhD antigen are established. The initial maternal immunoglobulin (Ig)M anti-D production is short lived with a rapid change to an IgG response. Memory B lymphocytes then await a new anti-

genic exposure in the subsequent pregnancy. If stimulated by the RhD antigen on fetal erythrocytes, these plasma cells can rapidly proliferate and produce IgG antibodies and an increase in the maternal titer. Maternal IgG crosses the placenta and destroys any RhD-positive erythrocytes, resulting in fetal anemia.

Prevention of Rh Disease

Four different RhIg products are now available in the United States. Two (RhoGAM and BayRho-D) are processed by Cohn cold ethanol fractionation, which results in some contamination with IgA antibodies and other plasma proteins. These products must therefore be given by intramuscular injection. The two available RhIg preparations (Rhophlac and WinRho-SDF) are prepared by Sepharose column and ion-exchange chromatography, respectively. The resulting products contain only IgG and, therefore, administration can either be by the intravenous or intramuscular route. All available products undergo solvent detergent treatment to inactivate enveloped viruses; many manufacturers have added micropore filtration as an additional step to further reduce the chance for viral transmission. Thimerosal, a mercury-based preservative once found in all RhIg products, is no longer included in the manufacturing process.

Although once produced from the plasma of sensitized women, the decreasing prevalence of Rh disease has necessitated that the plasma source for RhIg be derived from RhD-negative male donors that undergo repeated injections of RhD-positive red cells. Several monoclonal anti-D antibodies are now being studied in clinical trials and may soon replace the current plasma-derived polyclonal products (4, 5). Because RhIg is a blood derivative, all patients should be informed of its source and give informed consent for its use. Although most RhIg is issued from hospital blood banks, various manufacturers' products can be purchased by private physicians for use in their offices. A recall by one manufacturer in the late 1990s because of inadequate doses in the prefilled syringes warrants that careful records of lot numbers be

225

documented in the patient's medical chart and a general clinic logbook. All pregnant patients should undergo antibody screening at the first prenatal visit. Patients that are determined to be weak Rh-positive (previously Du-positive) are not at risk for Rh alloimmunization and, therefore, do not require RhIg. If there is no evidence of anti-D alloimmunization in the RhD-negative woman, 300 mcg of RhIg should be administered intramuscularly at 28 weeks of gestation. This practice has been reported to reduce the incidence of antenatal alloimmunization from 2% to 0.1% (6). The American Association of Blood Banks recommends that a repeat antibody screen be obtained before antenatal RhIg is administered, although the incidence of alloimmunization before 28 weeks of gestation is very low. The cost-effectiveness of this practice has been questioned by the American College of Obstetricians and Gynecologists (7). Maternal sensitization occasionally does occur by 28 weeks of gestation, and by not screening for the antibody, the clinician loses the opportunity of detecting the hemolytic disease. It would therefore appear prudent to repeat the antibody screening. The maternal blood sample can be drawn and the RhIg injection can be given at the same office visit. Although the administration of the exogenous anti-D antibodies will eventually result in a weakly positive titer, this will not occur in the short interval of several hours because of the slow absorption from the intramuscular site. Although there are no data to provide guidance, some experts recommend that a second dose of RhIg be given if delivery has not occurred by 40 weeks of gestation.

Although not well studied, additional indications for the antepartum administration of RhIg include spontaneous abortion, elective abortion, ectopic pregnancy, genetic amniocentesis, chorion villous sampling, and fetal blood sampling. A dose of 50 mcg of RhIg is effective until 12 weeks of gestation because of the small volume of red cells in the fetoplacental circulation. From a practical sense, most hospitals and offices do not stock this dose of RhIg; therefore, a standard dose of 300 mcg is often given. Evidence for the use of RhIg in other scenarios that breach the fetoplacental barrier is lacking. Such events as hydatidiform mole, threatened abortion, fetal death in the second or third trimester, blunt trauma to the abdomen, and external cephalic version also require administration of RhIg.

Because the half life of RhIg is approximately 24 days, 15–20% of patients receiving it at 28 weeks of gestation will have a very low anti-D titer (usually 2 or 4) detected at the time of admission for labor at term (7). If umbilical cord blood typing reveals an RhD-positive infant, 300 mcg of RhIg should be administered within 72 hours of delivery. This amount is sufficient to protect

from sensitization caused by a fetomaternal hemorrhage of 30 mL of fetal whole blood. Approximately 1 in 1,000 deliveries will be associated with an excessive fetomaternal hemorrhage; only 50% of these deliveries will be identified on the basis of risk factors. Routine screening of all women at the time of delivery for excessive fetomaternal hemorrhage should therefore be undertaken. A qualitative yet sensitive test for fetomaternal hemorrhage, the rosette test, is first performed. Results return as positive or negative. A negative result warrants administration of a standard dose of RhIg. If the rosette test results are positive, a Kleihauer–Betke test or fetal cell stain using flow cytometry is undertaken. The percentage of fetal blood cells is multiplied by a factor of 50 to estimate the volume of the fetomaternal hemorrhage. Because this calculation includes an inaccurate estimation of the maternal blood volume, the blood bank will typically indicate that additional vials of RhIg should be administered over the calculated amount. No more than five units of RhIg should be administered by the intramuscular route in one 24-hour period. This recommendation is based on the number and volume of injections that are required to administer this amount of RhIg using prefilled syringes. Should a large dose of RhIg be necessary, an alternative method would be to give the entire calculated dose intravenously in divided increments (maximum dose for each increment: 3,000 international units or 600 mcg) every 8 hours. If RhIg is inadvertently omitted after delivery, some protection has been shown with administration within 13 days; recommendations have been made to administer it as late as 28 days after delivery (8). If delivery occurs less than 3 weeks from the administration of RhIg used for antenatal indications, such as amniocentesis for fetal lung maturity or external cephalic version, a repeat dose is unnecessary unless a large fetomaternal hemorrhage is detected at the time of delivery. Despite the widespread acceptance of similar guidelines, studies from Scotland have revealed that two thirds of rhesus alloimmunized cases are secondary to antepartum sensitization, whereas an additional 13% are caused by failure to administer RhIg for the usual obstetric indications (9).

If a patient is undergoing initial blood typing at delivery and a weak Rh-positive result (formerly Du positive) is obtained, this result may be secondary to a large fetomaternal hemorrhage causing a mixed field agglutination reaction and a false interpretation of the maternal blood type. A standard test for fetomaternal hemorrhage should be performed. If none is detected, then the weak rhesus-positive typing can be considered valid, and RhIg is not required. The administration of RhIg after a postpartum tubal ligation is controversial. The possibility of a new partner in conjunction with the availability of in vitro fertilization would seem to make the use of RhIg in these situations prudent. In addition, RhD sensitization would limit the availability of blood products if the patient later required a transfusion. RhIg is not effective once alloimmunization to the RhD antigen has occurred.

Diagnostic Approach

Genetics

In 1946, the concept of three genes that encode for the three major rhesus antigen groups—D, C/c, and E/e—was proposed (8). Some 45 years later, the Rh locus was localized to the short arm of chromosome one (10). Only two genes were identified—an RhD gene and an RhCE gene. Production of two distinct proteins from the latter gene probably occurs as a result of alternative messenger RNA splicing. A single C to G transition in exon 5 of the RhCE gene results in formation of the e antigen instead of the E antigen (11). One nucleotide difference (cytosine to thymine) in exon 2 of the RhCE gene results in a single amino acid change of a serine to proline. This causes the expression of the C antigen as opposed to the c antigen (12). These discoveries have resulted in major changes in the management of the RhD-sensitized pregnancy. In the case of a heterozygous father, amniocentesis can be used to detect the RhD-negative fetuses that will be noted in 50% of cases. In such situations, additional maternal or fetal testing is unwarranted because the maternal antibody will not affect the fetus. Because the RhC/c and E/e antigens are inherited in a closely linked fashion to RhD, blood banks can employ antisera to these antigens along with gene frequency tables based on ethnicity to determine the paternal zygosity at the RhD locus. In addition, mathematic modeling has been proposed to modify the incidence of heterozygosity based on the paternal history of RhD-positive offspring

(13). As an example, a white partner who undergoes serologic testing with the following results—anti-D, positive; anti-C, negative; anti-c, positive; anti-E, negative; and anti-e, positive—would be considered Dce. If he had never fathered an RhD-positive child in the past, his chance of being heterozygous is 94% (Table 18-1). A history of previous RhD-positive offspring would decrease his chances of being heterozygous. Note that very different results for the same serologic findings cited in the above example occur if the male patient is not white. In the future, paternal zygosity testing will not use serology but instead will use quantitative polymerase chain reaction (PCR) performed on genomic DNA extracted from white blood cells (14).

First described in 1993, amniocentesis is now accepted as the primary modality that is used in the United States to test the fetal blood type in cases of a heterozygous paternal genotype (15). Chorion villus biopsy has been employed, but this practice should be discouraged in patients who wish to continue the pregnancy if the fetus is found to be RhD positive. Disruption of the chorionic villi during the procedure can result in fetomaternal hemorrhage and an anamnestic response in maternal titer, thereby worsening the fetal disease. When amniocentesis is used for fetal typing, all attempts should be made to avoid transplacental passage of the needle to prevent this same phenomenon from occurring.

One must understand that these techniques assess the fetal genotype (DNA analysis of fetal cells in the amniotic fluid) and not the fetal phenotype (expression of the RhD antigen on the fetal red cells as determined by serology). Ultrasound-guided umbilical blood sampling can be used for serologic typing of the fetus but is associated with a fourfold or more rate of perinatal loss compared with amniocentesis. Extensive experience with the use of amniocentesis for determining the fetal blood type

Table 18-1. Percentage of Paternal Heterozygosity Based Ethnic Background, Number of Previous Rhesus D-Positive Offspring, and Blood Type

Number of RhD-positive infants	White						Black						Hispanic					
	0	1	2	3	4	5	0	1	2	3	4	5	0	1	2	3	4	5
Blood type																		
DCce	90	82	69	53	36	22	41	26	15	8	4	2	85	74	59	42	26	15
DCe	9	5	2	1	0.6	0.3	19	11	6	3	1	0.7	5	2	1	0.6	0.3	0.1
DCEe	90	82	69	53	36	22	37	23	13	7	4	2	85	74	59	42	26	15
DcE	13	7	4	2	0.9	0.5	1	0.5	0.3	0.1	0.1	0	2	0.9	0.5	0.2	0.1	0.1
DCcEe	11	6	3	2	0.8	0.4	10	5	1	0.7	0.3	12	6	3	2	0.8	0.4	
Dce	94	89	80	66	50	33	54	37	23	13	7	4	92	85	74	59	42	26

Moise KJ, Jr. Management of Rhesus Alloimmunization in Pregnancy. Obstet Gynecol 2002;100:600–11.

has revealed rare discrepancies between fetal genotype and phenotype. In the event of a PCR result that reveals an RhD-negative fetus when the fetus is RhD positive by serology, usual surveillance techniques would not be employed, and fetal loss can occur. In a review of reports of 500 amniocenteses in which four different sets of oligonucleotide primers were used, this occurred in 1.5% of cases (16). The overall sensitivity and specificity of PCR typing were 98.7% and 100%, respectively, and the positive and negative predictive values were 100% and 96.9% (16). The most likely cause for inconsistencies is either erroneous paternity or a rearrangement of the paternal RhD gene locus. Such rearrangements have been documented in approximately 2% of individuals (17). Checking paternal blood (the source of the fetal RhD gene) with the same primers used on the amniotic fluid verifies that a gene rearrangement is not a potential source of error. For this reason, most laboratories offering fetal red cell antigen typing on amniotic fluid cells require an accompanying paternal blood sample. In one study of serial titers in patients with RhD alloimmunization who subsequently delivered RhD-negative offspring, serial maternal titers rose by fourfold in less than 2% of cases (18). Therefore, if paternity is unknown or the patient's partner is not available, a repeat maternal antibody titer should be obtained 4–6 weeks later as a confirmatory strategy. If a fourfold increase in antibody titer is noted, then an RhD-negative PCR result on amniotic fluid is suspect. Repeat amniocentesis to evaluate the Δ optical density $(OD)_{450}$ or fetal blood sampling to determine the fetal RhD status using serologic techniques should be considered.

An RhD pseudogene has been described in 69% of South African blacks and 21% of African Americans (19). In this situation, the pregnant patient is RhD negative on serologic testing, but the entire RhD gene is present on her chromosomes. Because the fetus inherits one of its RhD genes from its mother, amniotic PCR testing would, therefore, yield a false-positive result—the fetus is RhD-negative by serology but RhD-positive by genotype. This could lead to unnecessary intervention with its inherent risks. For this reason, a maternal blood sample also should accompany the amniotic fluid sent for fetal RhD testing in an effort to rule out the presence of a maternal RhD pseudogene. If the maternal sample is positive for this variant, then fetal testing for the gene also should be undertaken (Fig. 18-1).

Free fetal DNA can be found in maternal plasma in the first trimester of pregnancy. Apoptosis of placental trophoblasts, either in situ or once they enter the maternal circulation, is the likely source. For this reason, free fetal DNA is cleared rapidly after delivery. Since the first report of the use of free fetal DNA to determine the fetal RhD status (20), numerous series have been published

that indicate a 94–100% accuracy in determining the RhD status of the fetus (21, 22). The assay is routinely used in clinical practice in England and Europe, although it is not yet available in the United States.

Maternal Titer

The maternal titer is the first step in the evaluation of the RhD-sensitized patient. Old methodologies using albumin or saline should no longer be employed. The human antiglobulin titer (indirect Coombs) is used to determine the degree of alloimmunization. By convention, titer values are reported as the integer of the greatest tube dilution with a positive agglutination reaction (ie, a titer of 16 is equivalent to a dilution of 1:16). Variation in results between laboratories is not uncommon because many commercial laboratories use enhancing media to avoid missing low titer samples. However, in the same laboratory, the titer should not vary by more than one dilution. Thus, an initial titer of 8 that returns 16 may not represent a true increase in the amount of antibody in the maternal circulation. A critical titer is defined as the titer associated with a significant risk for fetal hydrops. When this finding is present, further testing is required with more invasive techniques. This titer will vary with institutions based on the correlation with clinical outcome of hemolytic disease of the newborn; however, in most centers, a critical value for anti-D antibodies between 8 and 32 is used.

In Europe and the United Kingdom, the amount of circulating anti-D antibodies is compared with an international standard and reported in international units per milliliter. A threshold value of 15 international units/mL has been recommended for invasive testing because only mild hemolytic disease of the newborn is usually noted at lower anti-D levels (23).

Ultrasonography

Ultrasonography plays a key role in the management of the alloimmunized pregnancy. It should be used early in the pregnancy to establish the correct gestational age because this parameter becomes important in determining such normative laboratory values as amniotic fluid bilirubin levels (ΔOD_{450}). A variety of ultrasound parameters have been used in an attempt to determine when fetal anemia is present. These have included placental thickness, umbilical vein diameter, hepatic length, splenic perimeter, and polyhydramnios (24). Most of these parameters have not proved to be reliable in clinical practice. Fetal hydrops can be detected and usually is heralded by the onset of ascites. Late findings include pleural effusions and scalp edema. Hydrops fetalis should be considered end-stage hemolytic disease because the fetal hemoglobin is often one third of normal or less in

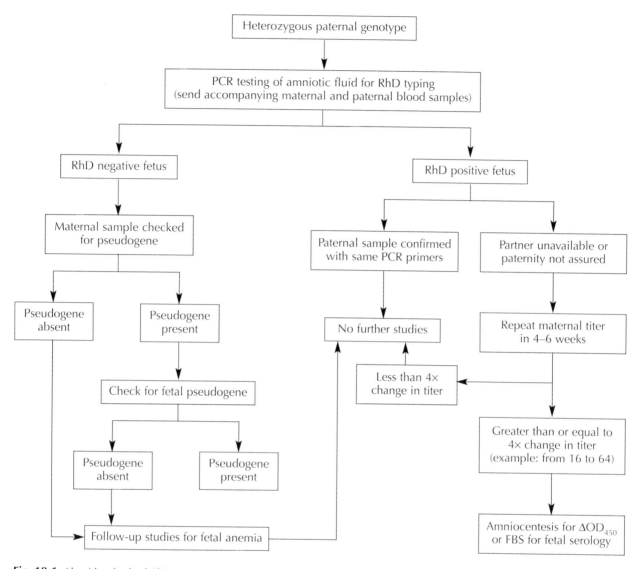

Fig. 18-1. Algorithm for fetal RhD testing in the case of a heterozygous paternal phenotype. Abbreviations: FBS, fetal blood sampling; OD optical density; PCR, polymerase chain reaction. (Moise KJ, Jr. Management of Rhesus Alloimmunization in Pregnancy. Obstet Gynecol 2002;100:600–11.)

these situations. In the first study to propose that Doppler ultrasound assessment of the peak velocity in the fetal middle cerebral artery could accurately determine if the fetus was anemic (25), a value above 1.5 multiples of the median (MoM) for gestational age detected all cases of moderate to severe anemia with a false-positive rate of only 12% (Fig. 18-2). In a more recent study, middle cerebral artery Doppler ultrasonography was compared with amniocentesis for ΔOD_{450} in 165 fetuses at risk for hemolytic disease of the fetus/newborn in 10 centers (26). The positive and negative predictive rates for severe anemia were 80% and 89%, respectively, and those for amniocentesis were 73% and 80%, respectively.

Technically, the determination of the peak middle cerebral artery velocity is relatively straightforward. The

anterior wing of the sphenoid bone at the base of the skull is located; color or power Doppler ultrasonography is then used to locate the middle cerebral artery vessel. The angle of insonation is maintained as close to zero as possible by positioning the ultrasound transducer on the maternal abdomen. The middle cerebral artery vessel closer to the maternal abdominal wall is usually studied, although the posterior vessel will give equivalent results (27). Angle correction software is not employed. The Doppler ultrasound gate is then placed in the proximal middle cerebral artery as the vessel arises from the carotid siphon. Measurements in the more distal aspect of the vessel will be inaccurate because reduced peak velocities will be obtained (27). The fetus should be in a quiescent state during the Doppler ultrasound exam-

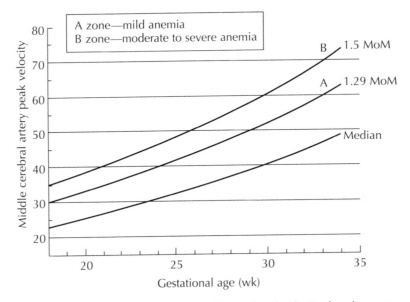

Fig. 18-2. Middle cerebral artery Doppler ultrasound peak velocities based on gestational age. Abbreviation: MoM, multiples of the median. (Moise KJ, Jr. Management of rhesus alloimmunization in pregnancy. Obstet Gynecol 2002;100:600–11.)

ination as accelerations of the fetal heart rate can result in a false elevation in the peak velocity, especially late in the third trimester (28). Measurements can be initiated as early as 18 weeks of gestation and should be repeated at 1–2 week intervals depending on the rate of increase in the values after three weekly values have been obtained (29).

After 35 weeks of gestation, there appears to be a higher false-positive rate in the detection of fetal anemia (30). Therefore, late in gestation, a normal middle cerebral artery velocity can be monitored with repeat measurements. If an elevated value is noted, amniocentesis for ΔOD_{450} and fetal lung maturity test should be undertaken to determine if delivery is indicated. Because a learning curve is associated with performing middle cerebral artery Doppler ultrasonography, a center with minimal experience with this technique initially should perform these assessments in conjunction with serial amniocenteses for ΔOD_{450} (31). In addition, serial amniocenteses may prove useful if a perinatal center with staff skilled in middle cerebral artery Doppler ultrasonography is not within geographic proximity.

Amniocentesis

Since it was first introduced to clinical practice by Liley (32) in 1961, the spectral analysis of amniotic fluid at 450 nm (ΔOD_{450}) has been used to measure the level of bilirubin, an indirect indicator of the degree of fetal hemolysis. The original Liley curve was divided into three zones and remains useful after 27 weeks of gestation. Extrapolation of Liley curves to earlier gestational ages underestimates the level of fetal disease and thus

should not be used. A modified curve for such gestations has been proposed by Queenan et al and involves four zones instead of three (Fig. 18-3) (33). A comparative study found this curve to be more predictive for fetal anemia compared with Liley's curve (26). If amniocentesis is used to monitor fetal disease, serial procedures are undertaken at 10-day to 2-week intervals and continued until delivery to follow trends in the ΔOD_{450} values. As mentioned earlier, all attempts should be made to avoid transplacental passage of the needle because this can lead to fetomaternal hemorrhage and an increase in maternal antibody titer. An increasing or plateauing trend of ΔOD_{450} values that reaches the intrauterine transfusion zone of the Queenan curve necessitates investigation by fetal blood sampling. After 37 weeks of gestation, fetal lung maturity testing can be assessed; in the presence of studies that confirm maturity, induction of labor can be considered in lieu of subsequent amniocentesis.

Fetal Blood Sampling

Ultrasound-directed fetal blood sampling (also percutaneous umbilical blood sampling, cordocentesis, and funipuncture) allows direct access to the fetal circulation to obtain important laboratory values such as hematocrit level, direct Coombs' test result, fetal blood type, reticulocyte count, and total bilirubin level. Serial fetal blood samplings have been proposed as one method of following alloimmunized pregnancies after a maternal critical titer is reached. However, because this procedure is associated with a 1–2% rate of fetal loss, it usually is reserved for patients with elevated ΔOD_{450} values or elevated peak

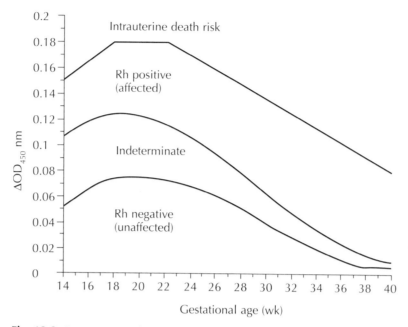

Fig. 18-3. Queenan curve for D optical density$_{450}$ values. Abbreviation: OD, optical density. (Reprinted from Queenan JT, Tomai TP, Ural SH, King JC. Deviation in amniotic fluid optical density at a wavelength of 450 nm in Rh-immunized pregnancies from 14 to 40 weeks' gestation: A proposal for clinical management. Am J Obstet Gynecol 1993;168:1370–6. Copyright © 1993, with permission from Elsevier.)

middle cerebral artery Doppler ultrasound velocities. When used in this context, blood should be available for intravascular intrauterine transfusion if fetal anemia is detected (hematocrit level less than 30% or less than two standard deviations for gestational age).

Clinical Management

The use of available diagnostic tools varies based on the history of fetal or neonatal hemolytic disease (Figs. 18-4, 18-5). As a general rule, the patient's first RhD-sensitized pregnancy involves minimal fetal or neonatal disease; subsequent gestations are associated with a worsening degree of anemia. The rarity of this condition warrants consideration of consultation or referral to a maternal–fetal medicine specialist.

First Affected Pregnancy

Once sensitization to the RhD antigen is detected, assessments of maternal titers are repeated every month until approximately 24 weeks of gestation and thereafter repeated every 2 weeks. Paternal blood is drawn to determine RhD status and zygosity. In cases of a heterozygous paternal phenotype, once a critical titer is reached (usually 32), an amniotic fluid sample along with maternal and paternal blood samples are sent to a DNA reference laboratory at the time of amniocentesis to determine the fetal RhD status. In the case of an RhD-negative paternal

blood type or fetal RhD-negative genotype at amniocentesis, further maternal and fetal monitoring is unwarranted as long as paternity is assured.

If there is evidence of an RhD-positive fetus (homozygous paternal phenotype, or RhD-positive fetus by PCR testing of amniotic fluid), serial middle cerebral artery Doppler ultrasonography is undertaken at 1–2 week intervals. In addition, antenatal testing (nonstress test or biophysical profile) should be initiated after 32 weeks of gestation. If the middle cerebral artery values remain less than or equal to 1.5 MoM, induction of labor should be considered by 37–38 weeks of gestation. If a value greater than 1.5 MoM is noted after 35 weeks of gestation, amniocentesis should be performed to assess ΔOD_{450} values and fetal lung maturity. If pulmonary maturity is noted and the ΔOD_{450} value is not in the upper Rh-positive-affected zone or the intrauterine transfusion zone of the Queenan curve, induction should be considered in 2 weeks to allow fetal hepatic maturity to occur. This will decrease the need for prolonged neonatal bililight therapy or exchange transfusion.

If the results of amniocentesis indicate fetal pulmonary immaturity in conjunction with a ΔOD_{450} value below the upper Rh-positive-affected zone, consideration should be given to repeat amniocentesis in 10 days to 2 weeks. If serial amniocenteses are used to assess the fetal status, the procedures are repeated at 10-day to 2-week intervals. In the case of an increasing or plateau-

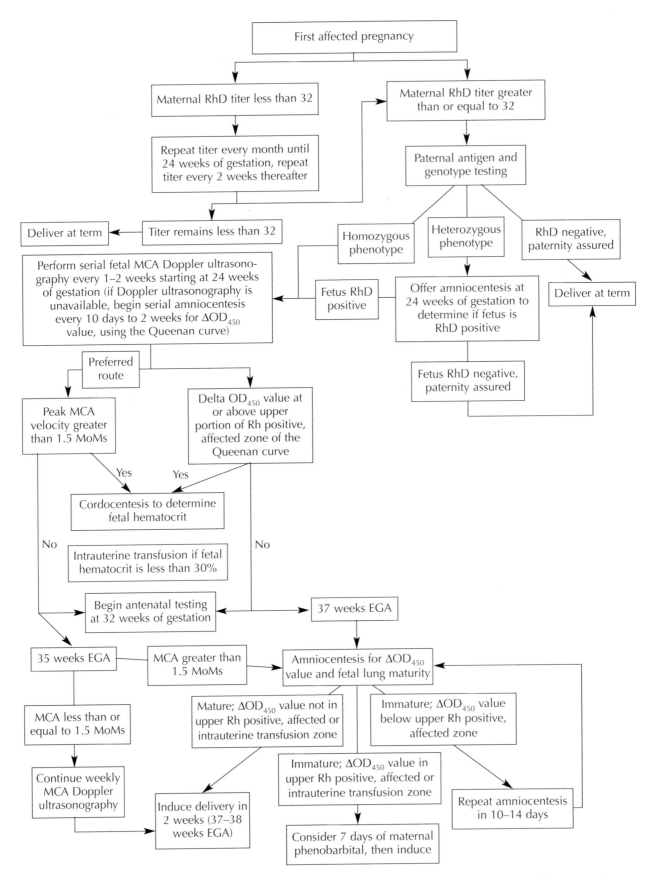

Fig. 18-4. Algorithm for the clinical management of the first RhD alloimmunized pregnancy. Abbreviations: EGA, estimated gestational age; MCA, middle cerebral artery; MoM, multiples of the median; OD, optical density.

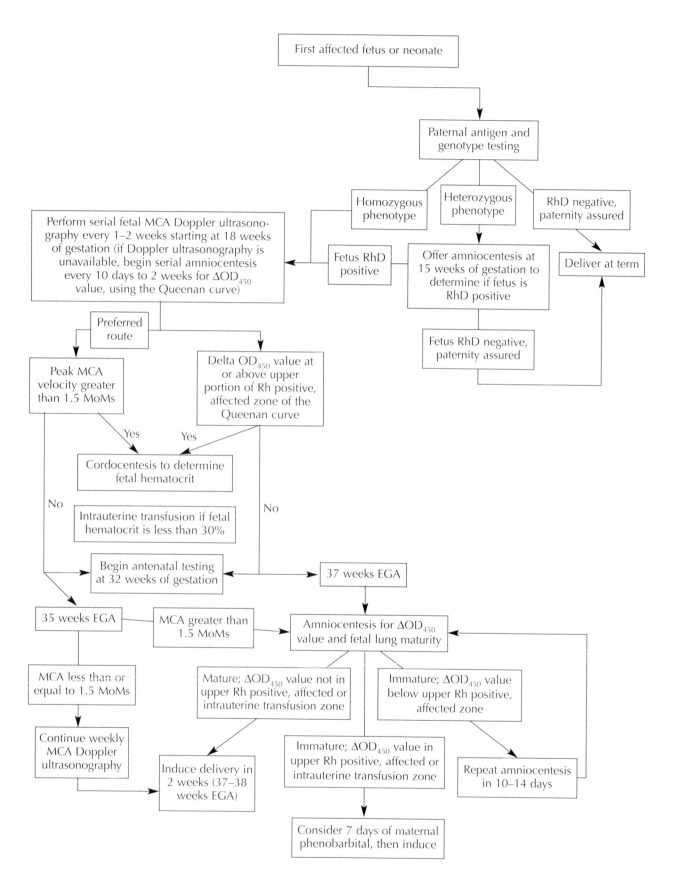

Fig. 18-5. Algorithm for the clinical management of RhD alloimmunized pregnancy with a history of a previously affected fetus or neonate. Abbreviations: EGA, estimated gestational age; MCA, middle cerebral artery; MoM, multiples of the median; OD, optical density.

ing ΔOD_{450} values trend into the intrauterine transfusion zone of the Queenan curve, fetal blood sampling is undertaken with blood readied for intrauterine transfusion if the fetal hematocrit level is less than 30%. If no increase in the ΔOD_{450} values is detected, the last amniocentesis should be performed at 37 weeks of gestation. If testing indicates fetal lung maturity, induction at 38–39 weeks of gestation would appear warranted in lieu of additional amnioceteses.

Previously Affected Fetus or Infant

If there is a history of a previous perinatal loss related to hemolytic disease of the fetus/newborn, a previous need for intrauterine transfusion, or a previous need for neonatal exchange transfusion, the patient should be referred to a perinatal center with experience in the management of the severely alloimmunized pregnancy. In these cases, maternal titers are not predictive of the degree of fetal anemia. In the case of a heterozygous paternal phenotype, amniocentesis should be performed at 15 weeks of gestation to determine the fetal RhD status. Most centers are now using serial middle cerebral artery Doppler ultrasound measurements to monitor these pregnancies at risk for fetal hemolytic disease. Testing should begin at 18 weeks of gestation and be repeated every 1–2 weeks. Alternatively, if expertise in middle cerebral artery Doppler ultrasonography is not available, serial amnioceteses for measurement of ΔOD_{450} can be used with the Queenan curve for reference values. If a peak middle cerebral artery Doppler ultrasound velocity greater than 1.5 MoM or an increasing ΔOD_{450} value into the intrauterine transfusion zone of the Queenan curve is found, fetal blood sampling is performed with blood readied for intrauterine transfusion if the fetal hematocrit level is found to be less than 30%.

Therapeutic Approach

Intrauterine Transfusion

Historically, intraperitoneal transfusion was the mainstay of fetal therapy for almost 20 years after its introduction by Liley in 1963 (34). With the advent of real-time ultrasonography for guidance, direct access to the fetal circulation by puncturing the umbilical cord at its placental insertion became commonplace. As a result, direct intravascular transfusion has replaced the intraperitoneal transfusion in most centers. Compared with intraperitoneal transfusion, intravascular transfusion is clearly advantageous to the hydropic fetus in which absorption of cells from the peritoneal cavity is compromised. Some centers continue to incorporate the intraperitoneal transfusion in conjunction with the intravascular transfusion; many European centers prefer to use the intrahepatic portion of the umbilical vein as the site of intravascular transfusion.

The source of red cells for intrauterine transfusion is typically a blood type O, RhD-negative, cytomegalovirus-negative donor. Cells are packed to a hematocrit of 75–85% to prevent volume overload. Units are irradiated to prevent graft-versus-host reaction and processed through a leukocyte-poor filter. Some centers prefer to use maternal blood as the source of red cells (35). Advantages include the potential to decrease the risk for sensitization to new red cell antigens associated with exposure to donor units. In addition, a fresh unit can be routinely acquired. Repeated maternal donations are possible with additional folate and iron supplementation. Such donations produce a maternal reticulocytosis that enhances the average life-span of the donor red cells. This practice can potentially decrease the total number of intravascular transfusions that are necessary. Patients must still undergo rigorous U.S. Food and Drug Administration testing for infectious markers with each donation. In addition, washing of the cells is required to remove any maternal serum containing anti-D antibodies.

At the start of the intravascular transfusion procedure, an initial fetal hematocrit level is determined after puncture of the umbilical cord near the placental insertion. A paralyzing agent is usually administered to cause cessation of fetal movement, although this may be omitted in cases of anterior placentation. Our center uses vecuronium at a dose of 0.1 mg/kg of estimated fetal weight. The total amount of red cells to transfuse will depend on the initial fetal hematocrit level, gestational age, and hematocrit level of the donor unit. If the donor unit has a hematocrit level of approximately 75%, the estimated fetal weight in grams using ultrasonography can be multiplied by a factor of 0.02 to determine the volume of red cells to be transfused to achieve a hematocrit increment of 10% (36). A final target hematocrit level of 40–50% is used; a decrease of approximately 1% per day can be anticipated between transfusions. In the extremely anemic fetus, the initial hematocrit level should not be increased by more than fourfold to allow the fetal cardiovascular system to compensate for the acute change in viscosity (37). A repeat procedure is undertaken 48 hours later to normalize the fetal hematocrit level in cases of severe fetal anemia. Hydrops will usually reverse rapidly after one or two intravascular transfusions; placentomegaly is the last feature of the hydropic state to reverse. If the fetus is not severely anemic at the first intrauterine transfusion, subsequent procedures are scheduled at 14-day intervals until suppression of fetal erythropoiesis is noted on Kleihauer–Betke test results. This usually occurs by the third intrauterine transfusion. Thereafter, the interval for repeat procedures can be determined based on the decrease in the hematocrit level for the individual fetus, usually a 3–4 week interval. The middle cerebral artery peak systolic velocity may be used to time the second intrauterine transfusion (38). A modified threshold of 1.32 MoM (instead of 1.5 MoM) should be used to detect moderate-to-severe anemia. After the second transfusion, the timing of subsequent transfusions cannot be accurately determined using the middle cerebral artery Doppler ultrasonography. This may be because of the rheology of the transfused red cells that replace most of the fetal red cell population.

During the era of intraperitoneal transfusions, fetuses were routinely delivered at 32 weeks of gestation and often suffered complications of prematurity such as hyaline membrane disease and the need for neonatal exchange transfusions for the treatment of hyperbilirubinemia. As experience with intravascular transfusion became widespread, delivery was done at later gestational ages. Most authorities will now perform the final intrauterine transfusion at up to 35 weeks of gestation, with delivery anticipated at 37–38 weeks of gestation (39). Such a practice allows maturation of both the pulmonary and hepatic enzyme systems, virtually eliminating the need for neonatal exchange transfusions. After a viable gestational age is attained, performing the transfusion in immediate proximity to the labor and delivery suite appears prudent so that operative delivery can be undertaken if fetal distress should occur. The administration of oral phenobarbital to the mother may be considered 7–10 days before delivery. This practice has been proposed to induce hepatic maturity and allow for improved conjugation of bilirubin. One retrospective study has demonstrated a reduction in the need for neonatal exchange transfusions for hyperbilirubinemia (40).

Short-Term Outcome

Perinatal survival after intrauterine transfusion varies by center and the experience of the operator. Clearly, intervention before the appearance of hydrops fetalis is preferable. In one review series, the overall survival rate was noted to be 84% (41). The survival rate of nonhydropic fetuses (92%) was markedly improved over those with hydrops (70%). Suppression of erythropoiesis is not uncommon after several intravascular transfusions. These infants are born with a virtual absence of reticulocytes, with their blood volume being almost entirely comprised of donor red cells. Because exchange transfusion is rarely required, passively acquired maternal antibodies remain in the neonatal circulation for weeks. As a result, the infant may need several top-up red cell transfusions for a 1–3 month period. (42). Neonatal hemat-

ocrit and reticulocyte counts should be assessed weekly. Threshold hematocrit values of less than 30% in the symptomatic infant or less than 20% in the asymptomatic infant have been suggested for transfusion. A neonatal trial with subcutaneous erythropoietin, administered three times per week, revealed a decreased need for top-up transfusions (43).

Long-Term Outcome

Advances in treatment techniques of the fetus with severe hemolytic disease of the fetus/newborn now allow more moribund and severely anemic fetuses to survive. Several investigations have not found hydrops fetalis to be associated with any difference in neurologic outcome compared with the nonhydropic fetus (44). Cerebral palsy and developmental delay is more common in fetuses with hemolytic disease of the fetus/newborn when compared with unaffected infants, although a normal outcome can be expected in more than 90% of cases (45). A review of the cases of cerebral palsy reveals that the mean gestational age at delivery was 33.5 weeks; 80% of cases underwent emergency cesarean delivery. Sensorineural hearing loss is more frequent in infants affected by hemolytic disease of the fetus/newborn, probably because of their prolonged exposure to elevated levels of bilirubin and its toxic effect on the developing eighth cranial nerve (44).

Future Treatment

Clearly, selective maternal immunomodulation is the most promising next breakthrough for the treatment of severe hemolytic disease of the fetus/newborn. Purposeful immunization to paternal leukocytes exhibits a protective effect in the prevention of fetal anemia in a rabbit model (46). Investigation in a transgenic mouse model has indicated that the intranasal administration of specific RhD epitope peptides could be used to ameliorate an established anti-D response, thereby preventing severe hemolytic disease of the fetus or newborn in a subsequent pregnancy (47).

Summary

Great advances in the treatment of red cell sensitization have markedly diminished perinatal loss. Despite this diminished loss, an estimated 200 fetuses die each year in the United States, secondary to hemolytic disease of the fetus/newborn or the complications of treatment (25, 41). Free fetal DNA testing and serial middle cerebral artery Doppler ultrasonography have now replaced amniocentesis in the identification of the fetus at risk for hemolytic disease. In the future, maternal immunotherapy may supplant intrauterine transfusion.

References

1. Chavez GF, Mulinare J, Edmonds LD. Epidemiology of Rh hemolytic disease of the newborn in the United States. JAMA 1991;265:3270–4.

2. Martin JA, Hamilton BE, Sutton PD, Ventura SJ, Menacker F, Munson ML. Births: final data for 2003. National Vital Statistics Reports 2003;54:1–116.

3. Bowman JM, Pollock JM, Penston LE. Fetomaternal transplacental hemorrhage during pregnancy and after delivery. Vox Sang 1986;51:117–21.

4. Kumpel BM. Monoclonal anti-D development programme. Transpl Immunol 2002;10:199–204.

5. Bichler J, Spycher MO, Amstutz HP, Andresen I, Gaede K, Miescher S. Pharmacokinetics and safety of recombinant anti-RhD in healthy RhD-negative male volunteers. Transfus Med 2004;14:165–71.

6. Bowman JM. The prevention of Rh immunization. Transfus Med Rev 1988;2:129–50.

7. American College of Obstetricians and Gynecologists. Prevention of RhD alloimmunization. ACOG Practice Bulletin 4. Washington, DC: ACOG;1999.

8. Bowman JM. Controversies in Rh prophylaxis. Who needs Rh immune globulin and when should it be given? Am J Obstet Gynecol 1985;151:289–94.

9. Hughes RG, Craig JI, Murphy WG, Greer IA. Causes and clinical consequences of Rhesus (D) haemolytic disease of the newborn: a study of a Scottish population, 1985-1990. Br J Obstet Gynaecol 1994;101:297–300.

10. Cherif-Zahar B, Mattei MG, Le Van Kim C, Bailly P, Cartron JP, Colin Y. Localization of the human Rh blood group gene structure to chromosome region 1p34.3–1p36.1 by in situ hybridization. Hum Genet 1991;86:398–400.

11. Carritt B, Kemp TJ, Poulter M. Evolution of the human RH (rhesus) blood group genes: a 50 year old prediction (partially) fulfilled. Hum Mol Genet 1997;6:843–50.

12. Avent ND. Fetal genotyping. In: Hadley A, Soothill P, editors. Alloimmune disorders in pregnancy anaemia, thrombocytopenia, and neutropenia in the fetus and newborn. Cambridge: Cambridge University Press; 2002.

13. Kanter MH. Derivation of new mathematic formulas for determining whether a D-positive father is heterozygous or homozygous for the D antigen. Am J Obstet Gynecol 1992;166:61–3.

14. Chiu RW, Murphy MF, Fidler C, Zee BC, Wainscoat JS, Lo YM. Determination of RhD zygosity: comparison of a double amplification refractory mutation system approach and a multiplex real-time quantitative PCR approach. Clin Chem 2001;47:667–72.

15. Bennett PR, Le Van Kim C, Colin Y, Warwick RM, Cherif-Zahar B, Fisk NM, et al. Prenatal determination of fetal RhD type by DNA amplification. N Engl J Med 1993;329:607–10.

16. Van den Veyver IB, Moise KJ, Jr. Fetal RhD typing by polymerase chain reaction in pregnancies complicated by rhesus alloimmunization. Obstet Gynecol 1996;88:1061–7.

17. Simsek S, Faas BH, Bleeker PM, Overbeeke MA, Cuijpers HT, van der Schoot CE, et al. Rapid Rh D genotyping by polymerase chain reaction-based amplification of DNA. Blood 1995;85:2975–80.

18. Hopkins DF. Maternal anti-Rh(D) and the D-negative fetus. Am J Obstet Gynecol 1970;108:268–71.

19. Singleton BK, Green CA, Avent ND, Martin PG, Smart E, Daka A, et al. The presence of an RHD pseudogene containing a 37 base pair duplication and a nonsense mutation in africans with the Rh D-negative blood group phenotype. Blood 2000;95:12–8.

20. Lo YM. Fetal RhD genotyping from maternal plasma. Ann Med 1999;31:308–12.

21. Gautier E, Benachi A, Giovangrandi Y, Ernault P, Olivi M, Gaillon T, et al. Fetal RhD genotyping by maternal serum analysis: a two-year experience. Am J Obstet Gynecol 2005;192(3):666–9.

22. Zhou L, Thorson JA, Nugent C, Davenport RD, Butch SH, Judd WJ. Noninvasive prenatal RHD genotyping by real-time polymerase chain reaction using plasma from D-negative pregnant women. Am J Obstet Gynecol 2005;193:1966–71.

23. Nicolaides KH, Rodeck CH. Maternal serum anti-D antibody concentration and assessment of rhesus isoimmunisation. BMJ 1992;304:1155–6.

24. Whitecar PW, Moise KJ, Jr. Sonographic methods to detect fetal anemia in red blood cell alloimmunization. Obstet Gynecol Surv 2000;55:240–50.

25. Mari G, for the Collaborative Group for Doppler Assessment of the Blood Velocity in Anemic Fetuses. Noninvasive diagnosis by Doppler ultrasonography of fetal anemia due to maternal red-cell alloimmunization. N Engl J Med 2000;342:9–14.

26. Oepkes D, Seaward PG, Vandenbussche FP, Windrim R, Kingdom J, Beyene J, et al. Doppler ultrasonography versus amniocentesis to predict fetal anemia. N Eng J Med 2006;355(2):156–64.

27. Abel DE, Grambow SC, Brancazio LR, Hertzberg BS. Ultrasound assessment of the fetal middle cerebral artery peak systolic velocity: A comparison of the near-field versus far-field vessel. Am J Obstet Gynecol 2003;189:986–9.

28. Sallout BI, Fung KF, Wen SW, Medd LM, Walker MC. The effect of fetal behavioral states on middle cerebral artery peak systolic velocity. Am J Obstet Gynecol 2004;191:1283–7.

29. Detti L, Mari G, Akiyama M, Cosmi E, Moise KJ, Jr., Stefor T, et al. Longitudinal assessment of the middle cerebral artery peak systolic velocity in healthy fetuses and in fetuses at risk for anemia. Am J Obstet Gynecol 2002;187:937–9.

30. Zimmerman R, Carpenter RJ, Jr., Durig P, Mari G. Longitudinal measurement of peak systolic velocity in the fetal middle cerebral artery for monitoring pregnancies complicated by red cell alloimmunisation: a prospective multicentre trial with intention-to- treat. BJOG 2002;109:746–52.

31. Mari G. Middle cerebral artery peak systolic velocity: is it the standard of care for the diagnosis of fetal anemia? J Ultrasound Med 2005;24:697–702.

32. Liley AW. Liquor amnii analysis in the management of pregnancy complicated by rhesus sensitization. Am J Obstet Gynecol 1961;82:1359–70.

33. Queenan JT, Tomai TP, Ural SH, King JC. Deviation in amniotic fluid optical density at a wavelength of 450 nm in Rh-immunized pregnancies from 14 to 40 weeks' gesta-

tion: a proposal for clinical management. Am J Obstet Gynecol 1993;168:1370–6.

34. Liley AW. Intrauterine transfusion of foetus in haemolytic disease. BMJ 1963;2:1107–9.

35. Gonsoulin WJ, Moise KJ, Jr., Milam JD, Sala JD, Weber VW, Carpenter RJ, Jr. Serial maternal blood donations for intrauterine transfusion. Obstet Gynecol 1990;75:158–62.

36. Giannina G, Moise KJ, Jr., Dorman K. A simple method to estimate the volume for fetal intravascular transfusion. Fetal Diagn Ther 1998;13:94–7.

37. Radunovic N, Lockwood CJ, Alvarez M, Plecas D, Chitkara U, Berkowitz RL. The severely anemic and hydropic isoimmune fetus: changes in fetal hematocrit associated with intrauterine death. Obstet Gynecol 1992; 79:390–3.

38. Detti L, Oz U, Guney I, Ferguson JE, Bahado-Singh RO, Mari G. Doppler ultrasound velocimetry for timing the second intrauterine transfusion in fetuses with anemia from red cell alloimmunization. Am J Obstet Gynecol 2001;185:1048–51.

39. Klumper FJ, van Kamp IL, Vandenbussche FP, Meerman RH, Oepkes D, Scherjon SA, et al. Benefits and risks of fetal red-cell transfusion after 32 weeks gestation. Eur J Obstet Gynecol Reprod Biol 2000;92:91–6.

40. Trevett TN, Jr., Dorman K, Lamvu G, Moise KJ, Jr. Antenatal maternal administration of phenobarbital for the prevention of exchange transfusion in neonates with hemolytic disease of the fetus and newborn. Am J Obstet Gynecol 2005;192:478–82.

41. Schumacher B, Moise KJ, Jr. Fetal transfusion for red blood cell alloimmunization in pregnancy. Obstet Gynecol 1996;88:137–50.

42. Saade GR, Moise KJ, Belfort MA, Hesketh DE, Carpenter RJ. Fetal and neonatal hematologic parameters in red cell alloimmunization: predicting the need for late neonatal transfusions. Fetal Diagn Ther 1993;8:161–4.

43. Ovali F, Samanci N, Dagoglu T. Management of late anemia in Rhesus hemolytic disease: use of recombinant human erythropoietin (a pilot study). Pediatr Res 1996; 39:831–4.

44. Hudon L, Moise KJ, Jr., Hegemier SE, Hill RM, Moise AA, Smith EO, et al. Long-term neurodevelopmental outcome after intrauterine transfusion for the treatment of fetal hemolytic disease. Am J Obstet Gynecol 1998;179: 858–63.

45. Moise KJ, Whitecar PW. Antenatal therapy for haemolytic disease of the fetus and newborn. In: Hadley A, Soothill P, editors. Alloimmune disorders in pregnancy: anaemia, thrombocytopenia and neutropenia in the fetus and newborn. Cambridge: Cambridge University Press; 2002.

46. Whitecar PW, Farb R, Subramanyam L, Dorman K, Balu RB, Moise KJ, Jr. Paternal leukocyte alloimmunization as a treatment for hemolytic disease of the newborn in a rabbit model. Am J Obstet Gynecol 2002;187:977–80.

47. Hall AM, Cairns LS, Altmann DM, Barker RN, Urbaniak SJ. Immune responses and tolerance to the RhD blood group protein in HLA-transgenic mice. Blood 2005;105: 2175–9.

CHAPTER 19

Placenta Previa, Placenta Accreta, and Vasa Previa

YINKA OYELESE AND JOHN C. SMULIAN

Placenta Previa

The term placenta previa refers to a placenta that overlies or is proximate to the internal os of the cervix. The placenta normally implants in the upper uterine segment. In placenta previa, the placenta either totally or partially lies within the lower uterine segment. Traditionally, placenta previa has been categorized into four types (Fig. 19-1):

1. Complete placenta previa—the placenta completely covers the internal os.
2. Partial placenta previa—the placenta partially covers the internal os. Thus, this scenario occurs only when the internal os is dilated to some degree.
3. Marginal placenta previa—the placenta just reaches the internal os, but does not cover it.
4. Low-lying placenta—the placenta extends into the lower uterine segment but does not reach the internal os.

Clinical Importance

Morbidities associated with placenta previa include antepartum bleeding (relative risk [RR], 9.81, 95% confidence interval [CI], 8.92–10.79), need for hysterectomy (RR, 33.26, 95% CI, 18.19–60.89), morbid adherence of the placenta, intrapartum hemorrhage (RR, 2.48, 95% CI, 1.55–3.98), postpartum hemorrhage (RR, 1.86, 95% CI, 1.46–2.36), blood transfusion (RR, 10.05, 95% CI, 7.45–13.55), septicemia (RR, 5.5, 95% CI, 1.31–23.54), and thrombophlebitis (RR, 4.85, 95% CI, 1.50–15.69) (1). In the United States, maternal mortality occurs in 0.03% of cases of placenta previa (2). Women with placenta previa may suffer considerable emotional distress because of recurrent bleeding along with hospitalizations that frequently occur in the second half of pregnancy. Placenta previa also is associated with an increase in preterm birth and perinatal mortality and morbidity (3). There is a higher rate of congenital malformations among women with placenta previa, although the precise mechanisms for these are unclear (3).

Incidence and Risk Factors

Placenta previa complicates approximately 0.3–0.5% of pregnancies (2). A U.S. population-based study for the years 1979–1987 found the overall annual incidence of placenta previa to be 4.8 per 1,000 deliveries (0.48%) (2). In several studies, it has been found that risk factors for

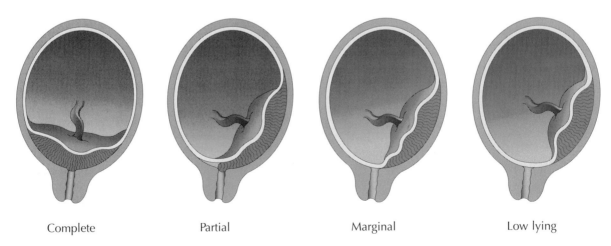

| Complete | Partial | Marginal | Low lying |

Fig. 19-1. Types of placenta previa. (Oyelese Y, Smulian JC. Placenta previa, placenta accreta, and vasa previa. Obstet Gynecol 2006;107:927–941.)

placenta previa include a history of prior cesarean delivery, termination of pregnancy or uterine surgery, smoking, increased age, multiparity, cocaine use, and multiple pregnancy (4–9). The likelihood of placenta previa increases in a dose-response fashion with a greater number of prior cesarean deliveries and with greater parity, from RR 4.5, 95% CI, 3.6–5.5 in women with one prior cesarean delivery to RR 44.9, 95% CI, 13.5–149.5 in women with four prior cesarean deliveries (7).

Pathophysiology

It is unclear why some placentas implant in the lower uterine segment rather than in the fundus (10). It does appear that uterine scarring may predispose to placental implantation in the lower segment. With the progression of pregnancy, more than 90% of these low-lying placentas identified early in pregnancy will appear to move away from the cervix and out of the lower uterine segment. Although the term "placental migration" has been used, most authorities do not believe the placenta moves (10). Rather, it is believed that the placenta grows preferentially toward a better-vascularized fundus (trophotropism), whereas the placenta overlying the less well-vascularized cervix may undergo atrophy (10). In some cases, this atrophy leaves vessels running through the membranes, unsupported by placental tissue or cord (vasa previa) (10). In cases in which the atrophy is incomplete, a succenturiate lobe may develop. The apparent movement of the placenta also may be caused by the development of the lower uterine segment. Contractions and cervical effacement and dilations that occur in the third trimester cause separation of the placenta, which leads to small amounts of bleeding. This bleeding may stimulate further uterine contractions that, in turn, stimulate further placental separation and bleeding. Rarely is this type of initial bleeding a major problem, although it may be a reason for hospitalization. In labor, as the cervix dilates and effaces, there is usually placental separation and unavoidable bleeding.

Diagnostic Approach

The classic clinical presentation of placenta previa is painless bleeding in the late second trimester or early third trimester. However, some patients with placenta previa will experience painful bleeding, possibly the consequence of uterine contractions or placental separation, whereas others will experience no bleeding at all before labor. Placenta previa also may lead to an unstable lie or malpresentation in late pregnancy.

Most cases of placenta previa are diagnosed during routine ultrasonography in asymptomatic women, usually during the second trimester. Although transabdominal ultrasonography frequently is used for placental location, this technique lacks some precision in diagnosing placenta previa (11–12). In numerous studies, the accuracy of transvaginal ultrasonography for the diagnosis of placenta previa has been demonstrated, uniformly finding that transvaginal ultrasonography is superior to transabdominal ultrasonography for this indication (Fig. 19-2) (11–12). False-positive and false-negative rates for the diagnosis of placenta previa using transabdominal ultrasonography range from 2% to 25% (11). In one study of 131 women believed to have a placenta previa because of results of transabdominal ultrasonography it was found that anatomic landmarks crucial for accurate diagnosis were poorly recognized in 50% of the cases (11). In 26% of the cases of suspected placenta previa, the initial diagnosis was changed because it was incorrect, based on the results of transvaginal ultrasonography.

The superiority of transvaginal ultrasonography over transabdominal ultrasonography can be attributed to several factors:

1. The transabdominal approach requires bladder filling, which results in approximation of the anterior and posterior walls of the lower uterine segment, with the result that a normally situated placenta may falsely appear to be a placenta previa.
2. Vaginal probes are closer to the region of interest, typically of higher frequency, and therefore obtain higher resolution images than transabdominal probes.
3. The internal cervical os and the lower placental edge frequently cannot be imaged adequately by the transabdominal approach. The position of the internal os is assumed rather than seen.
4. The fetal head may obscure views of the lower placental edge when using the transabdominal approach, and a posterior placenta previa may not be adequately imaged.

The improved accuracy of transvaginal ultrasonography over transabdominal ultrasonography means that fewer false-positive diagnoses are made; thus, the rate of placenta previa is significantly lower when using transvaginal ultrasonography than when using transabdominal ultrasonography (11–13). In one study, during routine transvaginal ultrasonography, an incidence of placenta previa of only 1.1% was found at 15–20 weeks of gestation, considerably lower than the incidence of second trimester placenta previa of 15–20% reported by previous investigators using transabdominal ultrasonography (13–14). In numerous studies the safety of transvaginal ultrasonography for the diagnosis of placenta previa has been demonstrated (12–15). There are two main reasons why this imaging technique does not lead

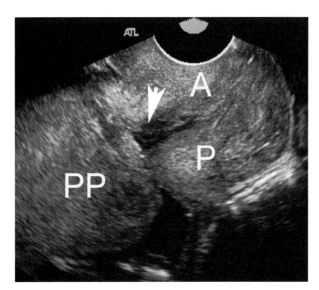

Fig. 19-2. Transvaginal ultrasonogram of a complete placenta previa. Abbreviations: A, anterior lip of cervix; P, posterior lip of cervix; PP, placenta previa. (Oyelese Y, Smulian JC. Placenta previa, placenta accreta, and vasa previa. Obstet Gynecol 2006; 107:927–941.)

to an increase in bleeding (15): 1) the vaginal probe is introduced at an angle that places it against the anterior fornix and anterior lip of the cervix, unlike a digital examination, during which articulation of the hand allows introduction of the examining finger through the cervix (Fig. 19-3) (15); and 2) the optimal distance for visualization of the cervix is 2–3 cm from the cervix, so the probe is generally not advanced sufficiently to make contact with the placenta (15). Nonetheless, the examination should be performed by personnel experienced in transvaginal ultrasonography, and the transvaginal probe should always be inserted carefully, with the examiner looking at the monitor to avoid putting the probe in the cervix.

Translabial ultrasonography has been suggested as an alternative to transvaginal ultrasonography and has been shown to be superior to transabdominal ultrasonography for placental location (16). However, because transvaginal ultrasonography is accurate, safe, and well tolerated, it should be the imaging mode of choice.

In several studies, it has been demonstrated that the majority of placentas that are in the lower uterine segment in the second trimester will no longer be in the region of the cervix by the time of delivery (Table 19-1) (13, 17–21). Persistence to term can be predicted based on whether the placenta overlaps the internal os in the second trimester and to what extent (13, 17–21). The later in pregnancy that placenta previa is diagnosed, the higher the likelihood of persistence to delivery (22). Women who at 20 weeks of gestation have a low-lying

placenta that does not overlie the internal os will not have a placenta previa at term and need no further ultrasound examinations for placental location. However, the presence of a low-lying placenta in the second trimester is a risk factor for developing a vasa previa, and, in these cases, ultrasonography should be performed later in pregnancy to exclude that condition.

Management

In the past, suspected placenta previa was managed by vaginal examination and immediate cesarean delivery if placenta previa was confirmed. It was believed that the first bleed (usually occurring in the early third trimester) would lead to maternal death. However, in one study it was shown that, in the absence of interference, this almost never happened and that the high perinatal mortality from placenta previa was primarily caused by prematurity, which could be reduced considerably by conservative expectant management and delivery as close to term as possible (23).

Women who present with bleeding in the second half of pregnancy should have an ultrasound examination (preferably by the transvaginal approach) for placental location before any attempt to perform a digital examination. Digital vaginal examination with a placenta previa may provoke catastrophic hemorrhage and should not be performed.

It is reasonable to hospitalize women with placenta previa while they are having an acute bleeding episode or uterine contractions. One to two wide-bore intravenous cannulas should be inserted and blood taken for a full blood count and type test and for screening. In the absence of massive bleeding or other complications, coagulation studies are not helpful. The blood bank must be capable of making available at least four units of compatible packed red blood cells and coagulation factors at short notice. Rh immune globulin should be administered to Rh-negative women. A Kleihauer-Betke test for quantification of fetal–maternal transfusion also should be performed in Rh-negative women because the mother may require increased doses of Rh immune globulin.

In small studies a benefit of tocolytic therapy has been suggested for women with placenta previa who are having contractions (24–25). Contractions may lead to cervical effacement and changes in the lower uterine segment, provoking bleeding that, in turn, stimulates contractions, creating a vicious cycle. In one small randomized study using the β-adrenergic ritodrine, a significant prolongation in pregnancy and higher birth weights were found in women treated with ritodrine compared with women treated with placebo (24). One retrospective study reported that use of intravenous magnesium sulfate or oral or subcutaneous terbutaline

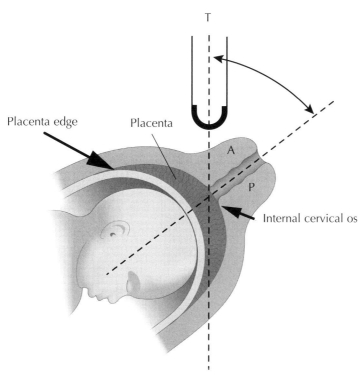

Fig. 19-3. Diagram demonstrating the technique for transvaginal ultrasonography of placenta previa. Abbreviations: A, anterior lip of cervix; P, posterior lip of cervix; T, transvaginal transducer. (Oyelese Y, Smulian JC. Placenta previa, placenta accreta, and vasa previa. Obstet Gynecol 2006;107:927–941.)

Table 19-1. Studies of Second Trimester Transvaginal Ultrasonography in the Prediction of Placenta Previa at Delivery.

Author	Gestational Age at Ultrasonography (wk)	Number of Women	Incidence of Placenta Previa at First- or Second- Trimester Ultrasonography (n [%])	Incidence at Delivery (n [%])
Becker (17)	20–23	8,650	99 (1.1)	28 (0.32)
Taipale (21)	18–23	3,969	57 (1.5)	5 (0.14)
Hill (19)	9–13	1,252	77 (6.2)	4 (0.31)
Mustafa (20)	20–24	203	8 (3.9)	4 (1.9)
Lauria (13)	15–20	2,910	36 (1.2)	5 (0.17)
Rosati (18)	10–16	2,158	105 (4.9)	8 (0.37)

Oyelese Y, Smulian JC. Placenta previa, placenta accreta, and vasa previa. Obstet Gynecol 2006;107:927–941.

in women with symptomatic placenta previa was associated with greater prolongation of pregnancy and higher birth weight than in women who were not treated with tocolytics (25). Thus, cautious use of tocolytics in women with placenta previa who are having contractions, when both mother and fetus are stable, appears reasonable.

Steroids should be administered in women between 24 weeks and 34 weeks of gestation, generally at the time of admission for bleeding, to promote fetal lung maturation. The patient and her family should have a neonatology consultation so that the treatment of the infant after birth may be discussed. In women who have a history of cesarean delivery or uterine surgery, a detailed ultrasonography should be performed to exclude placenta accreta. Because prematurity is the main cause of perinatal mortality associated with placenta previa, it is desirable to prolong gestation as long as safely possible.

Therefore, before 32 weeks of gestation, moderate-to-severe bleeding when there is no maternal or fetal compromise may be managed aggressively with blood transfusions, rather than resorting to delivery (26). When the patient has had no further bleeding for 48 hours, she may be considered for discharge as long as there are appropriate home conditions to allow outpatient management. Specifically, the patient should have access to a telephone, have a responsible adult and transportation available at all times, and live within a reasonable distance from a hospital. She should return to the hospital immediately if she experiences bleeding or contractions. Although there are no data to support the efficacy of avoidance of intercourse and excessive activity, common sense suggests that these should be avoided. Similarly, bedrest is often advised, but there is no evidence that this practice is beneficial.

Outpatient Versus Inpatient Management

Whether women with placenta previa should be treated as inpatients or outpatients has been a matter of controversy. A few retrospective studies have addressed this issue and have found no difference in outcomes, whether patients received care in the hospital or at home, and found that outpatient management may be associated with lower costs (27–28). These studies concluded that outpatient management of selected women with placenta previa was safe. However, in another retrospective study, an increase in the rate of perinatal mortality, lower gestational age at delivery, increased neonatal hospitalization duration, and neonatal morbidity among women who were treated as outpatients was found when compared with those treated expectantly as inpatients (29). In one of the few prospective randomized studies dealing with placenta previa, 53 women with placenta previa at gestational ages between 24 weeks and 36 weeks, who had been initially stabilized in hospital, were randomized to inpatient or outpatient management, and no significant difference in outcomes was found (30). Thus, women who are stable and asymptomatic and who are reliable and have quick access to a hospital may be considered for outpatient management.

Cerclage

In one study 25 women who were admitted to the hospital with symptomatic placenta previa at 24–30 weeks of gestation were randomized to cerclage or no cerclage and found a higher mean birth weight and gestational age at delivery and fewer neonatal complications in the cerclage group (31). Women with cerclage had lower hospitalization costs and fewer bleeding episodes. However, in a later study, 39 women with placenta previa at 24–30 weeks of gestation were randomized to cerclage or no cerclage and no statistically significant differences in gestational age at delivery, prolongation of pregnancy, or amount of blood lost were found between the two groups (32). In view of the lack of convincing data to support cerclage in these women, cerclage should not be performed for treatment of placenta previa.

Mode of Delivery

There is consensus that a placenta previa that totally or partially overlies the internal cervical os requires cesarean delivery. However, the mode of delivery when the placenta lies in proximity to the internal os is more controversial. In three small retrospective studies using transvaginal or translabial ultrasonography the role of ultrasonography in determining the optimal mode of delivery for women whose placentas were in proximity to the internal cervical os was evaluated (33–35). In all 3 studies it was found that women in whom the distance between the lower placental edge and the internal cervical os was greater than 2 cm could safely have a vaginal delivery. Conversely, among women with a placenta–internal os distance less than 2 cm, most required cesarean delivery, usually for bleeding. However, in none of these studies were the clinicians blinded to the results of the scan, and this may have influenced obstetric management. Furthermore, these studies had relatively small numbers. Nonetheless, the available evidence suggests that women with placenta previa should have transvaginal ultrasonography in the late third trimester and those with a placental edge to internal os distance of less than 2 cm should give birth by cesarean delivery. Many women with a placenta–internal os distance of less than 2 cm who undergo a trial of labor almost invariably experience significant bleeding during labor, necessitating cesarean delivery. Consequently, it is now the practice of some health care clinicians to have these women give birth by elective cesarean delivery. Women whose placentas are 2 cm or more from the os undergo a normal labor. It is important to realize that, in women with a placenta that extends into the noncontractile lower uterine segment who have a vaginal delivery, there is potential for postpartum hemorrhage.

When there is an anterior placenta previa, there is a considerable likelihood of incising through the placenta during delivery. Incising the placenta could lead to significant maternal and fetal blood loss and also to difficulty with delivery, although it rarely constitutes a significant problem. Alternative strategies to avoid incision into the placenta include the use of a fundal vertical uterine incision, especially in women who have no desire for further childbearing (36). This may be especially useful when there is a complete placenta previa with a fetal transverse lie with the fetal back down. Ultrasonography before surgery for placental location enables the surgeon to plan the most appropriate incision (36). Generally, a lower segment transverse uterine incision is performed, incising the placenta when it is unavoidable. The infant is delivered as rapidly as possible, and the cord is clamped immediately to avoid hemorrhage from fetal vessels.

Timing of Delivery

As gestational age advances, there is an increased risk of significant bleeding, necessitating delivery. It is preferable to perform a cesarean delivery for placenta previa under controlled scheduled conditions rather than as an emergency. Therefore, in a stable patient, it is reasonable to perform a cesarean delivery at 36–37 weeks of gestation, after documentation of fetal lung maturity by amniocentesis. If the amniocentesis does not demonstrate lung maturity, the women should give birth by elective cesarean delivery at 38 weeks of gestation, without repeating the amniocentesis if they remain stable, or earlier if bleeding occurs or the patient goes into labor.

Anesthesia for Delivery

In the past, it was generally recommended that cesarean deliveries for placenta previa be performed using a general anesthetic (37). It was believed that this allowed more controlled surgery. At least two studies, including a prospective randomized trial, have found that cesarean deliveries for women with placenta previa performed using a general anesthetic were associated with significantly greater estimated blood loss and greater requirements for blood transfusion than those performed with a regional anesthetic, possibly because of increased uterine relaxation associated with general anesthetics (38, 39). Otherwise, there was no difference in the incidence of intraoperative or anesthetic complications between regional and general anesthetics. In a survey of anesthesiologists in the United Kingdom a wide variety of opinions regarding whether general or regional anesthetics should be used for cesarean delivery for women with placenta previa was found. However, anesthesiologists who performed more obstetric anesthesia were more likely to employ regional anesthetics (40). In another survey, it was found that 60% of the time anesthesiologists used regional anesthetics for cesarean delivery for women with placenta previa (37).

Placenta Accreta

Definition

Placenta accreta refers to a placenta that abnormally adheres to the uterus (Fig. 19-4). When the placenta invades the myometrium, the term placenta increta is used. Placenta percreta refers to a placenta that has invaded

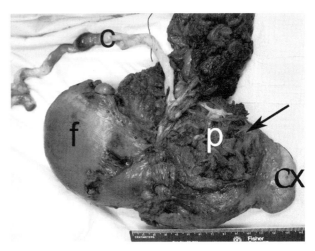

Fig. 19-4. Hysterectomy specimen demonstrating placenta accreta. Abbreviations: C, umbilical cord; CX, cervix; F, uterine fundus; P, placenta. (Oyelese Y, Smulian JC. Placenta previa, placenta accreta, and vasa previa. Obstet Gynecol 2006;107: 927–941.)

through the myometrium and serosa, sometimes into adjacent organs, such as the bladder. The term placenta accreta is often used interchangeably as a general term to describe all of these conditions.

Clinical Significance

Placenta accreta may lead to massive obstetric hemorrhage, resulting in such complications as disseminated intravascular coagulopathy, need for hysterectomy, surgical injury to the ureters, bladder, and other viscera, adult respiratory distress syndrome, renal failure, and even death (41–42). The average blood loss at delivery in women with placenta accreta is 3,000–5,000 mL (41). In several centers, placenta accreta has become the leading reason for cesarean hysterectomy (43). Rarely, placenta accreta may lead to spontaneous uterine rupture in the second or third trimester, resulting in intraperitoneal hemorrhage, a life-threatening emergency (44). Minor degrees of placenta accreta may occur, which may lead to slightly heavier postpartum bleeding, but may not require the aggressive management that is often employed with more extensive placenta accreta.

Incidence and Risk Factors

In one study, 155,670 deliveries at a hospital between 1985 and 1994 were reviewed and found that 62 deliveries (one in 2,510) were complicated by placenta accreta (45). The incidence of placenta accreta is increasing, primarily as a consequence of increasing cesarean delivery rates. In a recent study that examined the incidence of placenta accreta over a 20-year period (1982–2002), it was found that an incidence of 1 in 533 pregnancies (46). Placenta accreta occurs most frequently in women with one or more prior cesarean deliveries who have a placenta previa in the current pregnancy. In one study, it was found that, in the presence of a placenta previa, the risk of having placenta accreta increased from 24% in women with one prior cesarean delivery to 67% in women with three or more prior cesarean deliveries (47).

It has been proposed that the abnormality of the placental–uterine interface in women with placenta accreta will lead to leakage of fetal alpha-fetoprotein into the maternal circulation, resulting in elevated levels of maternal serum alpha-fetoprotein (MSAFP) (48). In one review of 44 cases of women who had cesarean hysterectomies, 9 of the 20 women (45%) with placenta accreta had elevated MSAFP levels (between 2.7 and 40.3 multiples of the median [MoM]), whereas the controls all had MSAFP levels within normal limits (less than 2 MoM) (49). Similarly, results from another study found elevated second-trimester MSAFP levels (between 2.3 and 5.5 MoM) in 45% of 11 women with placenta accreta, whereas none of the controls who had placenta previa without accreta had elevated MSAFP levels (48). Although these studies are small, the results suggest that women with elevated MSAFP levels with no other obvious cause should be considered at increased risk of placenta accreta.

Pathophysiology

Placenta accreta is thought to be caused by an absence or deficiency of Nitabuch's layer or the spongiosus layer of the decidua (10). This may be the consequence of failure of reconstitution of the endometrium–decidua basalis after repair of a cesarean incision. Histology usually shows that the trophoblast has invaded the myometrium without intervening decidua (10). This becomes a problem at delivery when the placenta does not separate and massive bleeding ensues (Fig. 19-5).

Diagnostic Approach

It is important to diagnose placenta accreta prenatally to allow effective management planning to minimize morbidity. This diagnosis is usually determined by ultrasonography or magnetic resonance imaging (MRI). Placenta accreta should be suspected in women who have both a placenta previa and a history of cesarean delivery or other uterine surgery (41, 50). Vigilance is particularly indicated when the placenta is anterior and overlies the cesarean scar.

ULTRASONOGRAPHY

The efficacy of ultrasonography in the diagnosis of placenta accreta has been documented in several studies (50–52). In a recent review, the ultrasonographic features suggestive of placenta accreta were described (50). These

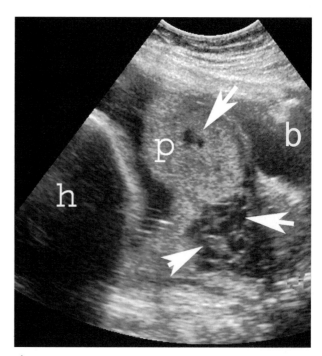

Fig. 19-5. Grayscale ultrasonogram of placenta percreta. Abbreviations: B, bladder; H, fetal head; P, placenta. (Oyelese Y, Smulian JC. Placenta previa, placenta accreta, and vasa previa. Obstet Gynecol 2006;107:927–941.)

include irregularly shaped placental lacunae (vascular spaces) within the placenta, thinning of the myometrium overlying the placenta, loss of the retroplacental "clear space," protrusion of the placenta into the bladder, increased vascularity of the uterine serosa–bladder interface, and, on Doppler ultrasonography, turbulent blood flow through the lacunae (Fig. 19-5) (Fig. 19-6) (51). Previously in another study, findings showed that, at 15–20 weeks of gestation, the presence of lacunae in the placenta was the most predictive ultrasound sign of placenta accreta, with a sensitivity of 79% and a positive predictive value of 92% (51). These lacunae may give the placenta a "moth-eaten" or "Swiss cheese" appearance (Fig. 19-5). The risk of placenta accreta increases with an increased number of lacunae (52). Obliteration of the retroplacental "clear space," which is the finding most commonly thought to be associated with placenta accreta, had only a 57% sensitivity and a false-positive rate of 48.4% (51). After 20 weeks of gestation, the sensitivity of these findings increased, with values of 93% and 80% for lacunae and obliteration of the retroplacental clear space, respectively (51). The ultrasound appearance of apparent bulging into the bladder may occur in cases of placenta accreta without increta or percreta (50). Thus, this finding may not reliably differentiate between cases in which the placenta has invaded the bladder and cases in which it has not (50).

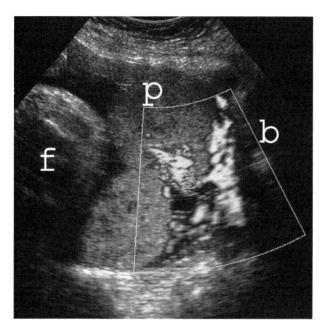

Fig. 19-6. Color Doppler ultrasonagram of placenta percreta. Abbreviations: B, bladder wall; F, fetus; P, placenta. (Oyelese Y, Smulian JC. Placenta previa, placenta accreta, and vasa previa. Obstet Gynecol 2006;107:927–941.)

Power and color Doppler ultrasonography are often used for the diagnosis of placenta accreta, demonstrating turbulent flow through placental lacunae (Fig. 19-6) (53). However, in most cases this imaging mode does not significantly improve the diagnosis over that achieved by grayscale ultrasonography alone. Thus, in most clinical situations, Doppler ultrasonography should not be the primary technique used to diagnose placenta accreta.

In a retrospective review of images of first-trimester ultrasonograms of cases of placenta accreta it was found that, in all the cases, the gestational sac was in the lower uterine segment and that the gestational sac was abnormally close to the uterine scar, suggesting attachment to the scar (54). This finding in the first trimester, in women with a prior cesarean delivery, should lead to a suspicion of placenta accreta.

MAGNETIC RESONANCE IMAGING

In several articles the use of MRI was described in the diagnosis of placenta accreta (55–57). Most were retrospective, limited to a few cases, and lacked pathologic correlation (56). Although most study results have suggested reasonable diagnostic accuracy of MRI for placenta accreta, it appears that MRI is no more sensitive than ultrasonography for diagnosing placenta accreta (50, 57). Ultrasonography is readily available in most centers, whereas MRI is costly and relatively inaccessible. Therefore, ultrasonography is the primary imaging mode for diagnosing accreta. However, when there is a

posterior placenta accreta, ultrasonography may be less than adequate, and MRI may be superior to ultrasonography for this specific indication (50, 57).

Therapeutic Approach

Ideally, placenta accreta is treated by total abdominal hysterectomy. In addition, there is almost universal consensus that the placenta should be left in place; attempts to detach the placenta frequently result in massive hemorrhage. However, the physician should be aware that focal placenta accreta may exist that may not require such aggressive therapy. It is better to perform surgery for placenta accreta under elective, controlled conditions rather than as an emergency without adequate preparation. Therefore, scheduled delivery at 36–37 weeks of gestation, after documentation of fetal lung maturity by amniocentesis, seems reasonable. If amniocentesis fails to document fetal lung maturity, the patient, if stable, should have a cesarean delivery by 38 weeks of gestation or earlier if she bleeds or goes into labor. In a study comparing emergency with elective peripartum hysterectomy, it was found that women in the emergency hysterectomy group had greater intraoperative blood loss, were more likely to have intraoperative hypotension, and were more likely to receive blood transfusions than women who had elective obstetric hysterectomies (58).

Prevention of complications ideally requires a multidisciplinary team approach. The patient should be counseled preoperatively about the need for hysterectomy and the likely requirement for transfusion of blood and blood products (59). Although scheduled delivery should be the goal, contingency plans should be made for possible emergent delivery, if necessary. It is important that delivery be performed by an experienced obstetric surgeon, with other surgical specialists such as urologists and gynecologic oncologists readily available if required. It is not unusual for the lower uterine segment to be markedly enlarged and vascular, with distortion of normal anatomy and tissue planes. Preoperative cystoscopy with placement of ureteric stents may help prevent urinary tract injury. A 3-way Foley catheter can be inserted in the bladder via the urethra, allowing simultaneous irrigation and drainage of the bladder during the surgery. In instances in which tissue plane identification is difficult because of adhesions or the invasive placenta, there is the option of distending the bladder to aid in its identification and then emptying it to avoid injury during surgery. Use of a vertical skin incision facilitates adequate exposure. Generally, a vertical incision in the uterus allows delivery of the infant while avoiding the placenta. There should be no attempt to detach the placenta from the uterine wall. The edges of the uterine incision should be oversewn for hemostasis, after which a total abdominal hysterectomy should be performed. Although some have advocated supracervical hysterectomy, in most cases the lower uterine segment is involved in the morbid adhesion and therefore needs to be removed.

It is important to minimize blood loss and ensure that the blood lost is replaced promptly and adequately (59). Because of the large volumes of blood that are typically lost, as well as the replacement with packed red blood cells, these patients are at risk of disseminated intravascular coagulopathy. Thus, coagulation factors should be replaced liberally, adequately, and quickly. Donor-directed blood transfusions and the use of a blood cell saver may reduce the need for transfusion with blood from another donor (59). Some centers use acute normovolemic hemodilution to reduce the need for blood (41). The role of experienced anesthesiology personnel who are skilled in obstetric anesthesia cannot be overemphasized, and they should be involved in preoperative assessment of the patient (59). Use of regional anesthesia in the management of placenta accreta has been shown to be safe.

BALLOON CATHETER OCCLUSION AND EMBOLIZATION

Balloon catheter occlusion or embolization of the pelvic vessels decreases blood flow to the uterus and potentially leads to reduced blood loss. This makes it possible to perform surgery under easier, more controlled circumstances, with less profuse hemorrhage (60–62). Two different approaches have been described. In one approach, several investigators preoperatively place occlusive balloon catheters in the internal iliac arteries. These catheters are inflated after delivery of the fetus, allowing surgery under controlled circumstances, and are deflated after the surgery. In the other approach, catheters with or without balloons are placed preoperatively in the internal iliac arteries, and embolization of the vessels is performed after delivery of the fetus and before hysterectomy. These studies are for the most part retrospective and limited by small numbers. In one study pelvic vessel embolization did not improve surgical outcomes in women who had the procedure when compared with women who did not have embolization (62). In another study, five cases of placenta accreta were reported in which prophylactic hypogastric artery balloon catheter embolization was performed after the cesarean delivery and before hysterectomy (61). Findings suggested that embolization was both effective and safe, but there was no comparison group. In another study, elective embolization resulted in improved outcomes when compared with embolizations done emergently (60). In some cases, occlusive balloon catheters are placed in the anterior branch of the internal iliac arteries

before surgery. After delivery of the infant, the balloons are inflated and embolization is performed before hysterectomy.

MANAGEMENT WITHOUT HYSTERECTOMY

Hysterectomy removes any prospect of future fertility and is associated with considerable morbidity and potential mortality, including that of surgical injury, given the distorted tissue planes and the need to operate in what is sometimes a blood-filled field. Recently, there has been some interest in attempting to conserve the uterus and avoid hysterectomy to minimize these complications and preserve fertility (63–66). Generally in these cases, the placenta is left in situ, with no attempt at removal. Adjunctive procedures include embolization of the internal iliac vessels, treatment with methotrexate, resection of the affected segment of the uterus, use of uterine compression sutures, and oversewing of the placental bed (63–66). A problem with several of these reports is that varying criteria are used for the diagnosis of placenta accreta and, in most cases, there was no pathologic confirmation of the diagnosis (56, 65). Thus, it is possible that some patients did not have a placenta accreta. Another problem is that in several cases the patients developed severe hemorrhage, necessitating either emergency surgical intervention or embolization (64, 67). It is preferable to deal with massive hemorrhage in a controlled setting with all resources available, rather than to have to deal with it as an emergency at an unpredictable time. Conservative management also carries the risk of intrauterine infection, which could potentially be life threatening. Nevertheless, conservative management may have a limited role in carefully selected patients who desire future fertility. It has been suggested that delayed surgery leads to a less vascular surgical field and may have potential benefits when there is bladder involvement (42). Women offered conservative management should be counseled extensively that the outcomes are unpredictable and that there is a significant risk of serious complications, including death. It is possible that conservative management will assume a more important role in the management of placenta accreta. However, at the present, this option cannot be recommended as a mainstay of therapy. Further studies are required to identify women who may be ideal candidates for conservative management and to define the risks associated with this approach.

METHOTREXATE THERAPY

Methotrexate, a folate antagonist, has been proposed as a conservative treatment for placenta accreta (63). Methotrexate acts primarily against rapidly dividing cells and therefore is effective against proliferating trophoblast. However, more recently, others have argued that, after delivery of the fetus, the placenta is no longer dividing and therefore methotrexate is of no value. In one study of suspected placenta accreta managed conservatively with methotrexate therapy, two of the three cases, uterine conservation was possible (68). However, the use of methotrexate did not prevent delayed hemorrhage. At least two reports have documented failed conservative treatment of placenta accreta with methotrexate (64, 67). No large studies have compared use of methotrexate with no use of methotrexate in the treatment of placenta accreta. Therefore, there are no convincing data for or against the use of methotrexate for accreta.

BLADDER INVOLVEMENT

The bladder is the most frequently involved extrauterine organ in placenta percreta. Bladder involvement is associated with significant morbidity (69–72). In a meta-analysis of 54 reported cases of placenta percreta with bladder involvement it was shown that predelivery hematuria was only present in 17 cases (31%) (73). Although cystoscopy was performed in 12 of these patients, it did not help in diagnosing in any of them. In 33% of the cases, the diagnosis was made prenatally by ultrasonography or MRI. The maternal morbidity was high, with 39 urologic complications. These included laceration of the bladder (26%), urinary fistula (13%), gross hematuria (9%), ureteral transaction (6%), and small capacity bladder (4%). Partial cystectomy was necessary in 24 cases (44%). There were three maternal deaths (5.6%) and 14 fetal deaths (25.9%).

Treatment of the patient with bladder involvement requires careful perioperative planning and should involve a urogynecologist, a urologist, or a gynecologic oncologist. Preoperative cystoscopy and placement of ureteric stents may aid in identification of the ureters, leading to a reduced risk of damage or injury to these structures. Involvement of the bladder may require resection of the bladder and, occasionally, of the ureters. Intentional cystotomy may be helpful in identifying the extent of involvement and location of the ureters (74).

Vasa Previa

Definition

Vasa previa refers to fetal vessels running through the membranes over the cervix and under the fetal presenting part, unprotected by placenta or umbilical cord (75). The condition usually results from a velamentous insertion of the cord into the membranes rather than the placenta (Fig. 19-7) or from vessels running between lobes of a placenta with one or more accessory lobes (75–76).

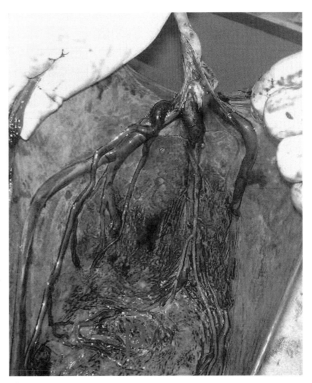

Fig. 19-7. Placenta after delivery showing vasa previa. (Oyelese Y, Smulian JC. Placenta previa, placenta accreta, and vasa previa. Obstet Gynecol 2006;107:927–941.)

Clinical Importance

Vasa previa is a condition that, if undiagnosed, is associated with a perinatal mortality rate of approximately 60% (77). The condition is important because, when the membranes rupture, spontaneously or artificially, the fetal vessels running through the membranes have a high risk of concomitant rupture, frequently resulting in fetal exsanguination and death (75, 78). Because the fetal blood volume is only approximately 80–100 mL/kg, loss of even small amounts of blood could prove disastrous to the fetus. Pressure on the unprotected vessels by the presenting part could lead to fetal asphyxia and death.

Incidence and Risk Factors

The estimated incidence of vasa previa is approximately 1 in 2,500 deliveries (75). Risk factors for the condition include a second-trimester low-lying placenta (even if the "low-lying" placenta or placenta previa resolves in the third trimester), pregnancies in which the placenta has accessory lobes, multiple pregnancies, and pregnancies resulting from in vitro fertilization (79–80).

Diagnostic Approach

Vasa previa is most commonly diagnosed when rupture of the membranes is accompanied by vaginal bleeding and fetal distress or death. The diagnosis is often confirmed only when the placenta is inspected after delivery. Until recently, most obstetricians have been resigned to the belief that the death of a fetus from a ruptured vasa previa is unavoidable. Very rarely, vasa previa may be diagnosed during a digital cervical examination when the examiner's fingers palpate fetal vessels running through the membranes. Use of an amnioscope in this situation may allow direct visualization of the vessels. When bleeding occurs in pregnancy or during labor, a test to determine the presence of fetal blood cells in the vaginal blood, such as the Apt test or Kleihauer-Betke test, may aid in the diagnosis of vasa previa (75). However, when acute bleeding occurs from a ruptured vasa previa, emergent delivery is frequently indicated, and there may be no time to test for fetal blood cells. Whenever bleeding accompanies rupture of the membranes in labor, especially if there are associated fetal heart rate decelerations, fetal bradycardia, or a sinusoidal fetal heart rate pattern, the obstetrician should have a high index of suspicion for a ruptured vasa previa (81, 82). Usually in these situations, immediate cesarean delivery is indicated. Even when the neonate has lost a considerable amount of blood, immediate transfusion may be lifesaving (83).

In numerous reports and studies it has been demonstrated that vasa previa can be diagnosed prenatally with ultrasonography (75, 84). The grayscale ultrasound appearance of vasa previa is of linear echolucent structures overlying the cervix (84). When color or power Doppler ultrasonography is used, flow can be demonstrated through these vessels, and pulsed Doppler ultrasonography will demonstrate a fetal umbilical arterial or venous waveform (Fig. 19-8). It is important to differenti-

ate a vasa previa from a funic presentation. In the latter, the vessels will move when the patient changes position, especially when the patient is placed in the Trendelenburg's position. Conversely, the vessels do not move when there is a vasa previa. Most prenatally diagnosed cases of vasa previa are detected incidentally in women who have transvaginal ultrasonography for evaluation of low-lying placentas. However, most cases of vasa previa in asymptomatic women can be diagnosed prenatally by routinely evaluating the placental cord insertion when an ultrasound examination is performed. Vaginal ultrasonography with color Doppler should be considered if the placental cord insertion cannot be identified or if there is a low-lying placenta or a suspected succenturiate placental lobe (76, 84, 85).

In at least four studies the use of ultrasonography in routine screening for vasa previa in large populations has been prospectively evaluated (76, 84–86). In these studies it was found that ultrasound identification of placental cord insertion was accurate and sensitive and added little or no extra time to the duration of the obstetric ultrasound examination. In all the prenatally diagnosed cases, the neonatal survival rate of infants without congenital malformations was 100%.

Therapeutic Approach

Good outcomes with vasa previa depend on prenatal diagnosis and cesarean delivery before rupture of the membranes. In a multicenter retrospective study of 155 cases of vasa previa, the impact of prenatal diagnosis on outcomes of pregnancies complicated by vasa previa was evaluated (77). In 61 of these cases, the diagnosis was determined prenatally. In the absence of prenatal diagnosis, the perinatal mortality rate was 56%, whereas 97% of fetuses survived with prenatal diagnosis (77). Among the survivors, when the condition was not diagnosed prenatally, the median 1-minute and 5-minute Apgar scores were only 1 and 4, respectively, compared with 8 and 9, respectively, when the condition was diagnosed prenatally (76). Two thirds of the women had a low-lying placenta in the second trimester. By the time of delivery, two thirds of these placentas were no longer low lying. In one third of the cases, the placenta was bilobed. The main predictors of survival were prenatal diagnosis and gestational age at delivery.

Consideration should be given to hospitalization at about 30–32 weeks of gestation and administration of corticosteroids to promote fetal lung maturation. Hospitalization allows proximity to the operating room for emergent cesarean delivery if the membranes rupture. Approximately 10% of women will have ruptured membranes before the onset of labor, so this risk is significant. However, in selected asymptomatic patients,

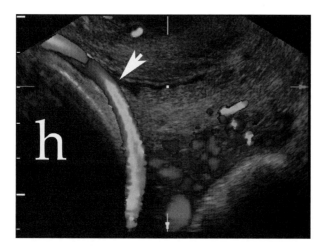

Fig. 19-8. Transvaginal ultrasonography with color Doppler showing the fetal vessels running over internal os of the cervix. Abbreviation: H, fetal head. (Oyelese Y, Smulian JC. Placenta previa, placenta accreta, and vasa previa. Obstet Gynecol 2006;107:927–941.)

there may be a role for outpatient management, especially if the patient has no signs of labor or uterine activity and has a long-closed cervix on transvaginal ultrasonography. Delivery should occur at an institution where there are adequate facilities for neonatal resuscitation that might include emergent blood transfusions. It is preferable that, before surgery, the surgeon is aware of the position of the fetal vessels and plans the incision to avoid lacerating these vessels. Three-dimensional ultrasonography with power Doppler angiography may be used to map out the fetal vessels and thereby make the optimal uterine incision (87, 88). It is desirable to deliver the fetus en caul, with intact membranes, avoiding incising the membranes.

Between 35 weeks and 36 weeks of gestation is the optimal time for cesarean delivery in women with vasa previa, with a reasonable tradeoff between prematurity with the risk of RDS and that of rupture of the membranes with the risk of fetal exsanguination and death (77). Although amniocentesis is generally recommended before elective cesarean delivery before 39 weeks of gestation in most conditions, in vasa previa, if the membranes rupture, the risks of fetal death or adverse outcome are so severe that it is justifiable to proceed with delivery by 36 weeks of gestation without amniocentesis documentation of lung maturity.

There is possibly no other condition in which prenatal diagnosis and appropriate perinatal management makes such a dramatic impact on the difference between survival and death for an otherwise healthy infant. Thus, especially because it adds little in terms of time to the routine obstetric ultrasonography, screening for vasa previa should be routine.

Summary

Achieving optimal outcomes with placenta previa, placenta accreta, and vasa previa depends on prenatal diagnosis and appropriate management at the time of delivery. Advances in ultrasonography have made it possible to diagnose all three conditions with reasonable accuracy, which allows appropriate management planning. Women with these conditions should be considered at high risk and should give birth at institutions with skilled personnel, adequate blood transfusion facilities, and good neonatal resources.

References

1. Crane JM, Van den Hof MC, Dodds L, Armson BA, Liston R. Maternal complications with placenta previa. Am J Perinatol 2000;17:101–5.

2. Iyasu S, Saftlas AK, Rowley DL, Koonin LM, Lawson HW, Atrash HK. The epidemiology of placenta previa in the United States, 1979 through 1987. Am J Obstet Gynecol 1993;168:1424–9.

3. Crane JM, van den Hof MC, Dodds L, Armson BA, Liston R. Neonatal outcomes with placenta previa. Obstet Gynecol 1999;93:541–4.

4. Ananth CV, Smulian JC, Vintzileos AM. The association of placenta previa with history of cesarean delivery and abortion: a metaanalysis. Am J Obstet Gynecol 1997;177:1071–8.

5. Barrett JM, Boehm FH, Killam AP. Induced abortion: a risk factor for placenta previa. Am J Obstet Gynecol 1981;141:769–72.

6. Ananth CV, Savitz DA, Luther ER. Maternal cigarette smoking as a risk factor for placental abruption, placenta previa, and uterine bleeding in pregnancy. Am J Epidemiol 1996;144:881–9.

7. Ananth CV, Wilcox AJ, Savitz DA, Bowes WA Jr, Luther ER. Effect of maternal age and parity on the risk of uteroplacental bleeding disorders in pregnancy. Obstet Gynecol 1996;88:511–6.

8. Macones GA, Sehdev HM, Parry S, Morgan MA, Berlin JA. The association between maternal cocaine use and placenta previa. Am J Obstet Gynecol 1997;177:1097–100.

9. Ananth CV, Demissie K, Smulian JC, Vintzileos AM. Placenta previa in singleton and twin births in the United States, 1989 through 1998: a comparison of risk factor profiles and associated conditions. Am J Obstet Gynecol 2003;188:275–81.

10. Benirschke K, Kaufmann P. Pathology of the human placenta. 4th ed. New York (NY): Springer; 2000.

11. Smith RS, Lauria MR, Comstock CH, Treadwell MC, Kirk JS, Lee W, et al. Transvaginal ultrasonography for all placentas that appear to be low-lying or over the internal cervical os. Ultrasound Obstet Gynecol 1997;9:22–4.

12. Leerentveld RA, Gilberts EC, Arnold MJ, Wladimiroff JW. Accuracy and safety of transvaginal sonographic placental localization. Obstet Gynecol 1990;76:759–62.

13. Lauria MR, Smith RS, Treadwell MC, Comstock CH, Kirk JS, Lee W, et al. The use of second-trimester transvaginal sonography to predict placenta previa. Ultrasound Obstet Gynecol 1996;8:337–40.

14. Varma TR. The implication of a low implantation of the placenta detected by ultrasonography in early pregnancy. Acta Obstet Gynecol Scand 1981;60:265–8.

15. Timor-Tritsch IE, Yunis RA. Confirming the safety of transvaginal sonography in patients suspected of placenta previa. Obstet Gynecol 1993;81:742–4.

16. Hertzberg BS, Bowie JD, Carroll BA, Kliewer MA, Weber TM. Diagnosis of placenta previa during the third trimester: role of transperineal sonography. AJR Am J Roentgenol 1992;159:83–7.

17. Becker RH, Vonk R, Mende BC, Ragosch V, Entezami M. The relevance of placental location at 20-23 gestational weeks for prediction of placenta previa at delivery: evaluation of 8650 cases. Ultrasound Obstet Gynecol 2001;17:496–501.

18. Rosati P, Guariglia L. Clinical significance of placenta previa detected at early routine transvaginal scan. J Ultrasound Med 2000;19:581–5.

19. Hill LM, DiNofrio DM, Chenevey P. Transvaginal sonographic evaluation of first-trimester placenta previa. Ultrasound Obstet Gynecol 1995;5:301–3.

20. Mustafa SA, Brizot ML, Carvalho MH, Watanabe L, Kahhale S, Zugaib M. Transvaginal ultrasonography in predicting placenta previa at delivery: a longitudinal study. Ultrasound Obstet Gynecol 2002;20:356–9.

21. Taipale P, Hiilesmaa V, Ylostalo P. Transvaginal ultrasonography at 18-23 weeks in predicting placenta previa at delivery. Ultrasound Obstet Gynecol 1998;12:422–5.

22. Dashe JS, McIntire DD, Ramus RM, Santos-Ramos R, Twickler DM. Persistence of placenta previa according to gestational age at ultrasound detection. Obstet Gynecol 2002;99:692–7.

23. MacAfee C. Placenta previa: study of 174 cases. J Obstet Gynecol Br Emp 1945;52:313–24.

24. Sharma A, Suri V, Gupta I. Tocolytic therapy in conservative management of symptomatic placenta previa. Int J Gynaecol Obstet 2004;84:109–13.

25. Besinger RE, Moniak CW, Paskiewicz LS, Fisher SG, Tomich PG. The effect of tocolytic use in the management of symptomatic placenta previa. Am J Obstet Gynecol 1995;172:1770–5; discussion 1775–8.

26. Cotton DB, Read JA, Paul RH, Quilligan EJ. The conservative aggressive management of placenta previa. Am J Obstet Gynecol 1980;137:687–95.

27. Droste S, Keil K. Expectant management of placenta previa: cost-benefit analysis of outpatient treatment. Am J Obstet Gynecol 1994;170:1254–7.

28. Mouer JR. Placenta previa: antepartum conservative management, inpatient versus outpatient. Am J Obstet Gynecol 1994; 170:1683–5; discussion 1685–6.

29. D'Angelo LJ, Irwin LF. Conservative management of placenta previa: a cost-benefit analysis. Am J Obstet Gynecol 1984;149:320–6.

30. Wing DA, Paul RH, Millar LK. Management of the symptomatic placenta previa: a randomized, controlled trial of inpatient versus outpatient expectant management. Am J Obstet Gynecol 1996;175:806–11.

31. Arias F. Cervical cerclage for the temporary treatment of patients with placenta previa. Obstet Gynecol 1988;71:545–8.

32. Cobo E, Conde-Agudelo A, Delgado J, Canaval H, Congote A. Cervical cerclage: an alternative for the management of placenta previa? Am J Obstet Gynecol 1998;179:122–5.

33. Oppenheimer LW, Farine D, Ritchie JW, Lewinsky RM, Telford J, Fairbanks LA. What is a low-lying placenta? Am J Obstet Gynecol 1991;165:1036–8.

34. Bhide A, Prefumo F, Moore J, Hollis B, Thilaganathan B. Placental edge to internal os distance in the late third trimester and mode of delivery in placenta praevia. BJOG 2003;110:860–4.

35. Dawson WB, Dumas MD, Romano WM, Gagnon R, Gratton RJ, Mowbray RD. Translabial ultrasonography and placenta previa: does measurement of the os-placenta distance predict outcome? J Ultrasound Med 1996;15:441–6.

36. Boehm FH, Fleischer AC, Barrett JM. Sonographic placental localization in the determination of the site of uterine incision for placenta previa. J Ultrasound Med 1982;1:311–4.

37. Parekh N, Husaini SW, Russell IF. Caesarean section for placenta praevia: a retrospective study of anaesthetic management. Br J Anaesth 2000;84:725–30.

38. Hong JY, Jee YS, Yoon HJ, Kim SM. Comparison of general and epidural anesthesia in elective cesarean section for placenta previa totalis: maternal hemodynamics, blood loss and neonatal outcome. Int J Obstet Anesth 2003;12:12–6.

39. Frederiksen MC, Glassenberg R, Stika CS. Placenta previa: a 22-year analysis. Am J Obstet Gynecol 1999;180:1432–7.

40. Bonner SM, Haynes SR, Ryall D. The anaesthetic management of Caesarean section for placenta praevia: a questionnaire survey. Anaesthesia 1995;50:992–4.

41. Hudon L, Belfort MA, Broome DR. Diagnosis and management of placenta percreta: a review. Obstet Gynecol Surv 1998;53:509–17.

42. O'Brien JM, Barton JR, Donaldson ES. The management of placenta percreta: conservative and operative strategies. Am J Obstet Gynecol 1996;175:1632–8.

43. Kastner ES, Figueroa R, Garry D, Maulik D. Emergency peripartum hysterectomy: experience at a community teaching hospital. Obstet Gynecol 2002;99:971–5.

44. deRoux SJ, Prendergast NC, Adsay NV. Spontaneous uterine rupture with fatal hemoperitoneum due to placenta accreta percreta: a case report and review of the literature. Int J Gynecol Pathol 1999;18:82–6.

45. Miller DA, Chollet JA, Goodwin TM. Clinical risk factors for placenta previa-placenta accreta. Am J Obstet Gynecol 1997;177:210–4.

46. Wu S, Kocherginsky M, Hibbard JU. Abnormal placentation: twenty-year analysis. Am J Obstet Gynecol 2005;192:1458–61.

47. Clark SL, Koonings PP, Phelan JP. Placenta previa/accreta and prior cesarean section. Obstet Gynecol 1985;66: 89–92.

48. Zelop C, Nadel A, Frigoletto FD Jr, Pauker S, MacMillan M, Benacerraf BR. Placenta accreta/percreta/increta: a cause of elevated maternal serum alpha-fetoprotein. Obstet Gynecol 1992;80:693–4.

49. Kupferminc MJ, Tamura RK, Wigton TR, Glassenberg R, Socol ML. Placenta accreta is associated with elevated maternal serum alpha-fetoprotein. Obstet Gynecol 1993;82:266–9.

50. Comstock CH. Antenatal diagnosis of placenta accreta: a review. Ultrasound Obstet Gynecol 2005;26:89–96.

51. Comstock CH, Love JJ Jr, Bronsteen RA, Lee W, Vettraino IM, Huang RR, et al. Sonographic detection of placenta accreta in the second and third trimesters of pregnancy. Am J Obstet Gynecol 2004;190:1135–40.

52. Finberg HJ, Williams JW. Placenta accreta: prospective sonographic diagnosis in patients with placenta previa and prior cesarean section. J Ultrasound Med 1992;11:333–43.

53. Chou MM, Ho ES, Lee YH. Prenatal diagnosis of placenta previa accreta by transabdominal color Doppler ultrasound. Ultrasound Obstet Gynecol 2000;15:28–35.

54. Comstock CH, Lee W, Vettraino IM, Bronsteen RA. The early sonographic appearance of placenta accreta. J Ultrasound Med 2003;22:19–23; quiz 24–6.

55. Thorp JM Jr, Wells SR, Wiest HH, Jeffries L, Lyles E. First-trimester diagnosis of placenta previa percreta by magnetic resonance imaging. Am J Obstet Gynecol 1998;178: 616–8.

56. Palacios Jaraquemada JM, Bruno CH. Magnetic resonance imaging in 300 cases of placenta accreta: surgical correlation of new findings. Acta Obstet Gynecol Scand 2005;84: 716–24.

57. Levine D, Hulka CA, Ludmir J, Li W, Edelman RR. Placenta accreta: evaluation with color Doppler US, power Doppler US, and MR imaging. Radiology 1997;205:773–6.

58. Chestnut DH, Dewan DM, Redick LF, Caton D, Spielman FJ. Anesthetic management for obstetric hysterectomy: a multiinstitutional study. Anesthesiology 1989;70:607–10.

59. Placenta accreta. ACOG Committee Opinion No. 266. American College of Obstetricians and Gynecologists. Obstet Gynecol 2002;99:169–70.

60. Alvarez M, Lockwood CJ, Ghidini A, Dottino P, Mitty HA, Berkowitz RL. Prophylactic and emergent arterial catheterization for selective embolization in obstetric hemorrhage. Am J Perinatol 1992;9:441–4.

61. Kidney DD, Nguyen AM, Ahdoot D, Bickmore D, Deutsch LS, Majors C. Prophylactic perioperative hypogastric artery balloon occlusion in abnormal placentation. AJR Am J Roentgenol 2001;176:1521–4.

62. Levine AB, Kuhlman K, Bonn J. Placenta accreta: comparison of cases managed with and without pelvic artery balloon catheters. J Matern Fetal Med 1999;8:173–6.

63. Arulkumaran S, Ng CS, Ingemarsson I, Ratnam SS. Medical treatment of placenta accreta with methotrexate. Acta Obstet Gynecol Scand 1986;65:285–6.

64. Butt K, Gagnon A, Delisle MF. Failure of methotrexate and internal iliac balloon catheterization to manage placenta percreta. Obstet Gynecol 2002;99:981–2.

65. Kayem G, Davy C, Goffinet F, Thomas C, Clement D, Cabrol D. Conservative versus extirpative management in cases of placenta accreta. Obstet Gynecol 2004;104:531–6.

66. Weinstein A, Chandra P, Schiavello H, Fleischer A. Conservative management of placenta previa percreta in a Jehovah's Witness. Obstet Gynecol 2005;105 suppl:1247–50.

67. Jaffe R, DuBeshter B, Sherer DM, Thompson EA, Woods JR Jr. Failure of methotrexate treatment for term placenta percreta. Am J Obstet Gynecol 1994;171:558–9.

68. Mussalli GM, Shah J, Berck DJ, Elimian A, Tejani N, Manning FA. Placenta accreta and methotrexate therapy: three case reports. J Perinatol 2000;20:331–4.

69. Silver LE, Hobel CJ, Lagasse L, Luttrull JW, Platt LD. Placenta previa percreta with bladder involvement: new considerations and review of the literature. Ultrasound Obstet Gynecol 1997;9:131–8.

70. Price FV, Resnik E, Heller KA, Christopherson WA. Placenta previa percreta involving the urinary bladder: a report of two cases and review of the literature. Obstet Gynecol 1991;78 suppl:508–11.

71. Pelosi MA, 3rd, Pelosi MA. Modified cesarean hysterectomy for placenta previa percreta with bladder invasion: retrovesical lower uterine segment bypass. Obstet Gynecol 1999;93 suppl:830–3.

72. Caliskan E, Tan O, Kurtaran V, Dilbaz B, Haberal A. Placenta previa percreta with urinary bladder and ureter invasion. Arch Gynecol Obstet 2003;268:343–4.

73. Washecka R, Behling A. Urologic complications of placenta percreta invading the urinary bladder: a case report and review of the literature. Hawaii Med J 2002;61:66–9.

74. Bakri YN, Sundin T. Cystotomy for placenta previa percreta with bladder invasion [letter]. Urology 1992;40:580

75. Oyelese KO, Turner M, Lees C, Campbell S. Vasa previa: an avoidable obstetric tragedy. Obstet Gynecol Surv 1999; 54:138–45.

76. Catanzarite V, Maida C, Thomas W, Mendoza A, Stanco L, Piacquadio KM. Prenatal sonographic diagnosis of vasa previa: ultrasound findings and obstetric outcome in ten cases. Ultrasound Obstet Gynecol 2001;18:109–15.

77. Oyelese Y, Catanzarite V, Prefumo F, Lashley S, Schachter M, Tovbin Y, et al. Vasa previa: the impact of prenatal diagnosis on outcomes. Obstet Gynecol 2004;103:937–42.

78. Oyelese KO, Schwarzler P, Coates S, Sanusi FA, Hamid R, Campbell S. A strategy for reducing the mortality rate from vasa previa using transvaginal sonography with color Doppler. Ultrasound Obstet Gynecol 1998;12: 434–8.

79. Francois K, Mayer S, Harris C, Perlow JH. Association of vasa previa at delivery with a history of second-trimester placenta previa. J Reprod Med 2003;48:771–4.

80. Schachter M, Tovbin Y, Arieli S, Friedler S, Ron-El R, Sherman D. In vitro fertilization is a risk factor for vasa previa. Fertil Steril 2002;78:642–3.

81. Antoine C, Young BK, Silverman F, Greco MA, Alvarez SP. Sinusoidal fetal heart rate pattern with vasa previa in twin pregnancy. J Reprod Med 1982;27:295–300.

82. Gantt PA, Bird JS Jr, Randall GW. Sinusoidal fetal heart rate pattern with vasa previa. J Tenn Med Assoc 1990;83: 393–4.

83. Schellpfeffer MA. Improved neonatal outcome of vasa previa with aggressive intrapartum management: a report of two cases. J Reprod Med 1995;40:327–32.

84. Lee W, Lee VL, Kirk JS, Sloan CT, Smith RS, Comstock CH. Vasa previa: prenatal diagnosis, natural evolution, and clinical outcome. Obstet Gynecol 2000;95:572–6.

85. Sepulveda W, Rojas I, Robert JA, Schnapp C, Alcalde JL. Prenatal detection of velamentous insertion of the umbilical cord: a prospective color Doppler ultrasound study. Ultrasound Obstet Gynecol 2003;21:564–9.

86. Nomiyama M, Toyota Y, Kawano H. Antenatal diagnosis of velamentous umbilical cord insertion and vasa previa with color Doppler imaging. Ultrasound Obstet Gynecol 1998;12:426–9.

87. Canterino JC, Mondestin-Sorrentino M, Muench MV, Feld S, Baum JD, Fernandez CO. Vasa previa: prenatal diagnosis and evaluation with 3-dimensional sonography and power angiography. J Ultrasound Med 2005;24: 721–5.

88. Oyelese Y, Chavez MR, Yeo L, Giannina G, Kontopoulos EV, Smulian JC, et al. Three-dimensional sonographic diagnosis of vasa previa. Ultrasound Obstet Gynecol 2004;24:211–5.

CHAPTER 20

Placental Abruption

YINKA OYELESE AND CANDE V. ANANTH

$\mathcal{P}$lacental abruption, defined as the premature separation of the placenta, complicates approximately 1% of births (1). Abruption is an important cause of vaginal bleeding in the second half of pregnancy and is associated with significant perinatal mortality and morbidity. The purpose of this review is to describe the epidemiology of placental abruption with particular emphasis on its incidence, temporal trends, and risk factors and to present an evidence-based approach to the diagnosis and management of the condition, with consideration of the severity of the abruption and the gestational age at which it occurs.

Study Selection

We carried out a MEDLINE search using the keywords "abruption," "abruptio," and "bleeding" and "pregnancy," limiting our search to publications in the English language between 1966 and 2006. Further studies were identified through cross-referencing. There are no randomized controlled studies that have specifically examined abruption, and most studies are observational (ie, cohort, case–control, or case series). Most large studies dealing with abruption have examined risk factors for the condition. Studies that have examined management strategies for the condition are typically limited by small numbers. The levels of available evidence for the diagnosis and management of abruption, based on the classification of the United States Task Force on "Levels of Evidence," are mainly II-1, II-2, and III.

Definition

Placental abruption is defined as premature separation of a normally implanted placenta. Although some degree of placental separation often occurs when there is a placenta previa, these cases are not conventionally considered abruptions in the true sense. Abruption may be "revealed," in which case blood tracks between the membranes and the decidua and escapes through the cervix into the vagina (Fig. 20-1). The less common "concealed"

abruption occurs when blood accumulates behind the placenta, with no obvious external bleeding (Fig. 20-1). Abruption may be total, involving the entire placenta, in which case it typically leads to fetal death, or partial, with only a portion of the placenta detached from the uterine wall.

Clinical Importance

Placental abruption is associated with a wide spectrum of clinical significance, varying from cases with minor bleeding and little or no consequences to massive abruption leading to fetal death and severe maternal morbidity. Abruption may be implicated in up to 10% of preterm births (1). The risk to the fetus depends on both the severity of the abruption and the gestational age at which the abruption occurs (Fig. 20-2) (Fig. 20-3), whereas the danger to the mother is posed primarily by the severity of the abruption. A U.S. population-based cohort study of 7,508,655 pregnancies found a perinatal mortality rate of 119 per 1,000 births among pregnancies complicated by abruption, compared with 8.2 per 1,000 among all other births (2). More recent U.S. data corroborate these previous findings (Fig. 20-3). This high perinatal mortality rate is largely caused by preterm delivery because approximately one half of the excess perinatal deaths are associated with early delivery (Fig. 20-2) (Fig. 20-3).

Although placental abruption is an important cause of spontaneous preterm birth, it also is often an indication for iatrogenic preterm delivery (1). Premature separation of the placenta before delivery may deprive the fetus of oxygen and nutrition, leading to long-term handicap among survivors. A case–control study of 29 neonates, delivered after abruption at a median gestational age of 29 weeks, found that 34% of them developed cystic periventricular leukomalacia, a 10-fold increase over controls (3). Similarly, the rate of intraventricular hemorrhage among the abruption cases was higher than that of controls (3).

Although preterm premature rupture of the membranes frequently precedes abruption, in some cases, pla-

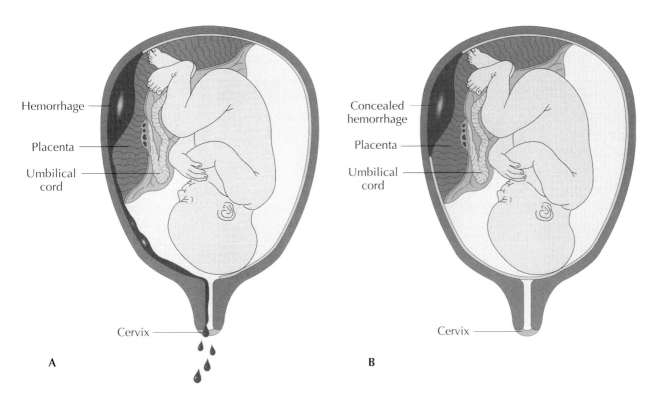

Fig. 20-1. Types of abruption. Revealed abruption: blood tracks between the membranes and escapes through the vagina and cervix **(A).** Concealed abruption: blood collects behind the placenta, with no evidence of vaginal bleeding **(B).** Illustration: John Yanson. (Modified from University Health Care at the University of Utah. High-risk pregnancy: bleeding in pregnancy/placenta previa/placental abruption. Available at: http://uuhsc.utah.edu/ healthinfo/pediatric/hrpregnant/bleed.htm. Retrieved October 18, 2006.)

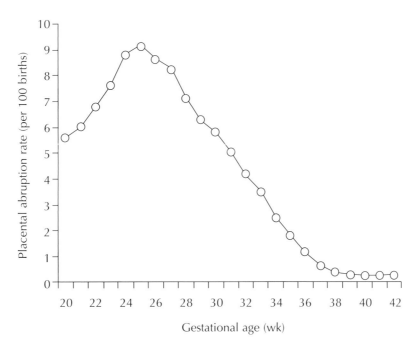

Fig. 20-2. Rates of abruption across gestation, United States, 2000–2002 (N=11, 635,328). (Oyelese Y, Ananth C. Placental abruption. Obstet Gynecol 2006;108: 1005–16.)

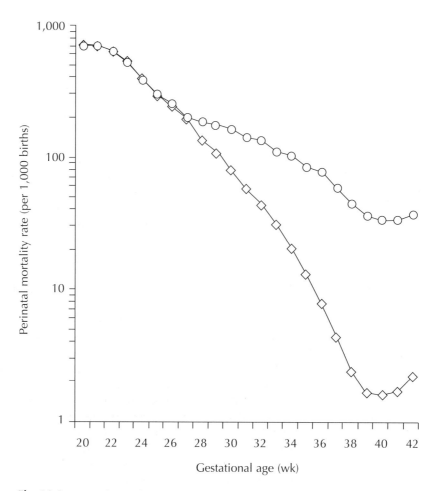

Fig. 20-3. Perinatal mortality in pregnancies with and without abruption across gestation, United States, 2000–2002 (N = 11,635,328). Circles represent pregnancies with abruption, and diamonds represent pregnancies without abruption. (Oyelese Y, Ananth C. Placental abruption. Obstet Gynecol 2006;108:1005–16).

cental abruption may cause weakening and premature rupture of the membranes (4). Placental abruption is associated with intrauterine growth restriction (5, 6). It appears that, in most cases, abruption is the end result of a chronic process and that both fetal growth restriction and abruption share a common cause. Maternal risks associated with abruption include, but are not limited to, disseminated intravascular coagulopathy, renal failure, obstetric hemorrhage, need for blood transfusions, hysterectomy, and less commonly, maternal death.

Incidence of Placental Abruption

Several epidemiologic cohort studies have found that placental abruption complicates approximately 1% of deliveries (2, 5 7–9). However, a subsequent pathologic examination of 7,038 consecutive placentas, disclosed evidence of abruption in 3.8% (10). Similarly, in the U.S. Collaborative Perinatal Project, a prospective cohort study of 55,908 pregnancies, disclosed evidence of abruption in 2.12% of pregnancies (11). When abruption is diagnosed by examination of the placenta by the pathologist, most cases are noted to have had an unremarkable obstetric history (12). Thus, there is significant discrepancy in the rates of diagnosis of abruption detected by clinicians and that experienced by pathologists (12). Because abruption diagnosed solely on the basis of pathology examination typically has no obvious clinical consequences, obstetricians should reserve the use of the term "abruption" for those cases diagnosed based on clinical findings. An obvious exception to this rule would be pregnancies with an adverse outcome in which examination of the placenta by the pathologist reveals evidence of an otherwise unrecognized abruption. Interestingly, the incidence of abruption is highest at 24–26 weeks gestation and decreases precipitously with advancing gestation (Fig. 20-2).

Temporal Trends in Placental Abruption

A recent evaluation of temporal trends in the rate of placental abruption among singleton births in the United Sates between 1979 and 2001 noted that the overall rate of abruption in the United Sates increased from 0.81% in 1979–1981 to 1% in 1999–2001—a relative increase of 23% (95% confidence interval, 22–24%) (8). There was a strong race disparity in the temporal trends in abruption risk; the rate of abruption increased among white women by 15% (from 0.82% to 0.94% between 1979–1981 and 1999–2001), and increased by 92% among black women (from 0.76% to 1.43% between 1979–1981 and 1999–2001) (8). These overall trends in placental abruption were similar in a Norwegian population, in which the frequency of placental abruption increased from 5.3 per 1,000 births in 1971 to 9.1 per 1,000 births in 1990 (9).

Risk Factors for Abruption

Risk factors for placental abruption are summarized in Table 20-1 (5, 7, 13–17). Other risk factors include trauma (18), thrombophilias (19), dysfibrinogenemia, hydramnios, advanced maternal age, and intrauterine infections. There is a dose–response relationship between the number of cigarettes smoked and the risk of abrup-

tion (13, 16). At least two recent population-based retrospective cohort studies have indicated that women who have a cesarean first birth have an increased risk of placental abruption in a second pregnancy when compared with women who had a vaginal first birth (20, 21).

Numerous case–control, cohort, and population-based studies have attempted to determine the association between abruption and thrombophilias (19, 22–24). Retrospective case–control studies that have examined the frequency of thrombophilias among women with abruption have mostly found increased rates of thrombophilias (19, 24). Conversely, those that have compared rates of abruption between thrombophilias and controls have generally found no significant differences (23). Prochaczka and colleagues (22), in a retrospective case–control study of 102 women with abruption, failed to show any difference in incidence of factor V Leiden carriage status between the cases and controls. Secondary analysis of a large National Institutes of Health-funded prospective cohort study also failed to find an association between maternal and fetal factor V Leiden carrier status and placental abruption in women with no history of thromboembolism (23). Mean levels of homocysteine are higher among patients with abruptions that among controls (24).

Bleeding in early pregnancy carries an increased risk of abruption in later pregnancy (25, 26). An elevated sec-

Table 20-1. Evidence and Strength of Association Linking Major Risk Factors With Placental Abruption Based on Published Studies

Risk Factors	Evidence	
	Strength	Relative Risk or Odds Ratio*
Maternal age and parity	+	1.1–3.7
Cigarette smoking	++	1.4–2.5
Cocaine and drug use	++	5–10
Multiple gestations	+++	1.5–3
Chronic hypertension	++	1.8–5.1
Mild and severe preeclampsia	++	0.4–4.5
Chronic hypertension with preeclampsia	++	7.8
Premature rupture of membranes	+++	1.8–5.1
Oligohydramnios	++	2.5–10
Chorioamnionitis	+	2.0–2.5
Dietary and nutritional deficiency	+/-	0.9–2
Male fetus	+/-	0.9–1.3

*These estimates are the ranges of Relative Risk or Odds Ratio found in independent studies.
Yeo L, Ananth CV, Vintzileos AM. Placental abruption. In: Sciarra J, editor. Gynecology and obstetrics. Vol. 2. Hagerstown (MD). Lippincott, Williams & Wilkins; 2003. ©2003 Lippincott Williams & Wilkins.

ond-trimester maternal serum alpha-fetoprotein may be associated with up to a 10-fold increased risk of placental abruption (27). Similarly, notching of the uterine artery waveform in the second trimester, a marker of impaired uteroplacental blood flow, carries an increased risk of abruption (28).

Perhaps the greatest determinant of abruption risk, however, is an abruption in a prior pregnancy (29). The recurrence risk of abruption in subsequent pregnancies was quantified in a meta-analysis (14). The risk increased 15- to 20-fold in subsequent pregnancies when an earlier pregnancy was complicated by abruption (14). The relative risk of recurrence was less than 9 in only 1 of the 11 studies examined (14).

Pathophysiology

The precise pathophysiology that leads to placental abruption is unknown in many cases. Abruption results from hemorrhage at the decidual–placental interface (12). It seems that acute vasospasm of small vessels may be the event that immediately precedes the placental separation. There may be thrombosis of the decidual vessels with associated decidual necrosis and venous hemorrhage (12). In some cases, abruption is an acute process. Shearing forces resulting from trauma may lead to acute placental separation (18) This also may be the mechanism by which abruption occurs when there is sudden uterine decompression resulting from membrane rupture with hydramnios or after delivery of a first twin. With cocaine use, acute vasoconstriction may lead to placental separation. However, it seems that in most cases, placental abruption may be the consequence of a long-standing process that probably dates back to the first trimester (12, 25). There is abundant support for this concept. A recent large cohort study of 34,271 women indicated that women with first-trimester low levels of pregnancy-associated plasma protein A (in the lowest fifth percentile) had an increased risk of placental abruption (30). A small case series of placental bed biopsies in 12 women with abruption demonstrated a lack of adequate trophoblastic invasion in seven (58%) of these women (31). These changes also are observed in placentas of women with preeclampsia, suggesting that the two conditions share some common causes (12). Indeed, abruption occurs frequently in the setting of preeclampsia (12). There also is an association of growth restriction with abruption, again implicating uteroplacental insufficiency as a possible causative factor (5). Placentas with abruption more often have evidence of chronic pathologic lesions than placentas from pregnancies without abruption (25). Furthermore, a prospective cohort study has found an association between notching of the

Doppler waveform of the uterine artery, a marker of impaired uteroplacental blood flow, at 20–24 weeks of gestation and the subsequent development of placental abruption (28). Thus, uteroplacental insufficiency seems to play a role in the cause of abruption (12). Bleeding in the first two trimesters of pregnancy is associated with an increased risk of subsequent placental abruption (25, 26). Thrombin is a potent uterotonic agent, and uterine contractions are frequently present. Histologic examination of placentas of women with preterm labor often have evidence of old placental bleeding, supporting the concept that thrombin production from placental abruption is implicated in a significant proportion of cases of spontaneous preterm birth (32).

Acute separation of the placenta deprives the fetus of oxygen and nourishment, with the consequence that the fetus frequently dies (12). The coagulation cascade is activated with consumption of coagulation factors and consequent disseminated intravascular coagulopathy (DIC). This risk is highest when there is such a large placental detachment as to cause fetal death. Hemorrhage associated with DIC leads to further consumption of coagulation factors, setting off a vicious circle. Bleeding may occur into the uterine myometrium, leading to a beefy, boggy uterus, called a Couvelaire uterus. When abruption is recent, pathologic examination frequently reveals fresh clot attached to the maternal surface of the placenta, whereas in older cases fibrin deposits at the site of the abruption and infarcts of the overlying placenta may be present (12). In such cases, there may be a depression in the maternal surface of the placenta (12). Microscopic examination reveals hemosiderin-laden macrophages and evidence of villous hemorrhage (12).

Clinical Presentation

The clinical presentation of abruption varies widely from totally asymptomatic cases to those in which there is fetal death with severe maternal morbidity. The classically described symptoms of placental abruption are vaginal bleeding and abdominal pain. It is important to realize, however, that severe abruption may occur with neither or just of one of these signs. The amount of vaginal bleeding correlates poorly with the degree of abruption. The severity of symptoms depends on the location of the abruption, whether it is revealed or concealed, and the degree of abruption. There is a correlation between the extent of placental separation and the risk of stillbirth, with stillbirth occurring in most cases in which there is greater than 50% placental separation (1, 12). Typically, uterine hypertonus is present with associated high-frequency, low-amplitude uterine contractions. The uterus frequently is tender and may feel hard on palpation.

Backache may be the only symptom, especially when the placental location is posterior. Acute fetal distress, and in cases in which more than 50% of the placenta has separated, fetal demise may occur. Rarely abruption can cause fetal death in the absence of other symptoms or signs. In some cases, evidence of abruption may be found on ultrasound examination of asymptomatic patients. Finally, abruption may present as idiopathic preterm labor.

A variety of fetal heart rate patterns have been described in association with abruption, including recurrent late or variable decelerations, reduced variability, bradycardia, or a sinusoidal fetal heart rate pattern. More infrequently, when concealed abruption is associated with fetal death, the first clinical sign may be of evidence of abnormal bleeding, the result of disseminated intravascular coagulopathy. In addition, maternal hypovolemic shock may occur. Labor typically proceeds fairly rapidly in cases of abruption. Placental abruption may be associated with acute tubular necrosis and acute cortical necrosis, leading to oliguria and renal failure. Although tubular necrosis may be caused by acute hypovolemia, it seems that cortical necrosis is the result of damage to the kidney, resulting from products of the coagulation cascade. Renal cortical necrosis may result in chronic renal failure.

Diagnosis

The diagnosis of abruption is a clinical one, and the condition should be suspected in women with vaginal bleeding or abdominal pain or both, a history of trauma, and otherwise unexplained preterm labor. The differential diagnosis includes all causes of abdominal pain and bleeding; specifically, placenta previa, appendicitis, urinary tract infections, preterm labor, fibroid degeneration, ovarian pathology, and muscular pain.

Ultrasonography

The ultrasound appearance of abruption depends, to a large extent, on the size and location of the bleeding (Fig. 20-4), as well as the duration between the abruption and the time the ultrasound examination was performed (33). In cases of acute revealed abruption, the examiner may detect no abnormal ultrasound findings. A retrospective cohort study of images in 57 cases of abruption found that the ultrasound appearance of abruption in the acute phase was hyperechoic to isoechoic when compared with the placenta (33). Later, as the hematomas resolved, they became hypoechoic within 1 week and sonolucent within 2 weeks. In some cases, only a thickened heterogenous placenta could be seen. Thus, it is important to realize that abruption may have a variety of

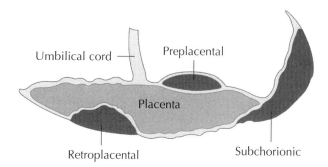

Fig. 20-4. Diagram showing the different sites at which ultrasonographic evidence of abruption may be observed. Subchorionic hematomas are thought to rise from marginal abruptions. "Preplacental hemorrhage" describes both subamniotic hematoma and massive subchorial thrombosis. Illustration: John Yanson. (Adapted from: Nyberg DA. Finberg HJ. Placenta, placental membranes, and umbilical cord. In: Nyberg DA, Mahony, BS, Pretorius DH. Diagnostic ultrasound of fetal anomalies. Chicago [IL]: Year Book Medical Publishers; 1990. Copyright 1990, with permission from Elsevier.)

ultrasound appearances (Fig. 20-4) (Fig. 20-5). The placenta may "jiggle" when sudden pressure is applied with the transducer, the so-called "jello" sign. (34), In a retrospective cohort study, researchers found that the sensitivity, specificity, and positive and negative predictive values of ultrasonography for placental abruption were 24%, 96%, 88%, and 53%, respectively (34). Thus, ultrasonography will fail to detect at least one half of cases of abruption. However, when the ultrasonogram seems to show an abruption, the likelihood that there is indeed an abruption is extremely high (34). Importantly, a negative ultrasonogram does not rule out an abruption. (34). In one study, ultrasound evidence of a clot was identified in only 25% of abruptions (35), whereas in another ultrasonography identified only 50% of abruptions confirmed by pathology (36). In a prospective cohort study of 73 patients presenting with vaginal bleeding in the second half of pregnancy, using 7 ultrasound parameters (Box 20-1), the sensitivity of ultrasonography for placental abruption was 80%, whereas the specificity was 92% (37). Positive and negative predictive values were 95% and 69%, respectively (37). However, no other studies have replicated this accuracy for the ultrasound diagnosis of abruption. Ultrasonography also may predict prognosis in abruption. In a retrospective review of 69 cases of abruption, fetal mortality correlated with the ultrasonographically estimated percentage of abruption and with the location, with the worst prognosis occurring in retroplacental abruptions (38). An important role of ultrasonography in evaluation of bleeding in the second half of pregnancy is placental location; if placenta previa is present, it is less likely that abruption is the cause of the bleeding. The ultrasonographer must be careful, how-

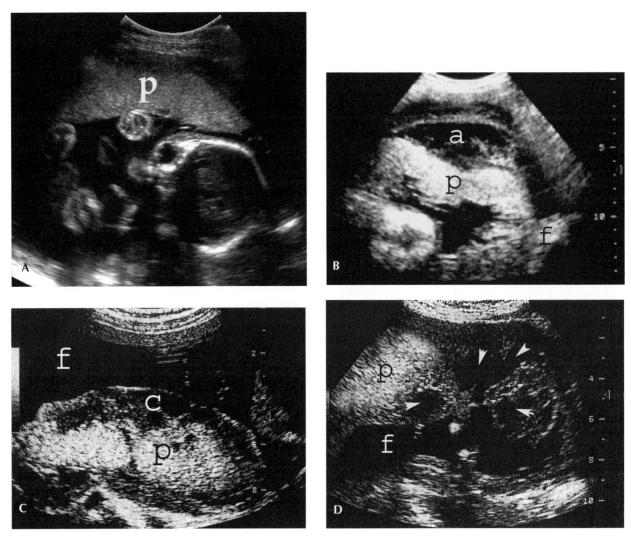

Fig. 20-5. Varying ultrasonographic appearances of normal placenta and placental abruption. **A.** Normal placenta (p). Note the retroplacental hypoechoic space. It is important not to mistake this for abruption. **B.** Large, retroplacental abruption (a) between the placenta (p) and the uterus. Fetus (f). This hypoechoic area is the typical appearance of abruption. **C.** Large, extensive ultrasonographic preplacental collection (c) beneath the chorionic plate, amniotic fluid (f), and placenta (p). **D.** Thickened placenta (p) with heterogenous appearance. The arrowheads point to areas of hemorrhage. (Panel **A**, Oyelese Y, Ananth C. Placental abruption. Obstet Gynecol 2006;108:1005–16 and Panels **B**, **C**, and **D**, Yeo L, Ananth CV, Vintzileos AM. Placental abruption. In: Sciarra J, editor. Gynecology and obstetrics. Vol. 2. Hagerstown [MD]. Lippincott, Williams & Wilkins; 2003. © 2003 Lippincott Williams & Wilkins.)

ever, not to mistake a clot over the cervix for placenta previa. The presence of a fundal placenta makes it unlikely that the mass covering the cervix is placenta. A clot may "jiggle" with movement of the fetus or ultrasound transducer (37).

Kleihauer–Betke Test

The Kleihauer–Betke test is frequently performed in women in whom abruption is suspected. A retrospective cohort study of the use of the Kleihauer–Betke test found no positive Kleihauer–Betke test results among the 27 placentas that showed evidence of abruption on pathologic examination (39). Nine percent of patients with no

evidence of abruption had positive Kleihauer–Betke test results. A retrospective case–control study comparing 100 low-risk women in the third trimester with 151 women of similar gestational ages who had undergone evaluation for abdominal trauma found that the incidence of positive Kleihauer–Betke test results were similar in the two groups (40). There was no association between a positive test result and abruption. Thus, the Kleihauer–Betke test has limited usefulness in the diagnosis of abruption. A negative test result should not be used to rule out abruption, nor does a positive test result necessarily confirm abruption. However, a Kleihauer–Betke test allows quantification of fetomaternal trans-

---

BOX 20-1

ULTRASOUND CRITERIA FOR DIAGNOSIS OF PLACENTAL ABRUPTION

1. Preplacental collection under the chorionic plate (between the placenta and amniotic fluid)
2. "Jello-like" movement of the chorionic plate with fetal activity
3. Retroplacental collection
4. Marginal hematoma
5. Subchorionic hematoma
6. Increased heterogenous placental thickness (more than 5 cm in a perpendicular plane)
7. Intraamniotic hematoma

Adapted from Yeo L, Ananth CV, Vintzileos AM. Placental abruption. In: Sciarra J, editor. Gynecology and obstetrics. Vol. 2. Hagerstown (MD): Lippincott Williams & Wilkins; 2003. © 2003 Lippincott Williams & Wilkins.

---

fusion to guide administration of Rh-immune globulin to Rh-negative women.

Management

The management of placental abruption depends on the presentation, the gestational age, and the degree of maternal and fetal compromise (Fig. 20-6). Because the presentation is widely variable, it is important to individualize management on a case-by-case basis. More aggressive management, desirable in cases of severe abruption, may not be appropriate in milder cases of abruption.

In cases of severe abruption with fetal death, regardless of gestational age, it is reasonable, as long as the mother's condition is stable and no other contraindications are present, to allow the patient to have a vaginal delivery. Typically, the uterus is contracting vigorously, and labor rapidly progresses. Amniotomy is frequently sufficient to speed up delivery. There is a significant risk of coagulopathy and hypovolemic shock. Intravenous access should be established, and blood and coagulation factors should be replaced aggressively. Meticulous attention should be paid the amount of blood loss; clinicians frequently underestimate this finding. Blood samples should be evaluated for complete blood count, coagulation studies, and type and crossmatch, and the blood bank should be informed of the potential for coagulopathy. A Foley catheter should be placed, and the hourly urine output should be monitored closely. It is prudent to involve an anesthesiologist in the patient's care early. When labor does not progress rapidly and when feto–pelvic disproportion, fetal malpresentation, or a prior classical cesarean delivery are present, cesarean delivery may be necessary to avoid worsening of the coagulopathy. In the presence of DIC bleeding from surgical incisions may be difficult to control, and it is important to stabilize the patient and to correct any coagulation derangement during surgery. After delivery, the patient should be monitored closely, with particular attention paid to vital signs, amount of blood loss, and urine output. In addition, the uterus should be observed closely to ensure that it remains contracted and is not increasing in size, and blood loss should be monitored closely. The uterus may be hypotonic, and occasionally hysterectomy may be necessary. Blood should be drawn for complete blood count and coagulation studies at regular intervals until the patient is stable. Some cases of abruption may be associated with severe preeclampsia, which may be masked because the patient may be normotensive because of hypovolemia. Thus, there should be a high index of suspicion for severe preeclampsia in patients with abruption not resulting from an obvious cause, such as trauma or cocaine use. In such cases, the patients may benefit from close volume status monitoring, early recognition of hypovolemia, and adequate blood replacement.

In cases of abruption at term or near term with a live fetus, prompt delivery is indicated. The main question is whether vaginal delivery can be achieved without fetal or maternal death or severe morbidity. In cases in which there is evidence of fetal compromise and delivery is not imminent, cesarean delivery should be performed promptly, because total placental detachment could occur without warning. When both maternal and fetal statuses are reassuring, conservative management, with the goal of vaginal delivery, is reasonable. Labor, if established, should be allowed to progress; otherwise induction of labor should be considered. Both mother and fetus should be monitored closely during labor. Should the fetal heart rate tracing become nonreassuring, with bradycardia, loss of variability, or persistent late decelerations, prompt cesarean delivery is indicated. Similarly, should maternal compromise occur, the fetus should be delivered promptly.

A few older retrospective cohort studies suggested that in cases of abruption in which the fetuses were alive outcomes with cesarean delivery were superior to those with vaginal delivery (41–43). In a case–control study in which the relationship between decision–delivery interval and perinatal outcome was examined in 33 patients with severe abruption and fetal bradycardia, longer decision–delivery intervals were associated with poorer perinatal outcomes (41). It must be emphasized that in the setting of significant abruption with fetal bradycardia, minutes may make a difference between survival and death.

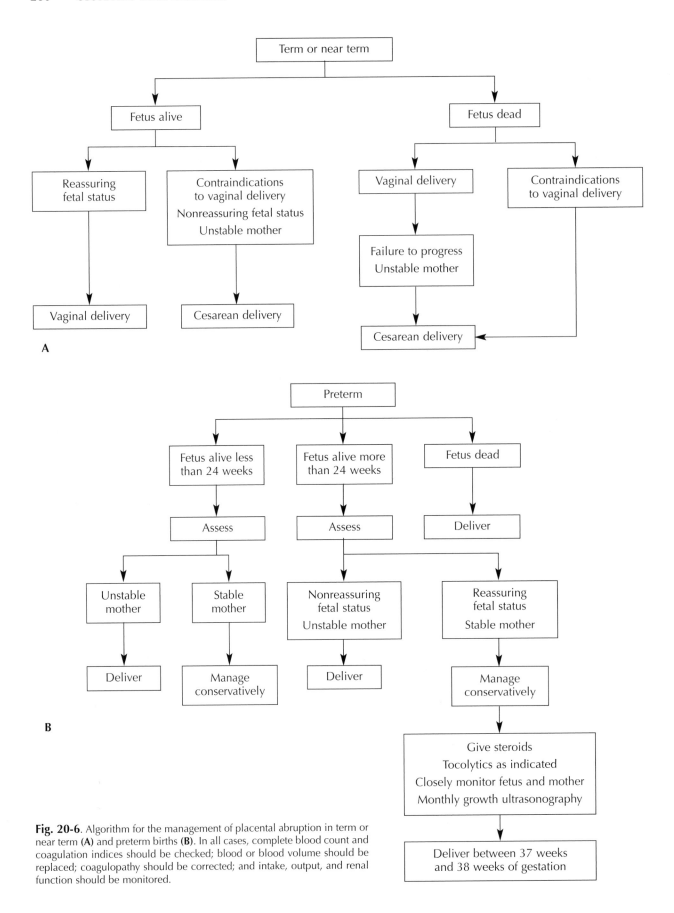

Fig. 20-6. Algorithm for the management of placental abruption in term or near term (**A**) and preterm births (**B**). In all cases, complete blood count and coagulation indices should be checked; blood or blood volume should be replaced; coagulopathy should be corrected; and intake, output, and renal function should be monitored.

At more preterm gestational ages (between 20–34 weeks of gestation), when partial placental abruption is present and the status of the mother and fetus is reassuring, the patient may be managed conservatively (44, 45). Preterm birth is the leading cause of perinatal death in women with abruption; to optimize perinatal outcomes, it is desirable, if possible, to prolong gestation. However, it cannot be overemphasized that these patients require extremely close monitoring, because there is a significant risk of fetal death. In cases in which the gestational age is between 24–34 weeks, steroids should be administered to promote fetal lung maturation. Patients should be delivered in a center with adequate neonatal facilities, and the parents should be counseled by a neonatologist regarding potential treatments and outcomes for the neonate. Prolonged hospitalization and monitoring may be necessary. It may be possible to discharge these patients to outpatient management if the fetal status is reassuring once they have remained stable for several days.

Abruption suspected on the basis of an incidental finding during an examination should be managed on a case-by-case basis. Thorough history taking and physical examination should be conducted to detect evidence of trauma, cocaine use, hypertension, preeclampsia, or any other predisposing factors. Subsequent management may follow the aforementioned recommendations, taking into consideration the gestational age and the state of maternal and fetal well-being. If ultrasonography suggests abruption in a term fetus, delivery is reasonable. With preterm gestations, if fetal status is reassuring, conservative management should be the goal (45). In a retrospective cohort study of conservative management of 40 cases of placental abruption in preterm gestations after 20 weeks of gestation, delivery was delayed until term in 33% of patients (45). The perinatal mortality rate was 22%, and all cases of perinatal death except one were attributable to extreme prematurity. Of those who delivered before term, 63% had at least one other risk factor (twins, advanced cervical dilation, rupture of membranes) that predisposed to preterm delivery.

In cases in which conservative management is chosen, initial hospitalization for further evaluation and assessment of fetal well-being is reasonable. Serial ultrasonography should be performed to evaluate progression or regression of the abruption.

Trauma in Pregnancy

Women who sustain trauma in pregnancy, such as those in motor vehicle accidents, are at risk of abruption (18). This usually is the result of shearing forces; it may occur even without direct abdominal trauma, and is independent of placental location (18). Current American College of Obstetricians and Gynecologists guidelines (18) recommend that women involved in trauma should undergo a minimum of 4 hours of fetal monitoring. This duration should be extended and further evaluation performed in the presence of uterine contractions or irritability, nonreassuring fetal heart rate tracing, uterine tenderness, vaginal bleeding, severe maternal trauma, or rupture of the membranes. When the results of fetal heart rate monitoring are nonreassuring, delivery is generally indicated, depending on gestational age and individual circumstances.

Screening for Thrombophilias

In women with abruption without a known cause, such as trauma or cocaine use, screening for congenital or acquired thrombophilias should be considered. Thrombophilias that may be associated with abruption include factor V Leiden, antithrombin III, prothrombin gene mutation, protein S and protein C deficiency, methyltetrahydrofolate reductase deficiency, lupus anticoagulant, and anticardiolipin antibodies. Women whose screening results are positive should be treated with heparin and aspirin in subsequent pregnancies or with vitamin B_6 and B_{12} in the case of methyltetrahydrofolate reductase deficiency.

Tocolysis

It is generally taught that tocolytics, especially β-sympathomimetics such as terbutaline, are contraindicated in the presence of vaginal bleeding because side effects such as tachycardia could mask the clinical signs of blood loss. However, a few retrospective cohort and case–control studies have been done to evaluate the use of tocolytics (including β-sympathomimetics) in the presence of bleeding in the second half of pregnancy, including patients with suspected stable placental abruptions (35, 45, 46). In one study of expectantly managed women with clinical evidence of placental abruption before 35 weeks of gestation, tocolysis was used when contractions were present (43). There were no intrauterine deaths, and a mean latency period to delivery of 12.4 days was achieved. Of these, in 23 cases delivery occurred within 1 week of admission, while in the remaining 20 patients, the mean time to delivery was 26.8 days. However, there was no comparison group. In a review of 236 cases of third-trimester bleeding, which included 131 cases of placental abruption, with a mean gestational age of 28.9 weeks at the time of first bleeding, tocolysis was used in 95 (73%) of these women (47). The mean time from bleeding until delivery was 18.9 days, the median time from bleeding until delivery was 7 days, and the neonatal mortality rate was 51 deaths per 1,000 live births. All cases of mortality were related to prematurity, and no adverse maternal or fetal effects of tocolysis occurred. Thus, it seems reasonable to use tocolytics with caution in women in a stable condition who have partial placental abruption but are remote from term (46). Because of the aforementioned concerns, magnesium sulfate may be a better choice than terbutaline as the first-line tocolytic in cases of stable suspected abruption.

Management in Subsequent Pregnancy

Women with an abruption are at approximately 10-fold increased risk of abruption in a subsequent pregnancy (48). In addition, they are at increased risk of other adverse pregnancy outcomes, including preterm birth and preeclampsia (48). Although no interventions have been shown to reduce this risk, some recommendations are possible. Women who smoke tobacco or use cocaine should be counseled about the adverse effects of exposure to these substances and encouraged to quit before the next pregnancy. Hypertension should be controlled before and during the subsequent pregnancy. Although no clear benefit in reducing recurrent abruption risk has been proved, it is reasonable to treat women with inherited thrombophilias with thromboprophylaxis, as indicated, in subsequent pregnancies. Because patients with abruption have an increased risk of impaired uteroplacental perfusion in subsequent pregnancies (48), it is reasonable to consider serial growth scans every 4 weeks in the second half of pregnancy. In cases in which the mother has had two or more prior abruptions, amniocentesis for lung maturity and delivery at about 37 weeks of gestation seems reasonable.

Summary

Placental abruption remains an important cause of perinatal mortality and morbidity. Perinatal mortality is determined by the severity of the abruption and the gestational age at which it occurs. Neither accurate prediction nor prevention of abruption is possible at present. Despite advances in medical technology, the diagnosis of abruption is still based on clinical considerations. When abruption does occur, there are some strategies that may help minimize the risks of morbidity and mortality associated with this condition. These strategies include early recognition and prompt delivery in cases in which the fetus is mature. When the mother's condition is stable remote from term, conservative management is appropriate to enable steroid administration, allow transfer to a center with facilities for care of the preterm infant, and in some cases, permit fetal maturation before delivery.

Close attention to maternal condition, with replacement of blood and blood products as indicated, may improve outcomes for the mother.

References

1. Ananth CV, Berkowitz GS, Savitz DA, Lapinski RH. Placental abruption and adverse perinatal outcomes. JAMA 1999;282:1646–51.

2. Ananth CV, Wilcox AJ. Placental abruption and perinatal mortality in the United States. Am J Epidemiol 2001;153: 332–7.

3. Gibbs JM, Weindling AM. Neonatal intracranial lesions following placental abruption. Eur J Pediatr 1994;153: 195–7.

4. Rosen T, Schatz F, Kuczynski E, Lam H, Koo AB, Lockwood CJ. Thrombin-enhanced matrix metalloproteinase-1 expression: a mechanism linking placental abruption with premature rupture of the membranes. J Matern Fetal Neonatal Med 2002;11:11–7.

5. Sheiner E, Shoham-Vardi I, Hallak M, Hadar A, Gortzak-Uzan L, Katz M, et al. Placental abruption in term pregnancies: clinical significance and obstetric risk factors. J Matern Fetal Neonatal Med 2003;13:45–9.

6. Ananth CV, Smulian JC, Srinivas N, Getahun D, Salihu HM. Risk of infant mortality among twins in relation to placental abruption: contributions of preterm birth and restricted fetal growth. Twin Res Hum Genet 2005;8: 524–31.

7. Salihu HM, Bekan B, Aliyu MH, Rouse DJ, Kirby RS, Alexander GR. Perinatal mortality associated with abruptio placenta in singletons and multiples. Am J Obstet Gynecol 2005;193:198–203.

8. Ananth CV, Oyelese Y, Yeo L, Pradhan A, Vintzileos AM. Placental abruption in the United States, 1979 through 2001: temporal trends and potential determinants. Am J Obstet Gynecol 2005;192:191–8.

9. Rasmussen S, Irgens LM, Bergsjo P, Dalaker K. The occurrence of placental abruption in Norway 1967-1991. Acta Obstet Gynecol Scand 1996;75:222–8.

10. Bernis K, Gille J. Placental pathology and asphyxia. In: Gluck L, editor. Intrauterine asphyxia and the developing fetal brain. Chicago (IL): Yearbook Medical Publishers; 1977.

11. Niswander K, Gordon M. The women and their pregnancies. Washington: (DC): U.S. Department of Health, Education, and Welfare, Public Health Service, National Institutes of Health; 1972.

12. Bernischke K, Kaufmann P. Pathology of the human placenta. 4th ed. New York (NY): Springer; 2000.

13. Ananth CV, Savitz DA, Luther ER. Maternal cigarette smoking as a risk factor for placental abruption, placenta previa, and uterine bleeding in pregnancy. Am J Epidemiol 1996;144:881–9.

14. Ananth CV, Savitz DA, Williams MA. Placental abruption and its association with hypertension and prolonged rupture of membranes: a methodologic review and meta-analysis. Obstet Gynecol 1996;88:309–18.

15. Ananth CV, Oyelese Y, Srinivas N, Yeo L, Vintzileos AM. Preterm premature rupture of membranes, intrauterine

infection, and oligohydramnios: risk factors for placental abruption. Obstet Gynecol 2004;104:71–7.

16. Ananth CV, Savitz DA, Bowes WA Jr, Luther ER. Influence of hypertensive disorders and cigarette smoking on placental abruption and uterine bleeding during pregnancy. Br J Obstet Gynaecol 1997;104:572–8.

17. Ananth CV, Smulian JC, Demissie K, Vintzileos AM, Knuppel RA. Placental abruption among singleton and twin births in the United States: risk factor profiles. Am J Epidemiol 2001;153:771–8.

18. ACOG educational bulletin. Obstetric aspects of trauma management. Number 251, September 1998 (replaces Number 151, January 1991, and Number 161, November 1991). American College of Obstetricians and Gynecologists. Int J Gynaecol Obstet 1999;64:87–94.

19. Kupferminc MJ, Eldor A, Steinman N, Many A, Bar-Am A, Jaffa A, et al. Increased frequency of genetic thrombophilia in women with complications of pregnancy [published erratum appears in N Engl J Med 1999;341:384]. N Engl J Med 1999;340:9–13.

20. Lydon-Rochelle M, Holt VL, Easterling TR, Martin DP. First-birth cesarean and placental abruption or previa at second birth(1). Obstet Gynecol 2001;97:765–9.

21. Getahun D, Oyelese Y, Salihu HM, Ananth CV. Previous cesarean delivery and risks of placenta previa and placental abruption. Obstet Gynecol 2006;107:771–8.

22. Prochazka M, Happach C, Marsal K, Dahlback B, Lindqvist PG. Factor V Leiden in pregnancies complicated by placental abruption. BJOG 2003;110:462–6.

23. Dizon-Townson D, Miller C, Sibai B, Spong CY, Thom E, Wendel G Jr, et al. The relationship of the factor V Leiden mutation and pregnancy outcomes for mother and fetus. Obstet Gynecol 2005;106:517–24.

24. Goddijn-Wessel TA, Wouters MG, van de Molen, EF, van de Molen EF, Spuijbroek MD, Steegers-Theunissen RP, et al. Hyperhomocysteinemia: a risk factor for placental abruption or infarction. Eur J Obstet Gynecol Reprod Biol 1996;66:23–9.

25. Ananth CV, Oyelese Y, Prasad V, Getahun D, Smulian JC. Evidence of placental abruption as a chronic process: associations with vaginal bleeding early in pregnancy and placental lesions. Eur J Obstet Gynecol Reprod Biol 2006; 128(1–2):15–21.

26. Weiss JL, Malone FD, Vidaver J, Ball RH, Nyberg DA, Comstock CH, et al. Threatened abortion: a risk factor for poor pregnancy outcome, a population-based screening study. Am J Obstet Gynecol 2004;190:745–50.

27. Katz VL, Chescheir NC, Cefalo RC. Unexplained elevations of maternal serum alpha-fetoprotein. Obstet Gynecol Surv 1990;45:719–26.

28. Harrington K, Cooper D, Lees C, Hecher K, Campbell S. Doppler ultrasound of the uterine arteries: the importance of bilateral notching in the prediction of pre-eclampsia, placental abruption or delivery of a small-for-gestational-age baby. Ultrasound Obstet Gynecol 1996;7:182–8.

29. Toivonen S, Heinonen S, Anttila M, Kosma VM, Saarikoski S. Obstetric prognosis after placental abruption. Fetal Diagn Ther 2004;19:336–41.

30. Dugoff L, Hobbins JC, Malone FD, Porter TF, Luthy D, Comstock CH, et al. First-trimester maternal serum PAPP-A and free-beta subunit human chorionic

gonadotropin concentrations and nuchal translucency are associated with obstetric complications: a population-based screening study (the FASTER Trial). Am J Obstet Gynecol 2004;191:1446–51.

31. Dommisse J, Tiltman AJ. Placental bed biopsies in placental abruption. Br J Obstet Gynaecol 1992;99:651–4.

32. Rana A, Sawhney H, Gopalan S, Panigrahi D, Nijhawan R. Abruptio placentae and chorioamnionitis-microbiological and histologic correlation. Acta Obstet Gynecol Scand 1999;78:363–6.

33. Nyberg DA, Cyr DR, Mack LA, Wilson DA, Shuman WP. Sonographic spectrum of placental abruption. AJR Am J Roentgenol 1987;148:161–4.

34. Glantz C, Purnell L. Clinical utility of sonography in the diagnosis and treatment of placental abruption. J Ultrasound Med 2002;21:837–40.

35. Sholl JS. Abruptio placentae: clinical management in nonacute cases. Am J Obstet Gynecol 1987;156:40–51.

36. Jaffe MH, Schoen WC, Silver TM, Bowerman RA, Stuck KJ. Sonography of abruptio placentae. AJR Am J Roentgenol 1981;137:1049–54.

37. Yeo L, Ananth C, Vintzileos A. Placenta Abruption. In: Sciarra J, editor. Gynecology and obstetrics. Hagerstown (MD): Lippincott, Williams & Wilkins; 2004.

38. Nyberg DA, Mack LA, Benedetti TJ, Cyr DR, Schuman WP. Placental abruption and placental hemorrhage: correlation of sonographic findings with fetal outcome. Radiology 1987;164:357–61.

39. Emery CL, Morway LF, Chung-Park M, Wyatt-Ashmead J, Sawady J, Beddow TD. The Kleihauer-Betke test. Clinical utility, indication, and correlation in patients with placental abruption and cocaine use. Arch Pathol Lab Med 1995;119:1032–7.

40. Dhanraj D, Lambers D. The incidences of positive Kleihauer-Betke test in low-risk pregnancies and maternal trauma patients. Am J Obstet Gynecol 2004;190:1461–3.

41. Kayani SI, Walkinshaw SA, Preston C. Pregnancy outcome in severe placental abruption. BJOG 2003;110:679–83.

42. Witlin AG, Sibai BM. Perinatal and maternal outcome following abruptio placentae. Hypertens Pregnancy 2001; 20:195–203.

43. Rasmussen S, Irgens LM, Bergsjo P, Dalaker K. Perinatal mortality and case fatality after placental abruption in Norway 1967-1991. Acta Obstet Gynecol Scand 1996; 75:229–34.

44. Bond AL, Edersheim TG, Curry L, Druzin ML, Hutson JM. Expectant management of abruptio placentae before 35 weeks gestation. Am J Perinatol 1989;6:121–3.

45. Combs CA, Nyberg DA, Mack LA, Smith JR, Benedetti TJ. Expectant management after sonographic diagnosis of placental abruption. Am J Perinatol 1992;9:170–4.

46. Saller DN Jr, Nagey DA, Pupkin MJ, Crenshaw MC Jr. Tocolysis in the management of third trimester bleeding. J Perinatol 1990;10:125–8.

47. Towers CV, Pircon RA, Heppard M. Is tocolysis safe in the management of third-trimester bleeding? Am J Obstet Gynecol 1999;180:1572–8.

48. Rasmussen S, Irgens LM, Dalaker K. Outcome of pregnancies subsequent to placental abruption: a risk assessment. Acta Obstet Gynecol Scand 2000;79:496–501.

CHAPTER 21

Venous Thromboembolism in Obstetrics and Gynecology

THOMAS C. KRIVAK AND KRISTIN K. ZORN

*I*n the United States, deep vein thrombosis (DVT) and pulmonary embolism, collectively referred to as venous thromboembolism, are diagnosed in more than 500,000 patients each year and are the cause of 200,000 deaths. Approximately 60,000 of those deaths occur in hospitalized patients annually (1–3). Virchow's triad of venous stasis, intimal damage, and hypercoagulability is present in many clinical scenarios in obstetrics and gynecology, increasing the risk for venous thromboembolism. The incidence of venous thromboembolism in the obstetric population ranges from 0.06% to 1.8% (2). In gynecologic surgery, DVT may occur in 14–40% of patients when no prophylaxis is used (3–8). Consideration, therefore, should be given to routine prophylaxis in some obstetric and most gynecologic settings.

Despite prophylaxis, venous thromboembolism will occur in some patients. Clinicians should have a low threshold to order diagnostic tests and initiate therapy in high-risk situations (9). Treatment goals include inhibition of further clot propagation, prevention of pulmonary embolism, and prevention of recurrent venous thromboembolism. In addition, long-term sequelae, such as postthrombotic syndrome, venous insufficiency, pulmonary hypertension, and right-sided heart failure may be avoided.

For this manuscript, a PubMed literature search was performed with the search criteria "DVT," "PE," "VTE," "gynecologic oncology," "gynecologic surgery," "obstetrics," "surgical complications," and "medical complications of pregnancy" from January 1973 to July 2006. Relevant articles were reviewed, with priority given to randomized trials and prospective studies. The Cochrane database also was searched using the previously listed terms.

Prevention Strategies

The important consideration when evaluating patients are: who needs prophylaxis, what to use as prophylaxis, and when to initiate and stop prophylaxis. Prevention should be the hallmark for all patients who are at risk for development of venous thromboembolism.

Patients Who Need Prophylaxis

Preoperative testing has been evaluated to identify patients who are at high risk for the development of venous thromboembolism. In an evaluation of coagulation parameters in patients with gynecologic malignancies, and specifically D-dimers, which are small molecules found in the circulation after fibrinolysis of thrombi, patients with elevated D-dimer and fibrinogen levels were at increased risk of transfusion, but there was no association with the development of venous thromboembolism (10). In another evaluation of preoperative D-dimer levels in patients undergoing gynecologic oncology surgery, an elevated D-dimer level was not predictive of subsequent venous thromboembolism (11). Therefore, preoperative evaluation is not recommended as a means of predicting venous thromboembolism risk. Instead, clinicians should rely on clinical factors that have been shown to correlate with risk for development of venous thromboembolism.

Box 21-1 lists risk factors for the development of venous thromboembolism, many of which are commonly encountered in the obstetric and gynecologic population (12–20). Pregnancy alone increases the risk of venous thromboembolism by five times when compared with nonpregnant controls (18–20). The physiologic changes associated with pregnancy that increase this risk include the presence of venous stasis, hypercoagulability state caused by the increased production of clotting factors, decreased thrombolysis, decreased protein S, increased platelet activation, and intimal damage associated with delivery. Malignancy predisposes patients to DVT through increased release of thromboplastin, increased activation of factor X, and decreased fibrinolysis (21). Perioperative blood transfusion also appears to increase DVT risk (22). Box 21-2 lists risk categories based on risk factors and type of surgery performed, with options for prophylaxis.

Methods of Prophylaxis

The ideal method for prevention of venous thromboembolism must be safe, effective, cost-effective, and acceptable for large-scale use by patients. Current prevention

264

BOX 21-1

RISK FACTORS FOR DEVELOPMENT OF DEEP VEIN THROMBOSIS

- Obesity (body mass index greater than 30)
- Malignancy
- Abdominal or pelvic surgery
- Age (older than 40 years)
- Pregnancy
- Smoking
- Chronic venous stasis
- History of deep vein thrombosis or pulmonary embolism
- Inherited thrombophilia
- Congestive heart failure
- Diabetes
- Varicose veins
- Estrogen use
- Trauma
- Malignancy
- Immobilization
- Selective estrogen receptor modulator use
- Pregnancy
- Thrombophilias
  —Factor V Leiden (homozygous)
  —Factor V Leiden (heterozygous)
  —Protein C deficiency
  —Protein S deficiency
  —Prothrombin gene mutation
  —Hyperhomocysteinemia
  —Antithrombin deficiency

Venous thromboembolism in obstetrics and gynecology. Obstet Gynecol 2007;109:761–77.

BOX 21-2

CATEGORIES OF DEEP VEIN THROMBOSIS IN SURGICAL PATIENTS

Low risk
- Minor surgery (eg, bilateral tubal ligation), no additional risk factors
- Prophylaxis—none typically required, may use graduated compression stockings or early ambulation

Intermediate risk
- Minor surgery, patients with additional risk factors
- Major surgery in patients 40–60 years old (eg, total abdominal hysterectomy), no additional risk factors
- Prophylaxis—pneumatic compression devices or low molecular weight heparin or subcutaneous unfractionated heparin

High risk
- Major surgery (eg, ovarian cancer debulking) in patients with additional risk factors
- Prophylaxis—low molecular weight heparin, subcutaneous unfractionated heparin three times per day, pneumatic compression devices

Very high risk
- Major surgery (eg, total pelvic exenteration), patients with multiple risk factors
- Patients with a history of venous thromboembolism
- Patients with known inherited thrombophilia
- Patients with known cancer
- Prophylaxis—low molecular weight heparin, once daily; subcutaneous unfractionated heparin, three times daily; consideration for dual prophylaxis with low molecular weight heparin and pneumatic compression devices or graduated compression stockings and low molecular weight heparin

Venous thromboembolism in obstetrics and gynecology. Obstet Gynecol 2007;109:761–77.

---

strategies include early ambulation, graduated compression stockings, pneumatic compression devices, and anticoagulants such as warfarin, subcutaneous unfractionated heparin, and low molecular weight heparin (1, 2, 21, 23–37). Figure 21-1 illustrates the coagulation cascade and where the pharmacologic agents have their specific effects. The use of a specific prophylactic regimen should be based on the clinician's assessment of the risk of the patient developing DVT. The cost-effectiveness of venous thromboembolism prophylaxis in gynecologic surgery has been studied. All of the methods studied, including the use of subcutaneous unfractionated heparin, low molecular weight heparin, and pneumatic compression devices, were cost-effective when compared with no therapy. The most cost-effective measure was the use of pneumatic compression devices (38).

Graduated compression stockings are placed over the lower extremity and have pressure differences throughout the stocking to decrease pooling of venous blood. Studies evaluating the use of graduated compression stockings have shown that this intervention may be effective in preventing venous thromboembolism in gynecologic surgery with few side effects (29). A prospective trial in the United Kingdom demonstrated that the use of graduated compression stockings in patients undergoing gynecologic surgery led to a decrease in DVT formation. In this study DVT was confirmed by ^{125}I-radiolabeled fibrinogen testing. Four patients in the control arm who did not receive DVT prophylaxis developed DVT compared with zero cases of DVT in the 104 patients who used graduated compression stockings (29). No adverse outcomes were noted to be caused by the graduated compression stockings.

Pneumatic compression devices, also called sequential compression devices, extend to either the knee or

Intrinsic pathway

Extrinsic pathway

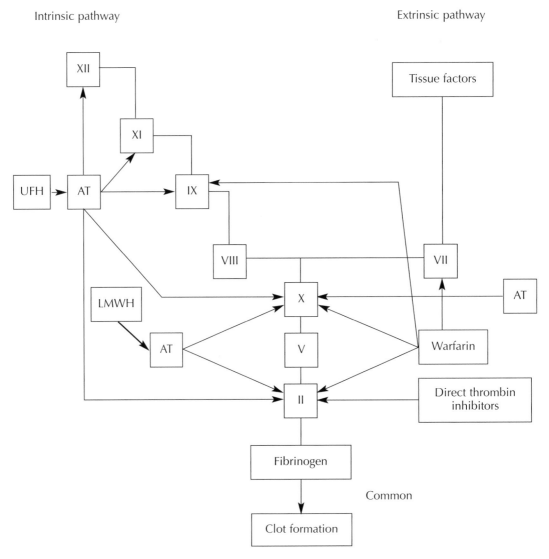

Fig. 21-1. Effects of anticoagulants on the coagulation cascade. Abbreviations: AT, antithrombin; LMWH, low molecular weight heparin; UFH, unfractionated heparin. (Originally published in Haines ST. Update on the prevention of venous thromboembolism. Am J Health-Syst Pharm 2004;7:S5–S11. Copyright © 2004, American Society of Health-System Pharmacists, Inc. All rights reserved. Reprinted with permission [R0635].)

thigh and have been used as DVT prophylaxis. The use of pneumatic compression devices decreases the risk of clot formation by stimulation of the release of fibrinolytic factors as well as by the mechanical compression and prevention of the pooling of venous blood. In a study of the use of perioperative pneumatic compression devices, it was found that patients using pneumatic compression devices at the time of anesthesia induction and for 24 hours postoperatively did not demonstrate any benefit in reduction of DVT when compared with patients not using prophylaxis (39). A follow-up study by the same group, however, used pneumatic compression devices placed intraoperatively and continued use postoperatively for 5 days. This trial demonstrated a benefit with a

reduction in DVT from 34% to 12.7% (40). This group also retrospectively studied which patients developed DVT despite the use of pneumatic compression devices. The risk factors identified included a history of prior DVT, cancer, and age greater than 60 years. Deep vein thrombosis risk increased with the presence of more risk factors (32). Together, the results of these studies indicate that pneumatic compression devices used at the time of induction of anesthesia and postoperatively for 5 days will decrease the risk of venous thromboembolism with few complications.

Pharmacologic agents that are used for DVT prevention include vitamin K antagonists (warfarin), unfractionated heparin, and low molecular weight heparin.

Unfractionated heparin is a mixture of polysaccharide chains with varying molecular weights, from 3,000 daltons to 30,000 daltons, that affect factor Xa and thrombin. Low molecular weight heparin consists of fragments of unfractionated heparin that have a predictable anticoagulant response and have a greater activity against factor Xa (4). Studies evaluating anticoagulant-based prophylaxis in gynecologic and general surgery consistently have had results demonstrating a benefit from pharmacologic prophylaxis (24, 41–48). In a meta-analysis of patients undergoing urologic, orthopedic, and general surgery, it was concluded that use of subcutaneous unfractionated heparin was effective in preventing DVT in moderate- and high-risk patients, with a slight increase in bleeding complications (43). No gynecologic surgery was included in the meta-analysis. The exact heparin dosage (twice daily versus three times daily) was not evaluated. In a 1978 study, the use of oral anticoagulation or subcutaneous unfractionated heparin in one arm of the study was examined, while a control arm received saline. In this study, patients were considered to be at intermediate risk for DVT because they underwent major gynecologic surgery. The patients were found to have equal rates of DVT in the oral anticoagulation group (6.3%) and subcutaneous unfractionated heparin arm (6.3%), compared with the control arm in which patients had a 23% rate of DVT (24).

The use of subcutaneous unfractionated heparin has been compared with no prophylaxis use for DVT prevention in patients who had gynecologic surgery. Twice daily doses of 5,000 units of subcutaneous unfractionated heparin decreased detection of DVT compared with the control group (29% versus 3%) (44). However, no benefit was found from the use of subcutaneous unfractionated heparin in gynecologic oncology patients. Patients were given 5,000 units of subcutaneous unfractionated heparin 2 hours before surgery and then postoperatively, twice daily, for 7 days. The authors concluded that no benefit from subcutaneous unfractionated heparin use might have been seen because the control group had an unusually low rate of venous thromboembolism (12.7%), making it difficult to show a statistically significant reduction in risk (46). In subsequent work, subcutaneous unfractionated heparin dosages were evaluated by randomizing patients to 5,000 units twice daily, 5,000 units three times daily, or no prophylaxis. A clinical benefit was seen in both groups using subcutaneous unfractionated heparin compared with the control arm. The authors concluded that, although both dosages were effective at decreasing DVT, they favored the three times daily regimen because of the lack of benefit from twice daily dosages in the previous study and the lack of increased complications with three times daily dosages

(47). The same group then compared the use of subcutaneous unfractionated heparin with the use of pneumatic compression devices in patients treated on the gynecologic oncology service at Duke University. The techniques showed similar efficacy with respect to prevention of venous thromboembolism (6.5% versus 4%, respectively); however, more bleeding complications were seen in the group that used subcutaneous unfractionated heparin (27). A follow-up study reported on 182 patients who were treated with 5,000 units of subcutaneous unfractionated heparin, given 2 hours preoperatively and every 12 hours postoperatively for 7 days. Although there were increases in intraoperative blood loss, wound hematomas, and transfusion requirements in patients who were treated with subcutaneous unfractionated heparin, these increases were not statistically significant. The authors concluded that use of both pneumatic compression devices and subcutaneous unfractionated heparin appear effective as methods of prophylaxis, but there may be increased bleeding complications with subcutaneous unfractionated heparin use (48).

Low molecular weight heparin was introduced as prophylaxis because of theoretical advantages such as decreased risk of bleeding complications and a once daily dosage (41, 42, 45, 49). In a randomized controlled trial, patients treated with low molecular weight heparin were compared with patients using postoperative pneumatic compression devices. The treatments were similar with respect to prevention of DVT, with two patients in the group using low molecular weight heparin and one patient in the group using pneumatic compression devices developing DVT. The group using low molecular weight heparin did not experience more bleeding episodes, leading to the conclusion that both methods are safe and effective for prevention of DVT (49). Subsequently, compliance and preference of patients using low molecular weight heparin was compared with patients using pneumatic compression devices. Patient compliance and satisfaction were not significantly different between the two methods (50).

Other trials have evaluated low molecular weight heparin use in general and gynecologic surgery. In a study of the use of low molecular weight heparin in patients undergoing abdominal surgery, patients were randomized between dalteparin, 2,500 units once daily, and subcutaneous unfractionated heparin, 5,000 units twice daily. There was no significant difference in the rate of DVT or bleeding episodes (42). In two reports, the experience of gynecologic patients who used different doses of low molecular weight heparin was described. In the first trial, a once-daily dose of 5,000 units of dalteparin was compared with a twice-daily dose of subcutaneous unfractionated heparin. The regimens were equally effective at preventing DVT. However, the group using low molecular weight heparin had more bleeding complications than the group using subcutaneous unfractionated heparin (41). The second study, however, did not show increased bleeding with the use of low molecular weight heparin, but it continued to demonstrate equal efficacy compared with the use of subcutaneous unfractionated heparin (45). The difference in bleeding between the two studies is most likely because of the higher dose of low molecular weight heparin the patients received in the initial study.

Anticoagulation therapy with unfractionated heparin and low molecular weight heparin has risks. The main risks include bleeding, osteoporosis (with prolonged therapy with unfractionated heparin), and heparin-induced thrombocytopenia (51, 52). The risks of bleeding with unfractionated heparin use appear to be higher because of unfractionated heparin-binding proteins and the unpredictable response in individual patients. Low molecular weight heparin use has been associated with less bleeding than unfractionated heparin use, with a more predictable patient response. Proper dosages of low molecular weight heparin in morbidly obese patients is not well studied. The development of heparin-induced thrombocytopenia is a potential life-threatening complication if not recognized. Patients treated with unfractionated heparin have approximately a 3% risk of heparin-induced thrombocytopenia. This risk appears to be lower in patients treated with low molecular weight heparin (51). A consensus among experts has evolved suggesting that the use of low molecular weight heparin is preferred over subcutaneous unfractionated heparin because of easier dosages, equivalent efficacy, and equivalent or decreased complication rates (53).

Randomized trials are lacking to describe the indications, risks, and complications of inferior vena cava (IVC) filter placement. In a review of IVC filter placement for prophylaxis in surgical patients, common indications for placement included the need for perioperative protection in patients at high risk for bleeding who are taking anticoagulants, an active DVT in patients requiring surgery, and an inability to provide anticoagulation for patients because of allergic reactions to heparins in the presence of an active DVT (36, 37). The contraindications for the use of heparin appear in Box 21-3; these patients may benefit from IVC filter placement. A single institution's experience with the use of IVC filter placement indicated that the prevalence of fatal pulmonary embolism was 3.7%; of major complications, 0.3%; of postfilter caval thrombosis, 2.7%. The authors concluded that IVC filter placement was safe and effective for prevention of life-threatening pulmonary embolism (36). Complications from IVC filter placement reported in additional studies

---

| **BOX 21-3** |

CONTRAINDICATIONS FOR HEPARIN THERAPY
- Active bleeding
- History of heparin-induced thrombocytopenia
- History of bleeding ulcer
- History of anaphylaxis to heparins
- Recent surgical procedure

Venous thromboembolism in obstetrics and gynecology. Obstet Gynecol 2007;109:761–77.

---

include filter migration, incomplete protection from pulmonary embolism, IVC perforation, worsening of lower extremity edema, and the need for anticoagulation (if possible) to protect against heightened DVT risk below the IVC filter (35–37).

Some investigators have started using "dual prophylaxis" in high-risk patients. Most often, heparin and pneumatic compression devices are used in combination, although early ambulation and graduated compression stockings also may be employed. A randomized trial compared the use of single prophylaxis with low molecular weight heparin to prophylaxis using low molecular weight heparin and graduated compression stockings. In another study, similar rates of venous thromboembolism were found in the two groups, and it was concluded that this combination of dual prophylaxis was not beneficial (31). However, in a cost-effectiveness analysis that evaluated combination prophylaxis in high-risk gynecologic oncology patients, it was demonstrated that low molecular weight heparin use combined with the use of pneumatic compression devices would be a cost-effective intervention in high-risk gynecologic oncology patients and merits evaluation in prospective trials (54). Dual prophylaxis has been studied in patients who have undergone colorectal surgery. A Cochrane review of that literature recommended the combination of graduated compression stockings used with low molecular weight heparin as prophylaxis in this high-risk group of patients (55).

Initiating and Stopping Prophylaxis

Initial trials investigating DVT formation demonstrated that 50% of DVT cases form during surgery whereas 25% occur within 72 hours after surgery (21). Therefore, it is important to initiate prophylaxis before induction of anesthesia in moderate- to high-risk patients. Graduated compression stockings and pneumatic compression devices may be placed on patients before they enter the operating room. Preoperative administration of low molecular weight heparin or subcutaneous unfractionated heparin in high-risk patients has been shown to have an acceptable complication rate (23–29, 38–49, 53,

56–58). An increased risk of operative bleeding and blood transfusion has not been consistently demonstrated throughout numerous studies, whereas the benefit of a reduction in DVT has been shown (23–29, 38–49, 53, 56–58). Surgeons must decide which patients may preoperatively receive subcutaneous unfractionated heparin or low molecular weight heparin based on the individual concerns for intraoperative bleeding and postoperative complications.

The duration of prophylaxis depends on the risk of development of DVT. Once patients are ambulatory, discontinuation of prophylaxis in most patients is acceptable at the time of discharge. The length of postoperative low molecular weight heparin prophylaxis has been evaluated in patients with known gynecologic malignancies. Enoxaparin, 40 mg, was given subcutaneously, once daily for either 1 week or 4 weeks postoperatively. A statistically significant decrease in the rate of venous thromboembolism from 12% to 4.8% was observed, favoring the 4-week arm. There were no significant differences in complications between the two groups in 2 months of follow-up (58).

The following summary lists recommendations for prophylaxis in gynecologic surgery:

1. Physicians should assess a patient's risk for venous thromboembolism based on clinical risk factors.
2. In patients at low risk for venous thromboembolism, early ambulation or a combination of graduated compression stockings and early ambulation may be used for prophylaxis.
3. In patients at intermediate risk for venous thromboembolism, early ambulation, graduated compression stockings, or pneumatic compression devices may be used for prophylaxis (but not typically both graduated compression stockings and pneumatic compression devices). Subcutaneous unfractionated heparin or low molecular weight heparin may be considered but carry a risk of complications.
4. In high-risk patients, early ambulation, graduated compression stockings or pneumatic compression devices, and subcutaneous unfractionated heparin or low molecular weight heparin may be used for venous thromboembolism prophylaxis.
5. In very high-risk patients, low molecular weight heparin or subcutaneous unfractionated heparin, three times daily, may be used. Dual prophylaxis with pneumatic compression devices and subcutaneous unfractionated heparin or low molecular weight heparin has not been proved to decrease the rate of DVT in gynecologic patients but may be considered in particularly high-risk situations such as known malignancy.

6. Postoperative prophylaxis for 4 weeks with low molecular weight heparin should be considered in patients with malignancy.
7. Although low molecular weight heparin has not been shown to be more efficacious than subcutaneous unfractionated heparin for DVT prophylaxis, ease of dosage and decreased side effects, such as heparin-induced thrombocytopenia, make the use of low molecular weight heparin more favorable.
8. Subcutaneous unfractionated heparin is still preferred in patients with renal failure.

The dosage of subcutaneous unfractionated heparin is 5,000 units every 8 hours, and the dosage of low molecular weight heparin (enoxaparin) is 40 mg every day.

Obstetric Management

Obstetric patients have venous stasis, increased blood volume, and changes in thrombosis and fibrinolysis that put them at risk for development of venous thromboembolism (33, 34). Women with a known thrombophilia, a history of previous venous thromboembolism, or a pregnancy complication requiring prolonged bed rest may be at particular risk (33). Prophylaxis is recommended during pregnancy for patients who have had a previous DVT during pregnancy, patients with an artificial heart valve, and patients with a known thrombophilia and prior DVT (59–61). Subcutaneous unfractionated heparin, intravenous unfractionated heparin, and low molecular weight heparin all have been shown to be safe during pregnancy (28, 34, 52, 62–64).

Patients with thrombophilia and a previous venous thromboembolism complication are at high risk for venous thromboembolism during pregnancy (5, 6, 61, 62). Currently, protein C deficiency, protein S deficiency, factor V Leiden mutation, and prothrombin G20210A mutation increase the risk of venous thromboembolism during pregnancy and merit prophylaxis. In a study of patients with a factor V Leiden or prothrombin G20210A mutation who had no prior venous thromboembolism, the patients did not appear to be at increased risk for venous thromboembolism during pregnancy (6). However, subsequently this group of patients was found to have an increased risk of venous thromboembolism during pregnancy and the puerperium (5). Patients with venous thromboembolism during pregnancy and no known risk factor should be referred for evaluation of a possible inherited thrombophilia (65).

In patients with prior DVT during pregnancy, the risk of recurrent DVT is approximately 5.6%. Antenatal prophylaxis should be used (34). If DVT occurred because of a transient risk factor that is no longer present and was not related to pregnancy, prophylaxis may be withheld. Women with a history of prior venous thromboembolism because of increased estrogen exposure (oral contraception) may be at increased risk for DVT during subsequent pregnancies. This group of patients should have prophylactic doses of subcutaneous unfractionated heparin or low molecular weight heparin initiated during the first trimester and continued for 6 weeks postpartum. In patients who had venous thromboembolism and were tested for thrombophilia and noted to have no genetic predisposition for venous thromboembolism, there were no episodes of recurrent venous thromboembolism. The authors concluded that withholding prophylaxis in this group of patients might be safe (66). A cost-effectiveness analysis demonstrated similar results. In this Markov model, prophylaxis was recommended only if the prior DVT was complicated by high-risk factors that were not considered to be transient (67).

Patients who are prescribed prolonged bed rest because of pregnancy complications are at risk for the development of DVT. There are little clinical data available regarding the use of low molecular weight heparin, subcutaneous unfractionated heparin, or pneumatic compression devices in this group of patients. Researchers have recommended against routine heparin prophylaxis because a retrospective analysis showed that the risk of DVT from prolonged bed rest is less than 1% whereas the risk of complications from heparin prophylaxis is at least 1% (4). No evaluation of pneumatic compression devices was included. The use of pneumatic compression devices or graduated compression stockings may be a low-risk alternative to heparin use for venous thromboembolism prophylaxis, but this issue has not been studied adequately.

Patients who undergo cesarean delivery are at increased risk when compared with patients who give birth vaginally (68–70). Studies evaluating different prophylaxis regimens have been underpowered, limiting their usefulness (68–70). In a published decision-tree analysis, the use of pneumatic compression devices was recommended in patients undergoing cesarean delivery because of concerns that heparin could cause unacceptable side effects such as postoperative bleeding and heparin-induced thrombocytopenia. The conclusion was that routine use of subcutaneous unfractionated heparin is not warranted for patients who have a cesarean delivery (70).

Therapy for pregnant patients with artificial heart valves is controversial because there are no randomized trials, and treatment recommendations based on expert opinions vary greatly. Reports of valvular thrombi and venous thromboembolism, occurring despite the use of therapeutic low molecular weight heparin, have raised concern for the use of this therapy in this subset of patients (71–74). One series examined 48 pregnancies in 37 women with mechanical heart valves. Two patients were treated with heparin and the remaining patients were treated with warfarin. In patients treated with heparin, two valvular thromboses occurred, requiring surgical intervention. The pregnancies ended in preoperative spontaneous abortions. There were no valvular complications in the patients treated with warfarin during pregnancy. The fetal outcomes in the patients treated with warfarin included 27 healthy infants, 2 stillbirths, 1 embryopathy, and 16 spontaneous abortions. The authors concluded that warfarin is preferable for prophylaxis in pregnant patients with mechanical heart valves (74). However, the high rate of fetal complications seen in patients treated with warfarin indicates that alternative therapy for patients with artificial heart valves should be considered. Some experts recommend the use of subcutaneous unfractionated heparin or low molecular weight heparin during the first and third trimesters of pregnancy, substituting warfarin during the second trimester to limit fetal exposure to warfarin (75). Warfarin crosses the placenta and can lead to fetal malformation and pregnancy loss (75, 76). The use of warfarin during pregnancy has been associated with nasal hypoplasia, stippled epiphyses, and central nervous system abnormalities. An alternative approach for anticoagulation in this group of patients includes conversion of treatment to subcutaneous unfractionated heparin, three times daily, or low molecular weight heparin, twice daily, with doses increasing throughout pregnancy (75). These treatment plans are obviously quite different. Therefore, it seems prudent to recommend that patients with artificial heart valves undergo extensive counseling with experts in maternal–fetal medicine and cardiology, ideally before pregnancy is attempted.

There are no randomized studies to guide the management of anticoagulation at the time of delivery. Expert opinions suggest that patients taking subcutaneous unfractionated heparin or low molecular weight heparin should be instructed to stop therapy when they go into labor to decrease bleeding complications and facilitate the use of epidural anesthesia. Scheduled induction after 37 weeks of gestation may assist in the timing of delivery and minimize bleeding complications. When induction is scheduled, patients should be instructed to stop anticoagulation therapy 24 hours before induction of labor. If spontaneous labor occurs, reversal of anticoagulation therapy may be accomplished with protamine sulfate in patients treated with unfractionated heparin and liberal use of fresh frozen plasma if bleeding complications occur in a patient treated with low molecular weight heparin.

There are no large clinical trials available to help guide the management of anticoagulation postpartum. Patients continue to be at increased risk for venous thromboembolism during the postpartum period and should be treated with subcutaneous unfractionated heparin, low molecular weight heparin, or warfarin. If anticoagulation therapy is indicated, therapy for patients taking prophylactic doses of subcutaneous unfractionated heparin or low molecular weight heparin may be initiated when the clinician's assessment of postpartum bleeding is acceptable (typically 4–8 hours after uncomplicated vaginal delivery and 24 hours after cesarean delivery). Patients who are at highest risk, such as patients with artificial heart valves, may have therapeutic doses of intravenous unfractionated heparin or low molecular weight heparin started 4–6 hours after delivery and then converted to prepregnancy anticoagulation.

The following summary lists recommendations for obstetric prophylaxis:

1. No randomized data exist to guide decisions regarding venous thromboembolism prophylaxis during pregnancy. Therefore, recommendations are largely based on retrospective studies and expert opinions.

2. Patients who are prescribed prolonged bed rest during pregnancy with no other risk factors may use graduated compression stockings. Routine use of heparin prophylaxis is not recommended.

3. Patients with a history of DVT and other known risk factors for venous thromboembolism should be treated with prophylactic doses of subcutaneous unfractionated heparin or low molecular weight heparin in subsequent pregnancies.

4. Patients with a history of previous DVT during pregnancy or associated with hormonal contraception should receive subcutaneous unfractionated heparin or low molecular weight heparin prophylaxis in subsequent pregnancies.

5. Pregnant patients with a known prior venous thromboembolism caused by estrogen exposure require prophylactic doses of subcutaneous unfractionated heparin or low molecular weight heparin initiated in the first trimester and continued for 6 weeks postpartum.

6. Pregnant patients with a known thrombophilia and history of previous venous thromboembolism should undergo prophylaxis with subcutaneous unfractionated heparin or low molecular weight heparin during pregnancy.

7. Routine prophylaxis with subcutaneous unfractionated heparin or low molecular weight heparin is not recommended in patients who have a cesarean delivery; early ambulation, graduated compression stockings, or pneumatic compression devices can be considered.

8. Patients with artificial heart valves should consult with experts, preferably before conception, regarding the management of anticoagulation during pregnancy.

9. Patients taking oral anticoagulants before pregnancy should be converted to subcutaneous unfractionated heparin or low molecular weight heparin when appropriate and receive the full dosage for therapeutic anticoagulation.

The prophylactic dosage of subcutaeous unfractionated heparin is 5,000 units every 12 hours or low molecular weight heparin (enoxaparin), 40 mg daily, at a fixed dose throughout pregnancy. The dosage may be adjusted and increased throughout pregnancy if activated partial thromboplastin time or factor Xa levels are monitored. For therapeutic treatment, the dosage of subcutaneous unfractionated heparin may be increased to 10,000 units two to three times per day, adjusting to maintain an activated partial thromboplastin time of 1.5–2, or low molecular weight heparin (enoxaparin) 30–80 mg every 12 hours.

Diagnosis

Clinical assessments of patients with suspected DVT are limited (2, 9). Patients may have no symptoms or symptoms that are nonspecific, such as lower extremity edema. Tests for evaluation for DVT include D-dimer testing, duplex Doppler ultrasonography, impedance plethysmography, and venography (77, 78).

D-dimer testing may be used as a complementary test with ultrasonography when evaluating patients for possible DVT. D-dimer testing has such a high sensitivity (85%) and an excellent negative predictive value that some investigators feel that a negative test result in combination with a low clinical pretest probability excludes DVT (79–82). However, the value of D-dimer test results during pregnancy or in the presence of malignancy is limited by the elevated levels that occur with these conditions, even in the absence of venous thromboembolism (83). In addition, the use of D-dimer testing in the postoperative period is of limited value because of tissue trauma and activation of fibrinolysis. D-dimer testing can be considered a screening tool but, in and of itself, an elevated level is not diagnostic of venous thromboembolism. In obstetric, oncology, and postoperative patients, a diagnostic test such as ultrasonography is advised.

Duplex Doppler ultrasonography can be used either in combination with D-dimer screening or alone to evaluate for the presence of DVT. Serial ultrasonography has been used to evaluate patients with clinical suspicion of DVT and initial negative compression ultrasound findings (84, 85). Impedance plethysmography and radiolabeled fibrinogen uptake testing were used in studies performed in the 1970s and 1980s. However, because of the complexity of these tests, they have been largely replaced in contemporary practice by compression ultrasonography. Venography has been the preferred technique for the diagnosis of venous thromboembolism. However, the high sensitivity of compression and duplex Doppler ultrasonography and the ease of performing these tests have limited the use of venography for the diagnosis of DVT. Venography remains useful for patients with persistent symptoms and negative noninvasive test results, who are at high risk for venous thromboembolism and have contraindications to anticoagulation therapy. Figure 21-2 is an algorithm for evaluating patients for suspected DVT.

As with DVT, pulmonary embolism is difficult to diagnose because patients may have few signs or nonspecific symptoms, delaying evaluation for pulmonary embolism (86–88). The signs and symptoms in patients with pulmonary embolism include shortness of breath, chest pain, tachycardia, tachypnea, fever, and anxiety.

Contrary to popular belief, low oxygen saturation is not a common presenting sign of pulmonary embolism unless it is a massive saddle embolus. Ultimately, untreated pulmonary embolism may lead to clot propagation, pulmonary hypertension, right-sided heart failure, and death (89). Laboratory studies and diagnostic tests to consider include arterial blood gas, complete blood count, chest X-ray, ventilation–perfusion scan, helical computed tomography (CT) scan, compression ultrasonography of lower extremities, and pulmonary angiography (90–96). Chest X-ray may not be diagnostic but assists in excluding differential diagnoses such as pleural effusions, pneumonia, pneumothorax, and pulmonary edema. Ventilation–perfusion scan should not be performed if an underlying abnormality is detected in the chest X-ray because of the high likelihood that it will be nondiagnostic. In this setting, helical CT scans can be helpful in not only evaluating patients for pulmonary embolisms but also assessing other pulmonary pathology such as pneumonia or effusion.

The sentinel study of the use of ventilation–perfusion scanning is the Prospective Investigation of Pulmonary Embolism Diagnosis Study, which evaluated the clinical utility of ventilation–perfusion scanning and

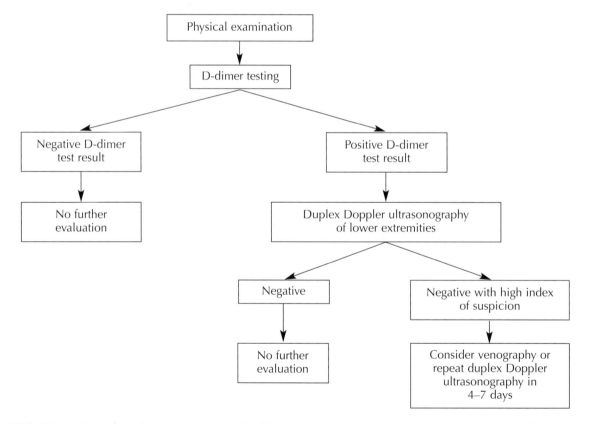

Fig. 21-2. Diagnostic algorithm for deep vein thrombosis. If the duplex Doppler ultrasonography results are positive, begin anticoagulation therapy with low molecular weight heparin or unfractionated heparin. If contraindications for anticoagulation exist, consider placement of an inferior vena caval filter. (Venous thromboembolism in obstetrics and gynecology. Obstet Gynecol 2007;109:761–77.)

additional tests in patients with suspected pulmonary embolism (95). The low-probability and high-probability categories for ventilation–perfusion scanning were found to correlate well with low and high rates of pulmonary embolism on angiography, respectively. Clinical follow-up and angiography confirmed that 12% of patients with low probability ventilation–perfusion scanning results had a pulmonary embolism. Patients with nondiagnostic ventilation–perfusion scanning results and normal ultrasound findings of the lower extremities have a low risk for development of pulmonary embolism (14). Patients with intermediate probability ventilation–perfusion scanning results and patients with low probability ventilation–perfusion scanning results but a high clinical suspicion and multiple risk factors for venous thromboembolism merit further testing, which would include helical CT scanning or pulmonary angiography.

Ventilation–perfusion scanning has been shown to have clinical use in obstetric patients (96, 97). In a report on 82 pregnant patients referred for ventilation–perfusion scanning during pregnancy from 1990 to 1995, no patient with a normal or low probability ventilation–perfusion scanning result developed a pulmonary embolism (96). Patients with intermediate- or high-probability results received anticoagulation with no adverse outcomes. The use of helical CT scans during pregnancy has been reported to expose the fetus to a lower dose of radiation than would be encountered with ventilation–perfusion scanning (98, 99). Helical CT scan sensitivity and specificity are high and have resulted in decreased use of pulmonary angiography (99). A cost-effectiveness analysis comparing the use of helical CT scanning, ventilation–perfusion scanning, and duplex Doppler ultrasonography favored the use of helical CT scanning. Increased sensitivity of helical CT scanning for detecting pulmonary embolism, decreased need for follow-up testing, and decreased need for pulmonary angiography were reported. The author concluded that helical CT scanning should be used early in the evaluation of patients with suspected pulmonary embolism (100). Figure 21-3 is a diagnostic algorithm for patients with suspected pulmonary embolism.

In patients in whom venous thromboembolism is being considered but who also are at risk for bleeding, the feasibility of withholding anticoagulation, with a single duplex Doppler ultrasonography performed in the nonpregnant patient population has been evaluated. Of the 445 patients evaluated with duplex Doppler ultrasonography of the deep veins from the inguinal ligament to the malleolus, DVT was diagnosed in 61. Of the 375 patients who completed 3 months of follow-up, DVT was diagnosed subsequently in only three. No adverse outcomes with respect to pulmonary embolism were noted in this prospective trial (101).

Treatment

Anticoagulation therapy is required in patients with symptomatic proximal DVT because untreated patients have a 50% chance of having an acute pulmonary embolism. Management may include subcutaneous unfractionated heparin, intravenous unfractionated heparin, low molecular weight heparin, warfarin, IVC filter placement, and thrombolytic therapy. Classic treatment for stable postoperative patients with newly diagnosed DVT consisted of intravenous unfractionated heparin followed by warfarin (102, 103). Nomograms have been developed to assist in determining the appropriate dosage of intravenous unfractionated heparin to keep the activated partial thromboplastin time approximately 1.5–2 times the upper limit of normal (104, 105). However, the cost, need for blood to be drawn frequently, and the complication rate associated with intravenous unfractionated heparin led to interest in low molecular weight heparin in the treatment of venous thromboembolism (55, 106–114).

Low molecular weight heparin was as effective as intravenous unfractionated heparin in numerous studies (55, 106–114). Low molecular weight heparin was easily administered, required less laboratory evaluation, and improved predictability of therapeutic anticoagulation. The use of low molecular weight heparin at home has been shown to be safe and effective, without increased morbidity (114). Patients with DVT or pulmonary embolism may receive therapeutic anticoagulation with low molecular weight heparin. Warfarin may be initiated at the same time.

The appropriate duration of anticoagulation after venous thromboembolism to decrease the rate of recurrent thrombosis has been evaluated in numerous studies (115–118). In one study, patients with their first episode of venography-confirmed proximal DVT were treated with warfarin for 4 weeks compared with 3 months. The conclusions were that patients with ongoing risk factors for development of DVT might require oral anticoagulation therapy for more than 3 months (115). Decreased thromboembolic complications occurred in patients with their first episode of DVT who were treated with oral anticoagulation therapy for 6 months when compared with 3 months of treatment. The authors concluded that the patients had a high rate of recurrent venous thromboembolism when anticoagulation was discontinued at 3 months and recommended prolongation of oral anticoagulation for longer than 3 months. The side effects of the prolonged oral anticoagulation included an increased risk of serious bleeding. However, this risk is not as great as the risk of a fatal complication from discontinuing anticoagulation therapy (116). In another study, patients treated with oral anticoagulation therapy after a second idiopathic venous thromboembolism were evaluated. The trial compared patients treated with anticoagulation therapy for 6 months with treatment that was continued indefinitely. The results showed a risk of recurrent venous thromboembolism in the 4-year follow-up period, which was 20.7% for the 3-month treatment group compared with 2.6% for the indefinite treatment group. The authors concluded that patients should be treated for longer than 6 months. In the patients receiving

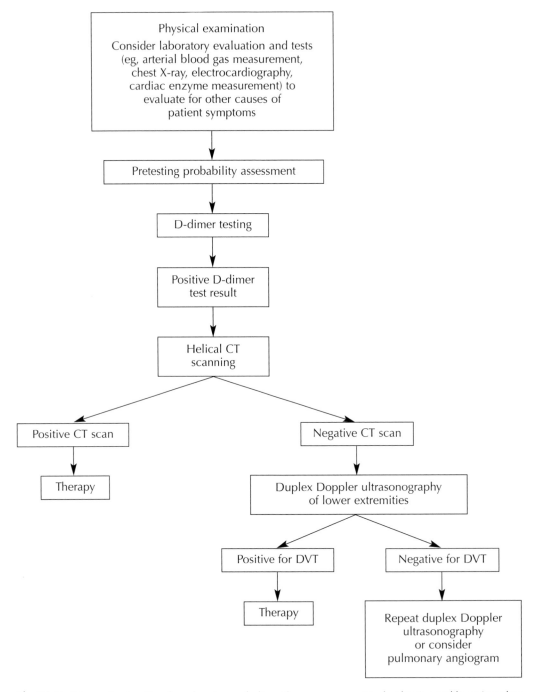

Fig. 21-3. Diagnostic algorithm for pulmonary embolism. Therapy may consist of unfractionated heparin or low molecular weight heparin, as well as supportive care (supplemental oxygen). If the patient is unstable, thrombolytic therapy may be considered. If contraindication for anticoagulation exists, consider placement of inferior vena caval filter. If the D-dimer test result is negative and pretest probability is low, duplex Doppler ultrasonography of lower extremities would be considered. Withhold anticoagulation therapy if both test results are negative. (Venous thromboembolism in obstetrics and gynecology. Obstet Gynecol 2007;109:761–77.)

lifelong anticoagulation, however, there was a tendency for bleeding complications to increase, making the appropriate time to stop warfarin a matter of debate (117).

Although not an actual treatment for venous thromboembolism, IVC filters may be used in the management of DVT to prevent pulmonary embolism in patients in whom adequate anticoagulation cannot be achieved. In patients with known DVT at the time of surgery, they can be placed during the preoperative period. Other candidates include patients who experience propagation of the clot while receiving anticoagulation therapy or who cannot tolerate anticoagulation therapy because of side effects (34–37). Side effects and complications from IVC filters include erosion and perforation of the IVC filter, migration of the filter, improper placement, arteriovenous fistula formation, filter infection, IVC filter occlusion, and worsening lower extremity edema (35, 36). Additional concerns are the risks of new DVT, failure to prevent all pulmonary embolisms, and the potential need for lifelong anticoagulation therapy. Temporary IVC filters have been developed to try to address some of these concerns. These filters need to be rotated periodically to prevent significant fibrin deposition, necessitating the removal of the filter. Studies have shown good results with few complications, but as a new technology, recommendations for the length of time they can remain in place are variable (35).

Thrombolytic therapy may be initiated in patients with massive pulmonary embolism who are candidates. This situation is unlikely to occur in obstetric and gynecologic patients because pregnancy and recent surgery are contraindications to thrombolysis. Given the complication rate, thrombolytics should be reserved for life-threatening pulmonary embolism and used only in consultation with critical care specialists in an intensive care setting. Thrombectomy may be used in patients with massive pulmonary embolism or DVT that has progressed to significant arterial insufficiency because of the large DVT.

Following is a summary of treatment recommendations for venous thromboembolism and pulmonary embolism in gynecology:

1. Unless contraindicated, patients with venous thromboembolism may be treated with therapeutic doses of intravenous unfractionated heparin or low molecular weight heparin while being converted to warfarin.
2. For the first episode of venous thromboembolism, patients should be treated with oral anticoagulation therapy for 6 months.
3. For patients with a DVT in the presence of malignancy, continuation of treatment with low molecular weight heparin for the duration of an active malignancy is preferred. If this is not possible

because of patient compliance or cost, patients should be treated with warfarin.
4. For patients experiencing a second episode of venous thromboembolism, lifelong treatment with warfarin is recommended.
5. Patients with contraindications for anticoagulation therapy may have an IVC filter placed in an attempt to limit the risk of pulmonary embolism after careful consideration of the long-term complications.
6. Low molecular weight heparin should be avoided in patients with renal failure.
7. In patients with life-threatening acute venous thromboembolism, catheter-directed thrombolysis or thrombectomy might be considered in consultation with critical care experts.

The dosage of intravenous unfractionated heparin should be regulated to achieve an activated partial thromboplastin time of 1.5–2 times the upper limit of normal. The dosage of low molecular weight heparin (enoxaparin) should be 1 mg/kg every 12 hours or 1.5 mg/kg daily, although most experts prefer twice-daily dosages whenever possible. This is the bridge to warfarin to maintain an international normalized ratio of 2–3.

Traditionally, pregnant patients with venous thromboembolism receive a loading dose of unfractionated heparin followed by a continuous infusion for 5–7 days, with subsequent conversion to subcutaneous unfractionated heparin (28, 34). As discussed previously, warfarin is avoided in pregnancy because of concerns regarding fetal loss and malformations. As in the general population, however, the use of low molecular weight heparin has gained popularity in obstetric patients. Many studies have shown that the use of low molecular weight heparin in pregnancy is safe and as effective as the use of unfractionated heparin (28, 104, 119). In one review, the authors concluded that the use of low molecular weight heparin should be the treatment of choice for pregnant patients with venous thromboembolism. This recommendation was based on equivalent efficacy, improved safety, and ease of delivery of low molecular weight heparin when compared with intravenous unfractionated heparin and subcutaneous unfractionated heparin (119). When venous thromboembolism occurs in pregnancy the proposed duration of anticoagulation therapy after venous thromboembolism in pregnancy is from 6 weeks to 3 months postpartum but, as with nonpregnant women, should total at least 6 months for the first episode. (34, 75).

Inferior vena cava filters may be used in some obstetric patients who are unable to tolerate anticoagulation therapy or who experience clot propagation while receiving appropriate therapy. The use of temporary IVC filters to assist in the intrapartum management of 17 patients who had been receiving heparin anticoagulation throughout pregnancy has been studied. Although a small series, the results are encouraging, with successful placement and removal of the filters without complications (120). Thrombectomy also has been reported during pregnancy to relieve severe symptoms such as arterial insufficiency associated with venous thromboembolism. This procedure did have significant side effects, with 5 fetal losses in 97 pregnancies. The use of this aggressive therapy should be limited to patients who are not responding to or are unable to tolerate anticoagulation therapy (121). Treatment of massive DVT or pulmonary embolism with the use of new agents such as thrombolytics has been performed only in special circumstances (75).

The following summary lists treatment recommendations for obstetric patients with venous thromboembolic complications:

1. Intravenous unfractionated heparin, subcutaneous unfractionated heparin, or low molecular weight heparin may be used to treat venous thromboembolism in pregnancy, but low molecular weight heparin is preferred.
2. Patients with newly diagnosed venous thromboembolism who have no underlying thrombophilia or other risk factors should receive anticoagulation therapy combined with oral warfarin given for 6 weeks to 3 months postpartum for a total of at least 6 months.
3. Thrombectomy should be used with great caution and only in emergent situations because of the fetal loss rate associated with this procedure and the success of low molecular weight heparin.
4. The use of IVC filters may be considered during pregnancy and delivery in patients with contraindications to anticoagulation therapy.

The dosage of intravenous unfractionated heparin should be regulated to achieve an activated partial thromboplastin time of 1.5–2 times the upper limit of normal, with conversion to subcutaneous unfractionated heparin and escalating administration of heparin throughout pregnancy to maintain an activated partial thromboplastin time of 1.5–2 times the upper limit of normal. Low molecular weight heparin may be used with doses of enoxaparin, 30–80 mg twice daily, throughout pregnancy. Treatment should convert to warfarin postpartum with a target international normalized ratio of 2–3.

References

1. American College of Obstetricians and Gynecologists. Prevention of deep vein thrombosis and pulmonary embolism. ACOG Practice Bulletin 21. Washington, DC: ACOG; 2000.
2. Gherman RB, Goodwin TM, Leung B, Bryne JD, Hethumumi R, Montoro M. Incidence, clinical characteristics, and timing of objectively diagnosed venous thromboembolism during pregnancy. Obstet Gynecol 1999;94:730–4.
3. Bonnar J. Can more be done in obstetrics and gynecologic practice to reduce morbidity and mortality associated with venous thromboembolism? Am J Obstet Gynecol 1999;180:784–91.
4. Carr MH, Towers CV, Eastenson AR, Pircon RA, Iriye BK, Adashek JA. Prolonged bedrest during pregnancy: does the risk of deep vein thrombosis warrant the use of routine heparin prophylaxis. J Matern Fetal Med 1997;6:264–7.
5. Gerhardt A, Scharf RE, Beckmann MW, Struve S, Bender HG, Pillany M, et al. Prothrombin and factor V mutations in women with a history of thrombosis during pregnancy and the puerperium. N Engl J Med 2000;342:374–80.
6. Dizon-Townson D, Miller C, Sibai B, Spong CY, Thom E, Wendel G, et al. The relationship of the factor V Leiden mutation and pregnancy outcomes for mother and fetus. Obstet Gynecol 2005;106:517–24.
7. Ginsberg JS, Chan WS, Bates SM, Kaatz S. Anticoagulation of pregnancy women with mechanical heart valves. Arch Intern Med 2003;163:694–8.
8. Toglia MR, Weg JG. venous thromboembolism during pregnancy. New Engl J Med 1996;335:108–14.
9. Goodacre S, Sutton AJ, Sampson FC. Meta-analysis: the value of clinical assessment in the diagnosis of deep venous thrombosis. Ann Intern Med 2005;143:129–39.
10. Myers ER, Clarke-Pearson DL, Olt GJ, Soper JT, Berchuck A. Preoperative coagulation testing on a gynecologic oncology service. Obstet Gynecol 1994;83:438–44.
11. Olt GJ, Greenberg C, Synan I, Coleman RE, Clarke-Pearson D. Preoperative assessment of fragment D-dimer as a predictor of postoperative venous thrombosis. Am J Obstet Gynecol 1990;162:772–5.
12. Anderson AA, Spencer FA. Risk factors for venous thromboembolism. Circulation 2003;107:I9–I16.
13. Heit JA, Silverstein MD, Mohr DN, Petterson TM, O'Fallon M, Melton J. Risk factors for deep vein thrombosis and pulmonary embolism: a population-based case-control study. Arch Intern Med 2000;160:809–15.
14. Tutschek B, Struve S, Goecke T, Pillny M, Zotz R, Gerhardt A, et al. Clinical risk factors for deep vein thrombosis in pregnancy and the puerperium. J Perinat Med 2002;30:367–70.
15. Cook D, Crowther M, Meade M, Rabbat C, Griffith L, Schiff D, et al. Deep venous thrombosis in medical-surgical critically ill patients: Prevalence, incidence, and risk factors. Crit Care Med 2005;33:1565–71.
16. Danilenko-Dixon DR, Heit JA, Silverstein MD, Yawn BP, Petterson TM, Lohse CM, et al. Risk factors for deep vein thrombosis and pulmonary embolism during pregnancy or postpartum: a population-based case control study. Am J Obstet Gynecol 2001;184:104–10.
17. Simpson EL, Lawrenson RA, Nightingale AL, Farmer RDT. Venous thromboembolism in pregnancy and puerperium: incidence and additional factors from a London peritoneal database. BJOG 2001;108:56–60.

18. Lindqvist P, Dahlback BD, Marsal K. Thrombotic risk during pregnancy: a population study. Obstet Gynecol 1999;94:595–9.

19. Stein PD, Hull RD, Kayali F, Olson RE, Alshab AK, Meyers FA, et al. Venous thromboembolism in pregnancy: 21-year trends. Am J Med 2004;164:2260–5.

20. Chisaka H, Utsunomiya H, Okamura K, Yaegashi N. Pulmonary embolism following gynecologic surgery and cesarean section. Int J Gynaecol Obstet 2004;84:47–53.

21. Davis JD. Prevention, diagnosis and treatment of venous thromboembolism of gynecologic surgery. Am J Obstet Gynecol 2001;184:759–75.

22. Abu-Rustum NR, Richard S, Wilton A, Lev G, Sonoda Y, Hensley ML, et al. Transfusion utilization during adnexal or peritoneal cancer surgery: effects on symptomatic venous thromboembolism and survival. Gynecol Oncol 2005;99:320–6.

23. Wasowicz-Kemps DK, Biesma DH, Van Leeuwen S, Ramshorst RV. Prophylaxis of venous thromboembolism in general gynecologic day surgery in the Netherlands. J Thromb Haemost 2006;4:269–71.

24. Taberner DA, Poller L, Burslem RW, Jones JB. Oral anticoagulants by the British comparative thromboplastin versus low-dose heparin in prophylaxis of deep vein thrombosis. Br Med J 1978;1:272–4.

25. Bergqvist D. Low molecular weight heparin for the prevention of venous thromboembolism after abdominal surgery. Br J Surg 2004;91:965–74.

26. Cyrkowicz A. Reduction in fatal pulmonary embolism and venous thrombosis by perioperative administration of low molecular weight heparin: gynecological ward retrospective analysis. Eur J Obstet Gynecol Reprod Biol 2002;100:223–6.

27. Clarke-Pearson DL, Synan IS, Dodge R, Soper JT, Berchuck A, Coleman RE. A randomized trial of low-dose heparin and intermittent pneumatic calf compression for the prevention of deep venous thrombosis after gynecologic oncology surgery. Am J Obstet Gynecol 1993;168:1146–54.

28. Lepercq J, Conrad J, Borel-Derlon A, Darmon JY, Boudignat O, Francoual C, et al. Venous thromboembolism during pregnancy: a retrospective study of enoxaparin safety in 624 pregnancies. BJOG 2001;108:1134–40.

29. Turner GM, Cole SE, Brooks JH. The efficacy of graduated compression stockings in the prevention of deep vein thrombosis after major gynaecologic surgery. Br J Obstet Gynaecol 1984;91:588–91.

30. Bergqvist D. Assessment of the risk and the prophylaxis of venous thromboembolism in surgical patients. Pathophysiol Haemost Thromb 2004;33:358–61.

31. Schulz SL, Stechemesser B, Seeberger U, Meyer D, Kesselring C. Graduated compression stockings for the prevention of venous thromboembolism in surgical patients in the age of low molecular weight heparin. J Thromb Haemost 2005;3:2363–5.

32. Clarke-Pearson DL, Dodge RK, Synan I, McClelland RC, Maxwell GL. Venous thromboembolism prophylaxis: patients at high risk to fail intermittent pneumatic compression. Obstet Gynecol 2003;101:157–63.

33. National Institutes of Health Consensus Development conference. Prevention of venous thromboembolism and pulmonary embolism. JAMA 1986;245:744–9.

34. American College of Obstetricians and Gynecologists. Thromboembolism in pregnancy. ACOG Practice Bulletin 19. Washington, DC: ACOG; 2000.

35. Sarani B, Chun A, Venbrux A. Role of optional (retrievable) IVC filters in surgical patients at risk for venous thromboembolic disease. J Am Coll Surg 2005;201:957–64.

36. Athanasoulis CA, Kaufman JA, Halpern EF, Waltman AC, Geller SC, Fan CM. Inferior vena caval filters: review of a 26-year single-center clinical experience. Radiology 2000;216:54–66.

37. Rutherford RB. Prophylactic indications for vena cava filters: a critical appraisal. Semin Vasc Surg 2005;18:158–65.

38. Maxwell GL, Myers ER, Clarke-Pearson DL. Cost-effectiveness of deep vein thrombosis prophylaxis in gynecologic oncology surgery. Obstet Gynecol 2000;95:206–14.

39. Clarke-Pearson DL, Creasman WT, Coleman RE, Synan IS, Hinshaw WM. Perioperative external pneumatic calf compression as thromboembolism prophylaxis in gynecologic oncology: report of a randomized controlled trial. Gynecol Oncol 1984;18:226–32.

40. Clarke-Pearson DL, Synan IS, Hinshaw WM, Coleman RE, Creasman WT. Prevention of postoperative venous thromboembolism by external pneumatic calf compression in patients with gynecologic malignancy. Obstet Gynecol 1984;63:92–8.

41. Borstad E, Urdal K, Handeland G, Abildgaard U. Comparison of low molecular weight heparin vs unfractionated heparin in gynecologic surgery. Acta Obstet Gynecol Scand 1988;67:99–103.

42. Kakkar VV, Cohen AT, Edmonson RA, Phillips MJ, Cooper DJ, Das SK, et al. Low molecular weight versus standard heparin for the prevention of venous thromboembolism after major abdominal surgery. Lancet 1993;341:259–65.

43. Collins R, Scrimgeour A, Yusuf S, Peto R. Reduction in fatal pulmonary embolism and venous thrombosis by perioperative administration of subcutaneous heparin: overview of results of randomized trials in general, orthopedic, and urologic surgery. N Engl J Med 1988;318:1162–73.

44. Ballard RM, Bradley-Watson PJ, Johnstone FD, Kenney A, McCarthy TG. Low doses of subcutaneous heparin in the prevention of deep vein thrombosis after gynaecologic surgery. J Obstet Gynaecol Br Commonw. 1973;80:469–72.

45. Borstad E, Urdal K, Handeland G, Abildgaard U. Comparison of low molecular weight heparin vs unfractionated heparin in gynecologic surgery II: reduced dose of low molecular weight heparin. Acta Obstet Gynecol Scand 1992;71:471–5.

46. Clarke-Pearson DL, Coleman RE, Synan IS, Hinshaw W, Creasman WT. Venous thromboembolism prophylaxis in gynecologic oncology: a prospective, controlled trial of low-dose heparin. Am J Obstet Gynecol 1983;145:606–13.

47. Clarke-Pearson DL, DeLong E, Synan IS, Soper JT, Creasman WT, Coleman RE. A controlled trial of two low-dose heparin regimens for the prevention of postoperative deep vein thrombosis. Obstet Gynecol 1990;75: 684–9.

48. Clarke-Pearson DL, DeLong ER, Synan IS, Creasman WT. Complications of low-dose heparin prophylaxis in gynecologic oncology surgery. Obstet Gynecol 1984;64: 689–93.

49. Maxwell GL, Synan I, Dodge R, Carroll B, Clarke-Pearson DL. Pneumatic compression versus low molecular weight heparin in gynecologic oncology surgery: a randomized trial. Obstet Gynecol 2001;98:989–95.

50. Maxwell GL, Synan I, Hayes P, Clarke-Pearson DL. Preference and compliance in postoperative thromboembolism prophylaxis among gynecologic oncology patients. Obstet Gynecol 2002;100:451–5.

51. Lindhoff-Last E, Nakov R, Misselwitz F, Breddin HK, Bauersachs R. Incidence and clinical relevance of heparin-induced antibodies in patients with deep vein thrombosis treated with unfractionated or low-molecular-weight heparin. Br J Haemotol 2002;118:1137–42.

52. Dahlman TC. Osteoporotic fractures and the recurrence of thromboembolism during pregnancy and the puerperium in 184 women undergoing thromboprophylaxis with heparin. Am J Obstet Gynecol 1993;168:1265–70.

53. Geerts WH, Pineo GF, Heit JA, Bergqvist D, Lassen MR, Colwell CW, et al. Prevention of venous thromboembolism: the Seventh ACCP Conference on Antithrombotic and Antithrombolytic Therapy. Chest 2004;126: 338S–400S.

54. Dainty L, Maxwell Gl, Clarke-Pearson DL, Meyers ER. Cost-effectiveness of combination thromboembolism prophylaxis in gynecologic oncology surgery. Gynecol Oncol 2004;93:366–73.

55. Wille-Jorgensen P, Rasmussen MS, Andersen BR, Borly L. Heparins and mechanical methods for thromboprophylaxis in colorectal surgery (Cochrane Review) In: The Cochrane Library, Issue 3, 2006. Oxford: Update Software.

56. Clarke-Pearson DL, Synan IS, Coleman RE, Hinshaw W, Creasman WT. The natural history of postoperative venous thromboemboli in gynecologic oncology: a prospective study of 382 patients. Am J Obstet Gynecol 1984;148:1051–4.

57. Gould MK, Dembitzer AD, Doyle RL, Hastie TJ, Garber AM. Low-molecular-weight heparins compared with unfractionated heparin for treatment of acute deep venous thrombosis: a meta-analysis of randomized, controlled trials. Ann Intern Med 1999;130:800–9.

58. Bergqvist D, Agnelli G, Cohen AT, Eldor A, Nilsson PE, Le Moigne-Amrani A, et al. Duration of prophylaxis against venous thromboembolism with enoxaparin after surgery for cancer. N Engl J Med 2002;346:975–80.

59. Weiss N, Bernstein PS. Risk factor scoring for predicting venous thromboembolism in obstetric patients. Am J Obstet Gynecol 2000;182:1073–10.

60. Martinelli I, DeStefano V, Taioli E, Paciaroni K, Rossi E, Mannucci PM. Inherited thrombophilia and first venous thromboembolism during pregnancy and puerperium. Thromb Haemost 2002;87:791–95.

61. Adachi T, Hashiguchi K, Arai Y, Ohta H. Clinical study of venous thromboembolism during pregnancy and puerperium. Semin Thromb Hemost 2001;27:149–53.

62. Nelson-Piercy C, Letsky EA, de Swiet M. Low-molecular-weight heparin for obstetric thromboprophylaxis: experience of sixty-nine pregnancies in sixty-one women at high risk. Am J Obstet Gynecol 1997;176: 1062–8.

63. Gates S, Brocklehurst P, Ayers S, Bowler U. Thromboprophylaxis and pregnancy: two randomized controlled pilot trials that used low-molecular weight heparin. Am J Obstet Gynecol 2004;191:1296–1303.

64. Sephton V, Farquharson RG, Topping J, Quenby SM, Cowan C, Back DJ, et al. A longitudinal study of maternal dose response to low molecular weight heparin in pregnancy. Obstet Gynecol 2003;101:1307–11.

65. Gallus AS. Management options for thrombophilias. Semin Thrombo Hemost 2005;31:118–26.

66. Brill-Edwards P, Ginsberg JS, Gent M, Hirsch J, Burrows R, Kearon C, et al. Safety of withholding heparin in pregnant women with a history of venous thromboembolism. N Engl J Med 2000;343:1439–44.

67. Johnston JA, Brill-Edwards P, Ginsberg JS, Pauker SG, Eckman MH. Cost-effectiveness of prophylactic low molecular weight heparin in pregnant women with a prior history of venous thromboembolism. Am J Med 2005;118:503–14.

68. Burrows RF, Gan ET, Gallus AS, Wallace EM, Burrows EA. A randomized double-blind placebo controlled trial of low molecular weight heparin as prophylaxis in preventing venous thrombolic events after caesarean section: a pilot study. BJOG 2001;108:835–9.

69. Jacobsen AF, Drolsum A, Klow NE, Dahl GF, Qvigstad E, Sandset PM. Deep vein thrombosis after elective cesarean section. Thromb Res 2004;113:283–8.

70. Quinones JN, James DN, Stamilio DM, Cleary KL, Macones GA. Thromboprophylaxis after cesarean delivery: a decision analysis. Obstet Gynecol 2005;106:733–40.

71. Lev-Ran O, Kramer A, Gurevitch J, Shapira I, Mohr R. Low-molecular-weight heparin for prosthetic heart valves: treatment failure. Ann Thorac Surg 2000;69: 264–6.

72. Rowan JA, McCowan LM, Raudkivi PJ, North RA. Enoxaparin treatment in women with mechanical heart valves during pregnancy. Am J Obstet Gynecol 2001;185: 633–7.

73 Safety of Lovenox in pregnancy. ACOG Committee Opinion No. 276. American College of Obstetricians and Gynecologists. Obstet Gynecol 2002;100:845–6.

74. De Santo LS, Romano G, Della Corte A, Tizzano F, Petraio A, Amarelli C, et al. Mitral mechanical replacement in young rheumatic women: analysis of long-term survival, valve-related complications, and pregnancy outcomes over a 3707-patient-year follow-up. J Thorac Cardiovasc Surg 2005;130:13–9.

75. Bates SM, Greer IA, Hirsch J, Ginsberg JS. Use of antithrombotic agents during pregnancy: the Seventh ACCP Conference on Antithrombotic and Thrombolytic Therapy. Chest 2004;126;627S–44S.

76. Stevenson RE, Burton OM, Ferlauto GJ, Taylor HA. Hazards of oral anticoagulants during pregnancy. JAMA 1980;243:1549–51.

77. Kearon C, Ginsberg JS, Douketis J, Crowther MA, Turpie AG, Bates SM, et al. A randomized trial of diagnostic strategies after proximal vein ultrasonography for suspected deep venous thrombosis: d-dimer testing compared with repeated ultrasonography. Ann Intern Med 2005;142:490–6.

78. Kearon C, Julian JA, Math M, Newman TE, Ginsberg JS. Noninvasive diagnosis of deep venous thrombosis. An Internal Med 1998;128:663–77.

79. Subramaniam RM, Chou T, Heath R, Allen R. Importance of pretest probability score and D-dimer assay before sonography for lower limb DVT. AJR Am J Roentgenol 2006;186:206–12.

80. Kearon C, Ginsberg JS, Douketis J, Tripe AG, Bates SM, Lee AY, et al. An evaluation of D-dimer in the diagnosis of pulmonary: a randomized trial. Ann Intern Med 2006;144:812–21.

81. Linkins LA, Bates SM, Ginsberg JS, Kearon C. Use of different D-dimer levels to exclude venous thromboembolism depending on clinical pretest probability. J Thromb Haemost 2004;2:1256–60.

82. Wells PS, Anderson DR, Rodger M, Forgie M, Kearon C, Dreyer J, et al. Evaluation of D-dimer in the diagnosis of suspected deep-venous thrombosis. N Engl J Med 2003; 349:1227–35.

83. Ghirardini G, Battioni M, Bertellini C, Colombini R, Colla R, Rossi G. D-dimer after delivery in uncomplicated pregnancies. Clin Exp Obstet Gynecol 1999;26:211–2.

84. Huisman MV, Buller HR, Cate JW, Vreeken J. Serial impedance plethysmography for suspected deep venous thrombosis in outpatients: the Amsterdam General Practitioner Study. N Engl J Med 1986;314:823–8.

85. Stein PD, Hull RD, Pineo G. Strategy that includes serial noninvasive tests for diagnosis of thromboembolic disease in patients with suspected acute pulmonary embolism based on data from PIOPED. Arch Intern Med 1995;155:2101–4.

86. Martino MA, Borges E, Williamson E, Siegfried S, Cantor AB, Lancaster J, et al. Pulmonary embolism after major abdominal surgery in gynecologic oncology. Obstet Gynecol 2006;107:666–71.

87. Raskob GE, Hull RD. Diagnosis of pulmonary embolism. Curr Opin Hematol 1999;6:280–4.

88. Bates S. Treatment and prophylaxis of venous thromboembolism during pregnancy. Thromb Res 2002;108: 97–106.

89. Goldhaber SZ, Visani L, De Rosa M. Acute pulmonary embolism: clinical outcomes in the International Cooperative Pulmonary Embolism Registry (ICOPER). Lancet 1999;353:1386–9.

90. Nijkeuter M, Ginsberg JS, Huisman MV. Diagnosis of deep vein thrombosis and pulmonary embolism in pregnancy: a systematic review. J Thromb Haemost 2006;4: 496–500.

91. The PIOPED investigators. Value of the ventilation/perfusion scan in acute pulmonary embolism: Results of the prospective investigation of pulmonary embolism diagnosis (PIOPED). JAMA 1990;263:2753–9.

92. Roy PM, Colombet I, Durieux P, Chatellier G, Sors H, Meyer G. Systematic review and meta-analysis of strategies for the diagnosis of suspected pulmonary embolism. BMJ 2005;331: 259.

93. Chan WS, Ginsberg JS. Diagnosis of deep vein thrombosis and pulmonary embolism in pregnancy. Thromb Res 2002;107:85–91.

94. Worsley DF, Alavi A. Comprehensive analysis of the results of the PIOPED Study. J Nucl Med 1995;36: 2380–7.

95. Stein PD, Hull RD, Pineo G. Strategy that includes serial noninvasive leg tests for diagnosis of thromboembolic disease in patients with suspected acute pulmonary embolism based on data from PIOPED. Arch Intern Med1995;155:2101–4.

96. Balan KK, Critchley M, Vedavathy KK, Smith ML, Vinjamuri S. The value of ventilation-perfusion imaging in pregnancy. Br J Radiol 1997;70:338–40.

97. Chan WS, Ray JG, Murray S, Coady GE, Coates G, Ginsberg JS. Suspected pulmonary embolism in pregnancy: clinical presentation, results of lung scanning, and subsequent maternal and pediatric outcomes. Arch Intern Med 2002;162:1170–5.

98. Patel S, Kazerooni EA. Helical CT for the evaluation of acute pulmonary embolism. AJR Am J Roentgenol 2005;185:135–49.

99. Winer-Muram HT, Boone JM, Brown HL, Jennings SG, Mabie WC, Lombardo GT. Pulmonary embolism in pregnant patients: fetal radiation dose with helical CT. Radiology 2002;224:487–92.

100. Doyle NM, Ramirez MM, Mastrobattista JM, Monga M, Wagner LK, Gardner MO. Diagnosis of pulmonary embolism: a cost-effective analysis. Am J Obstet Gynecol 2004;191:1019–23.

101. Stevens SM, Elliott CG, Chan KJ, Egger MJ, Ahmed KM. Withholding anticoagulation after a negative result on duplex ultrasonography for suspected deep venous thrombosis. Ann Intern Med 2004;140:985–91.

102. Hull RD, Raskob GE, Rosenbloom D, Panja AA, Brill-Edwards P, Ginsberg JS, et al. Heparin for 5 days as compared with 10 days in the initial treatment of proximal venous thrombosis. N Engl J Med 1990;322:1260–4.

103. Bates SM, Ginsberg JS. Treatment of deep vein thrombosis. N Engl J Med 2004;351:268–77.

104. Cruickshank MK, Levine MN, Hirsh J, Roberts R, Siguenza M. A standard nomogram for the management of heparin therapy. Arch Intern Med 1991;151:333–7.

105. Raschke RA, Reilly BM, Guidry JR, Fontana JR, Srinivas S. The weight-based heparin dosing nomogram compared with a "standard care" nomogram. Ann Intern Med 1993;119:874–81.

106. Buller HR, Agnelli C, Hull RD, Hyers TM, Prins MH, Raskob GE. Antithrombotic therapy for venous thromboembolic disease: the Seventh ACCP Conference on Antithrombotic and Thrombolytic Therapy. Chest 2004: 126:401S–28S.

107. Kirchmaier CM, Wolf H, Schafer H, Ehlers B, Breddin HK. Efficacy of a low molecular weight heparin administered intravenously or subcutaneously in comparison

with intravenous unfractionated heparin in the treatment of deep venous thrombosis. Int Angiol 1998;17: 135–45.

108. Gould MK, Dembitzer AD, Sanders GD, Garber AM. Low-molecular-weight heparins compared with unfractionated heparin for the treatment of acute deep venous thrombosis: a cost-effectiveness analysis. Ann Intern Med 1999;130:789–99

109. The Columbus Investigators. Low-molecular-weight heparin in the treatment of patients with venous thromboembolism. N Engl J Med 1997;337:657–62.

110. Mismetti P, Quenet S, Levine M, Merli G, Decousus H, Derobert E, et al. Enoxaparin in the treatment of deep vein thrombosis with or without pulmonary embolism: an individual patient data meta-analysis. Chest 2005;128:2203–10.

111. Breddin HK, Hach-Wunderle V, Nakov R, Kakkar VV, CORTES investigators. Effects of a low-molecular-weight heparin on thrombus regression and recurrent thromboembolism in patients with deep-vein thrombosis. N Engl J Med 2001;344:626–31.

112. Merli G, Spiro TE, Olsson CG, Abildgaard U, Davidson BL, Eldor A, et al. Subcutaneous enoxaparin once or twice daily compared with intravenous unfractionated heparin for treatment of venous thromboembolic disease. Ann Intern Med 2001;134:191–202.

113. Simonneau G, Sors H, Charbonnier B, Page Y, Laaban JP, Azarian R, et al. A comparison of low-molecular-weight heparin with unfractionated heparin for acute pulmonary embolism. N Engl J Med 1997;337:663–9.

114. Levine M, Gent M, Hirsh J, Leclerc J, Anderson D, Weitz J, et al. A comparison of low-molecular-weight heparin administered primarily at home with unfractionated heparin administered in the hospital for proximal deep vein thrombosis. N Engl J Med 1996;334:677–81.

115. Levine M, Hirsh J, Gent M, Turpie AG, Weitz J, Ginsberg J, et al. Optimal duration of oral anticoagulation therapy: a randomized trial comparing four weeks with three months of warfarin ion patients with proximal deep vein thrombosis. Thromb Haemost 1995;74:606–11.

116. Kearon C, Gent M, Hirsh J, Weitz J, Kovacs MJ, Anderson DR, et al. A comparison of three months of anticoagulation with extended anticoagulation for a first episode of idiopathic venous thromboembolism. N Engl J Med 1999;340:901–7.

117. Schulman S, Granqvist S, Holmstrom M, Carlson A, Lindmarker P, Nicol P, et al. The duration of oral anticoagulation therapy after a second episode of venous thromboembolism. N Engl J Med 1997;336:393–8.

118. Schulman S, Rhedin AS, Lindmarker P, Carlsson A, Larfars G, Nicol P, et al. A comparison of six weeks with six months of oral anticoagulant therapy after a first episode of venous thromboembolism. N Engl J Med 1995;332:1661–5.

119. McColl MD, Greer IA. Low-molecular-weight heparin for the prevention and treatment of venous thromboembolism in pregnancy. Curr Opin Pulm Med 2004;10: 371–5.

120. Kawamata Z, Chiba Y, Tanaka R, Higashi M, Nishigami K. Experience of temporary inferior vena cava filters inserted in the perinatal period to prevent pulmonary embolism in pregnant women with deep vein thrombosis. J Vasc Surg 2005;41:652–6.

121. Pillny M, Sandmann W, Luther B, Muller BT, Tutschek B, Gerhart A, et al. Deep vein thrombosis during pregnancy and after delivery: indications for and results of thrombectomy. J Vasc Surg 2003;37:528–32.

PART IV

INFECTIONS

CHAPTER 22

Urinary Tract Infections in Pregnancy

JEANNE S. SHEFFIELD AND F. GARY CUNNINGHAM

$\mathcal{U}$rinary tract infections are the most common bacterial infection in pregnant and nonpregnant women and are responsible for 10% of all antepartum admissions (1). Every year in the United States cystitis is diagnosed in approximately 10% of women, and this is associated with direct costs of $1.6 billion dollars (2). During their lifetime, more than one half of women will have a urinary infection and up to one half of these women have another infection within a year (3). In approximately 3–5% of women, there are multiple recurrences over many years (4).

In most women, these infections are limited to the lower urinary tract and are manifest by asymptomatic bacteriuria. Cystitis is the most common symptomatic infection and is characterized by dysuria, urgency, and frequency concomitant with pyuria and bacteriuria. Although cystitis is usually uncomplicated, the upper urinary tract may become involved by ascending infection. Pyelonephritis is infection of the renal parenchyma and pelvicaliceal system and it arises either *de novo* from asymptomatic renal bacteriuria or from ascending bladder infection. Renal infections are more common in the setting of obstruction from urinary tract malformations, urolithiasis, and pregnancy-induced changes. Recurrent and chronic infections with the same organism are usually termed relapses or persistent infections. Infection after a symptomatic cure, or that is caused by a second pathogen, is defined as reinfection. Acute urethritis, caused predominantly by *Neisseria gonorrhoeae* and *Chlamydia trachomatis* usually occurs concomitantly with cervicitis.

Pathophysiology

Urinary infection in women results from complex interactions between host and microorganism. Most commonly, infection arises from perineal and periurethral bacteria that gain entrance to the bladder. Such extension of colonization or infection most probably is associated with physiological trauma such as sexual intercourse, urethral massage, or catheterization. Ascending infection may then involve the ureters, pyelocaliceal system, and renal parenchyma. Rarely, renal infection may result from bacteremia or lymphatic spread.

Host Factors

Women are anatomically predisposed to bacterial colonization. The external third of the short urethra often is colonized by pathogens from normal vaginal flora. Intercourse increases the risk of infection because of meatal trauma, urethral massage, and probably changes in vaginal flora. Women who use a diaphragm with spermicidal agents for contraception also are at increased risk, presumably secondary to changes in the vaginal flora and possibly trauma from the diaphragmatic ring. An increased risk of infection accrues with age, likely because of the hypoestrogenic state associated with vaginal mucosal atrophy, impaired voiding, and changes in hygiene. There are other risk factors, including medical conditions such as diabetes, obesity, and sickle cell trait; anatomical congenital abnormalities; urinary tract calculi; and neurological or anatomical disorders that require indwelling or repetitive bladder catheterization.

One of the most important risk factors for symptomatic infection, especially acute pyelonephritis, is pregnancy-induced physiological changes in the urinary system (Fig. 22-1). Dilation of the ureters and renal calyces is evident as early as 12 weeks of gestation and is thought to be caused by progesterone-induced relaxation of their muscular layers. More importantly, as the uterus enlarges, it begins to compress the ureters at the pelvic brim, particularly on the right side (5, 6). Vesicoureteral reflux may first appear or worsen during gestation in some women, particularly multiparous women. Anatomical changes in bladder position in late pregnancy also may render it more susceptible to infection. Bladder and urethral trauma, periurethral tears, large vulvar lacerations, and epidural analgesia for labor and delivery predispose to urinary retention and the need for catheterization.

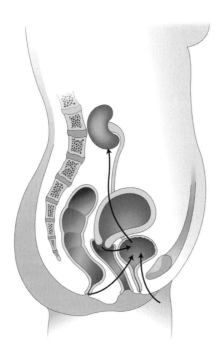

Fig. 22-1. Routes of infection in the urinary tract. Arrows depict the ascending nature of infection, from the bladder and urethra up the ureters to the kidneys. (Modified from American College of Obstetricians and Gynecologists. Urogynecology: an illustrated guide for women. Washington, DC: ACOG; 2004. Illustration: John Yanson.)

Bacterial Factors

Urinary infections in pregnant women are caused by a number of bacterial species, most of which are from the normal perineal flora. Specific serogroups of "uropathogenic" *Escherichia coli* are the most commonly identified organisms (7). These serogroups have a number of virulence factors specific for colonization and invasion of urinary epithelium. Some of these include adhesions such as P-fimbria and S-fimbria, which enhance binding to vaginal and uroepithelial cells. These adhesions also bind to erythrocyte membranes, inhibiting serum bactericidal activity by expression of the *dra* gene cluster associated with ampicillin resistance (8). (Fig. 22-2) Other *E coli* serogroups express an increase in K antigen production, which helps protect the microorganism from leukocyte phagocytosis. Greater adherence of type I fimbriated *E coli* to uroepithelial cells in diabetes may be related to impaired cytokine secretion and blunted leukocyte response (9). A complete list of identifiable virulence factors is beyond the scope of this review.

Although the overwhelming majority of urinary infections are caused by these strains of *E coli*, most of the remainder are caused by *Enterobacter*, *Enterococcus*, *Proteus mirabilis* and *Klebsiella* species. These latter organisms also are associated with structural abnormali-

ties or renal calculi. *Staphylococcus saprophyticus* was isolated from 3% of nonpregnant reproductive-aged women with pyelonephritis (10). Gram-positive organisms, including group B streptococci, are increasingly isolated in certain populations, including pregnant women (11). Patients with indwelling catheters also are susceptible to fungal infections. Anaerobic bacteria and mycoplasma may play a greater role in urinary infections than previously reported, although data are limited.

Lower Urinary Tract Infections

Asymptomatic Bacteriuria

The prevalence of bacteriuria in pregnant women is reported to be as high as 7% (12); most of these women are asymptomatic. Bacteriuria is diagnosed by using a clean-voided, midstream urine sample. For research purposes, significant bacteriuria is defined as isolation of a single microorganism with at least 100,000 organisms per mL (colony-forming units per mL). Some authors recommend using a colony count of 10,000/mL or greater to increase the sensitivity of the test. In the clinical setting, most consider a colony count of 100,000 colony-forming units per mL or greater to be clinically significant and thus require treatment (13, 14). Newer, alternative testing methods such as urine dipstick testing to screen for asymptomatic bacteriuria have not been found to be as sensitive as urine culture and are not currently recommended as a first-line screening method.

Depending on the population, the incidence of asymptomatic bacteriuria during pregnancy ranges from 2% to 7%. Bacteriuria typically is present at the time of the first prenatal visit and, after an initial negative urine culture result, less than 1% of women develop acute

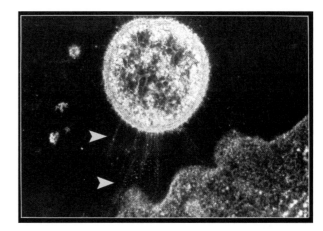

Fig. 22-2. Transmission of electron microscopy showing fimbriated Escherichia coli adhering to a transitional cell (X 180,000, original magnification). Arrows show the pili. (Modified from Roberts JA. Pathophysiology of pyelonephritis. Infect Surg 1986;Nov:633.)

cystitis (15). If asymptomatic bacteriuria is not treated, one fourth of these women subsequently develop acute pyelonephritis. For these reasons, the American College of Obstetricians and Gynecologists and the American Academy of Pediatrics (16) recommend routine screening for bacteriuria at the first prenatal visit, with eradication to prevent serious renal infections during pregnancy. There is little evidence that asymptomatic bacteriuria has a significant clinical impact on other significant adverse pregnancy outcomes (17).

Treatment for asymptomatic bacteriuria is usually empirical, and determination of in vitro susceptibilities is not necessary. A number of antimicrobial regimens have proved effective. These regimens are listed in Table 22-1 with their relative costs. Although it is doubtful that 3-day exposures are harmful to the fetus, some clinicians recommend against the use of fluoroquinolone derivatives as first-line treatment because of conflicting data regarding human and animal toxicity. For resistant infection, however, use of these drugs is certainly reasonable. We have found that nitrofurantoin macrocrystals, 100 mg at bedtime for 10 days is usually effective and has a high compliance rate. To date, there is limited resistance to nitrofurantoin, and it remains the most commonly prescribed drug for urinary tract infections in pregnancy. Regardless of the regimen chosen, recurrent asymptomatic bacteriuria is identified in at least 30% of women (15). For women with either persistent bacteriuria or those with frequent recurrences, suppressive therapy with nitrofurantoin, 100 mg at bedtime for the remainder of the pregnancy may be indicated.

Acute Cystitis

Acute bladder infection is usually uncomplicated and accompanied by varying degrees of dysuria, frequency, and urgency. Patients also may complain of suprapubic pain and fullness. Although acute cystitis may irritate the lower uterine segment and incite preterm contractions, there is no evidence that bladder infection causes preterm labor. Diagnosis is based on the clinical findings and confirmed by urine studies. Urinary dipstick testing is fast and convenient. A finding of either nitrite or leukocyte esterase is considered a positive result, with a sensitivity of 75% and specificity of 82% (3, 18, 19). Urine culture is indicated in symptomatic women not responding to standard therapy who occasionally may have a resistant pathogen. The distal urethra and peri-urethral-colonized areas may contaminate a midstream clean-voided urine specimen but with lower colony counts. A urine culture should be obtained by catheterization in problematic cases. Some cases of persistent lower-tract symptoms with a "sterile" urine culture may be caused by epithelial infection with *C trachomatis* (5).

Table 22-1. Treatment Regimens for Uncomplicated Urinary Infections in Women and the Relative Cost of Each Regimen.*

Single-Dose Treatment	
Ampicillin, 2 g	$
Amoxicillin, 3 g	$
Nitrofurantoin, 200 mg	$
Trimethoprim-sulfamethoxazole, 320/1600 mg	$

3-Day Course	
Amoxicillin, 500 mg 3 times daily	$
Ampicillin, 250 mg 4 times daily	$
Cephalexin, 250 mg 4 times daily	$$$
Nitrofurantoin, 50 mg 4 times daily; 100 mg twice daily	$$
Trimethoprim-sulfamethoxazole, 160/800 mg twice daily	$$
Ciprofloxacin, 250 mg twice daily	$$$
Levofloxacin, 250 mg daily	$$$

Other	
Nitrofurantoin, 100 mg at bedtime for 7–14 days	$$$
Nitrofurantoin, 100 mg 4 times daily for 7–14 days	$$$$

Treatment Failures	
Nitrofurantoin, 100 mg at bedtime for 21 days	$$$$

Suppression for Bacterial Persistence or Recurrence	
Nitrofurantoin, 100 mg at bedtime for remainder of pregnancy	N/A

$, less than or equal to $5; $$, $5–$15; $$$,$15–30; $$$$, more than $30.

* Based on generic average wholesale price (Redbook Pharmacy's Fundamental Reference, 2004 edition. Montvale [NJ]: Thompson PDR; 2004.)

Cunningham FG, Leveno KJ, Bloom SL, Hauth JC, Gilstrap LC, Wenstrom KD. Renal and urinary tract disorders. In: Cunningham FG, Leveno KJ, Bloom SL, Hauth JC, Gilstrap LC, Wenstrom KD, editors. Williams Obstetrics. 22nd ed. New York (NY): McGraw-Hill; 2005. p. 1095–9. Copyright © 2005. Reprinted with permission of The McGraw-Hill Companies.

In most cases, uncomplicated bacterial cystitis responds quickly to therapy. The 3-day regimens shown in Table 22-1 are effective in 90% of women (3). In pregnant women with cystitis, single-dose therapy is not recommended. Any of the 3-day or longer treatment regimens shown in Table 22-1 are effective, with the same caveats for fluoroquinolone derivatives as discussed for asymptomatic bacteriuria. Recently, it has been recommended that β-lactams not be used to treat urinary infections because of increasing resistance among the common uropathogens (3).

Recurrent Cystitis

Recurrent urinary infections, both symptomatic and asymptomatic, are common in women, occurring in up to 35% of those with an initial episode. During pregnancy, at least, a "test-of-cure" urine culture is performed 1–2 weeks after completing therapy, and a different treatment regimen is used if the result is positive. Use of antibiotics, including nitrofurantoin, ciprofloxacin, trimethoprim, or norfloxacin, has been shown to decrease the recurrence risk by 95% or more when used in a prophylactic regimen (3).

Cranberry or lingonberry juice has been shown in randomized trials to decrease the risk of recurrent urinary infections. This is because the proanthocyanidins inhibit attachment of the urinary pathogens to the uroepithelium (3). Approximately 200–750 mL of juice or an equivalent dose in concentrated tablets has been found effective. Other proposed preventive measures such as wiping techniques, postcoital voiding, douching, and timing of voiding have not been shown to prevent recurrent infections (3).

Acute Pyelonephritis

Acute pyelonephritis is a clinical syndrome characterized by flank pain, chills and fever, and variable symptoms of dysuria, urgency, and frequency. It remains the most common serious medical complication of pregnancy (1). From most surveys, 1–2% of pregnant women are admitted for this condition, despite prenatal screening and treatment for bacteriuria. Renal infections may result in significant maternal morbidity and occasional mortality. At our institution, 12% of antepartum admissions to the obstetric intensive care unit are for sepsis caused by pyelonephritis (20). Acute renal infection is less common in early pregnancy, except in women with diabetes. As many as 80–90% of cases are reported to occur either in the latter two trimesters or in the puerperium (11). This observation is related to the increasing urinary tract obstruction with stasis caused by progesterone and uterine enlargement.

Clinical findings are similar to those for nonpregnant women. In more than one half of cases, pyelonephritis is unilateral and right sided, and it is left sided or bilateral in another 25% each. The right-sided predominance may be from obstruction caused by uterine dextrorotation, protection from obstruction provided on the left by the descending colon, or both. Onset of illness usually is abrupt with fever, chills, and aching pain in one or both lumbar regions. There frequently is anorexia, nausea, and vomiting, which worsen the dehydration resulting from fever. Tenderness usually can be elicited by percussion in one or both costovertebral angles, and urinalysis discloses bacteriuria that is confirmed by culture. Approximately 1 in 5 women will have bacteremia. *Escherichia coli* is by far the most common pathogen identified; however, gram-positive organisms, including group B Streptococci, account for approximately 10% of cases of acute pyelonephritis at our institution (11).

As many as 20% of pregnant women will develop evidence of multiple-system derangement from endotoxemia and sepsis syndrome (11, 18, 21–25). These disorders result from endothelial activation that is followed by capillary fluid extravasation with diminished perfusion. These vascular changes aggravate the dehydration from nausea, vomiting, and fever and resultant hypotension is common. Fortunately, most women respond to rapid fluid resuscitation with intravenous crystalloid solutions, and cardiac output is restored without the use of vasopressor drugs.

There are a number of sepsis-related derangements that are common. With early and aggressive fluid resuscitation, only approximately 5% of women have seriously diminished renal function (11). Before the concept of aggressive hydration, however, this number was 20% (21, 22). Although transient, renal dysfunction is important to recognize so that nephrotoxic drugs can be avoided. Anemia is common, and up to one fourth of women have a hematocrit decrease to less than 30 volumes percent. In severe cases, the hematocrit decreases as low as 20 volumes percent. Hemolysis is caused by the lipopolysaccharide in endotoxin and is associated with deranged erythrocyte morphology and elevated serum lactate dehydrogenase levels (23). With severe sepsis, activation of coagulation is common, with potentially serious, occasionally life-threatening complications (Fig. 22-3).

The most common serious manifestation of sepsis syndrome is acute respiratory insufficiency, which develops to varied degrees in up to 10% of pregnant women (11). Endotoxin injures endothelium and alters alveolar capillary membrane permeability. In its worst form, pulmonary injury causes severe acute respiratory distress syndrome as shown in Figure 22-4. Some women require 100% oxygen by nonrebreathing mask or with nasal continuous positive airway pressure. In some of these women, tracheal intubation and mechanical ventilation is necessary to maintain oxygenation (25).

Uterine activity stimulated by endotoxin is commonly seen. In one study, it was found that women had an average of 5.1 contractions per hour when admitted for pyelonephritis (26). This number decreased to 2 per hour by 6 hours. Even so, preterm labor is not common. When it is identified, care must be taken with tocolysis. Beta-agonist therapy increases the likelihood of respiratory insufficiency from alveolar flooding because of its sodium and fluid-retaining properties (27). The incidence of pulmonary edema has been shown to be 8% in women with pyelonephritis who were given β-agonists (28).

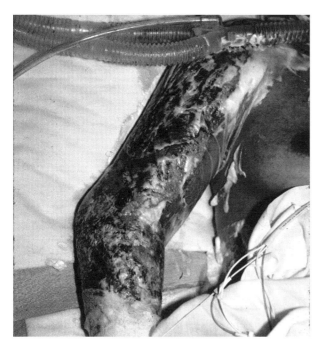

Fig. 22-3. Pregnant woman at 28 weeks of gestation admitted for severe pyelonephritis, sepsis syndrome, and preterm labor. Within 24 hours of delivering a liveborn infant, she developed purpura fulminans and was transferred to the burn intensive care unit. She sloughed 90% of her skin and died from dermal septicemia. (Sheffield JS, Cunningham FG. Urinary Tract Infection in Women. Obstet Gynecol 2005;106:1085–92.)

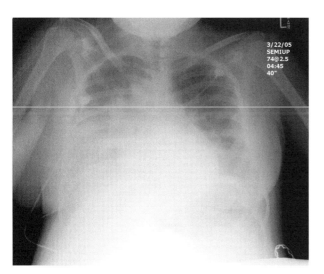

Fig. 22-4. A semiupright anteroposterior chest radiograph demonstrating diffuse bilateral parenchymal infiltrates and pleural effusion consistent with acute respiratory distress syndrome (courtesy of Dr. Diane Twickler). (Sheffield JS, Cunningham FG. Urinary Tract Infection in Women. Obstet Gynecol 2005;106:1085–92.)

Pregnant women with acute antepartum pyelonephritis should initially be assessed in the hospital (Box 22-1). During this time, hydration is paramount while laboratory studies and further clinical evaluation are performed. Women who cannot tolerate oral medications are hospitalized, as are women who appear very ill. Vigorous crystalloid infusion to ensure adequate urinary output is a mainstay of treatment. Because pulmonary edema is a possible risk of aggressive hydration in these women, careful monitoring with pulse oximetry should be performed. The diagnosis is confirmed promptly and intravenous antimicrobials are begun. Blood cultures have been shown to have limited utility in management (29). Urinary output, blood pressure, and temperature are monitored closely. High fever can be decreased with a cooling blanket or acetaminophen. This is especially important in early pregnancy because of possible teratogenic effects of hyperthermia.

Outpatient management of pyelonephritis in pregnancy is an option in those women who are able to tolerate oral intake with no evidence of sepsis, serious underlying medical illness, evidence of respiratory insufficiency, known renal or urologic disorders, or preterm labor (30, 31). These women need close follow-up that may include home-health care visits.

BOX 22-1

MANAGEMENT OF THE HOSPITALIZED PREGNANT WOMAN WITH ACUTE PYELONEPHRITIS.

1. Hospitalization
2. Urine studies
3. Hemogram, serum creatinine, and electrolytes
4. Monitor vital signs frequently, including urinary output; consider indwelling catheter
5. Intravenous crystalloid to establish urinary output 50 mL/hr
6. Intravenous antimicrobial therapy
7. Chest radiograph if there is dyspnea or tachypnea
8. Repeat hematology and chemistry studies at 48 hours if clinically relevant
9. Change antimicrobials if necessary when sensitivity results are available
10. Discharge when afebrile 24 hours; administer antimicrobials 10 days total therapy
11. Urine studies 1–2 weeks after therapy completed to "test for cure"

Lucas MJ, Cunningham FG. Urinary tract infections complicating pregnancy. In: Williams Obstetrics 19th ed. (suppl 5). Norwalk (CT): Appleton & Lange; 1994. Copyright © 1994. Reprinted with permission of McGraw-Hill Companies.

A number of antimicrobial regimens that may be used are detailed in Table 22-2. We initially give ampicillin plus gentamicin. In general, women will respond to therapy within 48 hours. For nonresponders, a search for obstruction or complicated infections should be undertaken. Renal ultrasonography is the best noninvasive method to evaluate for obstruction within the renal collecting system. The most common cause of obstruction is stones. In many cases, calculi are not seen with ultrasonography, and intravenous pyelography is used to identify an obstructing stone (32). The renal parenchyma also is visualized using ultrasonography, and pyelonephritis usually causes some renal enlargement. Intrarenal or perirenal abnormalities are better assessed with contrast-enhanced computed tomography. Parenchymal abnormalities appearing as an area of sharply demarcated attenuation signifies an intrarenal phlegmon also called lobar nephro-

Table 22-2. Intravenous and Oral Regimens for the Treatment of Acute Uncomplicated Pyelonephritis and the Relative Cost for Each Regimen.*

Outpatient Regimens (10–14 Days)	
Ciprofloxacin, 500 mg twice daily	$
Ciprofloxacin-XR, 1,000 mg once daily	$
Gatifloxacin, 400 mg once daily	$
Levofloxacin, 250 mg once daily	$
Ofloxacin, 400 mg twice daily	$
Amoxicillin–clavulanate, 875/125 mg twice daily	$
Trimethoprim-sulfamethoxazole DS, 160/800 mg twice daily	$
Intravenous Regimens	
Ciprofloxacin, 400 mg every 12 hours	$$$
Levofloxacin, 500 mg once daily	$$
Cefepime, 2 g every 8 hours	$$$$
Cefotetan, 2 g every 12 hours	$$$
Ticarcillin-clavulanate, 3.1 g every 6 hours	$$$
Trimethoprim-sulfamethoxazole, 2 mg/kg every 6 hours	$$
Ceftriaxone, 1–2 g every 12–24 hours	$$$$
Gentamicin, 3–5 mg/kg/day (once daily dosing acceptable)	$
Ampicillin, 2 g every 6 hours for suspected enterococcus	$$
Aztreonam, 2 g every 8 hours	$$$$
Cefotaxime, 2 g every 8 hours	$$$

$, less than or equal to $20; $$, $20–$60; $$$, $60–$100; $$$$, more than $100.

* Based on generic average wholesale price per day when available. (Redbook Pharmacy's Fundamental Reference. 2004 ed. Montvale (NJ): Thompson PDR; 2004.)

Sheffield JS, Cunningham FG. Urinary Tract Infection in Women. Obstet Gynecol 2005;106:1085–92

nia or focal or segmental pyelonephritis (Fig. 22-5) (33). These areas sometimes suppurate, and drainage may be necessary. In either case, there is a prolonged hospital course. Some women will be found to have a perinephric phlegmon or abscess. The latter is quite serious and drainage is frequently necessary. Once afebrile, women can be discharged to complete a 10-day course of therapy.

Recurrent bacteriuria develops in 30–40% of women after completion of therapy, and if untreated, one fourth of these women develop recurrent pyelonephritis (25). We recommend nitrofurantoin suppression, 100 mg at bedtime, after a single episode of pyelonephritis for the remainder of pregnancy to reduce the likelihood of recurrent infection (34). In our hospital, 3% of women develop recurrent pyelonephritis during the same pregnancy, and in almost every case, they were noncompliant with the suppression regimen (11).

Summary

Urinary tract infections are the most common bacterial infection encountered during pregnancy. Most infections are limited to the lower urinary tract and manifest as asymptomatic bacteriuria or cystitis. Upper urinary tract infection or pyelonephritis occurs in 1–2% of pregnant women and is a major cause of antepartum admissions. Pregnancy-induced changes, including dilation of the renal calyces and ureters and increased vesicoureteral reflux predispose the pregnant woman to urinary tract

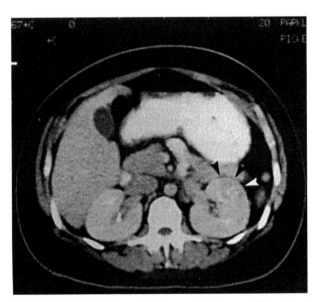

Fig. 22-5. Abdominal computed-tomographic scan with contract depicting lobar nephronia. The wedge-shaped nonenhanced area within the left kidney is indicated by arrowheads. (Sheffield JS, Cunningham FG. Urinary Tract Infection in Women. Obstet Gynecol 2005;106:1085–92.)

infections. Once infection is established, treatment is initially empirical. It is important for clinicians to be aware of common organisms and antibiotic resistance profiles at their institutions because this will determine initial treatment regimens. Urine culture results and antibiotic sensitivities will help focus treatment in the case of treatment failure or recurrent infection. Untreated asymptomatic bacteriuria will progress to acute pyelonephritis in one fourth of patients; thus, screening for asymptomatic bacteriuria is an important part of the prenatal laboratory evaluation. Pyelonephritis should be diagnosed and treated promptly because complications such as septic shock and respiratory insufficiency are not uncommon. Once the patient is afebrile for 24 hours while taking antimicrobial therapy, she may be discharged home to complete 10 days of total therapy. She is then given antimicrobial suppression for the remainder of pregnancy.

References

1. Bacak SJ, Callaghan WM, Dietz PM, Crouse C. Pregnancy-associated hospitalizations in the United States, 1999-2000. Am J Obstet Gynecol 2005;192:592–7.

2. Foxman B, Barlow R, D'Arcy H, Gillespie B, Sobel JD. Urinary tract infection: self-reported incidence and associated costs. Ann Epidemiol 2000;10:509–15.

3. Fihn SD. Acute uncomplicated urinary tract infection in women. N Engl J Med 2003;349:259–66.

4. Hooton TM. Recurrent urinary tract infection in women. Int J Antmicrob Agents 2001;17:259–68.

5. Schulman A, Herlinger H. Urinary tract dilatation in pregnancy. Br J Radiol 1975;48:638–45.

6. Faundes A, Bricola-Filho M, Pinto e Silva JC. Dilatation of the urinary tract during pregnancy: Proposal of a curve of maximal caliceal diameter by gestational age. Am J Obstet Gynecol 1998;178:1082–86.

7. Mulvey MA. Adhesion and entry of uropathogenic Escherichia coli. Cell Microbiol 2002;4:257–71.

8. Hart A, Nowicki BJ, Reisner B, Pawelczyk E, Goluszko P, Urvil P, et al. Ampicillin-resistant Escherichia coli in gestational pyelonephritis: increased occurrence and association with the colonization factor Dr adhesin. J Infect Dis 2001;183:1526–29.

9. Geerlings CE, Meiland R, van Lith EC, Brouwer EC, Gaastrra W, Hoepelman AI. Adherence of type 1-fimbriated Escherichia coli to uroepithelial cells: more in diabetic women than in control subjects. Diabetes Care 2002;25:405–9.

10. Scholes D, Hooton TM, Roberts PL, Gupta K, Stapleton AE, Stamm WE. Risk factors associated with acute pyelonephritis in healthy women. Ann Intern Med 2005;142:20–27.

11. Hill JB, Sheffield JS, McIntire DD, Cunningham FG, Wendel GD Jr. Acute pyelonephritis in pregnancy. Obstet Gynecol 2005;105:18–23.

12. Hooton TM, Scholes D, Stapleton AE, Roberts PL, Winter C, Gupta K, et al. A prospective study of asymptomatic bacteriuria in sexually active young women. N Engl J Med 2000;343:992–97.

13. Wilson ML, Gaido L. Laboratory diagnosis of urinary tract infections in adult patients. CID 2004;38:1150–8.

14. McNair RD, MacDonald SR, Dooley SL, Peterson LR. Evaluation of the centrifuged and Gram-stained smear, urinalysis, and reagent strip testing to detect asymptomatic bacteriuria in obstetric patients. Am J Obstet Gynecol 2000;182:1076–9.

15. Whalley P. Bacteriuria of pregnancy. Am J Obstet Gynecol 1967;97:723–38.

16. American Academy of Pediatrics, American College of Obstetricians and Gynecologists. Guidelines for Perinatal Care. 5th ed. Elk Grove Village (IL): AAP; Washington, DC: ACOG; 2002.

17. Smaill F. Antibiotics for asymptomatic bacteriuria in pregnancy (Cochrane Review). In: The Cochrane Library, Issue 2, 2001. Oxford: Update Software.

18. Cunningham FG, Hauth JC, Leveno KJ. Renal and urinary tract disorders. In: Williams Obstetrics. 22nd ed. New York (NY): McGraw-Hill; 2005. p. 1095-9.

19. Hurlbut TA III, Littenberg B. The diagnostic accuracy of rapid dipstick tests to predict urinary tract infection. Am J Clin Pathol 1991;96:582–8.

20. Zeeman GG, Wendel GD Jr, Cunningham FG. A blueprint for obstetric critical care. Am J Obstet Gynecol 2003;188:532–36.

21. Whalley PJ, Cunningham FG, Martin FG. Transient renal dysfunction associated with acute pyelonephritis of pregnancy. Obstet Gynecol 1974;46:174–7.

22. Gilstrap LC III, Cunningham FG, Whalley PJ. Acute pyelonephritis in pregnancy: an anterospective study. Obstet Gynecol 1981;57:409–13.

23. Cox SM, Shelburne P, Mason R, Guss S, Cunningham FG. Mechanisms of hemolysis and anemia associated with acute antepartum pyelonephritis. Am J Obstet Gynecol 1991;164:587–90.

24. Cunningham FG, Lucas MJ, Hankins GDV. Pulmonary injury complicating antepartum pyelonephritis. Am J Obstet Gynecol 1987;156:797–807.

25. Cunningham FG, Morris GB, Mickal A. Acute pyelonephritis of pregnancy: A clinical review. Obstet Gynecol 1973;42:112–17.

26. Millar LK, DeBuque L, Wing DA. Uterine contraction frequency during treatment of pyelonephritis in pregnancy and subsequent risk of preterm birth. J Perinat Med 2003;31:41–6.

27. Lamont RF. The pathophysiology of pulmonary edema with the use of beta-agonists. Br J Obstet Gynaecol 2000;107:439–44.

28. Towers C, Kaminskas CM, Garite TJ, Nageotte MP, Dorchester W. Pulmonary injury associated with antepartum pyelonephritis: can patients at risk be identified? Am J Obstet Gynecol 1991;164:974–78.

29. Wing DA, Park AS, DeBuque L, Millar LK. Limited clinical utility of blood and urine cultures in the treatment of acute pyelonephritis during pregnancy. Am J Obstet Gynecol 2000;182:1437–41.

30. Millar LK, Wing DA, Paul RH, Grimes DA. Outpatient treatment of pyelonephritis in pregnancy: a randomized clinical trial. Obstet Gynecol 1995;86:560–4.

31. Wing DA, Hendershott CM, Debuque L, Millar LK. Outpatient treatment of acute pyelonephritis in pregnancy after 24 weeks. Obstet Gynecol 1999;94:683–8.

32. Butler EL, Cox SM, Eberts E, Cunningham FG. Symptomatic nephrolithiasis complicating pregnancy. Obstet Gynecol 2000;96:753–6

33. Cox SM, Cunningham FG. Acute focal pyelonephritis (lobar nephronia) complicating pregnancy. Obstet Gynecol 1988;71:510–11.

34. Van Dorsten JP, Lenke RR, Schifrin BS. Pyelonephritis in pregnancy: the role of in-hospital management and nitrofurantoin suppression. J Reprod Med 1987;32:897–900.

CHAPTER 23

Perinatal Infections Caused by Group B Streptococci

Ronald S. Gibbs, Stephanie Schrag, and Anne Schuchat

*I*n the universe of perinatal infections, the increase of group B streptococci (GBS) has been meteoric. Although the first cases of human infection with GBS were reported in the 1930s, this organism was virtually unknown to clinicians until 1964, when the first study of perinatal GBS infections was published (1). By the 1970s, GBS emerged dramatically as the leading cause of neonatal infection, with initial case fatality rates of 20–50%. Also, GBS was recognized as one of the most important causes of maternal uterine infection and septicemia (2–4).

In the preprevention era, active surveillance for invasive neonatal GBS disease indicated that approximately 6,100 early-onset cases and 1,400 late-onset cases occurred annually in the United States (5, 6). During the 1980s and early 1990s, early-onset neonatal GBS disease incidence remained fairly constant, ranging from 1.5 to 2 cases per 1,000 live births. As prevention implementation increased in the mid-1990s, disease incidence declined by 70% to a rate of 0.5 cases per 1,000 live births (6, 7). From 1999 to 2001, the rate of early onset GBS sepsis remained stable, averaging 0.47 cases per 1,000 live births. Based on active multistate surveillance data for 2004, the rate of early onset decreased to 0.34 cases per 1,000 live births, and the rate of late onset disease decreased to 0.38 cases per 1,000 live births (8).

Approximately one decade after GBS emerged as a leading infectious cause of neonatal mortality, clinical trials demonstrated that giving women intravenous penicillin or ampicillin during labor was highly effective at preventing newborn disease (9). In contrast, prenatal treatment of women to try to eradicate GBS genital colonization before labor was not effective (10, 11). Despite identification of intrapartum chemoprophylaxis as an effective intervention, controversy continued to surround methods of identifying candidates for chemoprophylaxis. Competing strategies included 1) monitoring women for known obstetric risk factors (fever, preterm labor, prolonged membrane rupture) during labor, and 2) performing culture-based screening of women before labor to identify women colonized with GBS. Screening propo-

nents also disagreed about the best time to perform screening, given the transient nature of GBS colonization in some women, and the lack of affordable, practical, reliable rapid tests at the time of labor. In 1992, the American Academy of Pediatrics (AAP) recommended a culture-based screening approach at 26–28 weeks of gestation (12). That same year, the American College of Obstetricians and Gynecologists (ACOG) suggested a risk-based approach and called for more evaluation of a culture-based screening approach before such a strategy could be recommended (13). In 1995, The Centers for Disease Control and Prevention (CDC) convened a meeting of experts, including representatives of ACOG and AAP, to come to agreement on prevention guidelines.

In 1996, the first national consensus guidelines were released (14–16). These guidelines presented culture-based screening and the risk-based approach as equally acceptable alternatives. Screening under these guidelines was recommended at 35–37 weeks of gestation. By bringing key organizations together in a united prevention effort, these guidelines set the stage for more detailed evaluation of effective strategies for identifying chemoprophylaxis candidates. Based on new evidence from a large retrospective cohort study, new national prevention guidelines from CDC, AAP, and from ACOG were released in 2002 (4, 17). These guidelines recommend a single prevention strategy, namely, universal antenatal culture-based screening at 35–37 weeks of gestation.

Group B Streptococci

In 1933, Lancefield reported her classic taxonomic classification of β-hemolytic streptococci. The most common groups causing human infection are: A *(Streptococcus pyogenes)*, B *(S. agalactiae)*, and D, which includes enterococci. Groups C and G are occasionally causes of infection in humans. Group B streptococci are facultative, gram-positive diplococci, with approximately 99% of strains showing β (complete) hemolysis on blood agar plates (Fig. 23-1). Several serotypes of GBS have been

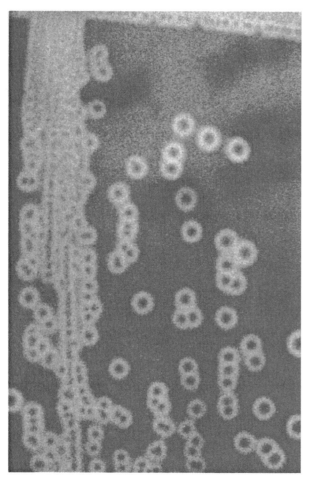

Fig. 23-1. Colonies of group B streptococci on a blood agar plate. Note the zone of clear homolysis. (Sweet RL, Gibbs RS. Atlas of infectious diseases of the female genital tract. Philadelphia [PA]: Lippincott Williams & Wilkins 2005. Copyright © 2005. Lippincott Williams & Wilkins.)

identified. The predominant types causing disease are Ia, Ib, II, III, and more recently, V. Among genital isolates from pregnant women, the distribution has been reported as Ia, 38%; Ib, 11%; II, 7%; III, 26%; and V, 18% (3). The distribution of isolates from cases of early neonatal sepsis is very similar to that of genital isolates from pregnant women. However, in cases of late-onset neonatal disease, isolates are predominantly type III. One representative study showed Ia, 23%; Ib, 5%; II, 2%; III, 64%; and V, 14% (with 2% of strains being nontypeable) (3).

Epidemiology of Group B Streptococci Perinatal Infection

Maternal Colonization

The lower gastrointestinal tract and vagina are often colonized with GBS. Longitudinal studies suggest transient, intermittent, or chronic colonization can occur. Recent studies in college-aged women found new acquisition was quite frequent among sexually active women (18). Group B streptococci can be isolated from swabs of the vagina, rectum, or both sites, and swabbing both lower vagina and rectum is recommended to increase the sensitivity of prenatal screening.

Cross-sectional studies in the United States have found GBS colonization rates to be higher in African-American women compared with whites or Asians (19), and international reports confirm racial or ethnic differences are likely after accounting for methodologic differences (20, 21). An estimated 20–30% of all pregnant women are GBS carriers, and it is likely that GBS colonizes virtually every woman at some point. Because colonization can be intermittent or transient, culture status can vary between pregnancies, and screening during each subsequent pregnancy is advised. The predictive value of prenatal screening improves with shorter intervals between culture and delivery (22, 23), so that prenatal screening at 35–37 weeks of gestation currently is recommended in the United States. (Chemoprophylaxis at delivery should be based on the 35–37 week culture even if cultures were obtained earlier.)

Neonatal Disease

In newborns, GBS can cause sepsis, pneumonia, meningitis, and less frequently, focal infections such as osteomyelitis, septic arthritis, or cellulitis (Fig. 23-2). Early-onset disease occurs within the first week of life, with most of these cases evident on the day of birth or within 72 hours. Late-onset disease occurs after the first week, and cases are relatively evenly distributed through 90 days of age. Now that early-onset disease rates have declined, the ratio of early- to late-onset GBS neonatal disease is approximately 1:1. Clinical presentations of early- and late-onset disease overlap, although 24% of late-onset disease presented as meningitis compared with only 6% of early-onset disease (6). Surveillance during the 1990s suggested case fatality ratios of 4.7% for early-onset and 2.8% for late-onset disease. (6). Although survival has improved in recent years, it remains lowest for preterm infants. For infants at more than 37 weeks of gestation with GBS sepsis, survival is very good at 98%, but for preterm infants the survival is lower at 90% for cases at 34–36 weeks of gestation and 70% for cases at less than 33 weeks of gestation (6). It is these suboptimal outcomes that prompted the search for effective prevention strategies.

Risk factors for early-onset disease have been well described (24–26) and include maternal GBS colonization, prolonged rupture of membranes, preterm delivery, GBS bacteriuria during pregnancy, birth of a previous infant with invasive GBS disease, maternal chorioamnionitis as evidenced by intrapartum fever, young mater-

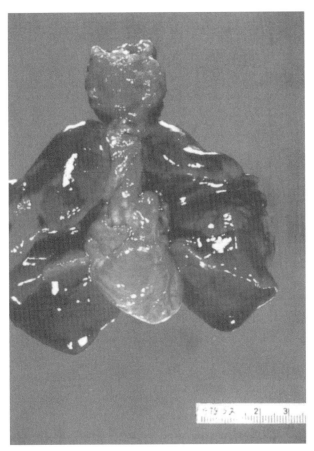

Fig. 23-2. Neonatal autopsy showing congenital pneumonia caused by group B streptococci. (Sweet RL, Gibbs RS. Atlas of infectious diseases of the female genital tract. Philadelphia [PA]: Lippincott Williams & Wilkins 2005. Copyright © 2005. Lippincott Williams & Wilkins.)

nal age, African-American race, Hispanic ethnicity, and low levels of antibody to type-specific capsular polysaccharide antigens. Although many of these factors occur in concert, multivariate analyses have demonstrated that African-American race, maternal age, and gestational age are independent predictors of early-onset disease risk.

Until recently little data existed on risk factors for late-onset disease although, as in early-onset cases, preterm gestation, maternal race, and young age each were associated with disease by multivariate analysis (25). Maternal GBS colonization is also a strong risk factor for neonatal GBS disease in the late-onset period (27). Because meningitis can occur in up to one third of late-onset cases, risk of long-term neurologic sequelae seems to be higher among survivors of late-onset disease compared with early-onset.

Maternal Disease

In the mother, GBS can cause urinary tract infection, chorioamnionitis, endometritis and bacteremia. GBS

also is a cause of some stillbirths related to infection. In urinary tract infections in pregnant and nonpregnant women, the most common isolates are *Escherichia coli* and then other aerobic, gram-negative rods collectively accounting for 80–90% of cases. Gram-positive infections, including enterococci, *Staphylococcus saprophyticus*, and GBS are responsible for the remainder (28).

Clinically evident chorioamnionitis also is referred to clinically as amnionitis, intrapartum infection, amniotic fluid infection, and clinical intraamniotic infection (29). When amniotic fluid has been cultured from such cases, polymicrobial results are usually reported. In one large study, GBS were isolated from the amniotic fluid in 15% of cases (30). Similarly, endometritis is polymicrobial. When the endometrium was cultured through a triple lumen catheter (to minimize contamination from cervical vaginal organisms), one study found GBS in 16% of cases (31). Group B streptococci are isolated in 2–15% of infected abdominal wounds after cesarean delivery (32–34).

Among obstetric patients with bacteremia, GBS are isolated from approximately 15% (35). Overall, in cases of bacteremia (including pyelonephritis), GBS were the second most common isolate (n = 31) after *E coli* (n = 55). At the time of evaluation, patients with GBS bacteremia had a mean temperature of 39°C, and half of the women had no localizing signs. The mean white blood count was 16,700/mm^3. Among postpartum women, fever occurred early, with 80% being evaluated within 24 hours of delivery. The antecedent infection was endometritis in 81% of cases, and chorioamnionitis in the remaining 19%. Although most patients responded well to antibiotic therapy, cases of fatal infection, abdominal abscess, necrotizing fasciitis, and meningitis have been reported (3, 35).

Overall, bacterial infection is estimated to be the cause of 9–15% of stillbirths (36). Infection seems to be a more common cause of early stillbirth (less than 28 weeks of gestation) than of stillbirth at term. A recent review identified GBS as a "common cause of stillbirth" (37). Although stillbirths caused by GBS seem to have decreased substantially in the United States (perhaps associated with screening programs), in other countries such as Sweden, GBS are the most common bacterial infections associated with stillbirth (37). One study from 1961 isolated GBS from internal tissues at autopsy in 9.3% of consecutive stillborn infants (38).

Diagnosis

Although definitive microbiologic identification is done by serologic detection of the group B antigen, presumptive tests are used in clinical laboratories and include the CAMP test, bile esculin reaction, and bacitracin sensitivity (3). Presumptive identification of GBS, based on colonial morphology and Gram stain, can often be determined within 24 hours of plating on blood agar. A final report usually is available within 48 hours.

To optimize yield of GBS from rectogenital tract specimens, it is necessary to use selective media to suppress the growth of competing bacteria. Commercially available selective media include Todd-Hewitt broth (a nutritive broth for gram-positive organisms) supplemented with either gentamicin plus nalidixic acid or colistin plus nalidixic acid (4). The 2002 CDC guidelines provide directions for collecting and processing these specimens (Box 23-1). These guidelines continue to recommend a rectogenital specimen to obtain optimal yield of GBS. However, in one recent comparison, the rates of culture positivity were similar in vaginoperianal, anorectal, and perianal specimens (rates of positivity were 26.5%, 27.2%, and 28.7%, respectively) (39).

Usual laboratory media such as blood agar are satisfactory for recovery of group B streptococci from endometrial, amniotic fluid, urine, and blood specimens. In addition, blood specimens are incubated in nutrient broth media. Amniotic fluid and endometrial specimens may also be placed in nutrient media.

There has been intense interest in tests for rapid identification of group B streptococci. These tests include Gram stain, immunofluorescent antibody, colorimetric assay using starch serum media, and antigen detection (including coagglutination, latex agglutination, and enzyme immunoassay). None of these tests provides sufficient sensitivity and sufficient positive predictive value from genital specimens (40). More recently, a polymerase chain reaction (PCR) test reported excellent results, with sensitivity of 97% (32:33), specificity of 100% (79:79), positive predictive value of 100% (32:32), and negative predictive value of 98.8% (79:80) when compared with conventional anovaginal cultures. The reported laboratory turnaround time was 40–100 minutes for these PCR methods (41). This past year, U.S. Food and Drug Administration approval of an intrapartum rapid PCR test that has strong sensitivity and specificity (compared with GBS culture methods) increases the possibility that some centers may consider shifting from a late antenatal screening policy to an intrapartum screening policy. Centers considering this shift will need to conduct implementation research to determine whether "real world" implementation of this test allows for sufficiently rapid turnaround of results so that the proportion of GBS-positive women who can receive adequate intrapartum prophylaxis (eg, more than 4 hours for penicillin or ampicillin) is similar to that of late antenatal culture-based screening. Systems also will need to be in place for women at high risk of penicillin anaphylaxis to continue

to receive antenatal culture, thus allowing sufficient time for GBS susceptibility testing. It remains to be seen, however, whether these tests will perform equally well and whether turnaround times are sufficient in routine practice, given decreased laboratory staffing at night and the round-the-clock nature of obstetric services (42).

Therapy

In Vitro Susceptibility of Group B Streptococci and Recommended Chemoprophylaxis Agents

Resistance to penicillin or ampicillin has not been detected in GBS. Thus penicillin, because of its narrow spectrum of activity, remains the agent of choice for GBS prophylaxis, with ampicillin an alternative (4, 17). Detection of penicillin resistance in a GBS isolate should be viewed as a sentinel event of importance requiring laboratory confirmation. If confirmed by a local laboratory, the CDC should be notified for confirmatory testing.

Resistance to clindamycin and erythromycin increased among GBS isolates in the 1990s and is now recognized as an international phenomenon. The prevalence of resistance in the United States, Canada, Germany, Spain, and Taiwan ranged from 7% to 30% for erythromycin and from 3% to 15% for clindamycin from 1998–2005 (43–51). In 2003, 37% of invasive GBS isolates from multistate active surveillance were resistant to erythromycin and 17% to clindamycin. Resistance of GBS to macrolides (antibiotics including erythromycin and clindamycin) may either be constitutive or inducible. In one study, determination of resistance phenotypes among 37 isolates resistant to erythromycin showed roughly 40% constitutive resistance and 40% showed inducible resistance, with only about 20% susceptible to clindamycin. However, only 14% of isolates with inducible resistance were identified as clindamycin resistant by traditional testing (ie, determination of minimal inhibitors). These developments have important implications in antibiotic recommendations. (Testing for induction of clindamycin resistance has been reported by the CDC for erythromycin-resistant isolates of S aureus. The test is called the "D test" (52). Some clinical laboratories have applied the D test to GBS isolates to determine whether the isolates are able to induce clindamycin resistance. However, the current CDC guidelines do not recommend use of the D test in selecting antibiotic usage in patients who cannot take penicillin). Resistance to cefoxitin, a second-generation cephalosporin sometimes used for broad-spectrum treatment of endometritis or chorioamnionitis, also has been detected (47).

Box 23-1

PROCEDURES FOR COLLECTING AND PROCESSING CLINICAL SPECIMENS FOR GROUP B STREPTOCOCCAL CULTURE AND PERFORMING SUSCEPTIBILITY TESTING TO CLINDAMYCIN AND ERYTHROMYCIN

Procedure for collecting clinical specimens for culture of GBS at 35–37 weeks of gestation

- Swab the lower vagina (vaginal introitus), followed by the rectum (ie, insert swab through the anal sphincter) using the same swab or two different swabs. Cultures should be collected in the outpatient setting by the health care provider or the patient herself, with appropriate instruction. Cervical cultures are not recommended and a speculum should not be used for culture collection.
- Place the swab(s) into a nonnutritive transport medium. Appropriate transport systems (eg, Amies or Stuart's without charcoal) are commercially available. If vaginal and rectal swabs were collected separately, both swabs can be placed into the same container of medium. Transport media will maintain GBS viability for up to 4 days at room temperature or under refrigeration.
- Specimen labels should clearly identify that specimens are for GBS culture. If susceptibility testing is ordered for penicillin-allergic women, specimen labels should also identify the patient as penicillin allergic and should specify that susceptibility testing for clindamycin and erythromycin should be performed if GBS is isolated.

Procedure for processing clinical specimens for culture of GBS

- Remove swab(s) from transport medium.* Inoculate swab(s) into a recommended selective broth medium, such as Todd–Hewitt broth supplemented with either gentamicin (8 mcg /mL) and nalidixic acid (15 mcg /mL) or with colistin (10 mcg/mL) and nalidixic acid (15 mcg/mL). Examples of appropriate commercially available options include Trans-Vag broth supplemented with 5% defibrinated sheep blood or Lossy Inhomogeneous Medium broth.†
- Incubate inoculated selective broth for 18–24 hours at 35–37°C in ambient air or 5% CO_2. Subculture the broth to a sheep blood agar plate (eg, tryptic soy agar with 5% defibrinated sheep blood).

- Inspect and identify organisms suggestive of GBS (ie, narrow zone of beta hemolysis, gram-positive cocci, catalase negative). Note that hemolysis may be difficult to observe, so typical colonies without hemolysis also should be further tested. If GBS is not identified after incubation for 18–24 hours, reincubate and inspect at 48 hours to identify suspected organisms.
- Various streptococcus grouping latex agglutination tests or other tests for GBS antigen detection (eg, genetic probe) may be used for specific identification, or the CAMP test may be employed for presumptive identification.

Procedure for clindamycin and erythromycin disk susceptibility testing of isolates, when ordered for penicillin-allergic patients‡

- Use a cotton swab to make a suspension from 18–24-hour growth of the organism in saline or Mueller–Hinton broth to match a 0.5 McFarland turbidity standard.
- Within 15 minutes of adjusting the turbidity, dip a sterile cotton swab into the adjusted suspension. The swab should be rotated several times and pressed firmly on the inside wall of the tube above the fluid level. Use the swab to inoculate the entire surface of a Mueller–Hinton sheep blood agar plate. After the plate is dry, use sterile forceps to place a clindamycin (2 mcg) disk onto half of the plate and an erythromycin (15 mcg) disk onto the other half.
- Incubate at 35°C in 50% CO_2 for 20–24 hours.
- Measure the diameter of the zone of inhibition using a ruler or calipers. Interpret according to National Committee for Clinical Laboratory Standards guidelines for *Streptococcus* species other than *Streptococcus pneumoniae* (2002 breakpoints‡: clindamycin: greater than or equal to 19 mm is susceptible, 16–18 mm is intermediate, less than or equal to 15 mm is resistant; erythromycin: greater than or equal to 21 mm is susceptible, 16–20 mm is intermediate, less than or equal to 15 mm is resistant).

*Before inoculation step, some laboratories may choose to roll swab(s) on a single sheep blood agar plate or colistin and nalidixic acid sheep blood agar plate. This should be done only in addition to, and not instead of, inoculation into selective broth. The plate should be streaked for isolation, incubated at 35–37°C in ambient air or 5% CO_2 for 18–24 hours and inspected for organisms suggestive of GBS as described above. If suspected colonies are confirmed as GBS, the broth can be discarded, thus shortening the time to obtaining culture results.

†Source: Fenton LJ, Harper MH. Evaluation of colistin and nalidixic acid in Todd–Hewitt broth for selective isolation of GBS. J Clin Microbiol 1979;9:167–9. Although Trans-Vag medium is often available without sheep blood, direct comparison of medium with and without sheep blood has shown higher yield when blood is added. The LIM broth also may benefit from the addition of sheep-blood, although the improvement in yield is smaller and sufficient data are not yet available to support a recommendation.

‡Source: Table 2H, Ferraro MJ. Performance standard for antimicrobial susceptibility testing, M100–S12. Wayne (PA): NCCLS; 2002. The National Committee for Clinical Laboratory Standards recommends disk diffusion (M-2) or broth microdilution testing (M-7) for susceptibility testing of GBS. Commercial systems that have been cleared or approved for testing of streptococci other than S pneumoniae may also be used. Penicillin susceptibility testing is not routinely recommended for GBS, because penicillin-resistant isolates have not been confirmed to date.

Abbreviation: GBS, group B streptococcus

Centers for Disease Control and Prevention. Prevention of Perinatal Group B Streptococcal Disease. MMWR 2002;51(RR-11):4.

These resistance trends, along with evidence for activity against GBS and ability to penetrate into the amniotic fluid, were taken into account when first- and second-line agents for GBS chemoprophylaxis were recommended by the CDC, AAP, and ACOG in 2002 (Box 23-2). Particular care must be taken in selecting a prophylactic agent for colonized women at high risk of penicillin anaphylaxis. Because of the possibility of inducible resistance, the 2002 guidelines recommend that clindamycin or erythromycin be used only if a given patient's GBS isolate was shown to have in vitro susceptibility to both. If there is in vitro resistance to either in a patient at high risk for penicillin anaphylaxis, vancomycin should be used. Because maternal administration of erythromycin provides subtherapeutic concentrations in both the fetal serum and amniotic fluid, there are concerns regarding its use for prophylaxis of perinatal GBS infec-

tion. For women at high risk of penicillin allergy colonized by clindamycin-resistant or erythromycin-resistant isolates, the 2002 guidelines recommend vancomycin. Vancomycin is recommended even if an isolate shows in vitro resistance to either clindamycin or erythromycin because of concern regarding inducible resistance. Vancomycin use is generally restricted because of concerns about emerging vancomycin resistance, thus clinicians should take care to reserve vancomycin for highly penicillin-allergic women with isolates of unknown susceptibility and isolates with resistance to either erythromycin or clindamycin.

Maternal Infection

Because of its uniform activity, penicillin G remains the drug of choice for clinically evident maternal infection with GBS as well as for GBS prophylaxis. There have been

---

Box 23-2

RECOMMENDED REGIMENS FOR INTRAPARTUM ANTIMICROBIAL PROPHYLAXIS FOR PERINATAL GROUP B STREPTOCOCCI DISEASE PREVENTION*

Recommended	Penicillin G, 5 million units intravenously (initial dose), then 2.5 million units intravenously every 4 hours until delivery
Alternative	Ampicillin, 2 g intravenously (initial dose), then 1 g intravenously every 4 hours until delivery
If penicillin allergic†	
Patients not at high risk for anaphylaxis	Cefazolin, 2 g intravenously (initial dose), then 1 g intravenously every 8 hours until delivery
Patients at high risk for anaphylaxis‡	
Group B streptococci susceptible to clindamycin and erythromycin§	Clindamycin, 900 mg intravenously every 8 hours until delivery or Erythromycin, 500 mg intravenously every 6 hours until delivery
Group B streptococci resistant to clindamycin or erythromycin or susceptibility unknown	Vancomycin,‖ 1 g intravenously every 12 hours until delivery

*Broader-spectrum agents, including an agent active against group B streptococci, may be necessary for treatment of chorioamnionitis.

†History of penicillin allergy should be assessed to determine whether a high risk for anaphylaxis is present. Penicillin-allergic patients at high risk for anaphylaxis are those who have experienced immediate hypersensitivity to penicillin, including a history of penicillin-related anaphylaxis; other high-risk patients are those with asthma or other diseases that would make anaphylaxis more dangerous or difficult to treat, such as persons being treated with β-adrenergic blocking agents.

‡If laboratory facilities are adequate, clindamycin and erythromycin susceptibility testing should be performed on prenatal group B streptococci isolates from penicillin-allergic women at high risk for anaphylaxis.

§Resistance to erythromycin is often but not always associated with clindamycin resistance. If a strain is resistant to erythromycin but seems susceptible to clindamycin, it may still have inducible resistance to clindamycin.

‖Cefazolin is preferred over vancomycin for women with a history of penicillin allergy other than immediate hypersensitivity reactions, and pharmacologic data suggest it achieves effective intraamniotic concentrations. Vancomycin should be reserved for penicillin-allergic women at high risk for anaphylaxis.

Centers for Disease Control and Prevention. Prevention of Perinatal Group B Streptococcal Disease. MMWR 2002:51 (RR-11):10.

national or regional shortages of penicillin G (48), and regionally practitioners encounter difficulties obtaining this preferred antibiotic for both treatment and prevention. Ampicillin is widely used and is an acceptable alternative. The usual dose of penicillin G is 5 million units, intravenously initially, then 2.5 million units, intravenously every 4–6 hours. Note that for prevention of GBS perinatal infections, the dosing interval is every 4 hours until delivery (4). For ampicillin, the usual adult dose is 2 g, intravenously initially, then 1 g, intravenously every 4–6 hours. Again, note that for GBS prophylaxis the dose interval is every 4 hours until delivery (4).

In clinical practice, therapy of genitourinary infection in pregnant and puerperal women is most often initiated empirically before culture results are available. In view of the polymicrobial nature of chorioamnionitis and the lack of a rapid, reliable test to detect specific organisms in a given case, treatment recommendations for this common infection are for empiric, broad-spectrum (usually combination) intravenous antibiotic therapy and for delivery. The antibiotic regimen should include an antibiotic with excellent activity against GBS. One traditional regimen is intravenous ampicillin (such as 2 g, intravenously every 6 hours) plus intravenous gentamicin (1.5 mg/kg every 8 hours) (49). Therapy should be initiated as soon as possible during labor once clinical chorioamnionitis has been diagnosed. Intrapartum treatment not only controls maternal illness but also treatment the fetus in utero and decreases overall neonatal sepsis (49).

As with chorioamnionitis, treatment of postpartum endometritis is directed at the polymicrobial pathogens, including GBS. Here, also, therapy should be empiric and broad spectrum. Intravenous therapy is used initially for postpartum endometritis in hospitalized patients at the University of Colorado. Many parenteral regimens of either single or combination antibiotic therapy have achieved very good results in endometritis overall. These have included regimens with activity against not only GBS but also other aerobes as well as anaerobes (50).

In obstetric patients with GBS bacteremia, response to appropriate intravenous therapy usually is prompt (51), but meningitis, abscess, and fatal sepsis have been reported. In contrast, when GBS septicemia occurs in nonobstetric adult patients, it is often in individuals with serious underlying conditions, and the mortality rate is high.

Neonatal Infection

Newborns with suspected sepsis initially are treated empirically with intravenous ampicillin and an intravenous aminoglycoside, a combination that includes activity against GBS as well as other common neonatal pathogens. If bacteremia is present without meningitis, this initial treatment is recommended for 48–72 hours

(until culture results are available). If GBS are the sole isolate, then therapy with intravenous penicillin G is continued to complete a total course of 10 days. If meningitis is present, intravenous ampicillin and intravenous gentamicin are continued until the cerebrospinal fluid is sterile, and then intravenous penicillin G is continued to complete the minimum course of 14 days (3).

Prevention of Perinatal Group B Streptococci Infection

Several clinical trials have demonstrated that use of intravenous antibiotics during the intrapartum period is highly effective at preventing early-onset neonatal GBS infections. Use of intrapartum prophylaxis also has been shown to be cost-effective in the United States (53–55). To date, this is the only effective intervention available against perinatal GBS disease. However, competing and evolving strategies for identifying chemoprophylaxis candidates have posed a challenge to prophylaxis implementation. Universal prophylaxis for deliveries is not advisable because only a small percentage of women in labor are at risk of transmitting GBS to their newborns, and universal prophylaxis would lead to vast overuse of intrapartum antibiotics. A recent, large, multistate retrospective evaluation of the effectiveness of the two recommended strategies in the 1990s found that late antenatal culture-based screening for GBS was greater than 50% more effective than the alternative risk-based approach at preventing neonatal early-onset GBS disease (56). This benefit derived largely from the identification and prophylaxis of culture-positive women who did not present with risk factors (18% of delivering women in the population-based retrospective study) as well as improved compliance with the screen-based approach. These findings were the basis of new perinatal GBS disease prevention guidelines released by the CDC, AAP, and ACOG in 2002 that recommend universal late antenatal screening of all pregnant women (4, 17). Multistate data from 2003 show a 34% decline in early-onset disease incidence in the year after issuance of these new guidelines (57).

Recommendations for Prophylaxis

The indications for prophylaxis under this universal prenatal screening strategy are shown in Figure 23-3. In addition to women who have a positive GBS screening culture result in the current pregnancy, as in past guidelines, women who had a previous infant with invasive GBS disease or who have any level of GBS bacteriuria during the pregnancy should receive intrapartum prophylaxis. Additionally, any women with unknown culture status at the time of labor should receive intrapartum antibiotic prophylaxis if they present with the

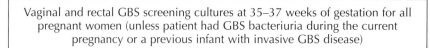

Vaginal and rectal GBS screening cultures at 35–37 weeks of gestation for all pregnant women (unless patient had GBS bacteriuria during the current pregnancy or a previous infant with invasive GBS disease)

Intrapartum prophylaxis indicated

- Previous infant with invasive GBS disease
- GBS bacteriuria during current pregnancy
- Positive GBS screening culture during current pregnancy (unless a planned cesarean delivery, in the absence of labor or amniotic membrane rupture, is performed)
- Unknown GBS status (culture not done, incomplete, or results unknown) and any of the following items:
  —Delivery at less than 32 weeks of gestation*
  —Amniotic membrane rupture for 18 hours or longer
  —Intrapartum temperature greater than or equal to 38°C (100.4°F)†

Intrapartum prophylaxis not indicated

- Previous pregnancy with a positive GBS screening culture (unless a culture was also positive during the current pregnancy)
- Planned cesarean delivery performed in the absence of labor or membrane rupture (regardless of maternal GBS culture status)
- Negative vaginal and rectal GBS screening culture in late gestation during the current pregnancy, regardless of intrapartum risk factors

Fig. 23-3. Indications for intrapartum antibiotic prophylaxis to prevent perinatal group B streptococci disease under a universal prenatal screening strategy based on combined vaginal and rectal cultures collected at 35–37 weeks of gestation from all pregnant women. *If onset of labor or rupture of amniotic membranes occurs at less than 37 weeks of gestation and there is a significant risk for preterm delivery (as assessed by the clinician), a suggested algorithm for GBS prophylaxis management is provided. †If amnionitis is suspected, broad-spectrum antibiotic therapy that includes an agent known to be active against GBS should replace GBS prophylaxis. Abbreviation: GBS, group B streptococcus. (Centers for Disease Control and Prevention. Prevention of Perinatal Group B Streptococcal Disease. MMWR 2002;51[RR-11]:8.)

risk factors outlined in Figure 23-3. Figure 23-3 also outlines some common circumstances in which intrapartum prophylaxis is not indicated. Women undergoing a planned cesarean delivery in the absence of labor or membrane rupture do not require GBS prophylaxis. This recommendation was based on evidence that the risk of neonatal early-onset disease was sufficiently low in this circumstance and that the potential risks associated with intrapartum antibiotics outweighed the benefits.

Recommended antibiotics for intrapartum prophylaxis are given in Box 23-2. Emerging resistance to erythromycin and clindamycin have shaped these recommendations. A key change for obstetricians is the need to get a detailed history from colonized women who report penicillin allergy to determine whether they are at high risk for anaphylaxis. Among penicillin-allergic patients, women at high risk for anaphylaxis are defined as those who have experienced immediate hypersensitivity to penicillin, including a history of penicillin-related anaphylaxis, and those with other conditions (such as asthma or treatment with β-adrenergic blocking agents) that would make anaphylaxis more dangerous or difficult to treat.

Preterm Premature Rupture of Membranes

Preterm premature rupture of the membranes places the fetus or newborn at double risk for GBS sepsis, based on the combination of prematurity and prolonged membrane rupture. Although the 2002 CDC Guidelines provide a sample algorithm (Fig. 23-4), specifics of the management are left to the individual provider because no data are available to recommend one approach. In addition, based on meta-analyses and expert opinion, it is now recommended that patients with preterm premature rupture of the membranes receive antibiotics in certain circumstances for the additional rationale of delaying delivery and preventing maternal or neonatal complications such as chorioamnionitis, neonatal infection, and neonatal sepsis (58–63). Proposed guidelines are summarized in Box 23-3.

Bacteriuria

Newborns whose mothers had GBS bacteriuria during pregnancy have been shown to have a higher risk of early-onset GBS disease, possibly because women with

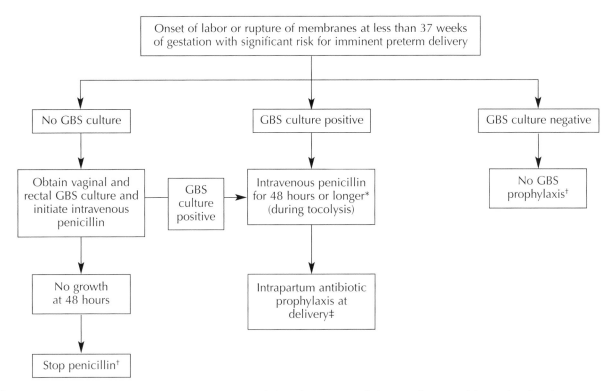

Fig. 23-4. Sample algorithm for group B streptococci prophylaxis for women with threatened preterm delivery. This algorithm is not an exclusive course of management. Variations that incorporate individual circumstances or institutional preferences may be appropriate. *Penicillin should be continued for a total of at least 48 hours, unless delivery occurs sooner. At the physician's discretion, antibiotic prophylaxis may be continued beyond 48 hours in a GBS culture-positive woman if delivery has not yet occurred. For women who are GBS culture positive, antibiotic prophylaxis should be reinitiated when labor likely to proceed to delivery occurs or recurs. †If delivery has not occurred within 4 weeks, a vaginal and rectal GBS screening culture should be repeated and the patient should be managed as described, based on the result of the repeat culture. §Intrapartum antibiotic prophylaxis. Abbreviation: GBS, group B streptococcus. (Centers for Disease Control and Prevention. Prevention of Perinatal Group B Streptococcal Disease. MMWR 2002;51[RR-11]:12.)

bacteriuria are more likely to have heavy colonization with GBS. Consequently, the 2002 GBS prevention guidelines recommend that all women with GBS bacteriuria, defined as GBS isolated from the urine at any level (even less than 10^5 colony-forming units), should receive intrapartum prophylaxis. Consequently, these women do not require late antenatal screening. In terms of antepartum antibiotics, women with symptomatic or asymptomatic urinary tract infections caused by GBS should receive antibiotic therapy according to the obstetric standard of care for managing urinary tract infections. When there is low level GBS bacteriuria (less than 100,000/mL) in an asymptomatic pregnant woman, there is currently no recommendation about treatment. In one small survey, it was reported that 77% (of 85) respondents would treat at the time of diagnosis, whereas 23% stated they would treat only during labor (65).

Alternative Antibiotic Approaches

There are no efficacy data to assess oral antibiotic approaches as alternatives to the intravenous regimens recommended by the 2002 CDC Guidelines. Requests for

such alternatives have come from practitioners caring for GBS-positive patients who, for example, refuse an intravenous catheter or who desire a home birth. Oral therapy, such as penicillin, ampicillin (66), or erythromycin (67) for 1 or more weeks in pregnancy still left 20–30% of women colonized at the end of therapy (3). Accordingly, there is no oral alternative regimen that is recommended for intrapartum prophylaxis.

Long-acting intramuscular penicillin, such as benzathine penicillin G, also has been evaluated during prenatal care (68, 69). A single dose of 4.8 million units of benzathine penicillin G significantly reduced maternal GBS rectovaginal colonization compared with those given no treatment, but 25% (7/28) of those treated remained culture positive at delivery (occurring at a mean of 19 days after treatment) (69). An earlier uncontrolled study also noted that a similar percent (28%) of women remained culture positive at delivery after treatment with 4.8 million units of benzathine penicillin G (68).

There are no data on the use of any intramuscular penicillin for intrapartum prophylaxis. Especially because many GBS-positive women deliver in less than 4 hours

---

Box 23-3

DETAILED SAMPLE ANTIBIOTIC ALGORITHM FOR PRETERM PREMATURE RUPTURE OF MEMBRANES

Premature rupture of membranes before viability (less than approximately 24 weeks of gestation)
- No GBS prophylaxis
- No antibiotics to prolong gestation (64)

Premature rupture of membranes at 24–32 weeks of gestation
- Obtain GBS anorectal culture
- Begin ampicillin, 2 g intravenously (initially), then 1–2 g intravenously every 4–6 hours* plus erythromycin, 250 mg intravenously every 6 hours for 48 hours. Then if patient still has not given birth, give amoxicillin, 250 mg orally every 8 hours plus erythromycin 333 mg orally every 8 hours until labor or to complete 7 days (64).
- If the GBS anorectal culture was negative before start of the antibiotic regimen, there is no need to give intrapartum antibiotics to prevent GBS perinatal infection (4).
- If the GBS anorectal culture was positive before the start of the antibiotic regimen, then our approach is to reculture for GBS while the patient is taking the ampicillin plus erythromycin regimen to determine whether colonization was suppressed (60). If the GBS culture remains positive, we retreat with the rationale of preventing ascending GBS infection and chorioamnionitis. There is no standard regimen, but our recommendation is to give intravenous ampicillin for an additional 5–7 days (4).

Premature rupture of membranes at more than 32 weeks of gestation
- Do not give antibiotic regimen to prolong delivery (64).
- If GBS anogenital culture status is unknown (ie, gestation is less than 35–37 weeks), obtain GBS anorectal culture.
- If the GBS culture status is positive or unknown, give intravenous penicillin G for 48 hours. Approximately 48 hours after completion of this, reculture, and if GBS remains positive, treat for another 48 hours to prevent ascending infection and chorioamnionitis (60).
- If GBS culture result is negative, then discontinue antibiotics at this juncture.

General recommendations
- Regardless of the management strategy used, patients at 24 weeks of gestation or longer with a positive GBS culture or unknown GBS status also should receive intrapartum antibiotic chemoprophylaxis for GBS when labor ensues.
- If clinical chorioamnionitis develops, broad-spectrum therapy should be started empirically in recognition of the polymicrobial cause of this infection.
- The accuracy of GBS anorectal cultures in predicting colonization status at delivery is most predictive if collected within 5 weeks of delivery. If a patient remains undelivered for 4 weeks after her screening culture, she should be screened again, especially if the initial culture was negative.

* One suggested dose interval for ampicillin is 2 g every 6 hours (64). However, another suggested dose interval is 2 g initially and then 1 g every 4 hours (4).

Abbreviation: GBS, group B streptococcus.

Gibbs RS, Schrag S, Schuchat A. Perinatal infections due to group B streptococci. Obstet Gynecol. 2004 Nov;104(5 Pt 1):1062–76.

---

after admission, the intravenous approach is recommended to achieve therapeutic levels as rapidly as possible. When given intravenously in usual doses, such as 5 million units, penicillin G achieves peak levels of 400 mcg/mL within a few minutes in maternal serum. In comparison, when penicillin G is given intramuscularly in the usual dose, such as 1 million units, peak serum concentrations are achieved in 15–30 minutes, but these peaks are only 12 mcg/mL (70). Accordingly, there is no intramuscular regimen that is recommended for intrapartum prophylaxis.

Measures to Improve Compliance

Both the 1996 and 2002 CDC Guidelines for prevention of perinatal GBS infection are complex, and noncompliance occurs frequently. With the risk-based approach, noncompliance occurred in up to 39% of cases, often those at highest risk, such as those in preterm labor (56). Compliance with the screen-based approach was better, but still, intrapartum prophylaxis was missed in about 14% of patients. In two studies, each conducted at a single institution, culture results were available at the time of delivery in 90–95%, and antibiotics were given to known GBS-positive patients in 93–94% (after excluding elective cesarean delivery) (71, 72) In one report, intrapartum antibiotics had been given for 2 hours or longer in 87% of cases, and in the other report they had been given for 4 hours or longer in 75% of cases, but factors beyond the control of the obstetrician (such as precipitous delivery) were noted often. Culturing before 35 weeks of gestation or after 37 weeks of gestation was noted in 17.5% and 12.6% of cases, respectively (72).

In every facility with obstetric deliveries, care providers must be vigilant to avoid noncompliance. One measure used at the University of Colorado Hospital is to note each patient's GBS status (positive, negative, or unknown) on the labor and delivery board so that active decisions are made for every patient.

Every effort should be made to have GBS culture results available in the hospital where the patient will give birth, as well as at the site of prenatal care. In a multistate review of births, this goal was achieved in approximately 95% of deliveries (56). When the GBS status is unknown, the 2002 CDC Guidelines recommend intrapartum prophylaxis only if there is a risk factor.

Use of antepartum prophylaxis for GBS eradication also should be monitored because this practice has not proved successful and is not recommended. A survey of obstetrician–gynecologists about practices in 2001 found that 22% reported prescribing antibiotics for GBS prenatal. Growing evidence that late antenatal exposure to β-lactam antibiotics, such as amoxicillin–clavulanic acid, may be associated with increased incidence of neonatal necrotizing enterocolitis lends further support to avoidance of this practice (59, 73).

Neonatal Approaches

Another strategy to prevent neonatal GBS infection is to give antibiotics to the neonate. Support for this approach has come from early retrospective studies and, more recently, from a prospective descriptive study (74, 75). However, current policy does not rely on this approach for two reasons: 1) single-dose prophylaxis to the neonate is not adequate, and most neonates who develop early-onset neonatal GBS sepsis are bacteremic within 1 hour of birth, and 2) a well-designed trial in low birth weight infants demonstrated that neonatal administration of antibiotics was ineffective at preventing bacteremia and reducing mortality (76). From the same hospital, a recent "before–after" study (77) assessed a combined intrapartum and neonatal protocol. Mothers were given intrapartum prophylaxis for risk factors and neonates for all asymptomatic mothers were given a single dose of penicillin G intramuscularly within one hour of birth. (Infants of women with chorioamnionitis were treated with ampicillin and gentamicin for at least 48

hours.) This regimen resulted in a rate of early-onset GBS sepsis of 0.4 per 1,000 liveborns. However, current guidelines do not recommend this approach, because its effectiveness has not been confirmed in other centers, and theoretically, it still has the disadvantages of each of its component strategies.

Remaining Clinical Questions

Group B Streptococci and Low Birth Weight or Preterm Birth

Women who have heavy colonization of the lower genital tract have a small, but significant, increase in risk for delivery of a low birth weight infant (odds ratio 1.2, 95% confidence interval 1.01–1.5) (78). However, there was no significant increase in other adverse outcomes, including preterm birth, for heavily colonized women. Other studies have not detected this increase consistently, perhaps because they were not large enough to detect this small difference. In a randomized clinical trial of erythromycin compared with placebo for up to 6 weeks in GBS-positive women, use of erythromycin was not effective in decreasing low birth weight or in decreasing preterm birth (67). The 2002 guidelines recommend not treating GBS-colonized women antepartum because it has no benefit and would expose approximately 1 million pregnant women per year in the United States to unnecessary antibiotics.

Adverse Effects of Antibiotics

Maternal anaphylaxis to penicillins or cephalosporins is possible, but the rate of life-threatening reactions is relatively low. Greater use of antibiotics in labor could potentially lead to more diagnostic testing of newborns whose mothers receive prophylaxis. However, one study showed that pediatricians have not been carrying out inappropriate testing and treatment in this setting (79).

The ecologic impact of large increases in antibiotic use in labor and delivery on the maternal and newborn bacterial flora remains a central concern, particularly that reductions of GBS cases would be followed by increased occurrence of other species, especially gram-negative organisms and penicillin- or ampicillin-resistant bacteria (80). Although one large study did identify a significant increase in the rate of early-onset *E coli* sepsis, this study was restricted to very low birth weight newborns (81), and the rate of total gram-negative bacterial sepsis actually declined despite the increase in *E coli* infections. Stable or decreasing rates of non-GBS sepsis have been reported in studies of the general population (82, 83).

Emergence of Resistant Organisms

Although GBS remain uniformly susceptible to penicillin, concerns have centered on whether increased use of penicillin or ampicillin for intrapartum prophylaxis will lead to increased illnesses associated with antibiotic-resistant organisms other than GBS. Even if an increasing proportion of perinatal infections are caused by ampicillin-resistant organisms, this increase may reflect community-wide changes rather than a direct relationship to intrapartum antimicrobial use. Proponents of penicillin have suggested its narrow spectrum, compared with that of ampicillin, might result in less selective pressure for the emergence of ampicillin resistant organisms. However, recent evaluation of vaginal colonization with Enterobacteriaceae among women randomly assigned to either intrapartum benzylpenicillin or ampicillin found that either agent led to significant increases in colonization with ampicillin-resistant organisms 36 hours postpartum (24% prepartum compared with 37% postpartum (84).

Obstetric Procedures in a Group B Streptococci-Positive Woman

Membrane sweeping (or stripping) among term patients has been shown to be an effective technique to hasten the onset of labor (85). A meta-analysis of available studies found no significant increases in overall perinatal or peripartum infection when women who had membrane sweeping were compared with those who did not have this procedure. However, because these studies did not report GBS status, there are no data to advise whether this procedure should or should not be avoided in GBS-positive women (84). Nevertheless, because the benefits of membrane sweeping are limited (such as a significantly greater likelihood of onset of labor within 48 hours), at the University of Colorado membrane sweeping is avoided in GBS-positive women. If there is an indication for delivery, there are many alternative interventions to membrane sweeping, such as the use of vaginal prostaglandin preparations.

Frequent vaginal examinations in labor and intrauterine fetal monitoring have been associated with chorioamnionitis and endometritis, but these factors also are confounding variables in women with complicated labors. Most studies have not randomly allocated patients to these procedures. In GBS-positive women, the obstetrician should not avoid appropriate vaginal examinations nor avoid indicated intrauterine fetal monitoring. Avoidance of these indicated procedures may actually prolong the labor and increase the risk of infection. In most circumstances, intrapartum prophylaxis will have been started at or before insertion of intrauterine fetal monitors.

Group B Streptococci and Stillbirth

There are few data for advising a patient who has experienced a stillbirth accompanied by evidence of GBS. Our practice at the University of Colorado is to determine whether there was weak evidence (such as simply a positive GBS genital culture) or whether there was strong evidence of causation between GBS and the stillbirth (such as intrauterine pneumonia on autopsy plus a positive culture of GBS from the lung, perhaps with a Gram stain showing gram-positive cocci in lung sections). For patients with the latter condition, screening for GBS in the genitourinary tract and then parenteral or oral antibiotic therapy during prenatal care may be offered in a subsequent pregnancy, although there is no evidence to support the efficacy of this regimen.

Future Research Issues

Vaccine Development

Because most maternal and neonatal GBS disease is caused by a small number of GBS serotypes, researchers began to explore development of vaccines shortly after GBS emerged. Immunization strategies hold promise to prevent a larger burden of disease, protecting against both early- and late-onset infections. Moreover, vaccination may prevent some adverse pregnancy outcomes associated with GBS, such as preterm delivery, spontaneous abortion, or stillbirth, particularly if vaccination of adolescent girls before pregnancy is a viable strategy. Additionally, immunization strategies would not contribute to emerging antimicrobial resistance among GBS. Promising capsular polysaccharide protein conjugate GBS vaccine candidates now exist. Phase I and II trials have been conducted in healthy, nonpregnant adults, and phase I safety and immunogenicity trials have been conducted in pregnant women yielding promising results (86–88). One obstacle in proceeding to phase III licensure trials is that large trials are needed in the context of intrapartum prophylaxis; use of immunologic correlates may be necessary. Liability concerns over researching a vaccine with an indication for use in pregnant women pose perhaps the larger obstacle and, to date, pharmaceutical company backing for phase III trials has not been obtained.

Disinfectants

In vitro studies have shown strong activity of some microbicides against GBS, and several clinical trials evaluating the disinfectant chlorhexidine have suggested that application to the birth canal during labor or wiping of the newborn at birth or both can reduce vertical transmission of GBS colonization from mother to newborn (89–91). There is suggestive evidence from some trials that chlorhexidine disinfection may also reduce neonatal GBS infections. A trial at a large hospital in Malawi found significant reductions in neonatal morbidity and mortality rates and maternal postpartum infections in the chlorhexidine arm of the trial (90). However, other studies have found no beneficial effects of chlorhexidine (92). Trials have used different methodologies that prevent direct comparisons, and without a pivotal trial, the efficacy against neonatal sepsis remains debatable. Although this intervention holds most promise for developing countries where intravenous intrapartum antibiotics are often not affordable or feasible, it also is of renewed interest in some developed countries, particularly to prevent emerging infection with ampicillin-resistant *E coli* (93).

Prevention of Late-Onset Neonatal Disease

As progress continues to be made in early-onset disease prevention, late-onset disease is now as common or more common than early-onset disease in many parts of the United States. Unfortunately, intrapartum prophylaxis has not led to decreases in late-onset disease (6). Potential interventions have not yet been identified because the baseline incidence of late-onset disease is below 0.5 cases per 1,000 live births and because the potential period for transmission is much longer than early-onset disease. Because late-onset disease represents a growing proportion of all neonatal GBS infections, future research should continue to explore risk factors and potential interventions.

Resources From the Centers for Disease Control and Prevention

Health communications tools and practical tools to assist with monitoring prevention are available from a recently designed web site (www.cdc.gov/groupbstrep). This web site has portals for clinicians, clinical microbiologists, the general public, and state health officials.

References

1. Eickhoff TC, Klein JO, Daly AK, Ingall D, Finland M. Neonatal sepsis and other infections due to group B beta-hemolytic streptococci. N Engl J Med 1964;271:1221–28.

2. Sweet RL, Gibbs RS. Group B Streptococci. In: Sweet RL, Gibbs RS. Infectious diseases of the female genital tract. 4th ed. Philadelphia (PA): Lippincott Williams & Wilkins; 2002. p. 31–46.

3. Edwards MS, Baker CJ. Group B streptococcal infections. In: Remington JS, Klein JO, editors. Infectious diseases of the fetus and newborn infant. 5th ed. Philadelphia (PA): W.B. Saunders; 2001. p. 1091–156.

4. Prevention of perinatal group B streptococcal disease. Revised guidelines from CDC. MMWR Recomm Rep 2002;51(RR-11):1–22.

5. Zangwill KM, Schuchat A, Wenger JD. Group B streptococcal disease in the United States, 1990: report from a multistate active surveillance system. MMWR CDC Surveill Summ 1992;41(SS-6):25–32.

6. Schrag SJ, Zywicki S, Farley MM, Reingold AL, Harrison LH, Lefkowitz LB, et al. Group B streptococcal disease in the era of intrapartum antibiotic prophylaxis. N Engl J Med 2000;342:15–20.

7. Early-onset group B streptococcal disease, United States, 1998-1999. MMWR Morb Mortal Wkly Rep 2000;49: 793–6.

8. Early-onset and late-onset neonatal group B streptococcal disease—United States, 1996–2004. Centers for Disease Control and Prevention (CDC). MMWR Morb Mortal Wkly Rep 2005;54(47):1205–8.

9. Boyer KM, Gotoff SP. Prevention of early-onset neonatal Group B streptococcal disease with selective intrapartum chemoprophylaxis. N Engl J Med 1986;314:1665–9.

10. Hall RT, Barnes W, Krishan L, Harris DJ, Rhodes PG, Fayez J, et al. Antibiotic treatment of parturient women colonized with group B streptococci. Am J Obstet Gynecol 1976;124:630–4.

11. Gardner SE, Yow MD, Leeds LJ, Thompson PK, Mason EO Jr, Clark DJ. Failure of penicillin to eradicate group B streptococcal colonization in the pregnant woman: a couple study. Am J Obstet Gynecol 1979;135:1062–5.

12. American Academy of Pediatrics Committee on Infectious Diseases and Committee on Fetus and Newborn. Guidelines for prevention of perinatal group B streptococcal (GBS) infection by chemoprophylaxis. Pediatrics 1992; 90:775–8.

13. American College of Obstetricians and Gynecologists. Group B streptococcal infections in pregnancy. ACOG Technical Bulletin 170. Washington, DC: ACOG; 1992.

14. American College of Obstetricians and Gynecologists. Prevention of early-onset group B streptococcal disease in newborns. ACOG Committee Opinion 173. Washington, DC: ACOG; 1996.

15. Revised guidelines for prevention of early-onset group B streptococcal (GBS) infection. American Academy of Pediatrics Committee on Infectious Diseases and Committee on Fetus and Newborn. Pediatrics 1997;99: 489–96.

16. Prevention of perinatal group B streptococcal disease: a public health perspective. MMWR Recomm Rep 1996;45 (RR-7):1–24.

17. Prevention of early-onset group B streptococcal disease in newborns. ACOG Committee Opinion No. 279. American College of Obstetricians and Gynecologists. Obstet Gynecol 2002;100:1405–12.

18. Meyn LA, Moore DM, Hillier SL, Krohn MA. Association of sexual activity with colonization and vaginal acquisition of group B Streptococcus in nonpregnant women. Am J Epidemiol. 2002;155:949–57.

19. Regan JA, Klebanoff MA, Nugent RP. The epidemiology of group B streptococcal colonization in pregnancy. Vaginal Infections and Prematurity Study Group. Obstet Gynecol 1991;77:604–10.

20. Stoll BJ, Schuchat A. Maternal carriage of group B streptococci in developing countries. Pediatr Infect Dis J 1998; 17:499–503.

21. Thinkhamrop J, Limpongsanurak S, Festin MR, Daly S, Schuchat A, Lumbiganon P, et al. Infections in international pregnancy study: performance of the optical immunoassay test for detection of group B streptococcus. J Clin Microbiol 2003;41:5288–90.

22. Yancey MK, Schuchat A, Brown LK, Ventura VL, Markenson GR. The accuracy of late antenatal screening cultures in predicting genital group B streptococcal colonization at delivery. Obstet Gynecol 1996;88:811–5.

23. Boyer KM, Gadzala CA, Kelly PD, Burd LI, Gotoff SP. Selective intrapartum chemoprophylaxis of neonatal group B streptococcal early-onset disease. II. Predictive value of prenatal cultures. J Infect Dis 1983;148:802–9.

24. Boyer KM, Gadzala CA, Burd LI, Fisher DE, Paton JB, Gotoff SP. Selective intrapartum chemoprophylaxis of neonatal group B streptococcal early-onset disease. I. Epidemiologic rationale. J Infect Dis 1983;148:795–801.

25. Schuchat A, Oxtoby M, Cochi S, Sikes RK, Hightower A, Plikaytis B, et al. Population-based risk factors for neonatal group B streptococcal disease: results of a cohort study in metropolitan Atlanta. J Infect Dis 1990;162:672–7.

26. Zaleznik DF, Rench MA, Hillier S, Krohn MA, Platt R, Lee ML, et al. Invasive disease due to group B streptococcus in pregnant women and neonates from diverse population groups. Clin Infect Dis 2000;30:276–81.

27. Lin FY, Weisman LE, Troendle J, Adams K. Prematurity is the major risk factor for late-onset group B streptococcus disease. J Infect Dis 2003;188:267–71.

28. Sweet RL, Gibbs RS. Urinary tract infection. In: Sweet RL, Gibbs RS. Infectious diseases of the female genital tract. 4th ed. Philadelphia (PA): Lippincott Williams & Wilkins; 2002. p. 413–48.

29. Sweet RL, Gibbs RS. Intraamniotic infection. In: Sweet RL, Gibbs RS. Infectious diseases of the female genital tract, 4th ed. Philadelphia (PA): Lippincott Williams & Wilkins; 2002. p. 516–27.

30. Sperling RS, Newton E, Gibbs RS. Intra-amniotic infection in low birth-weight infants. J Infect Dis 1988;157: 113–7.

31. Rosene K, Echenbach DA, Tompkins LS, Kenny GE, Watkins H. Polymicrobial early postpartum endometritis with facultative and anaerobic bacteria, genital mycoplasmas and Chlamydia trachomatis: treatment with piperacillin or cefoxitin. J Infect Dis 1986;153:1028–37.

32. Roberts S, Maccato M, Faro S, Pinell P. The microbiology of post-cesarean wound morbidity. Obstet Gynecol 1993; 81:383–6.

33. Emmons SL, Krohn M, Jackson M, Eschenbach DA. Development of wound infections among women undergoing cesarean section. Obstet Gynecol 1988;72:559–64.

34. Blanco JD, Gibbs RS. Infections following classical cesarean section. Obstet Gynecol 1980;55:167–9.

35. Blanco JD, Gibbs RS, Castaneda YS. Bacteremia in obstetrics: clinical course. Obstet Gynecol 1981;58:621–5.

36. Gibbs RS. The origins of stillbirth: infectious diseases. Semin Perinatol 2002;26:75–78 .

37. Goldenberg RL, Thompson C. The infectious origins of stillbirth. Am J Obstet Gynecol 2003;189:861–73.

38. Hood M, Janney A, Dameron G. Beta hemolytic streptococcus group B associated with problems of the perinatal period. Am J Obstet Gynecol 1961;82:809–18.

39. Orafu C, Gill P, Nelson K, Hecht B, Hopkins M. Perianal versus anorectal specimens: is there a difference in group B streptococcal detection? Obstet Gynecol 2002;99: 1036–9.

40. Yancey MK, Armer T, Clark P, Duff P. Assessment of rapid identification tests for genital carriage of group B streptococci. Obstet Gynecol 1992;80:1038–47.

41. Bergeron MG, Ke D, Menard C, Picard FJ, Gagnon M, Bernier M, et al. Rapid detection of group B streptococci in pregnant women at delivery. N Engl J Med 2000;343: 175–9.

42. Schuchat A. Neonatal group B streptococcal disease—screening and prevention. N Engl J Med 2000;343: 208–210.

43. Fernandez M, Hickman ME, Baker CJ. Antimicrobial susceptibilities of group B streptococci isolated between 1992 and 1996 from patients with bacteremia or meningitis. Antimicrob Agents Chemother 1998;42:1517–9.

44. Morales WJ, Dickey SS, Bornick P, Lim DV. Change in antibiotic resistance of group B streptococcus: impact on intrapartum management. Am J Obstet Gynecol 1999;181: 310–4.

45. Andrews JI, Diekema DJ, Hunter SK, Rhomberg PR, Pfaller MA, Jones RN, et al. Group B streptococci causing neonatal bloodstream infection: antimicrobial susceptibility and serotyping results from SENTRY centers in the Western hemisphere. Am J Obstet Gynecol 2000;183:859–62.

46. Bland ML, Vermillion ST, Soper DE, Austin M. Antibiotic resistance patterns of group B streptococci in late third trimester rectovaginal cultures. Am J Obstet Gynecol 2001;184:1125–6.

47. Berkowitz K, Regan JA, Greenberg E. Antibiotic resistance patterns of group B streptococci in pregnant women. J Clin Microbiol 1990;28:5–7.

48. Penicillin G availability, MMWR Morb Mortal Wkly Rep 2000;49:61.

49. Gibbs RS, Dinsmoor MJ, Newton ER, Ramamurthy RS. A randomized trial of intrapartum versus immediate postpartum treatment of women with intra-amniotic infection. Obstet Gynecol 1988;72:823–8.

50. Sweet RL, Gibbs RS. Postpartum infection. In: Sweet RL, Gibbs RS. Infectious diseases of the female genital tract. 4th ed. Philadelphia (PA): Lippincott Williams & Wilkins; 2002. p. 541–55.

51. Gibbs RS, Blanco JD. Streptococcal infections in pregnancy: a study of 48 bacteremias. Am J Obstet Gynecol 1981;140: 405–11.

52. Steward CD, Raney PM, Morrell AK, Williams PP, McDougal LK, Jevitt L, et al. Testing for induction of clindamycin resistance in erythromycin-sensitive isolates of Staphylococcus aureus. J Clin Micro 2005;43:1716–21.

53. Mohle-Boetani JC, Schuchat A, Plikaytis BD, Smith JD, Broome CV. Comparison of prevention strategies for neonatal group B streptococcal infection. A population based economic analysis. JAMA 1993;270:1442–8.

54. Rouse DJ, Goldenberg RL, Cliver SP, Cutter GR, Mennemeyer ST, Fargason CA Jr. Strategies for the prevention of early-onset neonatal group B streptococcal sepsis: a decision analysis. Obstet Gynecol 1994;83:483–94.

55. Mohle-Boetani JC, Lieu TA, Ray GT, Escobar G. Preventing neonatal group B streptococcal disease: cost-effectiveness in a health maintenance organization and the impact of delayed hospital discharge for newborns who received intrapartum antibiotics. Pediatrics 1999;103: 703–10.

56. Schrag SJ, Zell ER, Lynfield R, Roome A, Arnold KE, Craig AS, et al. A population-based comparison of strategies to prevent early-onset group B streptococcal disease in neonates. N Engl J Med 2002;347:233–9.

57. Diminishing racial disparities in early-onset neonatal group B streptococcal disease—United States 2000-2003. MMWR Morb Mortal Wkly Rep 2004;53:502–5.

58. Leitich H, Bodner-Adler B, Brunbauer M, Kaider A, Egarter C, Husslein P. Bacterial vaginosis as a risk factor for preterm delivery: a meta-analysis. Am J Obstet Gynecol 2003;189:139–47.

59. Kenyon SL, Taylor DJ, Tarnow-Mordi W; ORACLE Collaborative Group. Broad-spectrum antibiotics for preterm, prelabour rupture of fetal membranes: the ORACLE I randomised trial. Published erratum appears in: Lancet 2001;358:156. Lancet 2001;357:979–88.

60. Klein LL, Gibbs RS. Use of microbial cultures and antibiotics in the prevention of infection-associated preterm birth. Am J Obstet Gynecol 2004;190:1493–502.

61. Goldenberg RL, Hauth JC, Andrews WW. Intrauterine infection and preterm delivery. N Engl J Med 2000;342: 1500–7.

62. Hager WD, Schuchat A, Gibbs R, Sweet R, Mead P, Larsen JW. Prevention of perinatal group B streptococcal infection: current controversies. Obstet Gynecol 2000;96: 141–5.

63. Prophylactic antibiotics in labor and delivery. ACOG Practice Bulletin No. 47. American College of Obstetricians and Gynecologists. Obstet Gynecol 2003;102: 875–82.

64. Mercer BM, Miodovnik M, Thurnau GR. Antibiotic therapy for reduction of infant morbidity after preterm premature rupture of the membranes: a randomized controlled trial. National Institute of Child Health and Human Development Maternal–Fetal Medicine Units Network. JAMA 1997; 278:989–95.

65. Aungst M, King J, Steele A, Gordon M. Low colony counts of asymptomatic group B streptococcus bacteriuria: a survey of practice patterns. Am J Perinatol 2004;21:403–7.

66. Merenstein GB, Todd WA, Brown G, Yost CC, Luzier T. Group B beta hemolytic streptococcus: randomized controlled treatment at term. Obstet Gynecol 1980;55:315–8.

67. Klebanoff MA, Regan JA, Rao AV, Nugent RP, Blackwelder AC, Eschenbach DA, et al. Outcome of the Vaginal Infections and Prematurity Study: results of a clinical trial of erythromycin among pregnant women colonized with group B streptococci. Am J Obstet Gynecol 1995;172: 1540–5.

68. Weeks JW, Myers SR, Lasher L, Goldsmith J, Watkins C, Gall SA. Persistence of penicillin G benzathine in pregnant group B streptococcus carriers. Obstet Gynecol 1997; 90:240–3.

69. Bland ML, Vermillion ST, Soper DE. Late third-trimester treatment of rectovaginal group B streptococci with benzathine penicillin G. Am J Obstet Gynecol 2000;183: 372–6.

70. Sweet RL, Gibbs RS. Antimicrobial agents. In: Sweet RL, Gibbs RS. Infectious diseases of the female genital tract. 4th ed. Philadelphia (PA): Lippincott Williams & Wilkins:2002;609–60.

71. Pinette MG, Wax JR, Blackstone J, Cartin A, McCrann DJ. Culture-based group B streptococcal screening: adherence to current guidelines. J Reprod Med 2003;48:309–12.

72. Nemunaitis-Keller J, Gill P. Limitations of the obstetric group B streptococcus protocol. J Reprod Med 2003;48: 107–11.

73. Kenyon SL, Taylor DJ, Tarnow-Mordi W. Broad-spectrum antibiotics for spontaneous preterm labour: the ORACLE II randomised trial. ORACLE Collaborative Group. Lancet 2001;357:989–94.

74. Siegel JD, McCracken GH, Threlkeld N, Milvenan B, Rosenfeld CR. Single-dose penicillin prophylaxis against neonatal group B streptococcal infections: a controlled trial in 18,738 newborn infants. N Engl J Med 1980;303: 769–75.

75. Siegel JD, Cushion NB. Prevention of early-onset group B streptococcal disease: another look at single-dose penicillin at birth. Obstet Gynecol 1996;87:692–8.

76. Pyati SP, Pildes RS, Jacobs NM, Ramamurthy RS, Yeh TF, Raval DS, et al. Penicillin in infants weighing two kilograms or less with early-onset group B streptococcal disease. N Engl J Med 1983;308:1383–9.

77. Wendel GD Jr., Leveno KJ, Sanchez PJ, Jackson GL, McIntire DD, Siegel JD. Prevention of neonatal group B streptococcal disease: a combined intrapartum and neonatal protocol. Am J Obstet Gynecol 2002;186:618–26.

78. Regan JA, Klebanoff MA, Nugent RP, Eschenbach DA, Blackwelder WC, Lou Y, et al. Colonization with group B streptococci in pregnancy and adverse outcome: VIP Study Group. Am J Obstet Gynecol 1996;174:1354–60.

79. Balter S, Zell ER, O'Brien KL, Roome A, Noga H, Thayu M, et al. Impact of intrapartum antibiotics on the care and evaluation of the neonate. Pediatr Infect Dis J 2003; 22:853–7.

80. Moore MR, Schrag SJ, Schuchat A. Effects of intrapartum antimicrobial prophylaxis for prevention of group-B-streptococcal disease on the incidence and ecology of early-onset neonatal sepsis. Lancet Infect Dis 2003; 3:201–13.

81. Stoll BJ, Hansen N, Fanaroff AA, Wright LL, Carlo WA, Ehrenkranz RA, et al. Changes in pathogens causing early-onset sepsis in very-low-birth-weight infants. N Engl J Med 2002;347:240–7.

82. Baltimore RS, Huie SM, Meek JI, Schuchat A, O'Brien KL. Early-onset neonatal sepsis in the era of group B streptococcal prevention. Pediatrics 2001;108:1094–8.

83. Hyde TB, Hilger TM, Reingold A, Farley MM, O'Brien KL, Schuchat A; Active Bacterial Core surveillance (ABCs) of the Emerging Infections Program Network. Trends in incidence and antimicrobial resistance of early-onset sepsis: population-based surveillance in San Francisco and Atlanta. Pediatrics 2002;110:690–5.

84. Edwards RK, Clark P, Sistrom CL, Duff P. Intrapartum antibiotic prophylaxis 1: relative effects of recommended antibiotics on gram-negative pathogens. Obstet Gynecol 2002;100:534–9.

85. Boulvain M, Stan C, Irion O. Membrane sweeping for induction of labour (Cochrane Review). In: The Cochrane Library, Issue 3, 2001. Oxford: Update Software.

86. Kasper DL, Paoletti LC, Wessels MR, Guttormsen HK, Carey VJ, Jennings HJ, et al. Immune response to type III group B streptococcal polysaccharide-tetanus toxoid conjugate vaccine. J Clin Invest 1996;98:2308–14.

87. Baker CJ, Rench MA, McInnes P. Immunization of pregnant women with group B streptococcal type III capsular polysaccharide-tetanus toxoid conjugate vaccine. Vaccine 2003;21:3468–72.

88. Baker CJ, Edwards MS. Group B streptococcal conjugate vaccines. Arch Dis Child 2003;88:375–8.

89. Burman LG, Christensen P, Christensen K, Fryklund B, Helgesson AM, Svenningsen NW, et al. Prevention of excess neonatal morbidity associated with group B streptococci by vaginal chlorhexidine disinfection during labour: The Swedish Chlorhexidine Study Group. Lancet 1992;340: 65–9.

90. Taha TE, Biggar RJ, Broadhead RL, Mtimavalye LA, Justesen AB, Liomba GN, et al. Effect of cleansing the birth canal with antiseptic solution on maternal and newborn morbidity in Malawi: clinical trial. Br Med J 1997; 315:216–20.

91. Stray-Pedersen B, Bergan T, Hafstad A, Normann E, Grogaard J, Vangdal M. Vaginal disinfection with chlorhexidine during childbirth. Int J Antimicrob Agents 1999; 12:245–51.

92. Rouse DJ, Hauth JC, Andrews WW, Mills BB, Maher JE. Chlorhexidine vaginal irrigation for the prevention of peripartal infection: a placebo-controlled randomized clinical trial. Am J Obstet Gynecol 1997;176:617–22.

93. Facchinetti F, Piccinini F, Mordini B, Volpe A. Chlorhexidine vaginal flushings versus systemic ampicillin in the prevention of vertical transmission of neonatal group B streptococcus, at term. J Matern Fetal Neonatal Med 2002; 11:84–8.

CHAPTER 24

Genital Herpes Complicating Pregnancy

Zane A. Brown, Carolyn Gardella, Anna Wald, Rhoda Ashley Morrow, and Lawrence Corey

The prevalence of genital and neonatal herpes continues to increase (1). Approximately 1.6 million new cases of genital herpes occur annually (2), 22% of pregnant women are seropositive for herpes simplex virus (HSV)-2, and more than 2% of women acquire genital herpes during pregnancy (3). Given the high prevalence of HSV infection in women of reproductive age, obstetricians need to be able to diagnose and manage HSV in pregnancy and are in the unique position to prevent HSV transmission to the neonate.

The most devastating complication of genital HSV is infection of the neonate at the time of delivery. Neonatal HSV occurs in up to 1 in 3,200 live births (4), with an estimated incidence of 1,500 cases in the United States annually (5). Neonatal HSV causes disseminated or central nervous system (CNS) disease in approximately 50% of cases. Up to 30% of these infants will die, and up to 40% of survivors will have neurologic damage, despite antiviral therapy (5). The social and economic costs of the long-term care of infants with sequelae from neonatal herpes are substantial (6). Therefore, prevention of neonatal herpes infection remains critically important in decreasing the sequelae from this disease. This article will review genital HSV in pregnancy, emphasizing challenges in diagnosis and treatment of maternal infection in pregnancy and prevention of vertical transmission.

Epidemiology

A national survey conducted in the early 1990s showed that the seroprevalence of HSV-2 in the general U.S. population was 22%, an increase of 30% from 1978 (1, 7, 8). Consistent with that estimate, a recent study of suburban primary care offices showed an HSV-2 seroprevalence rate of 25.5% (9). Seroprevalence studies of pregnant women observed HSV-2 seroprevalence rates of 20–30% (3). Ten percent of pregnant women are at risk of HSV-2 acquisition from their partners, and most of these women are at unsuspected risk (10). Overall, 2% of women in a general obstetrics practice acquire HSV during pregnancy (3). For HSV-2 seronegative women with HSV-2

seropositive partners, the risk of HSV-2 acquisition in pregnancy is up to 20% (10).

Between 75% and 90% of HSV-2 infected persons are not aware of having the infection (1, 11–13). Most sexual transmission of HSV occurs during episodes of subclinical reactivation among persons with unrecognized infection (11, 14–17). Recent studies indicate that virtually all HSV-2 seropositive persons have virologically active infection with intermittent shedding from the genital mucosa, and most have mild (thus unrecognized and undiagnosed) disease (12). Among women, including pregnant women, these mild genital symptoms are frequently attributed to other genital conditions, such as recurrent yeast or urinary tract infections, bacterial vaginitis, and allergies to condoms, semen, spermicides, and pantyhose (12, 13, 18, 19).

Herpes simplex virus-2 seroprevalence data underestimate the actual prevalence of genital herpes because it does not include an increasing proportion of genital herpes caused by HSV-1 (20, 21). Herpes simplex virus-1 has emerged as a major cause of genital herpes, particularly among college-age individuals, in which up to 80% of new cases of genital HSV were caused by HSV-1 (21–23). Results of epidemiologic studies suggest that oral–genital contact is a risk factor for genital HSV-1 (20). Although clinical presentation of initial genital herpes is the same for HSV-1 and HSV-2, the differences in prognosis dictate the need to identify the viral type. The frequency of genital reactivation is much less with HSV-1, which rarely recurs symptomatically or asymptomatically after the first year of infection (24, 25). In contrast, genital HSV-2 continues to recur, often frequently, for many years (26).

Clinical Characteristics and Diagnosis of Herpes Simplex Virus in Pregnancy

The clinical manifestations of genital herpes cannot be relied on to diagnose infection or to differentiate a newly acquired infection from a reactivated infection (27). Approximately 70% of newly acquired HSV infections among pregnant women are asymptomatic or unrecognized (3, 10). The remaining 30% of women with new infections have clinical presentations that range from minimal lesions and mild discomfort to widespread genital lesions associated with severe local pain, dysuria, sacral paresthesia, tender regional lymph node enlargement, fever, malaise, and headache. Aseptic meningitis occurs less frequently, and disseminated disease is rare. Similarly, reactivations of genital herpes are most commonly unrecognized. In a study of 201 consecutive pregnant women, 177 gave no history of genital herpes although 30.4% were HSV-2 seropositive (28). The spectrum of clinically evident episodes varies from very mild episodes to severe symptoms that are clinically indistinguishable from a severe new infection (3, 27).

As such, providers should consider HSV when caring for women with subtle genital symptoms or with clinically unusual severe illness in pregnancy because both ends of the disease spectrum are easiest to miss. In all cases, the diagnosis of genital HSV infection requires laboratory confirmation, although antiviral therapy can be initiated based on clinical presentation. The Centers for Disease Control and Prevention recommends that both virologic tests and type-specific serologic tests for HSV be available in clinical settings that provide care for patients at risk for sexually transmitted infections (29). Isolation of HSV in cell culture is routinely done in patients who present with genital ulcers or other mucocutaneous lesions. However, the sensitivity of culture is relatively low, especially in recurrent lesions, and declines further as lesions begin to heal. Polymerase chain reaction (PCR) assays for HSV DNA are more sensitive, have become more widely commercially available, and can be used instead of viral culture (30–33). Both PCR and viral culture should be typed to determine whether HSV-1 or HSV-2 is the cause of the infection. As with culture, lack of HSV detection by PCR assay results does not indicate lack of HSV infection because viral shedding is intermittent. Thus, type-specific HSV serology is an important diagnostic tool for women who lack lesions at the time of presentation or whose cultures or PCR assay results are negative. If new infection is suspected and the HSV serology does not detect HSV antibodies and virus is not isolated from the lesion, repeat serologic testing in 6 weeks should be performed.

Rarely, new or recurrent HSV infection in pregnancy can cause disseminated disease, usually with prominent hepatitis or encephalitis, or it can cause postpartum endometritis. In such cases prompt diagnosis and initiation of therapy are critical to clinical outcome. Disseminated HSV should be considered in women who report a flulike prodrome, including fever that progresses to pneumonitis, hepatitis, or encephalitis, with or without characteristic skin lesions after midpregnancy

(34, 35). Herpes simplex virus hepatitis typically presents in the third trimester of pregnancy with fever, anicteric hepatic dysfunction, highly elevated transaminase levels, and abdominal tenderness. Mucocutaneous lesions may appear late or not at all, and the diagnosis is made only at autopsy in 25% of reported cases (36). Herpes simplex virus encephalitis should be considered in any pregnant woman with new onset seizures, change in mental status, or fever and headache (37). The diagnosis is confirmed with PCR assay of the cerebral spinal fluid. For postpartum women with persistent puerperal fever, despite use of antibiotics and anticoagulants, HSV endometritis should be considered and confirmed with endometrial biopsy for HSV PCR or culture (38, 39).

Based on serologic and viral detection test results, genital HSV is classified as primary, nonprimary first episode, or reactivation disease. Primary infection is characterized by isolation of HSV-1 or HSV-2 from genital secretions in the absence of HSV antibodies in serum. Nonprimary first episode disease is characterized by isolation of HSV-2 from genital secretions in the presence of HSV-1 antibodies in serum. Reactivation disease is characterized by isolation of HSV-1 or HSV-2 from the genital tract in the presence of HSV antibodies of the same serotype as the isolate. These categories are important in pregnancy because the risk of perinatal HSV transmission varies accordingly.

Type-Specific Herpes Simplex Virus Serologic Assays

Antibodies to HSV develop during the first several weeks after infection and persist indefinitely. Most of the immune response is type common for HSV-1 and HSV-2. However, the response to HSV-2 is distinguishable from HSV-1 because the surface glycoprotein G differs in size and epitope content between HSV-1 and HSV-2 (40). Serologic assays that detect antibodies to the HSV-1 glycoprotein G and the HSV-2 glycoprotein G and discriminate between HSV-1 and HSV-2 have been developed and are commercially available. These assays also permit the detection of HSV-2 infection occurring in the presence of HSV-1 antibodies or an HSV-1 infection occurring in the presence of HSV-2 antibodies (41, 42). The presence of type-specific HSV-2 antibody indicates genital infection because almost all HSV-2 infections are sexually transmitted. The presence of HSV-1 antibody alone is more difficult to interpret, especially in persons without a history of oral or genital herpes. Most people with HSV-1 antibody have oral HSV infection acquired in childhood, which may be asymptomatic. However, HSV-1 antibody may indicate genital HSV-1 infection, which also may be asymptomatic. Lack of symptoms in an HSV-1 seropositive person does not distinguish genital from orolabial or cutaneous infection.

Since 1999, several HSV glycoprotein G-based type-specific serologic tests have received U.S. Food and Drug Administration approval and are currently marketed (Table 24-1). The immunoblot test can detect antibodies to HSV-1 and HSV-2 on a single strip, whereas the enzyme-linked immunosorbent assay (ELISA) format provides separate plates for HSV-1 and HSV-2. Type-specific assays should replace the nonglycoprotein G-based HSV assays that are in widespread use and provide inaccurate results (43).

Assays differ in their operational characteristics. The finger-stick, point-of-care (office-based) diagnostic test can be done during the clinic visit (44–46). However, care must be taken in reading the color end point of these assays because variability in reading has been documented (47). Some assays are designed for use in hospital or reference laboratories, whereas others can be performed in clinical laboratories that are approved for moderately complex work (48). Choice of test should be driven by the availability of a high throughput laboratory and the volume of samples.

All of the type-specific assays are comparable in performance with the Western blot test (41, 45, 47–51). The sensitivities of these tests for detection of HSV-2 antibody vary from 93–100%, and false-negative results may occur, especially at early stages of infection. The specificities of these assays are 96% or greater. False-positive results can occur, especially in patients with a low likelihood of HSV infection. Repeat or confirmatory testing with a second glycoprotein G-based test may be indicated in some settings, especially if recent acquisition of genital herpes is suspected.

Treatment of Symptomatic Herpes Simplex Virus in Pregnancy

Primary or First-Episode Herpes Simplex Virus

Antiviral therapy is recommended for women with symptomatic primary or first-episode HSV infection during pregnancy (52). Oral antiviral medication for 7 days hastens lesion healing and reduces viral shedding. For women with disseminated HSV, pneumonitis, hepatitis, or complications of the CNS, intravenous acyclovir at a dose of 5–10 mg/kg body weight, administered every 8 hours until clinical improvement is observed, followed by oral antiviral therapy for at least 10 days of total therapy is recommended (29). Antiviral therapy should be initiated as soon as the diagnosis is suspected rather than waiting for laboratory confirmation. Early consultation

with an infectious diseases specialist may be advisable if disseminated HSV is suspected (Table 24-2). Clinicians should be aware that seroconversion may be delayed when first-episode HSV infection is treated with antiviral medications (53).

Recurrent Herpes Simplex Virus

Before labor, recurrent HSV does not appear to have an adverse effect on pregnancy outcomes (54). Therefore, treatment with antiviral medication is indicated only to relieve maternal symptoms. Generally, a 2- to 5-day course of oral antiviral medication will shorten the symptomatic period (29). For women with frequent or severe recurrences, daily suppressive therapy with antiviral medication may be indicated, especially after the first trimester (Table 24-2).

Antiviral Drug Choice and Safety in Pregnancy

Acyclovir is a nucleoside analog that is highly specific for HSV-infected cells. Once inside the infected cell, acyclovir is selectively activated by the viral thymidine kinase and specifically inhibits viral replication. Acyclovir crosses the placenta, is concentrated and excreted by the fetal kidney, and is found in the amniotic fluid and fetal tissue. Although it is concentrated in amniotic fluid, it does not appear to accumulate in the fetus (55). The bioavailability of oral acyclovir is only approximately 20%, and frequent doses are required to achieve therapeutic levels. The limited available data suggest that the physiologic changes that occur in late pregnancy do not significantly alter maternal acyclovir pharmacokinetics, which were similar to those reported for nonpregnant patients (55, 56).

Valacyclovir is a prodrug of acyclovir and requires hepatic metabolism to become active. It has the benefit of longer half-life, allowing for less frequent doses, which may improve compliance. Further, the bioavailability of acyclovir after the administration of oral valacyclovir is 3–5 times greater than that of oral acyclovir (56, 57). However, it is more expensive than acyclovir, and experience in pregnancy is limited because of its relatively recent introduction. Its mechanism of action is not different from that of acyclovir, but the consequences of higher levels of acyclovir in pregnancy are unknown. The efficacy of valacyclovir for episodic or suppressive therapy or for the suppression of viral shedding is comparable with that of acyclovir.

Famciclovir also is a prodrug that undergoes rapid biotransformation to penciclovir, the active antiviral compound. Like valacyclovir, it has a greater bioavailability than acyclovir and can be dosed less frequently than acyclovir. No studies directly address the use of famci-

Table 24-1. Glycoprotein G-Based Type-Specific Tests for Herpes Simplex Virus Antibody

Test	Manufacturer	FDA Approved	Antibodies Detected	Sensitivity (%)*	Specificity (%)*	Collection Method	Test Location	Median Time to Sero-conversion (Days)	Web Site	Telephone
HerpeSelect HSV-1 ELISA and Herpe-Select HSV-2 ELISA	Focus Diagnostics (Cyprus, CA)	Yes (2000)	HSV-1 HSV-2, respectively	HSV-1: 96 HSV-2: 100	HSV-1 95.2 HSV-2 96.1	Blood draw	Laboratories—best for high volume laboratories	21–23	http://www.herpeselect.com	800-505-0536
HerpeSelect HSV-1 and HSV-2 Immunoblot	Focus Diagnostics (Cyprus, CA)	Yes (2000)	HSV-1 and HSV-2	HSV-1: 100 HSV-2: 100	HSV-1 93.1 HSV-2 93.7	Blood draw	Laboratories—best for low volume laboratories	Not known	http://www.herpeselect.com	800-505-0536
biokitHSV-2 Rapid Test†	Biokit USA (Lexington, MA)	Yes (1999)	HSV-2	93–96	94–97	Finger stick	Provider office	13	http://www.biokitusa.com	800-926-3353
Captia HSV-1 ELISA, Captia HSV-2 ELISA	Trinity Biotech (Wicklow, Ireland)	Yes (2004)	HSV-1 HSV-2, respectively	HSV-1: (not available) HSV-2: 96	HSV-1: (not available) HSV-2: 98	Blood draw	Laboratories	14	http://www.trinitybiotech.com	800-325-3424
Western Blot	University of Washington (Seattle, WA)	No; "research gold standard"†	HSV-1 and HSV-2	Greater than 99	Greater than 99	Blood draw	University of Washington Virology Laboratory	42–47	http://depts.washington.edu/herpes/	206-598-6066

*The sensitivity and specificity of the HerpeSelect ELISA, Immunoblot, biokitHSV-2, and Captia ELISA were determined by comparison with Western blot tests. The sensitivity and specificity of the Western blot was determined using men and women (not selected for pregnancy status) with symptomatic established infections. Results for Captia HSV-1 ELISA have been determined but are not yet published.

†Formerly POCkit HSV-2 Rapid Test, also known as Surevue HSV-2 from Fisher Healthcare (Houston, TX).

Abbreviations: ELISA, enzyme-linked immunosorbent assay; FDA, U.S. Food and Drug Administration, HSV, herpes simplex virus.

Brown ZA, Gardella C, Wald A, Morrow RA, Corey L. Genital herpes complicating pregnancy. Obstet Gynecol 2005;106:845–56.

Table 24-2. Recommended Doses of Antiviral Medication for Herpes in Pregnancy

Indication	Acyclovir	Valacyclovir
Primary or first-episode HSV	400 mg orally, three times per day for 7–14 days	1 g twice per day for 7–14 days
Symptomatic recurrent HSV	400 mg orally, three times per day for 5 days	500 mg orally, twice per day for 5 days
Daily suppressive therapy	400 mg orally, three times per day from 36 weeks EGA to delivery	500 mg orally, twice per day from 36 weeks EGA to delivery

Abbreviations: EGA, estimated gestational age; HSV, herpes simplex virus.
Brown ZA, Gardella C, Wald A, Morrow RA, Corey L. Genital herpes complicating pregnancy. Obstet Gynecol 2005;106:845–56.

clovir in pregnancy, and therefore, at this time there is no recommended dose of famciclovir in pregnancy.

Antivirals frequently are used in pregnancy for the treatment or suppression of genital HSV. Acyclovir, valacyclovir, and famciclovir are designated "Pregnancy Category B." A registry of neonates exposed to acyclovir in utero found no significant teratogenic effects to the fetus (58). These data were sufficient to exclude a sevenfold increase in the risk of birth defects but could not address the risk of rare defects or those detected after the postnatal period (58). Based on acyclovir toxicity data in neonates undergoing treatment for neonatal herpes, potential neonatal complications of in utero exposure include renal insufficiency and neutropenia (59). Small studies of valacyclovir use in late pregnancy found no clinical or laboratory evidence of toxicity in participants or their infants over a 1-month or 6-month follow-up period (60).

Thus, limited data suggest the safety of antiviral medication in pregnancy. As with any medication used in pregnancy, consideration of the risk versus benefit in each clinical situation and open discussion with the patient should guide prescription. The maternal benefit from treating symptomatic HSV in pregnancy may outweigh potential fetal risk, especially in the case of symptomatic primary infection occurring in the latter half of pregnancy or frequent or severe recurrent disease after the first trimester.

Neonatal Herpes

Neonatal herpes is defined as the diagnosis of HSV infection in an infant within the first 28 days of life. It occurs in up to 1 in 3,200 live births in the Pacific Northwest (4), with an estimated incidence of 1,500 cases in the United States annually (5). More than 90% of cases are acquired intrapartum by contact with HSV in the maternal birth canal (4, 61–63). The major sites of viral entry are the eye, nasopharynx, or site of scalp trauma. Rarely, neonatal herpes results from intrauterine exposure to HSV related to transplacental or ascending infection (most commonly in the setting of primary infection), from

postnatal acquisition of HSV-1 from close contact with persons with orolabial herpes, or HSV-1 infection at another nongenital site, such as the finger (eg, herpetic whitlow) or the breast (64).

Neonatal HSV presents with a spectrum of disease that is classified based on clinical manifestations. Neonates with skin, eye, and mouth disease have limited viral dissemination without visceral involvement and account for 45% of cases since the advent of early antiviral therapy (65, 66). Almost one third of neonates with HSV are classified with CNS disease, characterized by seizures, lethargy, irritability, tremors, poor feeding, temperature instability, and bulging fontanelle. The remaining 25% of cases have disseminated infection that involves multiorgan systems and may result in death from severe coagulopathy, liver dysfunction, and pulmonary failure (5).

Factors that affect the severity of neonatal disease include prompt diagnosis and initiation of antiviral therapy. Polymerase chain reaction assay to detect HSV DNA in neonates has improved early diagnosis of disease. Although intravenous acyclovir has clearly reduced mortality and morbidity among neonates with skin, eye, and mouth disease, little progress has been made in reducing morbidity associated with disseminated or CNS disease. Despite early intervention with high-dose antiviral therapy, 30% of infants with disseminated disease die, and 40% of survivors of CNS disease have severe neurologic damage (5). Therefore, prevention of neonatal infection is critical.

Risk Factors

HERPES SIMPLEX VIRUS IN THE GENITAL TRACT AT THE TIME OF LABOR

The main mode of transmission to the neonate is exposure to infected maternal secretions at the time of passage through the birth canal. Isolation of HSV from the maternal genital tract at the time of labor is the primary risk factor for neonatal HSV, with an estimated relative risk for infection of more than 300 (4).

STAGE OF MATERNAL INFECTION

The second most-important risk factor for neonatal herpes is the stage of maternal infection. Overall, 60–80% of the cases of neonatal HSV occur from women who acquire genital herpes (approximately 75% of the time without symptoms) in the third trimester of pregnancy (3). The risk of neonatal herpes is 30–50% among women subclinically shedding virus at the time of labor as a result of having acquired genital herpes in the third trimester, compared with 3% among infants exposed to HSV from maternal symptomatic reactivation of genital herpes at the time of labor (4, 62, 63). The acquisition of genital HSV infection is associated with a high efficiency of transmission to the neonate because women with newly acquired infection in the third trimester of pregnancy do not have the 6–12 weeks necessary to develop type-specific homologous HSV antibody with which to transplacentally protect their neonate after intrapartum exposure. In addition, they also are likely to have high titers of virus in their genital secretions for many months after the initial infection (67). Therefore, the infant of a mother with acquisition of genital herpes in the third trimester of pregnancy is at double jeopardy; the infant lacks the protection of transplacental type-specific antibodies and is likely to be exposed to significantly greater amounts of virus in the genital secretions during parturition.

TYPE OF HERPES SIMPLEX VIRUS ISOLATED FROM THE GENITAL TRACT

Neonates exposed to genital HSV-1 at the time of delivery are more likely to become infected than those exposed to HSV-2, regardless of the stage of maternal infection (4). Thirty-one percent of neonates exposed to genital HSV-1 at the time of delivery became infected, compared with 3% of those exposed to HSV-2 (odds ratio 34.8, 95% confidence interval, 3.6–335, adjusted for first-episode versus reactivation HSV) (4). The mechanism of this observation is unclear, but it may explain, along with the increasing prevalence of genital HSV-1, the rising incidence of neonatal HSV-1 infection. However, infants exposed to HSV-1, in contrast to those exposed to HSV-2, are more likely to develop skin, eye, and mouth infection and less likely to develop CNS involvement (68).

INVASIVE OBSTETRIC PROCEDURES

The major sites of intrapartum viral entry include the neonatal eyes, nasopharynx, and break in the integument. Thus, any procedure that damages the neonatal skin in labor can facilitate transmission of HSV. Among neonates exposed to HSV at delivery, 10% of those delivered with the use of fetal scalp electrode, vacuum, or forceps were infected, compared with 2% of those who did not have invasive obstetric procedures (4).

Methods for Preventing Neonatal Herpes Simplex Virus

CESAREAN DELIVERY FOR WOMEN WITH HERPES SIMPLEX VIRUS IN THE BIRTH CANAL AT THE TIME OF LABOR

For women with genital lesions or prodromal symptoms suggestive of genital herpes, cesarean delivery is recommended to prevent neonatal infection (52). Although this has been recommended by The American College of Obstetricians and Gynecologists for decades, evidence for a benefit of cesarean delivery in preventing neonatal herpes is recent. Cesarean delivery significantly decreased, but did not completely eliminate, the risk of neonatal HSV among women with HSV detected in genital secretions at the time of labor (4). Cesarean delivery is likely to be more effective if done before rupture of membranes.

Some centers suggested that it is justifiably safe to allow an HSV-2 seropositive woman to give birth to her infant vaginally despite the presence of a genital herpetic lesion (69). This is based on the low risk of transmission to the neonate from a woman with established genital herpes (4). However, this observed low rate may reflect the practice of delivering women with lesions or symptoms at the time of labor by cesarean as well as the fetal protective effect of transplacental transmission of homologous antibody.

Currently, the standard of care in the United States is for women with symptomatic reactivation of genital herpes at the time of labor to have cesarean delivery. Based on our experience and available data, we feel that this standard of care should persist. In women with established genital HSV but without active genital lesions or prodromal symptoms at the time of labor, cesarean delivery is not indicated. Currently, physical examination is the main method to infer the presence of HSV in the genital tract at the time of labor. All women with known genital herpes should be questioned about genital symptoms and have a thorough examination of the cervix, vagina, and vulva at the time of admission in labor.

Physical examination to detect HSV in the genital tract has significant limitations. First, clinical diagnosis of genital herpes lacks sensitivity and specificity. Among women who underwent cesarean delivery for active genital herpes at the University of Washington, the positive predictive value of genital lesions for viral detection was 28% by culture and 47% by PCR (70). Thus, a significant portion of women who had cesarean delivery for active genital HSV did not have HSV detected in the genital tract by our current methods. Second, and perhaps more importantly, physical examination does not identify most women who transmit HSV to their infants because these women lack genital lesions (3, 4).

A clinically useful laboratory-based means of detecting HSV in the birth canal to inform the safest mode of delivery is not available currently. In the past, viral cultures of genital swabs collected in the late third trimester of pregnancy were used to predict women at risk of HSV transmission. However, results from prenatal specimens rarely correlated with culture results of swabs collected at the time of delivery (71). Therefore, this practice was abandoned in the late 1980s (52). Viral cultures or traditional HSV PCR to detect HSV from genital swabs collected at the time of labor are not clinically practical because results are not available before delivery. Until a valid rapid test to detect HSV in the genital tract at the time of labor becomes available, we continue to perform cesarean deliveries for women with genital lesions at the time of labor based on physical examination findings to prevent neonatal herpes.

Some specialists recommend cesarean delivery for women with newly acquired HSV in the third trimester of pregnancy to reduce the risk of neonatal HSV, regardless of symptoms or signs at the time of labor. Others recommend treatment with acyclovir, followed by suppressive therapy for the remainder of the pregnancy. Then, if type-specific antibodies are present by the time of delivery and the woman is without lesions, vaginal delivery is allowed. We believe that the latter approach is potentially risky because suppressive therapy may not completely eliminate viral shedding, and although type-specific antibodies are detectable, they may not provide sufficient passive immunity if quantities are low.

ANTIVIRAL SUPPRESSIVE THERAPY

In women with symptomatic genital herpes, antiviral suppressive medication initiated at 36 weeks of gestational age reduces the need for cesarean delivery for lesions and viral detection from the genital tract by both culture and PCR at the time of delivery (Table 24-2) (72–77). Although a study to prove that suppressive therapy prevents neonatal herpes is unlikely to be feasible, it is reasonable to prescribe suppressive therapy to women with symptomatic recurrent HSV to reduce the need for cesarean delivery for HSV lesions and to decrease neonatal viral exposure at the time of vaginal delivery (52). At this time, data are insufficient to recommend antiviral suppressive therapy to all asymptomatic HSV-2 seropositive pregnant women. However, after discussion of the potential risks and benefits, antiviral suppressive therapy in the last trimester of pregnancy may be a reasonable option for these patients.

The recommended doses of acyclovir and valacyclovir for HSV suppression in the third trimester of pregnancy are based on those used in the clinical trials published to date and are treatment doses in nonpregnant women. It is possible that lower doses of these medications in pregnancy may be equally effective given the similar pharmacokinetics of these drugs in pregnant and nonpregnant women. However, the pharmacokinetics data in pregnancy is limited, and to date, suppression trials have not been performed using the lower doses. Thus, the higher doses are recommended at this time (Table 24-2). Currently, there is no recommended dose of famciclovir in pregnancy.

PREVENT THE ACQUISITION OF HERPES SIMPLEX VIRUS BY PREGNANT WOMEN

Although the current recommendations of the American College of Obstetricians and Gynecologists do not include universal testing (52), the subject is controversial and widely debated. Given our current understanding of the risk of neonatal herpes, we believe that prevention of neonatal HSV will depend in large part on prevention of maternal acquisition of genital HSV in the third trimester of pregnancy.

There are three potential approaches to preventing maternal acquisition of HSV in late pregnancy. The first is to obtain a glycoprotein G-based (type-specific) HSV serologic assay at a prenatal visit between 24 weeks and 28 weeks of gestation when blood is routinely drawn for diabetes screening (Fig. 24-1). Screening at 24–28 weeks of gestation places the counseling and interventions in the third trimester of pregnancy, which is the time of greatest risk for subsequent neonatal HSV transmission if the mother should acquire genital herpes. For women who are identified as HSV-2 seropositive but unaware of their infection, this would provide adequate time to educate them about the significance of this finding and how to identify recurrences, particularly at the time of labor (19). It also would allow the patient and her provider time to formulate an appropriate labor and delivery plan.

Women who are seronegative (ie, without antibodies to either HSV-1 or HSV-2) or those who are HSV-1 seropositive but have no antibodies to HSV-2 should be counseled to avoid unprotected genital-to-genital contact during the third trimester of pregnancy. In addition, the women who are HSV seronegative also should be counseled to avoid oral–genital contact during this same period because approximately 30% of cases of neonatal HSV are caused by genital HSV-1 acquired by the mother in the last trimester of pregnancy (4).

The disadvantage to HSV serologically testing only women to determine HSV susceptibility is that it does

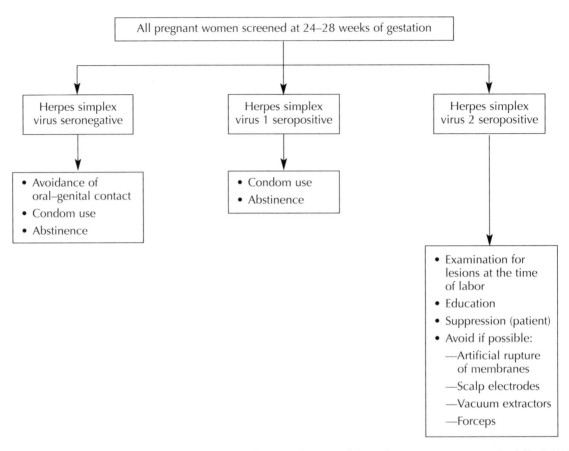

Fig. 24-1. Algorithm for testing and counseling women without involvement of the male partner. (Brown ZA, Gardella C, Wald A, Morrow RA, Corey L. Genital herpes complicating pregnancy. Obstet Gynecol 2005;106:845–56.)

not account for exposure status. That is, it does not determine whether the sexual partner has HSV. Without partner testing, a larger number of women will require counseling based on susceptibility to HSV alone, including those who are not at risk of acquisition because their partner is not infected. Women may be less likely to adhere to counseling messages because they believe that their partner is not infected with HSV. Those women who learn that they have HSV-2 infection may worry about transmitting the virus to their partners if the partner's status is unknown.

The second approach provides HSV serologic screening of pregnant couples to identify HSV susceptible women with serologically discordant partners (Fig. 24-2). Published studies indicate that only 15–25% of couples in early pregnancy are discordant in their HSV serologic status with the pregnant woman at risk (78). Therefore, this approach targets counseling toward those at highest risk for acquiring genital HSV. If the woman is HSV-2 susceptible and the partner has an HSV-2 infection, the couple should be advised to avoid genital contact during the third trimester of pregnancy. If this is not possible, then condoms should be used (79).

Additionally, the HSV-2 seropositive partner can be treated with suppressive antivirals in conjunction with condom use during the third trimester of her pregnancy (80). If the woman is HSV seronegative and the partner has only HSV-1 antibody, then oral–genital contact should be avoided in the third trimester of pregnancy. Because some HSV-1 seropositive men will have a genital rather than an oral HSV-1 infection, such HSV-1 discordant couples also should be counseled to either use condoms or avoid genital contact in the third trimester. The efficacy of these measures in pregnancy has not been determined.

If screening both partners is the preferred method, it may be most efficient to screen for HSV antibodies at 14–18 weeks of gestation, a time when maternal blood is drawn for screening for fetal neural tube defects and chromosomal disorders. This would allow ample time to approach the partners of susceptible women and to initiate appropriate interventions. There are some disadvantages to this "couples approach." The partner may refuse to participate in the screening or counseling process. It may also be difficult to identify a single sexual partner, or the partner may change during the course of the pregnancy.

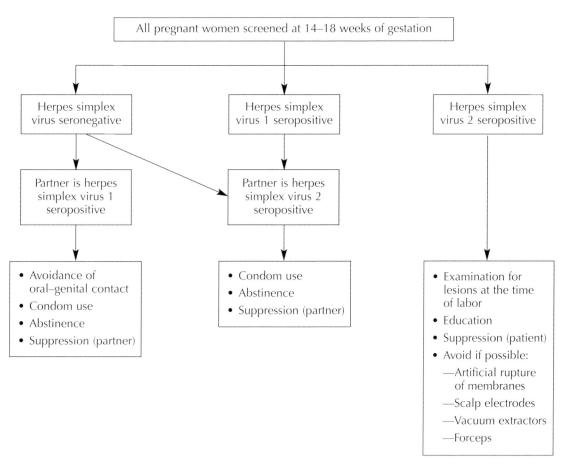

Fig. 24-2. Algorithm for testing and counseling women with involvement of the male partner. (Brown ZA, Gardella C, Wald A, Morrow RA, Corey L. Genital herpes complicating pregnancy. Obstet Gynecol 2005;106:845–56.)

The third approach is appropriate when serologic testing is either not available or economically not feasible. In these circumstances, it may be appropriate to advise all women to abstain from all forms of sexual contact in the third trimester of pregnancy. Because the frequency of sexual activity declines significantly with advancing gestation, particularly in the third trimester, this may not pose a hardship to many women and will obviate, in part, the need for serologic testing (81, 82). However, it lacks the objective certainty and credibility of a counseling recommendation based on a serologic test result. It also will fail to identify HSV-2 seropositive women and thereby fail to permit interventions for those with unrecognized genital herpes.

In our practice, since 1984, we have routinely screened all pregnant women early in pregnancy for HSV antibodies using the Western blot test. Women with HSV-2 are counseled regarding the signs of recurrence. For women without HSV-2 antibody, we inquire about the HSV status of the partner if this is known. If the partner has no history of genital herpes, we recommend serologic testing by the partner's primary care provider or at the public health clinic. If this is not acceptable or feasible, we counsel the patient according to the algorithm in Figure 24-1. If the partner has previously diagnosed genital HSV, the woman is counseled as outlined in Figure 24-2. Because neonatal HSV is relatively rare, studies to directly measure the benefit of such an approach in preventing neonatal HSV are difficult, if not impossible, to perform. However, we see little risk in this approach, and our experience with counseling women about their serologic test results has been positive, in accordance with published studies performed during pregnancy and in other settings (83–85).

Basic costs of these approaches can be measured indirectly, and information about cost-effectiveness relies on modeling the cost of various outcomes and expenditures. Two recently published cost–benefit analyses generated remarkably different results, with the estimated cost per quality-adjusted neonatal life year gained ranging from $18,680 to $155,988 (86, 87) Further research is required to understand the differences between the models.

AVOID UNNECESSARY INVASIVE PROCEDURES IN LABOR

Women with genital herpes but without lesions or symptoms at the time of labor may proceed with vaginal delivery. However, artificial rupture of membranes, fetal scalp electrodes, and vacuum or forceps delivery should be avoided in these women, except when critical to obstetric care, because these practices appear to increase the risk of HSV transmission (4).

Postpartum Recommendations

For women with known genital herpes or documented HSV-2 infection, the pediatricians who care for the neonates postpartum should be informed of the potential risk of neonatal herpes to allow enhanced observation of the neonates. The parents should be educated regarding the early signs of neonatal herpes and advised to set a low threshold for seeking medical care for the newborn after hospital discharge.

Women with active genital herpes at the time of delivery are not restricted from contact with the neonate but should wash their hands before contact. Women with active orolabial herpes should refrain from kissing the newborn at the face or site of skin break, such as a scalp electrode insertion site and also should wash their hands before contact with the neonate. In women with frequent symptomatic disease, antiviral suppressive therapy to decrease symptomatic lesions can be considered, or episodic therapy can be used. Antiviral suppressive therapy is not routinely recommended in women with asymptomatic oral HSV-1 infection. The risk of transmission by these women is likely to be low in these circumstances because asymptomatic viral shedding tends to occur at the oral mucosa rather than the lips (88). However, all women with orolabial HSV should be instructed to avoid biting their infants' nails because there have been case reports of herpetic whitlow resulting from this practice (89, 90).

Women with HSV of the breast should avoid nursing from the affected side. Antiviral suppressive therapy can be considered for these women.

The American Academy of Pediatrics considers use of acyclovir to be compatible with breastfeeding (91). Acyclovir is concentrated in breast milk, reaching peak levels approximately 3 hours after the initial maternal dose, with a half-life of 2–3 hours. The total dose received by infants of nursing mothers treated with acyclovir or valacyclovir reaches approximately 1 mg/d, which is approximately 1% of the effective neonatal dose (92–95). Because the dose is so low, we use suppressive antiviral therapy for breastfeeding women if such therapy is indicated for genital herpes or other mucocutaneous infection.

Summary

Pregnant women are routinely tested for many medical problems, including a number of sexually transmitted diseases. However, genital herpes, a prevalent sexually transmitted disease with significant consequences for pregnancy, is not routinely evaluated. Acquisition of HSV near term has been documented to be the most common cause of neonatal herpes infection, which can have devastating sequelae. The use of glycoprotein G-based serologic assays may be included in prenatal testing. For the prevention of neonatal HSV, testing would identify women at risk for acquiring genital HSV so that they may be counseled against unprotected coitus or oral–genital contact in the third trimester. Serologic testing also would identify HSV-2 seropositive women who are unaware they have previously acquired HSV-2 infection. Examination of these women for genital lesions at the time of admission in labor and avoidance of scalp electrodes, early artificial rupture of membranes, and instrumented deliveries may reduce the risk of fetal intrapartum HSV exposure. In addition, identifying HSV-2 seropositive, asymptomatic women who are unaware of their disease would result in education about their infection, the recognition of recurrences, and methods of avoiding transmission to sexual partners.

There is still much to be learned about the optimal strategies for management of genital herpes in the pregnant woman. Nevertheless, there is, at present, also much that can be done to initiate programs to reduce this potentially preventable cause of a devastating neonatal infection.

References

1. Fleming D, McQuillan G, Johnson R, Nahmias AJ, Aral SO, Lee FK, et al. Herpes simplex virus type 2 in the United States, 1976 to 1994. N Engl J Med 1997;337:1105–11.

2. Armstrong GL, Schillinger J, Markowitz L, Nahmias AJ, Johnson RE, McQuillan GM, et al. Incidence of herpes simplex virus type 2 infection in the United States. Am J Epidemiol 2001;153:912–20.

3. Brown ZA, Selke SA, Zeh J, Kopelman J, Maslow A, Ashley RL, et al. Acquisition of herpes simplex virus during pregnancy. N Engl J Med 1997;337:509–15.

4. Brown ZA, Wald A, Morrow RA, Selke S, Zeh J, Corey L. Effect of serologic status and cesarean delivery on transmission rates of herpes simplex virus from mother to infant. JAMA 2003;289:203–9.

5. Kimberlin DW. Neonatal herpes simplex infection. Clin Microbiol Rev 2004;17:1–13.

6. Mennemeyer ST, Cyr LP, Whitley RJ. Antiviral therapy for neonatal herpes simplex virus: a cost- effectiveness analysis. Am J Manag Care 1997;3:1551–8.

7. Stanberry L, Cunningham A, Mertz G, Mindel A, Peters B, Reitano M, et al. New developments in the epidemiology,

natural history and management of genital herpes. Antiviral Res 1999;42:1–14.

8. Nahmias A, Lee F, Beckman-Nahmias S. Sero-epidemiological and sociological patterns of herpes simplex virus infection in the world. Scand J Infect Dis Suppl 1990;69: 19–36.

9. Leone P, Fleming DT, Gilsenan AW, Li L, Justus S. Seroprevalence of herpes simplex virus-2 in suburban primary care offices in the United States. Sex Transm Dis 2004;31:311–6.

10. Kulhanjian J, Soroush V, Au D, Bronzan RN, Yasukawa LL, Weylman LE, et al. Identification of women at unsuspected risk of primary infection with herpes simplex virus type 2 during pregnancy. N Engl J Med 1992;326:916–20.

11. Bryson Y, Dillon M, Bernstein DI, Radolf J, Zakowski P, Garratty E. Risk of acquisition of genital herpes simplex virus type 2 in sex partners of persons with genital herpes: a prospective couple study. J Infect Dis 1993;167:942–6.

12. Wald A, Zeh J, Selke S, Warren T, Ryncarz AS, Ashley R, et al. Reactivation of genital herpes simplex virus type 2 infection in asymptomatic seropositive persons. N Engl J Med 2000;342:844–50.

13. Ashley RL, Wald A. Genital herpes: review of the epidemic and potential use of type-specific serology. Clin Microbiol Rev 1999;12:1–8.

14. Mertz GJ, Benedetti J, Ashley R, Selke SA, Corey L. Risk factors for the sexual transmission of genital herpes. Ann Intern Med 1992;116:197–202.

15. Mertz GJ, Schmidt O, Jourden JL, Guinan ME, Remington ML, Fahnlander A, et al. Frequency of acquisition of first episode genital infection with herpes simplex virus from symptomatic and asymptomatic source contacts. Sex Transm Dis 1985;12:33–9.

16. Mertz GJ, Coombs RW, Ashley R, Jourden J, Remington M, Winter C, et al. Transmission of genital herpes in couples with one symptomatic and one asymptomatic partner: a prospective study. J Infect Dis 1988;157:1169–77.

17. Langenberg A, Corey L, Ashley R, Leong W, Straus S. A prospective study of new infections with herpes simplex virus type 1 and type 2. N Engl J Med 1999;341:1432–8.

18. Fife KH, Bernstein DI, Tu W, Zimet GD, Brady R, Wu J, et al. Predictors of herpes simplex virus type 2 antibody positivity among persons with no history of genital herpes. Sex Transm Dis 2004;31:676–81.

19. Langenberg A, Benedetti J, Jenkins J, Ashley R, Winter C, Corey L. Development of clinically recognizable genital lesions among women previously identified as having "asymptomatic" HSV-2 infection. Ann Intern Med 1989; 110:882–7.

20. Lafferty WE, Downey L, Celum C, Wald A. Herpes simplex virus type 1 as a cause of genital herpes: impact on surveillance and prevention. J Infect Dis 2000;181:1454–7.

21. Roberts CM, Pfister JR, Spear SJ. Increasing proportion of herpes simplex virus type 1 as a cause of genital herpes infection in college students. Sex Transm Dis 2003;30: 797–800.

22. Ribes JA, Steele AD, Seabolt JP, Baker DJ. Six-year study of the incidence of herpes in genital and nongenital cultures in a central Kentucky medical center patient population. J Clin Microbiol 2001;39:3321–5.

23. Mertz GJ, Rosenthal SL, Stanberry LR. Is herpes simplex virus type 1 (HSV-1) now more common than HSV-2 in first episodes of genital herpes? Sex Transm Dis 2003;30: 801–2.

24. Wald A, Ericsson M, Krantz E, Selke S, Corey L. Oral shedding of herpes simplex virus type 2 [published erratum appears in Sex Transm Infect 2004;80:546]. Sex Transm Infect 2004;80:272–6.

25. Engelberg R, Carrell D, Krantz E, Corey L, Wald A. Natural history of genital herpes simplex virus type 1 infection. Sex Transm Dis 2003;30:174–7.

26. Wald A, Corey L, Cone R, Hobson A, Davis G, Zeh J. Frequent genital HSV-2 shedding in immunocompetent women: effect of acyclovir treatment. J Clin Invest 1997; 99:1092–7.

27. Hensleigh P, Andrews W, Brown Z, Greenspoon J, Yasukawa L, Prober C. Genital herpes during pregnancy: inability to distinguish primary and recurrent infections clinically. Obstet Gynecol 1997;89:891–5.

28. Brown Z, Benedetti J, Watts D, Selke S, Berry S, Ashley RL, et al. A comparison between detailed and simple histories in the diagnosis of genital herpes complicating pregnancy. Am J Obstet Gynecol 1995;172:1299–303.

29. Sexually transmitted diseases treatment guidelines 2002. Centers for Disease Control and Prevention. MMWR Recomm Rep 2002;51(RR-6):1–78.

30. Slomka MJ, Emery L, Munday PE, Moulsdale M, Brown DW. A comparison of PCR with virus isolation and direct antigen detection for diagnosis and typing of genital herpes. J Med Virol 1998;55:177–83.

31. Cone R, Hobson A, Brown Z, Ashley R, Berry S, Winter C, et al. Frequent detection of genital herpes simplex virus DNA by polymerase chain reaction among pregnant women. JAMA 1994;272:792–6.

32. Hobson A, Wald A, Wright N, Corey L. Evaluation of a quantitative competitive PCR assay for measuring of HSV DNA in genital tract secretions. J Clin Microbiol 1997;35: 548–52.

33. Wald A, Huang ML, Carrell D, Selke S, Corey L. Polymerase chain reaction for detection of herpes simplex virus (HSV) DNA on mucosal surfaces: comparison with HSV isolation in cell culture. J Infect Dis 2003;188: 1345–51.

34. Frederick DM, Bland D, Gollin Y. Fatal disseminated herpes simplex virus infection in a previously healthy pregnant woman: a case report. J Reprod Med 2002;47:591–6.

35. Young E, Chafizadeh E, Oliveira VL, Genta RM. Disseminated herpes virus infection during pregnancy. Clin Infect Dis 1996;22:51–8.

36. Kang AH, Graves CR. Herpes simplex hepatitis in pregnancy: a case report and review of the literature. Obstet Gynecol Surv 1999;54:463–8.

37. Dupuis O, Audibert F, Fernandez H, Frydman R. Herpes simplex virus encephalitis in pregnancy. Obstet Gynecol 1999;94:810–2.

38. Hollier LM, Scott LL, Murphree SS, Wendel GD Jr. Postpartum endometritis caused by herpes simplex virus. Obstet Gynecol 1997;89 suppl:836–8.

39. Hixson M, Collins JH. Postpartum herpes simplex endometritis: a case report. J Reprod Med 2001;46: 849–52.

40. Roizman B, Sears A. Herpes simplex viruses and their replication. In: Fields BN, Knipe DM, Howley PM, Chanock RM, Melnick JL, Monath TP, Roizman B, editors. Virology. 3rd ed. Philadelphia (PA): Lippincott-Raven; 1996. p 2231.

41. Ashley R. Performance and use of HSV type-specific serology test kits. Herpes 2002;9:38–45.

42. Ashley RL, Militoni J, Lee F, Nahmias A, Corey L. Comparison of Western blot (Immunoblot) and glycoprotein G-specific immunodot enzyme assay for detecting antibodies to herpes simplex virus types 1 and 2 in human sera. J Clin Microbiol 1988;26:662–7.

43. Morrow RA, Friedrich D. Inaccuracy of certain commercial enzyme immunoassays in diagnosing genital infections with herpes simplex virus types 1 or 2. Am J Clin Pathol 2003;120:839–44.

44. Ashley RL, Eagleton M, Pfeiffer N. Ability of a rapid serology test to detect seroconversion to herpes simplex virus type 2 glycoprotein G soon after infection. J Clin Microbiol 1999;37:1632–3.

45. Ashley RL, Wald A, Eagleton M. Premarket evaluation of the POCkit HSV-2 type-specific serologic test in culture-documented cases of genital herpes simplex virus type 2. Sex Transm Dis 2000;27:266–9.

46. Ashley-Morrow R, Nollkamper J, Robinson N, Bishop N, Smith J. Performance of Focus ELISA tests for herpes simplex virus type 1 (HSV-1) and HSV-2 antibodies among women in ten diverse geographic locations. Clin Microbiol Infect 2004;10:530–6.

47. Saville M, Brown D, Burgess C, Perry K, Barton S, Cowan F, et al. An evaluation of near patient tests for detecting herpes simplex virus type-2 antibody. Sex Transm Infect 2000;76:381–2.

48. Ribes JA, Hayes M, Smith A, Winters JL, Baker DJ. Comparative performance of herpes simplex virus type 2-specific serologic assays from Meridian Diagnostics and MRL diagnostics. J Clin Microbiol 2001;39:3740–2.

49. Eis-Hubinger AM, Daumer M, Matz B, Schneweis KE. Evaluation of three glycoprotein G2-based enzyme immunoassays for detection of antibodies to herpes simplex virus type 2 in human sera. J Clin Microbiol 1999; 37:1242–6.

50. Prince HE, Ernst CE, Hogrefe WR. Evaluation of an enzyme immunoassay system for measuring herpes simplex virus (HSV) type 1-specific and HSV type 2-specific IgG antibodies. J Clin Lab Anal 2000;14:13–6.

51. Ashley R, Cent A, Maggs V, Corey L. Inability of enzyme immunoassays to discriminate between infections with herpes simplex virus type 1 and 2. Ann Intern Med 1991; 115:520–6.

52. American College of Obstetricians and Gynecologists. Management of genital herpes in pregnancy. ACOG Practice Bulletin 8. Washington, DC: ACOG; 1999.

53. Bryson YJ, Dillon M, Lovett M, Acuna G, Taylor S, Cherry JD, et al. Treatment of first episodes of genital herpes simplex virus infections with oral acyclovir: a randomized double-blind controlled trial in normal subjects. N Engl J Med 1983;308:916–20.

54. Vontver LA, Hickok DE, Brown Z, Reid L, Corey L. Recurrent genital herpes simplex virus infection in pregnancy: infant outcome and frequency of asymptomatic recurrences. Am J Obstet Gynecol 1982;143:75–84.

55. Frenkel LM, Brown ZA, Bryson YJ, Corey L, Unadkat JD, Hensleigh PA, et al. Pharmacokinetics of acyclovir in the term human pregnancy and neonate. Am J Obstet Gyn 1991;164:569–76.

56. Kimberlin DF, Weller S, Whitley RJ, Andrews WW, Hauth JC, Lakeman F, et al. Pharmacokinetics of oral valacyclovir and acyclovir in late pregnancy. Am J Obstet Gynecol 1998;179:846–51.

57. Beutner KR. Valacyclovir: a review of its antiviral activity, pharmacokinetic properties, and clinical efficacy. Antiviral Res 1995;28:281–90.

58. Stone KM, Reiff-Eldridge R, White AD, Cordero JF, Brown Z, Alexander ER, et al. Pregnancy outcomes following systemic prenatal acyclovir exposure: Conclusions from the international acyclovir pregnancy registry, 1984-1999. Birth Defects Res A Clin Mol Teratol 2004;70:201–7.

59. Kimberlin D, Lin C-Y, Jacobs R, Powell DA, Corey L, Gruber WC, et al. Safety and efficacy of high-dose intravenous acyclovir in the management of neonatal herpes simplex virus infections. Pediatrics 2001;108:230–8.

60. Tyring SK, Baker D, Snowden W. Valacyclovir for herpes simplex virus infections: long-term safety and sustained efficacy after 20 years' experience with acyclovir. J Infect Dis 2002;186 suppl 1:S40–6.

61. Whitley RJ, Roizman B. Herpes simplex virus infections. Lancet 2001;357:1513–8.

62. Brown ZA, Benedetti J, Ashley R, Burchett S, Selke S, Berry S, et al. Neonatal herpes simplex virus infection in relation to asymptomatic maternal infection at the time of labor. N Engl J Med 1991;324:1247–52.

63. Boucher FD, Yasukawa LL, Bronzan RN, Hensleigh PA, Arvin AM, Prober CG. A prospective evaluation of primary genital herpes simplex virus type 2 infections acquired during pregnancy. Pediatr Infect Dis J 1990;9: 499–504.

64. Sullivan-Bolyai JZ, Fife KH, Jacobs RF, Z M, Corey L. Disseminated neonatal herpes simplex virus type 1 from a maternal breast lesion. Pediatrics 1983;71:455–7.

65. Kimberlin D, Lin C-Y, Jacobs R, Powell DA, Frenkel LM, Gruber WC, et al. Natural history of neonatal herpes simplex virus infections in the acyclovir era. Pediatrics 2001; 108:223–9.

66. Whitley R, Corey L, Arvin A, Lakeman FD, Sumaya CV, Wright PF, et al. Changing presentation of herpes simplex virus infection in neonates. J Infect Dis 1988;158:109–16.

67. Koelle DM, Benedetti J, Langenberg A, Corey L. Asymptomatic reactivation of herpes simplex virus in women after first episode of genital herpes. Ann Intern Med 1992;116:433–7.

68. Whitley R, Arvin A, Prober C, Corey L, Burchett S, Plotkin S, et al. Predictors of morbidity and mortality in neonates with herpes simplex infections. N Engl J Med 1991;324: 450–4.

69. van Everdingen JJ, Peeters MF, ten Have P. Neonatal herpes policy in The Netherlands: five years after a consensus conference. J Perinat Med 1993;21:371–5.

70. Gardella C, Brown ZA, Wald A, Morrow RA, Selke S, Krantz E, et al. Poor correlation between genital lesions

and detection of herpes simplex virus in women in labor. Obstet Gynecol 2005;106: 268–74.

71. Arvin A, Hensleigh P, Prober C, Au DS, Yasukawa LL, Wittek AE, et al. Failure of antepartum maternal cultures to predict the infant's risk of exposure to herpes simplex virus at delivery. N Engl J Med 1986;315:796–800.

72. Braig S, Luton D, Sibony O, Elinger C, Boissinot C, Blot, Oury JF. Acyclovir prophylaxis in late pregnancy prevents recurrent genital herpes and viral shedding. Eur J Obstet Gynecol Reprod Biol 2001;96:55–8.

73. Scott LL, Sanchez PJ, Jackson GL, Zeray F, Wendel GD Jr. Acyclovir suppression to prevent cesarean delivery after first episode genital herpes. Obstet Gynecol 1996;87: 69–73.

74. Brocklehurst P, Kinghorn G, Carney O, Helsen K, Ross E, Ellis E, et al. A randomised placebo controlled trial of suppressive acyclovir in late pregnancy in women with recurrent genital herpes infection. Br J Obstet Gynaecol 1998;105:275–80.

75. Scott LL, Hollier LM, McIntire D, Sanchez PJ, Jackson GL, WendelGDJr. Acyclovir suppression to prevent recurrent genital herpes at delivery. Infect Dis Obstet Gynecol 2002; 10:71–7.

76. Watts DH, Brown ZA, Money D, Selke S, Huang ML, Sacks SL, et al. A double-blind, randomized, placebo-controlled trial of acyclovir in late pregnancy for the reduction of herpes simplex virus shedding and cesarean delivery. Am J Obstet Gynecol 2003;188:836–43.

77. Sheffield JS, Hollier LM, Hill JB, Stuart GS, Wendel GD. Acyclovir prophylaxis to prevent herpes simplex virus recurrence at delivery: a systematic review. Obstet Gynecol 2003;102:1396–403.

78. Gardella C, Brown Z, Wald A, Selke S, Zeh J, Morrow RA, Corey L. Risk factors for herpes simplex virus transmission to pregnant women: a couples study. Am J Obstet Gynecol 2005;193:1891–9.

79. Casper C, Wald A. Condom use and the prevention of genital herpes acquisition. Herpes 2002;9:10–4.

80. Corey L, Wald A, Patel R, Sacks SL, Tyring SK, Warren T, et al. Once-daily valacyclovir to reduce the risk of transmission of genital herpes. N Engl J Med 2004;350(1):11–20.

81. Bartellas E, Crane JM, Daley M, Bennett KA, Hutchens D. Sexuality and sexual activity in pregnancy. BJOG 2000; 107:964–8.

82. von Sydow K. Sexuality during pregnancy and after childbirth: a metacontent analysis of 59 studies. J Psychosom Res 1999; 47:27–49.

83. Vonau B, Low-Beer N, Barton SE, Smith JR. Antenatal serum screening for genital herpes: a study of knowledge and attitudes of women at a central London hospital. Br J Obstet Gynaecol 1997;104:347–9.

84. Edmiston N, O'Sullivan M, Charters D, Chuah J, Pallis L. Study of knowledge of genital herpes infection and attitudes to testing for genital herpes among antenatal clinic attendees. Aust N Z J Obstet Gynaecol 2003;43:351–3.

85. Miyai T, Turner KR, Kent CK, Klausner J. The psychosocial impact of testing individuals with no history of genital herpes for herpes simplex virus type 2. Sex Transm Dis 2004;31:517–21.

86. Thung SF, Grobman WA. The cost-effectiveness of routine antenatal screening for maternal herpes simplex virus-1 and -2 antibodies. Am J Obstet Gynecol 2005;192:483–8.

87. Baker D, Brown Z, Hollier LM, Wendel G, Hulme L, Griffiths D, et al. Cost-effectiveness of herpes simplex virus type 2 serologic testing and antiviral therapy in pregnancy. Am J Obstet Gynecol 2004;191:2074–84.

88. Spruance SL. Pathogenesis of herpes simplex labialis: excretion of virus in the oral cavity. J Clin Microbiol 1984;19:675–9.

89. Feder Jr HM, Geller RW. Herpetic whitlow of the great toe. N Engl J Med 1992;326:1295–6.

90. Fischer RG, Livingood JC. Vesiculobullous lesion on the right fifth toe. Clinical Infectious Diseases 2005;40:579–80, 609–10.

91. American Academy of Pediatrics Committee on Drugs. The transfer of drugs and other chemicals into human milk. Pediatrics 2001;108(3):776–89.

92. Sheffield JS, Fish DN, Hollier LM, Cadematori S, Nobles BJ, Wendel GD Jr. Acyclovir concentrations in human breast milk after valaciclovir administration. Am J Obstet Gynecol 2002;186:100–2.

93. Meyer LJ, de Miranda P, Sheth N, Spruance S. Acyclovir in human breast milk. Am J Obstet Gynecol 1988;158:586–8.

94. Taddio A, Klein J, Koren G. Acyclovir excretion in human breast milk. Ann Pharmacother 1994;28:585–7.

95. Lau RJ, Emery MG, Galinsky RE. Unexpected accumulation of acyclovir in breast milk with estimation of infant exposure. Obstet Gynecol 1987;69 suppl:468–71.

CHAPTER 25

Human Immunodeficiency Virus Infection in Pregnancy

HOWARD MINKOFF

The acquired immunodeficiency syndrome (AIDS) epidemic continues to exact a horrific toll in the developing world. In the United States, however, the advent of effective therapies in the 1990s transformed human immunodeficiency virus (HIV) infection into a controllable disease for women and one that now infects only 1% of children exposed in utero. Women in the developed world rely on the expertise of their physicians to assure them of these improved outcomes. The most recent developments in the field will be summarized here in a fashion that should allow their integration into the practice of obstetrics. The focus of this work will be on the dual responsibilities of obstetricians, assuring the health of women and minimizing the risks of transmission. It must be emphasized that the standard of care for the management of HIV continues to evolve at a dizzying pace. In recognition of that fact, a web site has been created by the U.S. Department of Health and Human Services (www.aidsinfo.nih.gov), which provides a regularly updated, practical, and thorough guide to management of HIV. Those charged with the care of HIV-infected pregnant women should make frequent use of this site.

Human Immunodeficiency Virus Testing

Before any of the following new therapies can be provided to women, the HIV status of the women must be known. It is not uncommon for HIV serostatus to be determined for the first time during pregnancy. It is the responsibility of all clinicians charged with the care of pregnant women to be certain that serostatus is determined as early in pregnancy as possible. The Institute of Medicine has proposed an approach that is both simple and practical and should assure continued respect for patients' autonomy. In its report "Reducing the Odds" (1), the Institute of Medicine recommended an informed right of refusal approach to testing. Although such an approach would require that a prenatal patient be informed that she was going to be tested for the virus that causes AIDS and that she had the right to refuse such a test, a written affirmative consent would not be required. Thereby, the HIV test would still be offered with more consideration than that applied to the panel of other prenatal tests for which the "general care" consent generally suffices. However, the process of testing would not be so onerous as to dissuade physicians from offering it or to convey the sense that the test is reserved for women who in some way were perceived to be at special risk.

Despite the increasingly simple and straightforward approach recommended for prenatal testing, because approximately 15% of women infected with HIV receive no or minimal care and 20% do not initiate care until the third trimester, a number of women will still arrive in labor and delivery suites with unknown serostatus. In some circumstances, despite adequate care, women will not have been offered the test. There are compelling data to suggest that intrapartum and early neonatal prophylaxis, even in the absence of antepartum therapy, can reduce the risk of mother-to-child transmission (2). Therefore, efforts should be made during labor to rapidly discern the serostatus of those women whose results were not previously known. Although the current generation of rapid tests is highly reliable, they do not match the accuracy of the standard approach to prenatal testing (one or two enzyme-linked immunosorbent assays followed by a confirmatory Western blot test). However, they are sufficiently sensitive to identify women who should be offered therapy while confirmatory test results are pending. Patients should be informed that if the confirmatory test results are negative, then treatment of the infant would be discontinued. The Mother–Infant Rapid Intervention at Delivery study has demonstrated the acceptability and feasibility of offering counseling and rapid HIV-1 testing to women of unknown HIV-1 status who present while in labor (3). A model protocol on implementing rapid HIV testing at labor and delivery is available from the Center for Disease Control and Prevention (www.cdc.gov/hiv/rapid_testing). Rapid testing also can be used in settings other than labor and delivery. Its use in ambulatory care sites and emergency rooms can mitigate the loss to follow-up that often occurs when testing and counseling require separate visits spaced days or weeks apart. With rapid testing, results can be given to patients at the same time their blood is drawn. When using that approach, the obstetrician must establish a link with an individual who can offer posttest counseling to any individual found to be infected with HIV.

Treatment of Pregnant Women

Since the early years of the HIV epidemic, public health officials and obstetricians have echoed the refrain that pregnancy should not be a barrier to the most potent HIV therapies. Since the advent of highly active antiretroviral therapy in 1996, these therapies, though associated with serious side effects, have been shown to be very effective at keeping viral replication in check and to improve dramatically the prognosis and health of individuals infected with HIV. Thus, the first responsibility of obstetricians is to ensure that these medications are used appropriately in the setting of pregnancy. Toward that end, it is necessary to: 1) monitor women to know when highly active antiretroviral therapy should be instituted or altered, and 2) know the appropriate therapies to use in the setting of pregnancy. In this section, the standards for virologic, immunologic, and resistance monitoring will be outlined, and the medications that obstetricians should be prescribing to vouchsafe the health of their patients will be described.

Monitoring Virologic and Immunologic Status

Studies of the natural history of HIV infection have defined the relationship between shifts in viral load, progressive immunologic deterioration, and subsequent clinical decline. It is based on these data that algorithms for the initiation of antiretroviral therapy were devised. These management schemes have been modified over time as additional data have been developed that suggest that initiation of therapy can be delayed relative to the recommended start points from just a few years ago. More recent data have highlighted both the difficulty of sustaining long-term adherence to highly active antiretroviral therapy and the fact that no obvious clinical disadvantage has been associated with therapy that is initiated a bit farther into the course of disease.

The cornerstones of monitoring remain assessment of viral loads and CD4 counts. In the nonpregnant individual infected with HIV, treatment initiation is now recommended when the CD4 count falls below $350/mm^3$ or

when plasma HIV RNA levels exceed 100,000 copies per mL. Counseling regarding implementation of these guidelines must be individualized and, in addition to a discussion of immune and virological status, should include factors such as a woman's willingness and readiness to undertake a lifelong commitment to therapy; the potential benefits and risks of initiating therapy in asymptomatic individuals; and the likelihood, after counseling and education, of adherence to the prescribed treatment. These decisions, when made during pregnancy, take on yet another level of complexity.

Once a decision to begin therapy has been made, viral load monitoring provides a gauge of the success of the intervention. In pregnancy, that monitoring should occur monthly until the viral load is undetectable and thereafter every 2–3 months (Fig. 25-1). With appropriate therapy, viral load should be seen to drop by over one log within the first month of therapy and should eventually become undetectable. The speed with which that occurs will vary with the baseline load. The higher the load, the longer the time until undetectable levels are reached; however, in all circumstances, that goal should be achieved within 6 months. If that goal is not reached, or if after it is attained subsequent test results reveal a reemergence of detectable levels of virus beyond a transient low-level viremia, therapy must be deemed a failure and a decision will have to be made concerning a new approach.

Resistance Testing

Since pregnancy is not, *a priori*, a reason to modify HIV care, obstetricians must master an increasingly complex algorithm of diagnostic tests and therapeutic interventions. Resistance testing is now a standard component of HIV care. Most randomized trials of these technologies have demonstrated that those assigned to study arms with access to resistance test results have a greater reduction in viral load after the initiation of salvage therapy, although follow-up has generally been short (4). Currently, two types of testing are available, genotypic and phenotypic, each with distinct advantages and disadvantages. Phenotypic testing is a measure of the activity of the virus under set conditions, whereas genotyping is a measure of structure.

PHENOTYPIC TESTING

Phenotypic tests compare the ability of the virus to replicate in various concentrations of an antiretroviral drug with its ability to replicate in the absence of the drug (5). As such, they are somewhat analogous to bacterial sensitivity tests with which most physicians are familiar. Results are usually expressed as the amount of drug required to inhibit viral production in vitro by 50%,

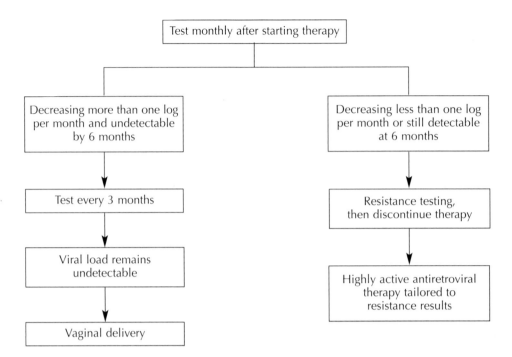

Fig. 25-1. Viral load monitoring.

although other levels such as 90% or 95% inhibition can be used. In general, if the amount of drug required to inhibit viral production by 50% is fourfold or greater for the patient's virus than the control strain, then the patient's strain is considered resistant.

GENOTYPIC TESTING

Genotypic testing seeks to detect mutations in the genes that control replication of the virus. These mutations result in the substitution of amino acids in the proteins produced. The significance of these point mutations is determined by correlating specific mutations with phenotypic resistance as measured by viral susceptibility assays and correlation with clinical response to therapy. In that manner, it can be determined if a given mutation can be expected to result in resistance to a specific agent.

Mutations can have adverse consequences in several ways. Primary mutations affect the binding of the drug to its target site, thus increasing the amount of drug necessary to inhibit the enzyme activity. However, the resultant mutant strain of the virus may be less able to replicate in the host and to induce immunologic compromise. Other, secondary mutations make that relatively less "fit" mutant virus more pathogenic. Thus, those secondary changes work by improving the ability of the virus with primary mutations to replicate and cause immunologic damage (ie, they restore fitness). The number of mutations required to cause a clinically relevant effect varies with the agent in question. Thus, the rate at

which resistance develops will depend on the number of mutations necessary to create a significant change in susceptibility. The life cycle of HIV predisposes to mutations because of the combination of the rapid turnover of HIV (107–108 rounds of replication per day) and the high error rate of reverse transcriptase when replicating the nearly 10,000 nucleotides present in the HIV genome. When incompletely suppressive drug regimens are used, they provide the evolutionary pressure that selects those mutations that cause resistance to antiretroviral agents.

CLINICAL APPLICABILITY

Certain limitations are present for both genotypic and phenotypic assays. Both types of assays require a plasma HIV RNA level above 1,000 copies per mL. In addition, the assays may not detect resistant species that constitute 20% or less of the population of circulating viruses. This issue may be especially important for evaluating resistance to drugs that a person took in the past but is no longer receiving. In that circumstance, the wild type virus (the nonmutant strain), being more fit, may have overgrown the mutant strain in the interim because the medication was discontinued. However, if the patient is reexposed to the offending agent, the resistant strain may again attain dominance. As a consequence, resistance testing is more useful for ruling out, than for ruling in, therapies to be used in a given patient. That is because the absence of resistance may merely reflect the reemergence of that wild type strain and the inability, in that circumstance, for the assays to detect the minority mutant strain.

Genotypic assays can usually be performed more rapidly than phenotypic assays, with results available in 1–2 weeks compared with several weeks for phenotypic assays, despite the use of recombinant assays. Genetic mutations that confer resistance may be detected before a change in susceptibility is detectable on phenotypic assays. However, the genetic basis for resistance must be understood before the impact of a specific mutation can be predicted. In addition, mutational interactions may make prediction of susceptibility difficult when multiple mutations are present. Cross resistance to other drugs within a class, such as protease inhibitors, can be difficult to predict based only on genotype. In clinical practice, most clinicians will rely on algorithms developed by panels of experts or on online databases. Obstetricians should interpret and act on these results in consultation with an expert in the field.

There are several defined circumstances in which clinicians should use these tests. The most common indication for testing is treatment failure. Treatment failure is defined as the failure to attain an undetectable level of virus or the persistent presence of virus after it had become undetectable. If it has been determined that failure has occurred, resistance testing should be performed before the failing regimen is discontinued. This is to prevent the overgrowth of wild type strain that might occur after the regimen is discontinued, such that resistant strains would not be detected even though they would be "lying in wait" for the reinstitution of some components of the regimen. Resistance testing also can be helpful in the setting of an individual who has recently seroconverted. It has been reported that a substantial percentage of new infections are with organisms that are resistant (6). If testing can be performed before a wild type virus overgrows the infecting strain, the clinician will have an opportunity to choose an initial regimen that will have a high probability of success against the infecting virus.

In pregnancy, any woman who is about to begin therapy, whether she has been using therapy in the past or not, should undergo resistance testing. Additionally, as with nonpregnant women, if the regimen is unsuccessful, then resistance testing is warranted. There are considerations that are unique to pregnancy and they relate to the fitness of resistance virus for mother-to-child transmission of HIV (ie, there is an open question as to whether resistant viruses are more or less likely to be transmitted). In general, zidovudine and other resistance mutations have not been associated with an increased risk of perinatal transmission. However, in one study, detection of zidovudine resistance was associated with transmission when adjustment was made for duration of rup-

tured membranes and total lymphocyte count (7). Although perinatal transmission of resistant virus has been reported (8), it appears to be unusual, and it is not clear that the mutant strains are more likely to be transmitted. In a multisite study of HIV-infected pregnant women (Women and Infants Transmission Study), it was reported that when a transmitting mother had a mixed viral population of wild type and low-level resistant viruses, only the wild type virus was found in the infant, suggesting that virus with low-level zidovudine resistance may be less transmissible (9).

Drug Therapy

As noted previously, in nonpregnant individuals infected with HIV, treatment initiation is recommended when the CD4 count falls below $350/mm^3$ or when plasma HIV RNA levels exceed 100,000 copies per mL. When that Rubicon has been crossed, the standard for treatment of HIV since 1996 has been highly active antiretroviral therapy. In pregnancy, the threshold for starting therapy is altered. Mother-to-child transmission rates are linked to viral loads, and rates start to climb well before viral loads of 100,000 copies are reached. Cesarean deliveries are recommended for women whose viral loads exceed 1,000 copies. For both those reasons, pregnant women should be informed of the advantages of initiating highly active antiretroviral therapy whenever their viral loads are above 1,000 copies (Fig. 25-2). Even women whose counts are below 1,000 will have lower rates of transmission if they take antiretroviral therapy during gestation, although in that circumstance, the advantage of highly active antiretroviral therapy over the simpler PACTG 076 zidovudine regimen is less clear. However, even in that circumstance, highly active antiretroviral therapy might lower the likelihood (already relatively low in women with undetectable virus) of development of resistance. Trials of highly active antiretroviral therapy versus zidovudine in the setting of counts below 1,000 have not been undertaken to date.

Highly active antiretroviral therapy consists of antiretroviral regimens that have been shown to result in a sustained virological response. Although the number of drug regimens that have been shown to achieve that goal continues to increase, a few broad categories of highly active antiretroviral therapy can be described. The original regimens described in 1996 included dual nucleoside reverse transcriptase inhibitors accompanied by a protease inhibitor. Currently, there are more than twenty nucleoside reverse transcriptase inhibitors, nonnucleoside reverse transcriptase inhibitors, protease inhibitors, and fusion inhibitors approved for therapy, so theoretically a large number of choices within these categories exist (Table 25-1). However, some of these medications

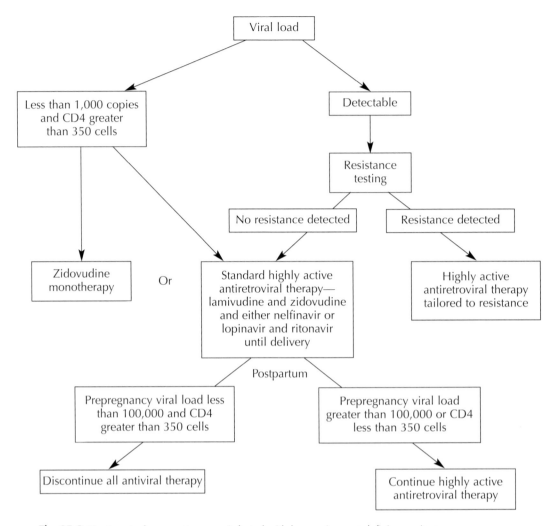

Fig. 25-2. Treatment of pregnant women infected with human immunodeficiency virus.

should not be used in combination. For example, zidovudine and stavudine have overlapping toxicities, didanosine and zalcitabine in combination have diminished efficacy, and didanosine and stavudine have recently been linked to several fatal cases of mitochondrial toxicity in pregnancy (10).

When initiating treatment, the clinician must bear in mind that choosing an appropriate second-line regimen is even more difficult than choosing an initial course of therapy. That fact should reinforce two rules regarding the initial decision to commence antiretroviral therapy of HIV-infected women: 1) adherence to therapy is crucial, and 2) the choice of a first-line course of therapy should always include a consideration of the possible need to deal with the failure of that regimen.

In regard to the first factor, adherence is the *sine qua non* of successful therapy. Haphazard or intermittent adherence with a drug regimen is a formula for the development of resistant virus. Even very brief drug holidays

have been associated with the replacement of wild strain virus with mutant strains that are resistant to therapeutic agents. Therefore, it is critical that time and effort are expended by health care providers to educate patients about the need to start treatment only after they are able to commit to rigorous and lifelong adherence to complex regimens. Additionally, providers must assist patients in developing the tools that will aid them in maintaining successful regimens.

With regard to factoring the possible need for future regimens into the choice of initial therapy, it is useful to choose a regimen that "spares" one class of antiretroviral agent. Thus, a regimen should spare protease inhibitors or nonnucleoside reverse transcriptase inhibitors or both. In fact, there are increasingly popular regimens that employ three nucleoside reverse transcriptase inhibitors alone. When those regimens are used, the patient is assured that if resistance develops, there are classes of drugs available to which the virus has not yet

Table 25-1. Preclinical and Clinical Data Relevant to the Use of Antiretrovirals in Pregnancy

Antiretroviral Drug	U.S. Food and Drug Administration Pregnancy Category*	Placental Passage (Newborn/Mother Drug Ratio)	Long-Term Animal Carcinogenicity Studies	Animal Teratogen Studies
Nucleoside and nucleotide analogue reverse transcriptase inhibitors				
Abacavir	C	Yes (rats)	Positive (malignant and nonmalignant tumors of liver, thyroid in female rats, and preputial and clitoral gland of mice and rats)	Positive (rodent anasarca and skeletal malformations at 1,000mg/kg [35 times human exposure] during organogenesis; not seen in rabbits)
Didanosine	B	Yes (human [0.5])	Negative (no tumors, lifetime rodent study)	Negative
Emtricitabine	B	Unknown	Not completed	Negative
Lamivudine	C	Yes (human [1])	Negative (no tumors, lifetime rodent study)	Negative
Stavudine	C	Yes (rhesus monkey [0.76])	Positive (mice and rats, at very high dose exposure, liver and bladder tumors)	Negative (but sternal bone calcium decreases in rodents)
Tenofovir DF	B	Yes (rat and monkey)	Positive (hepatic adenomas in female mice at high doses)	Negative (osteomalacia when given to juvenile animals at high doses)
Zalcitabine	C	Yes (rhesus monkey [0.30–0.50])	Positive (rodent, thymic lymphomas)	Positive (rodent—hydrocephalus at high dose)
Zidovudine	C	Yes (human [0.85])	Positive (rodent, noninvasive vaginal epithelial tumors)	Positive (rodent—near lethal dose)
Nonnucleoside reverse transcriptase inhibitors				
Delavirdine	C	Unknown	Positive (hepatocellular adenomas and carcinomas in male and female mice but not rats, bladder tumors in male mice)	Positive (rodent—ventricular septal defect)
Efavirenz	D	Yes (cynomolgus monkey, rat, rabbit [1])	Positive (hepatocellular adenomas and carcinomas and pulmonary alveolar and bronchiolar adenomas in female but not male mice)	Positive (cynomolgus monkey—anencephaly, anophthalmia, microphthalmos)
Nevirapine	C	Yes (human [1])	Positive (hepatocellular adenomas and carcinomas in mice and rats)	Negative
Protease inhibitors				
Amprenavir	C	Unknown	Positive (hepatocellular adenomas and carcinomas in male mice and rats)	Negative (but deficient ossification and thymic elongation in rats and rabbits)
Atazanavir	B	Unknown	Positive (hepatocellular adenomas in female mice)	Negative

(continued)

Table 25-1. Preclinical and Clinical Data Relevant to the Use of Antiretrovirals in Pregnancy *(continued)*

Antiretroviral Drug	U.S. Food and Drug Administration Pregnancy Category*	Placental Passage (Newborn/Mother Drug Ratio)	Long-Term Animal Carcinogenicity Studies	Animal Teratogen Studies
Protease inhibitors *(continued)*				
Fosamprenavir	C	Unknown	Positive (benign and malignant liver tumors in male rodents)	Negative (deficient ossification with amprenavir but not fosamprenavir)
Indinavir	C	Minimal (humans)	Positive (thyroid adenomas in male rats at highest dose)	Negative (but extra ribs in rodents)
Lopinavir and Ritonavir	C	Unknown	Positive (hepatocellular adenomas and carcinomas in mice and rats)	Negative (but delayed skeletal ossification and increase in skeletal variations in rats at maternally toxic doses)
Nelfinavir	B	Minimal (humans)	Positive (thyroid follicular adenomas and carcinomas in rats)	Negative
Ritonavir	B	Minimal (humans)	Positive (liver adenomas and carcinomas in male mice)	Negative (but cryptorchidism in rodents)
Saquinavir	B	Minimal (humans)	Negative	Negative
Tipranavir	C	Unknown	In progress	Negative (but decreased ossification and pup weights in rats at maternally toxic doses)
Fusion inhibitors				
Enfuvirtide	B	Unknown	Not done	Negative

*U.S. Food and Drug Administration Pregnancy Categories: A, adequate and well-controlled studies of pregnant women fail to demonstrate a risk to the fetus during the first trimester of pregnancy (and no evidence exists of risk during later trimesters); B, animal reproduction studies fail to demonstrate a risk to the fetus, and adequate but well-controlled studies of pregnant women have not been conducted; C, safety in human pregnancy has not been determined (animal studies are either positive for fetal risk or have not been conducted, and the drug should not be used unless the potential benefit outweighs the potential risk to the fetus); D, positive evidence of human fetal risk that is based on adverse reaction data from investigational or marketing experiences, but the potential benefits from the use of the drug among pregnant women might be acceptable despite its potential risks; X, studies among animals or reports of adverse reactions have indicated that the risks associated with the use of the drug for pregnant women clearly outweigh any possible benefit.

U.S. Department of Health and Human Services Panel on Antiretroviral Guidelines for Adults and Adolescents—A Working Group of the Office of AIDS Research Advisory Council (ORAC). Guidelines for the Use of Antiretroviral Agents in HIV-1-Infected Adults and Adolescents. Available at: http://aidsinfo.nih.gov/ContentFiles/AdultandAdolescentGL.pdf. Retrieved August 25, 2006.

been exposed and to which they are unlikely to have resistance.

The online recommendations for care of HIV-infected nonpregnant individuals (aidsinfo.nih.gov) includes "preferred" regimens, those that include a protease inhibitor or protease inhibitors (lopinavir and ritonavir coformulation) or a nonnucleoside reverse transcriptase inhibitor (efavirenz) in combination with one of several two nucleoside reverse transcriptase inhibitor combinations. A large amount of clinical outcome data support the use of a protease inhibitor in combination with two nucleoside reverse transcriptase inhibitors (11). Some of the protease inhibitors, such as

ritonavir, are less often used as first line therapy because of the difficulty many patients have in tolerating standard doses and because of the drug's many interactions. Other protease inhibitors create difficulties because of the large pill burden associated with their use. However, if a patient is first seen in pregnancy already successfully using one of these agents, there is no requirement to terminate her use of the agent, provided that she is tolerating it and that the regimen is effective.

A critical factor to recognize is that poor results often occur when antiretroviral regimens are instituted in the wake of virologic failure with a previous regimen. This fact suggests that the first regimen affords the best opportunity for long-term control of viral replication. Because the genetic barrier to resistance is greatest with protease inhibitors, many would consider a protease inhibitor in combination with two nucleoside reverse transcriptase inhibitors to be the preferred initial regimen. However, efavirenz in combination with two nucleoside reverse transcriptase inhibitors appears to be at least as effective as a protease inhibitor in combination with two nucleoside reverse transcriptase inhibitors in suppressing plasma viremia and increasing CD4+ T cell counts, and some have suggested that such a regimen is the preferred initial regimen because it may spare the toxicities of protease inhibitors for a considerable time (12). However, concerns about teratogenicity that have been demonstrated in animal models and neural tube defects in humans makes this a poor choice for use in early pregnancy. Abacavir in combination with two nucleoside reverse transcriptase inhibitors, a triple nucleoside reverse transcriptase inhibitors regimen, has been used with some success as well but may have short-lived efficacy when the baseline viral load is greater than 100,000 copies per mL. Certain individuals may have a genetic predisposition to a rash associated with abacavir use, a rash that can be a harbinger of a fatal reaction (13). In all circumstances, a rash signals the need to immediately discontinue therapy. Dual therapy with nucleoside reverse transcriptase inhibitors is less likely than highly active antiretroviral therapy regimens, to persistently suppress viremia to below detectable levels and should be used only if more potent treatment is not possible. Use of antiretroviral agents as monotherapy is contraindicated, except when there are no other options or, as noted previously, in pregnant women with very low viral loads when it is being used solely to reduce perinatal transmission.

Highly Active Antiretroviral Therapy Regimens

Although recommendations regarding antiviral therapy should not be modified a priori because of pregnancy, a few comments are deserving of note. First, zidovudine, the first agent clearly linked to significant reductions in rates of mother-to-child transmission of HIV, should be used whenever possible as a component of highly active antiretroviral therapy regimens. The current standard zidovudine regimen for adults is 200 mg, three times daily, or 300 mg, twice daily. Because the mechanism by which zidovudine reduces perinatal transmission is not known, it is theoretically possible that these dose regimens may not have equivalent efficacy to that observed in PACTG 076 when 100 mg, five times daily, was used. However, a regimen of two or three times daily has the advantage of probable enhanced adherence.

Second, the potential perinatal risks of agents must be considered when choosing a highly active antiretroviral therapy regimen. Nucleoside reverse transcriptase inhibitors were the first class of drug used for treatment of HIV, and there is a greater experience with their use than with other classes of drug, most of which is reassuring (14). These agents have been generally well tolerated and have not been shown to be teratogenic in humans. However, concerns have been raised about potential adverse effects on both mothers and infants related to the avidity of these drugs for mitochondria (5, 15). In the mother, clinical disorders associated with mitochondrial toxicity include neuropathy, myopathy, cardiomyopathy, pancreatitis, hepatic steatosis, and lactic acidosis.

Several cases of lactic acidosis, three of which were fatal and two of which were accompanied by pancreatitis, have been reported among pregnant or recently delivered women who had been taking didanosine and stavudine therapy, along with a variety of third agents, since before conception (10). Two cases of fatal liver failure in pregnant women taking zidovudine, lamivudine, and nelfinavir have been reported. These cases developed in late pregnancy and, in several cases, the presentation was similar to that seen with acute fatty liver of pregnancy, a condition that itself has been linked to mitochondrial fatty oxidation disorders in the fetus (homozygotic) and mother (heterozygotic) (16). Although these serious morbidities appear to be rare, providers caring for HIV-infected women receiving nucleoside reverse transcriptase inhibitor analogue agents should be aware of the risk and monitor patients accordingly. One approach would be to monitor hepatic enzyme levels during the last trimester and to aggressively investigate all new symptoms. In women with substantial elevations in transaminase levels above baseline or other new abnormalities, in the absence of other explanations for the abnormalities, such as preeclampsia, administration of nucleoside reverse transcriptase inhibitor agents should be discontinued, with either agents from another class of antiretroviral agents substituted or of all antiretroviral agents discontinued. In view of the reports of maternal deaths and toxicity associated with prolonged use of stavudine and didanosine in pregnancy, this combination should be used in pregnancy with caution and only if other nucleoside reverse transcriptase inhibitor agents cannot be used because of resistance or toxicity.

Concerns about mitochondrial toxicity also have been raised with regard to neonates by a French group who reported eight cases of infants uninfected with HIV who had abnormalities potentially related to mitochondrial dysfunction that developed after prophylactic nucleoside reverse transcriptase inhibitors therapy (both antenatally and neonatally) among 1,754 exposed fetuses (17). Mitochondrial abnormalities were not proved to be the cause of the abnormalities, but in response to these concerns, investigators from several large cohort studies in the United States reviewed all 353 deaths among more than 20,000 children born to women infected with HIV and found no deaths similar to those in the French cohort, although only 6% of the children had been exposed to the combination of zidovudine–lamivudine (18).

Other concerns that have been raised with regard to nucleoside reverse transcriptase inhibitors have included preterm births, mutagenesis, and febrile seizures. The reported association with prematurity emanated from a small European study (19). Larger American reviews have not confirmed this association. The concern about cancer arose on the basis of small animal models. A report from the National Cancer Institute suggested that mice exposed to high doses of zidovudine in utero had unexpectedly high rates of malignancies of the skin, lung, liver, and genital tract and that the frequency of tumors was higher in the zidovudine-exposed animals (20). Based on these findings, the National Institutes of Health convened a blue ribbon panel to review the findings. That panel concluded that even if the adverse outcomes seen in the animals did signal a risk from in utero exposure, the demonstrated benefits of the medication were such that the routine use of the PACTG 076 protocol should continue. Finally, with regard to nucleoside reverse transcriptase inhibitors, the French collaborative study reported on first febrile seizures among 4,426 children uninfected with HIV and found a significantly increased risk for those infants who had been exposed perinatally to nucleoside reverse transcriptase inhibitor therapy compared with unexposed infants ($P = .0198.$) (21).

Among the nonnucleoside reverse transcriptase inhibitors, efavirenz should not be used in the first trimester because of reported teratogenic effects in monkey models and reports of myelomeningoceles in humans (22). Nevirapine, the agent most widely used worldwide for prevention of mother-to-child transmission of HIV, should not be used in women who are relatively immune competent. A high risk of symptomatic, often rash-associated, nevirapine-related hepatotoxicity, which can be severe, life-threatening, and in some cases fatal, has been reported among women within the first 18 weeks of treatment with regimens including nevirapine at times when they were relatively immune competent (ie, CD4 counts generally greater than 250/mm^3) (23).

Among the protease inhibitors, indinavir may predispose to nephrolithiasis and hyperbilirubinemia, although evidence of harm to neonates has not been forthcoming. Protease inhibitors in general have been linked to abnormal glucose metabolism, but problems

particular to pregnancy in this regard have not been noted. Despite these concerns, pregnant women in the United States tend to receive highly active antiretroviral therapy as often as other women with similar immunologic status (24). All pregnant women taking antiretroviral therapy should have regular monitoring of liver functions and blood counts to detect toxicity as early as possible.

Prevention of Transmission of Human Immunodeficiency Virus

Background

Perinatal transmission is the most common cause of HIV infection in infants and children in the United States. It is responsible for more than 90% of pediatric AIDS cases and almost all new HIV infections in preadolescent children. In the absence of interventions, the reported frequency of mother-to-child transmission varies widely across the globe with rates ranging from 10% to 60%. That range reflects differences in patterns of breastfeeding, viral loads, and obstetric practices. Before the PACTG 076 regimen gained purchase as a standard approach in the United States, as many as 2,000 children each year were infected through birth. However, by the year 2000, only 174 pediatric AIDS cases were reported. That remarkable decrease reflects the development of interventions that were built on research detailing the timing and determinants of transmission. It is estimated that 70% of mother-to-child transmission occurs at delivery, and about 30% of transmissions occurs in utero. Approximately two of three in utero transmissions occur in the last 14 days before delivery. The possible mechanisms whereby the virus infects the fetus include microtransfusions during contractions, ascension through the cervix and vagina during parturition, or absorption of the virus through the infant's digestive tract. Studies demonstrating increased infection with increased duration of ruptured membranes (Fig. 25-3) and reduced rates with elective cesarean delivery provide supporting evidence of these phenomena (25).

Perhaps the factor that best predicts the likelihood of infection in the neonate is maternal viral load (26). Increasing geometric mean levels of plasma HIV-1 RNA are generally associated with increasing rates of perinatal transmission with the highest rate of transmission found among women whose HIV plasma level is more than 100,000 copies per mL. Conversely transmission is rare when viral loads are undetectable. The more effective a drug regimen is at reducing viral load, the greater the likelihood that it will succeed in preventing neonatal infection. However, even when analysis is limited to

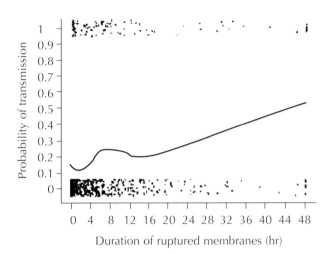

Fig. 25-3. Probability of human immunodeficiency virus type 1 transmission in relation to the duration of ruptured membranes. The dots at the top represent women who transmitted human immunodeficiency virus type 1 to their infants, and those at the bottom represent women who did not transmit human immunodeficiency virus type 1. Data on women whose membranes were ruptured for more than 48 hours are shown at the 48-hour mark. (Landesman S, Kalish L, Burns D, Minkoff H, Fox HE, Zorrilla C, et al. Obstetrical factors and the transmission of human immunodeficiency virus type 1 from mother to child. N Engl J Med 1996;334:1617–23. Copyright © 1996 Massachusetts Medical Society. All rights reserved.)

women with viral loads less than 1,000 copies per mL, those using antiretroviral therapy still have lower rates of transmission (27).

Factors other than viral load that have been linked to mother-to-child transmission include prolonged rupture of membranes, vaginal delivery, preterm birth, drug use and, perhaps most importantly from the international perspective, breastfeeding. In fact, in many parts of the world, it is estimated that breastfeeding can account for up to 50% of transmissions from mothers to children. However, randomized controlled trials of breastfeeding versus bottle-feeding in Africa have shown that the advantage of bottle-feeding in reducing neonatal deaths from AIDS is counterbalanced by increases in neonatal deaths from other illnesses, malnutrition, and dehydration (28). Interestingly, mothers in the breastfeeding arm fared less well in some of these trials (29). The probability of maternal death at 24 months after delivery was 10.5% in the breastfeeding group and 3.8% in the bottle-feeding group (*P* = .02).

Pharmaceutical Intervention

Because transmission correlates with viral load and because cesarean delivery is recommended whenever the load is greater than 1,000 copies, highly active antiretroviral therapy should be considered whenever the load

exceeds that threshold. Accordingly, most women will be appropriate candidates for highly active antiretroviral therapy during pregnancy. If highly active antiretroviral therapy is indicated, zidovudine should be incorporated into the regimen whenever possible. Although zidovudine is similar to other nucleoside reverse transcriptase inhibitors in many ways, it has the advantage of demonstrated efficacy in preventing mother-to-child transmission. The mechanism by which zidovudine achieved this effect is probably multifactorial. For example, placental passage of zidovudine is excellent, whereas other antiretroviral drugs have variable transplacental passage. That passage helps to assure inhibitory levels of the drug in the fetus during the birth process, resulting in preexposure prophylaxis. When deciding on drugs to be used in conjunction with zidovudine in a highly active antiretroviral therapy regimen, providers should be aware of the risks of individual agents.

Short-Course Therapies

Most mother-to-child transmission of HIV-1 infection occurs in the developing world. In those venues, the full PACTG 076 regimen is too costly and logistically complex to be implemented on a wide scale. Several studies have been performed that demonstrate that more abbreviated, affordable regimens may be substituted and will reduce transmission, albeit not to the level seen with a full course of therapy (30, 31). Evidence of benefit from extremely short regimens also has been reported from a retrospective review of transmission in New York State (2). When treatment was begun in the prenatal period, the rate of HIV transmission was 6.1% (95% confidence interval [CI], 4.1–8.9); when begun intrapartum, the rate was 10.0% (95% CI, 3.3–21.8); when begun within the first 48 hours of life, the rate was 9.3% (95% CI, 4.1–17.5); and when begun on day 3 of life or later, the rate was 18.4% (95% CI, 7.7–34.3). In the absence of zidovudine prophylaxis, the rate of HIV transmission was 26.6% (95% CI, 21.1–32.7). It should be noted that almost all of the successful postpartum interventions began within the first 24 hours postpartum.

Nevirapine also has been used as short-course therapy. Its extremely low price, rapid onset of action, and the rapid fall in viral load that occurs after use make it an attractive drug for peripartum use. In a Ugandan study, 626 women were randomized to receive either nevirapine, 200 mg orally at the onset of labor and 2 mg/kg to infants within 72 hours of birth, or zidovudine, 600 mg to the mother at the onset of labor and 300 mg every 3 hours until delivery and 4 mg/kg orally twice daily to infants for 7 days after birth. Almost all infants were breastfed. The estimated risks of HIV-1 transmission in the zidovudine and nevirapine groups were 10.4% and 8.2% at birth

($P = .35$), 21.3% and 11.9% by age 6–8 weeks ($P = .0027$), and 25.1% and 13.1% by age 14–16 weeks ($P = .0006$) (32). A concern about the widespread use of nevirapine for prevention of mother-to-child transmission in the developing world is that the same agent is commonly used in highly active antiretroviral therapy regimens. Thus, if resistance develops after use for prevention for mother-to-child transmission and the mother subsequently needs highly active antiretroviral therapy, its efficacy might be reduced. While resistance has in fact been reported after use for prevention of mother-to-child transmission prevention, there are some reports suggesting that resistant strains of virus are found increasingly less often as time passes after its pregnancy use.

In the United States, these short-course regimens may be particularly useful in the prevention of transmission from mothers who have not received treatment before labor because their HIV status was unknown. The public health service task force has recommended that one of the following four regimens be used during the intrapartum period if a woman infected with HIV with no prior therapy arrives in labor: 1) zidovudine in labor and 6 weeks to the neonate; 2) nevirapine, a single dose to the mother in labor and a single dose to the neonate; 3) zidovudine–lamivudine in labor and to the neonate for 1 week; and 4) both nevirapine as in regimen 2 and zidovudine as in regimen 1. If a regimen includes nevirapine, the health care provider should consider adding intrapartum ZDV/3TC and 3–7 days of ZDV/3TC postpartum to reduce nevirapine resistance.

Surgical Interventions

There had been speculation about a relationship between mode of delivery and perinatal transmission of HIV since early in the AIDS epidemic when it was recognized that most transmission occurred in the peripartum period. Data in support of that concept derived from studies comparing rates of transmission and duration of ruptured membranes (25), which, by highlighting relatively low rates of transmission in the setting of short intervals between rupture and delivery, suggested an important role for cesarean delivery.

Subsequent data from two prospective cohort studies, the French Perinatal Cohort (33) and the Swiss Neonatal HIV Study Group (34) demonstrated reduced rates of perinatal HIV-1 transmission among women who received zidovudine and underwent elective cesarean delivery. Around the time of those two reports, a meta-analysis using primary data from 15 prospective cohort studies, including more than 7,800 mother–child pairs, showed results similar to those in the previously cited studies (35). The rate of perinatal HIV-1 transmission in women undergoing elective cesarean delivery was 8.2% and 2% in those receiving no antiretrovirals and in those receiving zidovudine, respectively. Both rates were significantly decreased compared with either nonelective cesarean or vaginal delivery. Finally, in 1999, the results of a randomized trial of cesarean delivery, which had been performed in Europe, were reported (Table 25-2). The results were remarkably consistent with those that had been found by others (35).

In sum, all four of the previously cited studies indicate that, compared with other types of delivery, cesarean delivery performed before the onset of labor and before rupture of membranes (elective or scheduled cesarean delivery) significantly reduces the rate of perinatal HIV-1 transmission. On the basis of these data (35, 36), The American College of Obstetricians and Gynecol-

Table 25-2. Human Immunodeficiency Virus Type 1 Infection Status of Children According to Allocated and Actual Mode of Delivery*

	Infection Status		Odds Ratio (95% Confidence Interval)
	Negative	Positive	
Allocated mode			
Vaginal delivery	179 (89.5%)	21 (10.5%)	1*
Cesarean delivery	167 (98.2%)	3 (1.8%)	0.2 (0.1–0.6)
Actual mode			
Vaginal delivery	150 (89.8%)	17 (10.2%)	1*
Cesarean delivery	196 (96.5%)	7 (3.5%)	0.4 (0.2–0.9)
Elective	165 (97.6%)	4 (2.4%)	0.3 (0.1–0.8)
Emergency	31 (91.2%)	3 (8.8%)	1 (0.3–3.7)

*Reference category.

The European Mode of Delivery Collaboration. Elective cesarean section versus vaginal delivery in prevention of vertical HIV-1 transmission: a randomized clinical trial. Lancet 1999;353:1035–9. Copyright © 1999. Reprinted with permission from Elsevier.

ogists concluded that HIV-infected women should be offered scheduled cesarean delivery to reduce the rate of transmission beyond that which could be achieved with zidovudine alone (37). It also pointed out that data were insufficient to demonstrate a benefit for women with viral loads less than 1,000 copies per mL of plasma. They suggested that scheduled cesarean deliveries should be performed at 38 weeks of gestation, that amniocentesis should not be performed to avoid contamination of the amniotic cavity with viral antigen from maternal blood, and that prophylactic antibiotics be employed because of concerns of heightened risks of postoperative infectious morbidity.

Although not as compelling as the data just cited, there is some evidence that cesarean delivery could be beneficial even in the setting of viral loads less than 1,000 copies per mL (27). Those data come from a meta-analysis of studies that focused exclusively on women who had viral loads less than 1,000 copies per mL. In those women, antiretroviral therapy still played a major role in reducing transmission, decreasing rates from approximately 10% to approximately 1%. Cesarean delivery apparently lowered the rate from 6% to 1.5%, but there was no control in that analysis for the use of antiretroviral therapy. In the subset of women undergoing treatment, cesarean delivery lowered the transmission rate from 1.8% to 0%. In the era of highly active antiretroviral therapy, transmission rates are extremely low, independent of the mode of delivery. However, studies have not been sufficiently powered to clarify the relationship between highly active antiretroviral therapy, mode of delivery, and transmission rate (38). Women taking highly active antiretroviral therapy with HIV RNA levels above 1,000 copies per mL near delivery should be counseled regarding the potential benefits of scheduled cesarean delivery and the known risks of cesarean versus vaginal delivery. Until further data are available, elective cesarean delivery should continue to be recommended for women using highly active antiretroviral therapy with HIV RNA levels above 1,000 copies per mL near delivery. Pregnant women on antiretroviral therapy with HIV RNA levels below 1,000 copies per mL should be counseled regarding the low baseline rate of transmission, the uncertain benefits, and the known risks of elective cesarean delivery.

Although there are circumstances in which the role of cesarean delivery is clear, there are other clinical situations in which its utility is more controversial. For example, if a patient who had been scheduled for cesarean delivery experiences spontaneous rupture of membranes before delivery, the physician must balance the residual gain from shortening the period between rupture and delivery against the risks of surgery. The longer the time

since the membranes ruptured, the greater the percentage of eventual transmissions that will have occurred before a surgical procedure can be undertaken. However, if the interval has been relatively short (eg, less than 4 hours), the viral load is high (eg, more than 1,000 copies per mL), and delivery is not imminent, some advantage probably still accrues to the woman who undergoes cesarean delivery. Another difficult clinical situation involves the woman with preterm rupture of membranes remote from term. In that circumstance, the balance that must be struck is between the risks to the neonate from extreme prematurity and the risk from acquisition of HIV while the mother is undergoing expectant management. Although the former risks can be roughly quantified by reviewing institutional data related to prematurity, there are fewer empiric data on which to base estimates of the risk of acquisition of HIV in the setting of prolonged ruptured membranes and highly active antiretroviral therapy. Obviously, the closer the patient is to term, the greater the advantage to rapid delivery. At the extremes, management is simple. If the rupture occurs at 23 weeks of gestation and the viral load is undetectable, waiting would be prudent. Conversely, if the load is 100,000 copies per mL and the patient is at 36 weeks of gestation, then immediate delivery is obviously appropriate. In between those time points, the provider must consider a wealth of details, most important of which are the survival rate within their nursery at any given gestational age, the patient's viral load, and the antiretroviral regimen the patient is receiving. For example, in one report (39), if the patient had a viral load over 30,000 copies per mL and was on highly active antiretroviral therapy, the reported transmission rate was 4.8%, whereas among women with the same viral load on no therapy, it was 35%. The number of women on highly active antiretroviral therapy with that viral load was quite small (n = 21), and the manner in which prolonged rupture of membranes would affect those rates is unclear. However, those data suggest that if neonatal mortality is anticipated to be high (eg, over 50%), then an attempt at conservative management in conjunction with aggressive antiretroviral therapy might be justified.

Operative Morbidity

As with women uninfected with HIV, the key determinant of postpartum morbidity among women infected with HIV is mode of delivery, with women giving birth by cesarean delivery having higher rates of endometritis, fever, and bleeding (40). In the European Mode of Delivery Collaboration randomized trial, among pregnant women infected with HIV-1, no major complications occurred in either the cesarean or vaginal delivery group (41). However, postpartum fever occurred in two

(1.1%) of 183 women who gave birth vaginally and 15 (6.7%) of 225 women who gave birth by cesarean delivery ($P = 0.002$). Among the 497 women enrolled in the Pediatric AIDS Clinical Trials Group 185, only endometritis, wound infection, and pneumonia were increased among women who gave birth by scheduled or urgent cesarean delivery compared with vaginal delivery (42). Of note, complication rates were within the range previously reported for similar general obstetric populations. Most cesarean deliveries are now performed electively, to prevent mother-to-child transmission of HIV. In a more recent study, including a larger proportion of women undergoing scheduled cesarean delivery, fever was still increased after cesarean delivery when compared with vaginal delivery (40). Although the relative risk for postpartum complication was higher with section than for vaginal delivery, it was lower than it was for emergency cesarean delivery. Febrile morbidity was increased among women with low CD4$^+$ cell counts.

Differences between infected and uninfected women in postpartum morbidity have been reported by the European HIV in Obstetrics Group (43). Among subjects infected with HIV, minor complications (anemia, fever, wound infection, curettage, endometritis, urinary tract infection) occurred in 16.8% of women giving birth vaginally and 48.7% of those with giving birth by cesarean delivery, and major complications occurred in none of the women with vaginal delivery and 3.2% (5:158) of those with elective cesarean delivery. These frequencies were increased compared with matched women uninfected with HIV, but the relative difference between vaginal and cesarean deliveries was similar in women infected and women uninfected with HIV. The European HIV in Obstetrics Group study is one of many studies that have compared postoperative complications between women infected with HIV and similar women uninfected with HIV. Most of these studies reported an increased risk of one or more complications among the women infected with HIV. Most found increases in minor complications (eg, postoperative fever) but no difference in major complications (eg, sepsis or hemorrhage requiring transfusion). An increased risk of complications was seen among women infected with HIV with more advanced disease (34, 40). The liberal use of antibiotics in the setting of cesarean delivery and HIV infection would therefore seem reasonable.

Complication rates in most studies were within the range reported in populations of women uninfected with HIV-1 with similar risk factors and were not of sufficient frequency or severity to outweigh the potential benefit of reduced transmission among women at heightened risk of transmission. Women infected with HIV-1 should be counseled regarding the increased risks and potential benefits associated with cesarean delivery based on their HIV-1 RNA levels and current antiretroviral therapy.

Although clinicians will undoubtedly continue to confront nettlesome clinical scenarios for which only general guidelines can be offered, some recommendations, can be proffered with greater confidence.

Summary

In an editorial, Farmer noted that "Excellence without equity looms as the chief human-rights dilemma of health care in the 21st century" (44). No illness is more illustrative of that reality than HIV disease. For most of the world's health care providers, the hope of providing therapies that can temper the course of the illness remains illusory. American physicians don't confront the nightmare of therapies that are effective but out of reach, and American women are cared for in a system that should assure both excellence and access. Those blessings, however, place a unique burden on American obstetricians. They must recognize that although the institutional and fiscal barriers that bedevil health care providers in parts of the world where the pandemic rages are not insurmountable in our country, challenges remain. Human immunodeficiency virus disease is still an illness that demands the best physicians have to offer as scientists, clinicians, and human beings. Only by continuing the same level of commitment to patients that has transformed the diagnosis of HIV infection from one which engendered helpless dread to one which allows cautious hope can we look to a future in which there will be cures at home and opportunities to export our medical bounty abroad.

References

1. Institute of Medicine National Research Council. Reducing the odds: preventing perinatal transmission of HIV in the United States. Washington, DC: National Academy Press; 1999.

2. Wade N, Birkhead GS, Warren BL, Charbonneau TT, French PT, Wang L, et al. Abbreviated regimens of zidovudine prophylaxis and perinatal transmission of human immunodeficiency virus. N Engl J Med 1998;339:1409–14.

3. Bulterys M, Jamieson DJ, O'Sullivan MJ, Cohen MH, Maupin R, Nesheim S, et al. Mother-Infant Rapid Intervention At Delivery (MIRIAD) Study Group. Rapid HIV-1 testing during labor: a multicenter study. JAMA. 2004;292(2):219–23

4. Durant J, Clevenbergh P, Halfon P, Delgiudice P, Porsin S, Simonet P, et al. Drug-resistance in HIV-1 therapy: The VIRADAPT randomized control trial. Lancet 1999;353: 2195–9.

5. Watts H, Minkoff H. Managing pregnant patients. In: Dolin R, Masur H, Saag M, editors. AIDS therapy. 2nd ed. New York (NY): Churchill Livingstone; 2002.

6. Hirsch MS, Brun-Vezinet F, D'Auila RT, Hammer SM, Johnson VA, Kuritzkes DR, et al. Antiretroviral drug resistance testing in adult HIV-1 infection: Recommendations of an international AIDS Society-USA Panel. JAMA 2000;283:2417–26.

7. Welles SL, Pitt J, Colgrove R, McIntosh K, Chung PH, Colson A, et al. HIV-1 genotypic zidovudine drug resistance and the risk of maternal-infant transmission in the Women and Infants Transmission Study Group. AIDS 2000;14:263–71.

8. Johnson VA, Petropoulos CJ, Woods CR, Hazelwood JD, Parkin NT, Hamilton CD, et al. Vertical transmission of multi-drug-resistant human immunodeficiency virus type 1 (HIV-1) and continued evolution of drug resistance in an HIV-1-infected infant. J Infect Dis 2001;183:1688–93.

9. Colgrove RC, Pitt J, Chung PH, Welles SL, Japour AJ. Selective vertical transmission of HIV-1 antiretroviral resistance mutations. AIDS 1998;12:2281–8.

10. Bristol-Myers Squibb. Important drug warning. Available at: http://www.fda.gov/medwatch/safety/2001/zerit&videx_letter.htm. Retrieved March 3, 2003.

11. Gulick RM, Mellors JW, Havlir D, Eron JJ, Gonzalez C, McMahon D, et al. Treatment with indinavir, zidovudine, and lamivudine in adults with human immunodeficiency virus infection and prior antiretroviral therapy. N Engl J Med 1997;337:734–9.

12. Staszewski S, Morales-Ramirez J, Tashima KT, Rachlis A, Skiest D, Stanford J, et al. Efavirenz plus zidovudine and lamivudine, efavirenz plus indinavir, and indinavir plus zidovudine and lamivudine in the treatment of HIV-1 infection in adults. N Engl J Med 1999;341:1865–73.

13. Mallal S, Nolan D, Witt C, Masel G, Martin AM, Moore C, et al. Association between presence of HLA-B*5701, HLA-DR7, and HLA-DQ3 and hypersensitivity to HIV-1 reverse-transcriptase inhibitor abacavir. Lancet 2002;359:727–32.

14. Culnane M, Fowler M, Lee SS, McSherry G, Brady M, O'Donnell K, et al. Lack of long-term effects of in utero exposure to zidovudine among uninfected children born to HIV-infected women. Pediatric AIDS Clinical Trials Group Protocol 219/076 Teams. JAMA 1999;281:151–7.

15. Brinkman K, Ter Hofstede HJM, Burger DM, Smeitink JA, Koopmans PP. Adverse effects of reverse transcriptase inhibitors: Mitochondrial toxicity as common pathway. AIDS 1998;12:1735–44.

16. Ibday JA, Yang Z, Bennett MJ. Liver disease in pregnancy and fetal fatty acid oxidation defects. Mol Genet Metab 2000;71:182–9.

17. Blanche S, Tardieu M, Rustin P, Slama A, Barret B, Firtion G, et al. Persistent mitochondrial dysfunction and perinatal exposure to antiretroviral nucleoside analogues. Lancet 1999;354:1084–9.

18. The Perinatal Safety Review Working Group. Nucleoside exposure in the children of HIV-infected women receiving antiretroviral drugs: Absence of clear evidence for mitochondrial disease in children who died before 5 years of age in five United States cohorts. J Acquir Immune Defic Syndr 2000;25:261–8.

19. The European Collaborative Study and the Swiss Mother Child HIV Cohort Study. Combination antiretroviral therapy and duration of pregnancy. AIDS 2000;14:2913–20.

20. Olivero OA, Anderson LM, Diwan BA, Haines DC, Harbaugh SW, Moskal TJ, et al. Transplacental effects of 3′-azido-2′, 3′-dideoxythymidine (AZT): Tumorigenicity in mice and genotoxicity in mice and monkeys. J Natl Cancer Inst 1997;89:1602–8.

21. French Perinatal Cohort Study. Risk of early febrile seizures with perinatal exposure to nucleoside analogues. Lancet 2002;359:583–4.

22. Fundarao C, Genovese O, Rendeli C, Tamburrini E, Salvaggio E. Myelomeningocele in a child with intrauterine exposure to efavirenz. AIDS 2002;16:299–300.

23. Stern JO, Robinson PA, Love J, Lanes S, Imperiale MS, Mayers DL. A comprehensive hepatic safety analysis of nevirapine in different populations of HIV infected patients. J Acquir Immune Defic Syndr 2004;35(5):538–9.

24. Minkoff H, Ahdieh L, Watts HD, Greenblatt R, Schmidt J, Schneider M, et al. The relationship of pregnancy to the use of highly active antiretroviral therapy. Am J Obstet Gynecol 2001;184:1221–7.

25. Landesman S, Kalish L, Burns D, Minkoff H, Fox HE, Zorrilla C, et al. The relationship of obstetrical factors to the mother-to-child transmission of HIV-1. N Engl J Med 1996;334:1617–23.

26. Garcia PM, Kalish LA, Pitt J, Minkoff H, Quinn TC, Burchett SK, et al. Maternal levels of plasma human immunodeficiency virus type 1 RNA and the risk of perinatal transmission. N Engl J Med 1999;341:394–402.

27. Ioannidis JPA, Abrams EJ, Ammann A, Bulterys M, Goedert JJ, Gray L, et al. Perinatal transmission of human immunodeficiency virus type 1 by pregnant women with RNA virus loads 1000 copies/ml. J Infect Dis 2001;183:539–45.

28. Nduati R, John G, Mbori-Ngacha D, Richardson B, Overbaugh J, Mwatha A, et al. Effect of breastfeeding and formula feeding on transmission of HIV-1: A randomised clinical trial. JAMA 2000;238:1167–74.

29. Nduati R, Richardson BA, John G, Mbori-Ngacha D, Mwatha A, Ndinya-Achola J, et al. Effect of breastfeeding on mortality among HIV-1 infected women: A randomised trial. Lancet 2001;357:1651–5.

30. Dabis F, Msellati P, Meda N, Welffens-Ekra C, You B, Manigart O, et al. 6-month efficacy, tolerance and acceptability of a short regimen of oral zidovudine to reduce vertical transmission of HIV in breastfed children in Cote d'Ivoire and Burkina Faso: A double blind placebo controlled multicentre trial. Lancet 1999;353:786–92.

31. Wiktor SZ, Ekpini E, Karon JM, Nkengasong J, Maurice C, Severin ST, et al. Short course oral zidovudine for prevention of mother-to-child transmission of HIV-1 in Abidjan, Cote d'Ivoire: A randomized trial. Lancet 1999;353:781–5.

32. Guay LA, Musoke P, Fleming T, Bagenda D, Alen M, Nakabiito C, et al. Intrapartum and neonatal single-dose nevirapine compared with zidovudine for prevention of mother-to-child transmission of HIV-1 in Kampala, Uganda: HIVNET 012 randomised trial. Lancet 1999;354:795–802.

33. Mandelbrot L, Le Chenadec J, Berrebi A, Bongain A, Benifla JL, Delfraissy JF, et al. Perinatal HIV-1 transmission: Interaction between zidovudine prophylaxis and mode of delivery in the French Perinatal Cohort. JAMA 1998;280:55–60.

34. Kind C, Rudin C, Siegrisi CA, Wyler CA, Biedermann K, Lauper U, et al. Prevention of vertical HIV transmission: Additive protective effect of elective cesarean section and zidovudine prophylaxis. AIDS 1998;12:205–10.

35. The International Perinatal HIV Group. The mode of delivery and the risk of vertical transmission of human immunodeficiency virus type 1—a meta-analysis of 15 prospective cohort studies. N Engl J Med 1999;340:977–87.

36. The European Mode of Delivery Collaboration. Elective cesarean section versus vaginal delivery in prevention of vertical HIV-1 transmission: A randomised clinical trial. Lancet 1999;353:1035–9.

37. American College of Obstetricians and Gynecologists. Scheduled cesarean delivery and the prevention of vertical transmission of HIV infection. ACOG Committee Opinion No. 219. Washington, DC: ACOG; 1999

38. European Collaborative Study Mother-to-child transmission of HIV infection in the era of highly active antiretroviral therapy. Clin Infect Dis 2005:40(3):458–65.

39. Cooper ER, Chaurat M, Mofenson L, Hanson IC, Pitt J, Diaz C, et al. Combination antiretroviral strategies for the treatment of pregnant HIV-1-infected women and the prevention of perinatal HIV-1 transmission. J Acquir Immune Defic Syndr 2002;29:484–94.

40. Marcollet A, Goffinet F, Firtion G, et al. Differences in postpartum morbidity in women who are infected with the human immunodeficiency virus after elective cesarean delivery, emergency cesarean delivery, or vaginal delivery. Am J Obstet Gynecol 2002; 186(4):784–9

41. Elective caesarean-section versus vaginal delivery in prevention of vertical HIV-1 transmission: a randomised clinical trial. The European Mode of Delivery Collaboration. Lancet 1999;353(9158):1035–9.

42. Watts DH, Lambert JS, Stiehm ER, Bethel J, Whitehouse J, Fowler MG, Read J.Complications according to mode of delivery among human immunodeficiency virus-infected women with CD4 lymphocyte counts of less than or equal to 500/microL. Am J Obstet Gynecol 2000;183(1):100–7.

43. Fiore S, Newell ML, Thorne C. European HIV in Obstetrics Group. Higher rates of post-partum complications in HIV-infected than in uninfected women irrespective of mode of delivery. AIDS 2004;18:933–8

44. Farmer P. The major infectious diseases in the world—to treat or not to treat? N Engl J Med 2001;345:208–10.

LABOR AND DELIVERY

CHAPTER 26

Intrapartum Fetal Heart Rate Monitoring: Interpretation and Patient Management

ROGER K. FREEMAN

*B*efore the introduction of intrapartum electronic fetal heart rate (FHR) monitoring, most fetal deaths that occurred during labor were without warning. Although it was understood that fetal bradycardia detected by auscultation sometimes was associated with "fetal distress," most interventions that occurred because of fetal bradycardia resulted in the delivery of a fetus that appeared to be well oxygenated. In fact, an analysis of the collaborative project on auscultated FHR data concluded that there was "no reliable indicator of fetal distress in terms of fetal heart rate save in extreme degree" (1). Even though there were no reliable data to support a diagnosis of "fetal distress," it was commonly believed that the major cause of cerebral palsy was asphyxia occurring during the intrapartum period (2–6). Even in the mid-1970s it was believed that more than one half of the cases of mental retardation were caused by intrapartum asphyxia and that electronic FHR monitoring could potentially prevent it (7).

Early studies of electronic FHR monitoring largely compared its use with historical controls, and none of these studies were randomized. These early studies pointed to the benefit of electronic FHR monitoring relative to auscultated controls. One large analysis of these studies in the aggregate concluded that intrapartum fetal death was significantly less common in patients who were observed with electronic FHR monitoring than in those who had auscultation, which was practiced before electronic FHR monitoring (8). When the randomized controlled trials were undertaken in the 1970s and 1980s, the intrapartum fetal death rate did not differ in the auscultated control patients, but the auscultation was done with a one-on-one nurse listening every 15 minutes in the first stage of labor and every 5 minutes in the second stage of labor. Thus, it would appear that continuous electronic FHR monitoring and intensive auscultation are equivalent for the prevention of fetal death, and both are superior to the type of auscultation that was done before electronic FHR monitoring. It is probable that intensive monitoring by either electronic or auscultatory means

does decrease the intrapartum fetal death rate. A systematic MEDLINE search performed via PubMed using the search terms "electronic fetal monitoring" and "randomized controlled trial" from January 1, 1960, to August 31, 2002, disclosed no randomized controlled trials of electronic intrapartum fetal monitoring use without auscultation in the control group.

There were six randomized controlled trials comparing electronic FHR monitoring with intensive auscultation in term patients, and no difference was found with respect to perinatal mortality, Apgar scores, or neonatal intensive care unit admissions (9–14). Thus, it would appear that electronic FHR monitoring is equivalent to intensive auscultatory monitoring during labor because electronic FHR monitoring and intensive auscultatory monitoring both are better than nonintensive auscultatory monitoring in the prevention of intrapartum fetal death. It is interesting that there has been no reduction in the incidence of cerebral palsy since the introduction and nearly universal use of electronic FHR monitoring. Disappointment in the outcomes associated with electronic FHR monitoring may be related to a number of possibilities:

1. A large proportion of chronic asphyxial damage begins before labor and may not benefit from electronic FHR monitoring-prompted interventions occurring during labor.
2. Sudden acute total or near total asphyxia associated with such problems as prolapsed cord, ruptured uterus, ruptured vasa previa, sudden abruption, maternal cardiorespiratory collapse, and shoulder dystocia may not allow sufficient time for intervention before damage is done.
3. A larger proportion of surviving very low birth weight neonates undoubtedly contributes to the current pool of children with cerebral palsy.
4. The recently recognized contribution of infection producing a fetal inflammatory response may be responsible for a large percentage of patients who have abnormal electronic FHR monitoring patterns

and later develop cerebral palsy. It is unknown if there is a benefit from earlier intervention in such cases.

5. Because the amount of acute intrapartum asphyxia required to cause permanent neurologic damage is very near the amount that causes fetal death, the number of patients who develop cerebral palsy caused by acute intrapartum asphyxia proximate to birth is probably quite small.

Because of the difficulty in determining if intrapartum asphyxia causes cerebral palsy in a given case, The American College of Obstetricians and Gynecologists (ACOG) issued a technical bulletin in 1992 (15) concluding that, for perinatal asphyxia to be linked to a neurologic deficit in the child, all of the following criteria must be present: 1) profound umbilical artery metabolic or mixed acidemia (pH less than 7), 2) persistence of an Apgar score of 0–3 for longer than 5 minutes, 3) neonatal neurologic sequelae (eg, seizures, coma, hypotonia), and 4) multiorgan system dysfunction (eg, cardiovascular, gastrointestinal, hematologic, pulmonary, renal).

In 1995 the Task Force on Cerebral Palsy and Neonatal Asphyxia of the Society of Obstetricians and Gynaecologists of Canada issued a policy statement (16) in which they stated that the same criteria mentioned by ACOG must all be present, plus an umbilical artery base deficit of greater than or equal to 16 mmol/L. They stated that if all of these criteria are not present, we cannot conclude that hypoxic acidemia exists or has the potential to cause neurologic deficits during the intrapartum period.

The International Cerebral Palsy Task Force consensus statement was published in 1999 setting out a template with specific criteria required to implicate hypoxia proximate to birth as a cause of later cerebral palsy (17). In 2003, ACOG and the American Academy of Pediatrics published a joint document titled, *Neonatal Encephalopathy and Cerebral Palsy: Defining the Pathogenesis and Pathophysiology* (18). They modified the previously mentioned template and published the following criteria to define an acute intrapartum hypoxic event as sufficient to cause cerebral palsy:

1.1: Essential Criteria (must meet all four)
1. Evidence of a metabolic acidosis in fetal umbilical cord arterial blood obtained at delivery (pH less than 7 and base deficit greater than or equal to 12mmol/L)
2. Early onset of severe or moderate neonatal encephalopathy in infants born at 34 or more weeks of gestation
3. Cerebral palsy of the spastic quadriplegic or dyskinetic type

4. Exclusion of other identifiable etiologies such as trauma, coagulation disorders, infectious conditions, or genetic disorders
1.2: Criteria that collectively suggest an intrapartum timing (within close proximity to labor and delivery, eg, 0–48 hours) but are nonspecific to asphyxial insults
1. A sentinel (signal) hypoxic event occurring immediately before or during labor
2. A sudden and sustained fetal bradycardia or the absence of fetal heart rate variability in the presence of persistent, late, or variable decelerations, usually after a hypoxic sentinel event when the pattern was previously normal.
3. Apgar scores of 0–3 beyond 5 minutes
4. Onset of multisystem involvement within 72 hours of birth
5. Early imaging study showing evidence of acute nonfocal cerebral abnormality

Unfortunately, debates over causation of neurologic damage by intrapartum asphyxia usually take place in the courtroom. Nevertheless, it remains clear that approximately 10% of patients who later develop cerebral palsy have evidence of isolated intrapartum hypoxia. It also is clear that in some cases intervention may prevent or decrease the severity of cerebral palsy.

Animal studies show that patterns of late deceleration can be produced with induced fetal hypoxia. Early research showed that there is a rough correlation between metabolic acidosis and abnormal FHR patterns (19). Apgar scores have a poor correlation to abnormal FHR patterns. In fact, most fetuses with nonreassuring FHR patterns have Apgar scores of 7 or greater at 5 minutes (20). Fetal heart rate patterns are poor predictors of cerebral palsy, but patterns of late deceleration with decreased variability are seen more commonly in fetuses destined to develop cerebral palsy (21).

When FHR monitoring was first introduced, the following patterns were considered sufficient to require expeditious delivery: 1) persistent uncorrectable late deceleration, 2) persistent uncorrectable severe variable deceleration, and 3) uncorrectable prolonged deceleration. Since then, the significance of FHR variability has become more important, and there are some who say that as long as variability is present there is no need to intervene. Others say that if one waits until variability is lost it may be too late.

Numerous studies have been done to determine the reproducibility of FHR pattern interpretation between experienced physicians and, even in the same individual, at different times. The findings in these studies were disappointing in that there was poor agreement between individuals and even some inconsistency when the same individual was asked to repeat his or her readings.

It was because of the lack of agreement about pattern interpretation, as well as the high number of false-positive tracing results, that the National Institute of Child Health and Human Development decided to convene a conference on this subject. In 1997 the National Institute of Child Health and Human Development Research Planning Workshop on Fetal Monitoring (22) concluded that the following patterns are consistent with hypoxia that is predictive of current or impending fetal asphyxia so severe that the fetus is at risk for neurologic and other fetal damage or death:

1. Late decelerations with absent variability (Fig. 26-1)
2. Variable decelerations with absent variability (Fig. 26-2)
3. Sustained bradycardia with absent variability (Fig. 26-3)

They also concluded that patterns with all of the following characteristics confer a high probability of a normally oxygenated fetus (Fig. 26-4):

1. Normal baseline rate
2. Normal (moderate) FHR variability
3. Presence of FHR accelerations
4. Absence of FHR decelerations

There are FHR patterns that meet neither of the above ominous or reassuring criteria, and a consensus has not been developed for management of patients whose patterns are in between. The following problematic tracings are illustrated:

1. Late decelerations with moderate (normal) variability and accelerations (Fig. 26-5)
2. Variable decelerations with slow return or a late component (Fig. 26-6)
3. Absent variability with no decelerations associated with contractions (Fig. 26-7)
4. Fetal heart block (Fig. 26-8)
5. Fetal tachycardia without decelerations (Fig. 26-9)
6. Sinusoidal patterns (Fig. 26-10)
7. Blunted patterns (Fig. 26-11)
8. Check-mark pattern (Fig. 26-12)
9. Twins, one with absent variability and absent reactivity and one with reactive moderate (normal) variability (Fig. 26-13)

Although there is no agreement about the significance of these patterns, some of them are present in fetuses that subsequently develop neonatal encephalopathy and, later, cerebral palsy. Presently, only hypoxia is thought to be a cause of neurologic injury that may be alleviated by expeditious delivery. For this reason, a strategy that uses other means of fetal evaluation seems appropriate. Originally, fetal scalp blood sampling for pH analysis was used to assess fetuses with abnormal FHR patterns. When it was noted that the presence of accelerations, either spontaneous or evoked, can be considered evidence that the fetal pH is above 7.2, fetal scalp pH sampling fell into disfavor (23). More recently, fetal pulse oximetry has been introduced for use with these problematic FHR patterns, but its acceptance is still being evaluated (24–26). Additionally, some of the aforementioned patterns may reflect fetal central nervous system dysfunction, with or without hypoxia and acidosis; in such situations, FHR acceleration may not be present or evoked. Thus, fetal scalp blood pH sampling or fetal pulse oximetry may be helpful (Fig. 26-14).

Recently, the presence of infection has been found to be an important finding in fetuses that are destined to develop cerebral palsy. The fetal inflammatory response syndrome associated with maternal fever during labor, chorioamnionitis, and funisitis has been implicated as a cause of later cerebral palsy (27–29). It is believed that inflammatory cytokines can cause cerebral ischemia and neuronal necrosis, resulting in damage to the paraventricular area of premature fetal brains (30–34). These lesions appear as periventricular leukomalacia and intraventricular hemorrhage. The relation between chorioamnionitis and cerebral palsy in term fetuses has been demonstrated (35, 36). Cytokines also have been implicated in term fetuses (37). As knowledge of infectious causes of cerebral palsy increases, it may explain some of the reasons for the large percentage of cerebral palsy cases with unknown cause, and strategies for intervention may become evident. At this time, we do not know what FHR patterns are associated with fetal infection. In fact, it is possible that the cytokines elaborated in such cases could cause ischemia of the umbilical or uterine vessels and result in variable or late deceleration, and the fetus may become hypoxic and acidotic. There also is evidence that hypoxia and fetal inflammatory response syndrome may be additive if both are present (38). There are data to suggest that proinflammatory cytokines such as tumor necrosis factor α may be involved in a final common pathway to central nervous system damage with either hypoxia or fetal inflammatory response syndrome as the inciting cause (39). Figure 26-15 and Figure 26-16 illustrate interesting FHR patterns that were associated with later cerebral palsy in fetuses with infection.

Between completely reassuring patterns and patterns considered ominous by the National Institute of Child Health and Human Development task force, there are many FHR patterns that cannot be ignored and require another assessment by methods including fetal scalp stimulation, fetal scalp blood pH sampling, or fetal pulse oximetry. In addition, new knowledge about infection and inflammatory cytokines may point to possible explanations for cerebral palsy that were previously unappreciated and FHR patterns that are atypical. Presently, there are no strategies that have been shown to alter the outcome in cases of infection and the fetal inflammatory response syndrome.

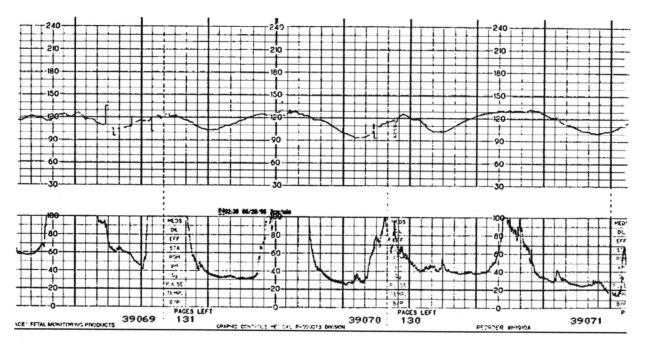

Fig. 26-1. Late deceleration with absent variability. (Modified from Freeman RK. Problems with intrapartum fetal heart rate monitoring interpretation and patient management. Obstet Gynecol 2002;100:813–26.)

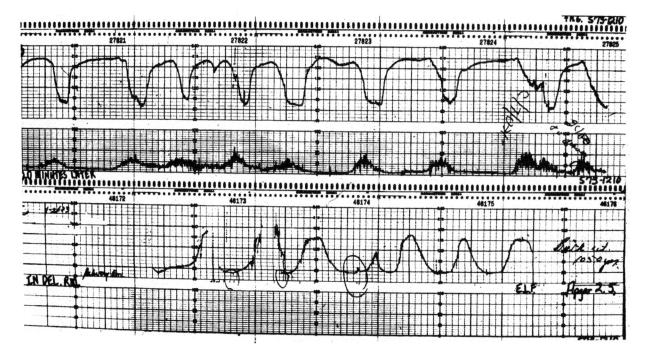

Fig. 26-2. Severe variable deceleration with absent variability. (Freeman RK. Problems with intrapartum fetal heart rate monitoring interpretation and patient management. Obstet Gynecol 2002;100:813–26.)

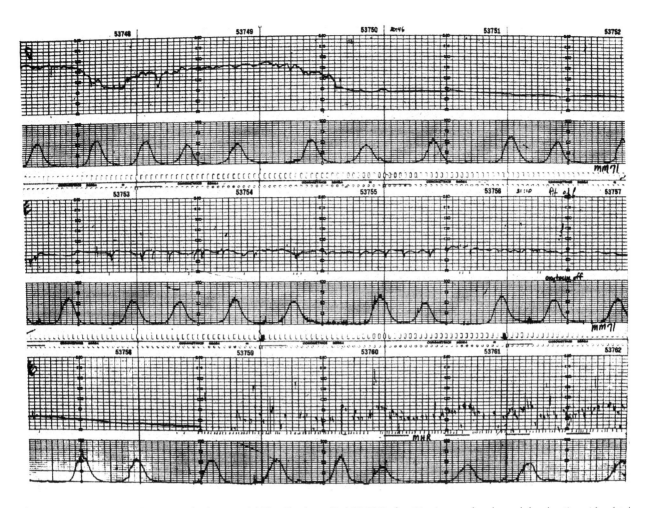

Fig. 26-3. Prolonged deceleration with absent variability. The fetus died (53759) after 18 minutes of prolonged deceleration. After fetal death occurred, the maternal heart rate was recorded from the fetal scalp electrode. (Freeman RK. Problems with intrapartum fetal heart rate monitoring interpretation and patient management. Obstet Gynecol 2002;100:813–26.)

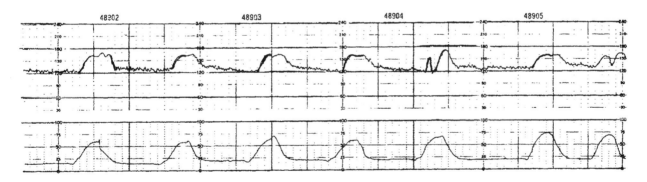

Fig. 26-4. Accelerations with uterine contractions are reassuring. (Freeman RK. Problems with intrapartum fetal heart rate monitoring interpretation and patient management. Obstet Gynecol 2002;100:813–26).

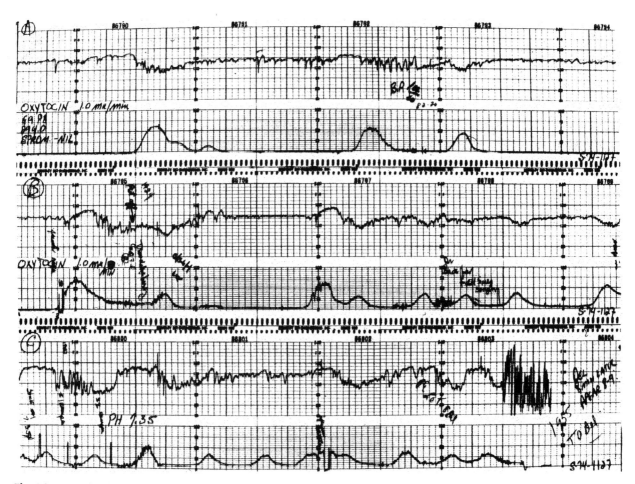

Fig. 26-5. Late decelerations with accelerations and moderate (normal) variability. Note that the fetal scalp blood pH level in the third panel is 7.35. (Freeman RK. Problems with intrapartum fetal heart rate monitoring interpretation and patient management. Obstet Gynecol 2002;100:813–26.)

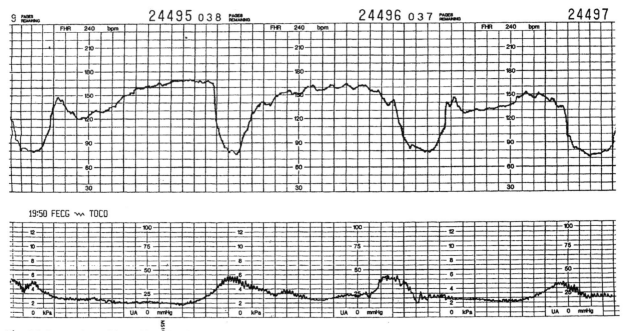

Fig. 26-6. Mixed variable and late decelerations. (Freeman RK. Problems with intrapartum fetal heart rate monitoring interpretation and patient management. Obstet Gynecol 2002;100:813–26.)

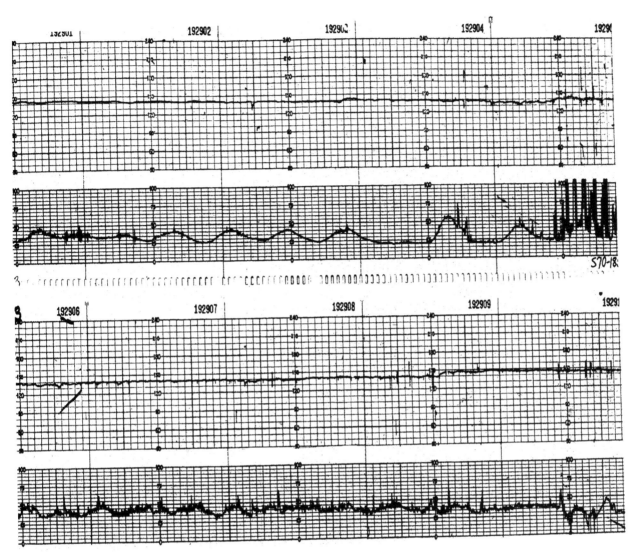

Fig. 26-7. Absent variability with no decelerations. (Freeman RK. Problems with intrapartum fetal heart rate monitoring interpretation and patient management. Obstet Gynecol 2002;100:813–26.)

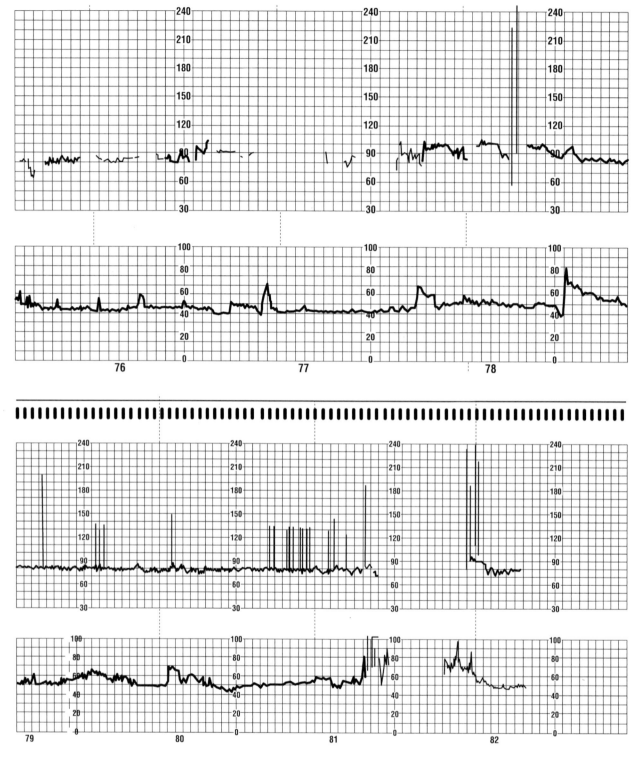

Fig. 26-8. This patient presented with no prenatal care and was noted to have a fetal heart rate of 60. Because it could not be determined if this was a prolonged deceleration, the fetus was delivered by cesarean delivery, resulting in a neonate with Apgar scores of 8 at 1 and 5 minutes. The neonatal electrocardiogram revealed a complete heart block. (Modified from Freeman RK. Problems with intrapartum fetal heart rate monitoring interpretation and patient management. Obstet Gynecol 2002;100:813–26.)

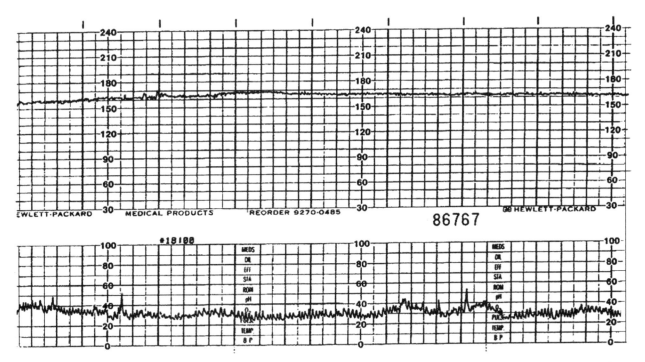

Fig. 26-9. Fetal tachycardia with absent variability. (Freeman RK. Problems with intrapartum fetal heart rate monitoring interpretation and patient management. Obstet Gynecol 2002;100:813–26.)

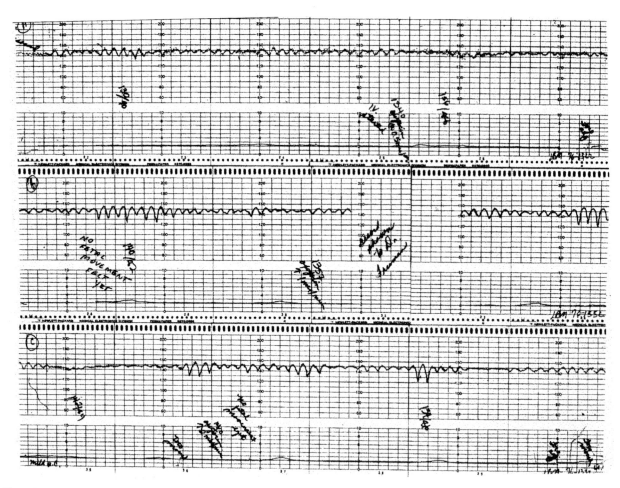

Fig. 26-10. Sinusoidal pattern in a fetus undergoing antepartum testing for maternal hypertension. The neonate had a hematocrit level of 9%. Of the maternal red blood cells, 3.5% were fetal, indicating a fetal maternal hemorrhage. The neonate had a difficult course but survived and developed normally. (Freeman RK. Problems with intrapartum fetal heart rate monitoring interpretation and patient management. Obstet Gynecol 2002;100:813–26.)

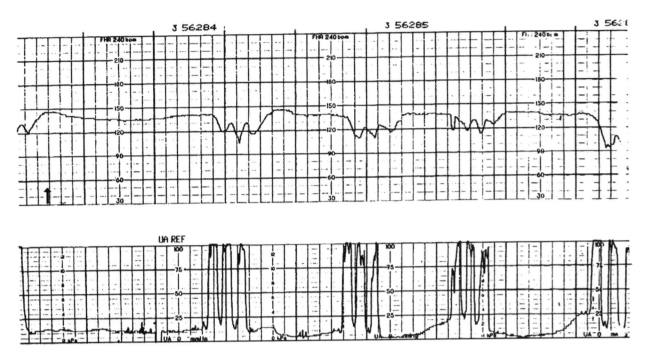

Fig. 26-11. Blunted variable decelerations with absent variability. (Modified from Freeman RK. Problems with intrapartum fetal heart rate monitoring interpretation and patient management. Obstet Gynecol 2002;100:813–26.)

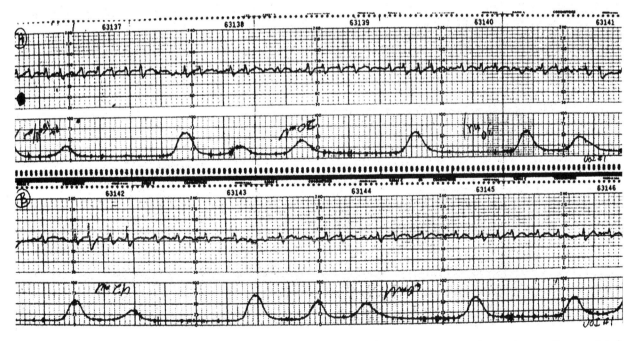

Fig. 26-12. Check-mark pattern in a fetus whose mother had undergone a cardiorespiratory arrest and was subsequently resuscitated. The newborn was born with a normal pH level but immediately began having seizures, and the child now has central nervous system damage. (Freeman RK. Problems with intrapartum fetal heart rate monitoring interpretation and patient management. Obstet Gynecol 2002;100:813–26.)

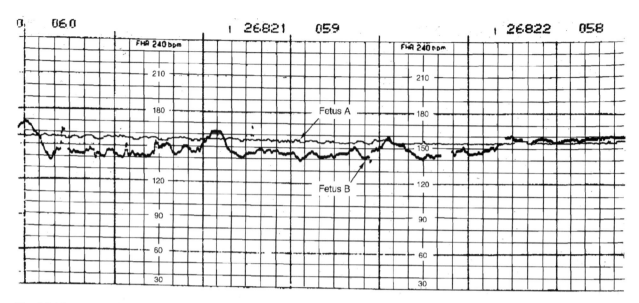

Fig. 26-13. Tracing of twins revealing an absent variability pattern in one twin (A) and a normal reactive pattern in the cotwin (B). (Freeman RK. Problems with intrapartum fetal heart rate monitoring interpretation and patient management. Obstet Gynecol 2002;100:813–26.)

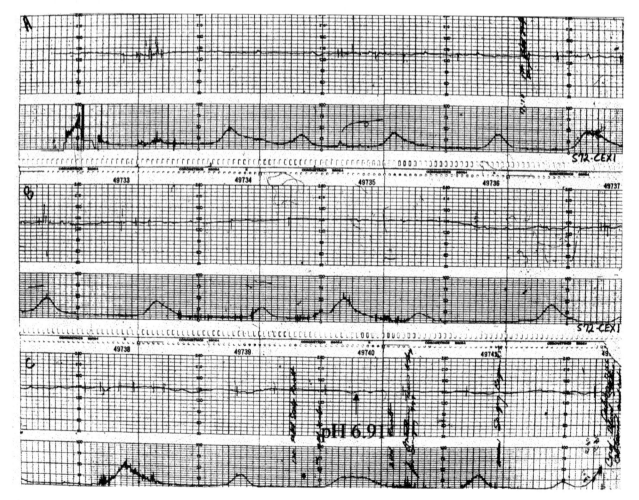

Fig. 26-14. An absent variability pattern with an unstable baseline but no periodic late or variable decelerations. Note the pH level of 6.91 in the middle of the third panel. (Freeman RK. Problems with intrapartum fetal heart rate monitoring interpretation and patient management. Obstet Gynecol 2002;100:813–26.)

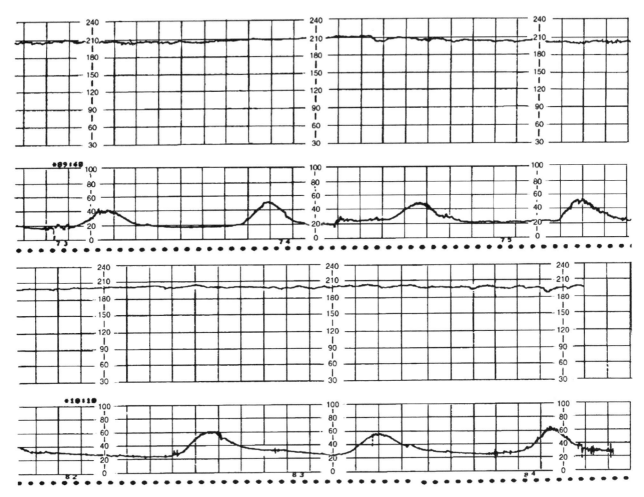

Fig. 26-15. Fetal tachycardia associated with maternal fever. The fetal scalp pH level was 7.23. This fetus had a difficult neonatal course, and the child now has central nervous system damage. There was evidence of chorioamnionitis and funisitis. (Modified from Freeman RK. Problems with intrapartum fetal heart rate monitoring interpretation and patient management. Obstet Gynecol 2002;100:813–26.)

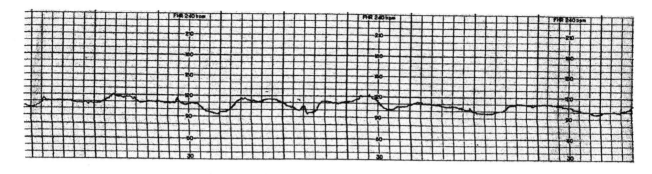

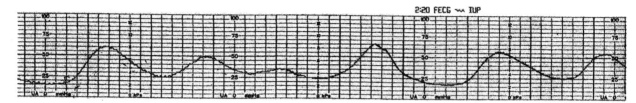

Fig. 26-16. This patient entered labor with a temperature of 38°C. The initial fetal heart rate pattern was tachycardia, but subsequently a blunted pattern developed. The cord pH level was 6.72, and the amniotic fluid culture indicated Staphylococcus aureus. The child developed spastic quadriparesis. (Freeman RK. Problems with intrapartum fetal heart rate monitoring interpretation and patient management. Obstet Gynecol 2002;100:813–26.)

References

1. Benson RC, Schubeck F, Deutschberger J, Weiss W, Berendes H. Fetal heart rate as a predictor of fetal distress: A report from the collaborative project. Obstet Gynecol 1968;32:259–66.

2. Little WJ. On the influence of abnormal parturition, difficult labours, premature birth and asphyxia neonatorum, on the mental and physical condition of the child, especially in relation to deformities. Trans Obstet Soc Lond 1862;3:293.

3. Lilienfeld AM, Pasamanick B. The association of maternal and fetal factors with the development of cerebral palsy and epilepsy. Am J Obstet Gynecol 1955;70:93.

4. Eastman NJ, DeLeon M. The etiology of cerebral palsy. Am J Obstet Gynecol 1955;69:950.

5. Eastman NJ, Kohl SG, Maisel JE, Kavaler F. The obstetrical background of 753 cases of cerebral palsy. Obstet Gynecol Surv 1962;17:459–500.

6. Steer CW, Bonney W. Obstetric factors in cerebral palsy. Am J Obstet Gynecol 1962;83:526.

7. Quilligan EJ, Paul RH. Fetal monitoring: Is it worth it? Obstet Gynecol 1975;45:96–100.

8. National Institutes of Health. Antenatal diagnosis. Report of a consensus development conference. NIH publication no. 79-1973. Bethesda (MD): National Institutes of Health; 1979.

9. Haverkamp AD, Thompson HE, McFee JG, Cetrulo C. The evaluation of continuous fetal heart rate monitoring in high risk pregnancy. Am J Obstet Gynecol 1976;125:310–20.

10. Haverkamp AD, Orleans M, Langendoerfer S, McFee J, Murphy J, Thompson HE. A controlled trial of the differential effects of intrapartum fetal monitoring. Am J Obstet Gynecol 1979;134:399–412.

11. Renou P, Chang A, Anderson I, Wood C. Controlled trial of fetal intensive care. Am J Obstet Gynecol 1976;126:470–6.

12. Kelso IM, Parsons RJ, Lawrence GE, Arora SS, Edmonds DK, Cooke ID. An assessment of continuous fetal heart rate monitoring in labor: A randomized trial. Am J Obstet Gynecol 1978;131:526–32.

13. Wood C, Renou P, Oates J, Farrell E, Beischer N, Anderson I. A controlled trial of fetal heart rate monitoring in a low-risk population. Am J Obstet Gynecol 1981;141:527–34.

14. McDonald D, Grant A, Sheridan-Pereira M, Boylan P, Chalmers I. The Dublin randomized control trial of intrapartum fetal heart rate monitoring. Am J Obstet Gynecol 1985;152:524–39.

15. American College of Obstetricians and Gynecologists. Fetal and neonatal neurologic injury. ACOG Technical Bulletin 163. Washington, DC: ACOG; 1992.

16. Policy statement of the Task Force on Cerebral Palsy and Neonatal Asphyxia of the Society of Obstetricians and Gynecologists of Canada (part I). J Soc Obstet Gynecol Can 1996;1267–79.

17. MacLennan A. A template for defining a causal relationship between acute intrapartum events and cerebral palsy—an international consensus statement. BMJ 1999;319:1054–9.

18. American Academy of Pediatrics, American College of Obstetricians and Gynecologists. Neonatal encephalopathy and cerebral palsy: defining the pathogenesis and pathophysiology. Washington, DC; 2003.

19. Kubli F, Hon E, Khazin A, Takemura H. Observations on fetal heart rate and pH in the human fetus during labor. Am J Obstet Gynecol 1969;104:1190–206.

20. Schifrin B, Dame L. Fetal heart rate prediction of Apgar score. JAMA 1972;219:1322–5.

21. Nelson KB, Dambrosia JM, Ting TY, Grether JK. Uncertain value of fetal heart rate monitoring in predicting cerebral palsy. N Engl J Med 1996;334:613–8.

22. National Institute of Child Health and Human Development Research Planning Workshop. Electronic fetal heart rate monitoring: Research guidelines for interpretation. Am J Obstet Gynecol 1997;177:1385–90.

23. Clark SL, Gimovsky ML, Miller FC. The scalp stimulation test: A clinical alternative to fetal scalp blood sampling. Am J Obstet Gynecol 1984;148:274–7.

24. Garite TJ, Dildy GA, McNamara H, Nageotte MP, Bohem FH, Dellinger EH. A multicenter controlled trial of fetal pulse oximetry in the intrapartum management of nonreassuring fetal heart rate patterns. Am J Obstet Gynecol 2000;183:1049–58.

25. East EC, Brennecke SP, King JF, Chan CF, Colditz PB: FOREMOST Study Group. The effect of intrapartum fetal pulse oximetry, in the presence of a nonreassuring fetal heart rate pattern, on operative delivery rates: a multicenter, randomized, controlled trial (the FOREMOST trial). Am J Obstet Gynecol 2006;194:606.e1–16

26. Fetal pulse oximetry. ACOG Committee Opinion No. 258. American College of Obstetricians and Gynecologists. Obstet Gynecol 2001;98:523–4.

27. Dammann O, Leviton A. Role of the fetus in perinatal infection and neonatal brain damage. Curr Opin Pediatr 2000;12:99–104.

28. Lieberman Richardson DK, Lang J, Frigoletto FD, Heffner LJ, Cohen A. Intrapartum maternal fever and neonatal outcome. Pediatrics 2000;105:8–13.

29. Impey L, Greenwood C, MacQuillan K, Reynolds M, Sheil O. Fever in labour and neonatal encephalopathy: A prospective cohort study. Br J Obstet Gynecol 2001;108:594–7.

30. Yoon BH, Jun JK, Romero R, Park KH, Gomez R, Choi JH. Amniotic fluid inflammatory cytokines (interlukin 6, interleukin 1B, and tumor necrosis factor a), neonatal white matter lesions, and cerebral palsy. Am J Obstet Gynecol 1997;177:19–26.

31. Yoon BH, Romero R, Park JS, Kim CJ, Kim SH, Choi JH, et al. Fetal exposure to an intra-amniotic inflammation and the development of cerebral palsy at the age of three years. Am J Obstet Gynecol 2000;182:675–81.

32. Naccasha N, Hinson R, Montag A, Ismail M, Bentz L, Mittendorf R. Association between funisitis and elevated interleukin-6 in cord blood. Obstet Gynecol 2001;97:220–4.

33. Dammann O, Leviton A. Maternal intrauterine infection, cytokines, and brain damage in the preterm newborn. Pediatr Res 1997;42:1–8.

34. Steinborn A, Niederhut A, Solbach C, Hildenbrand R, Sohn C, Kaufmann M. Cytokine release from placental endothelial cells, a process associated with pre-term labour in the absence of intrauterine infection. Cytokine 1999;11:66–73.

35. Grether JK, Nelson LB. Maternal infection and cerebral palsy in infants of normal birth weight. JAMA 1997;278:207–11.

36. Eschenbach DA. Amniotic fluid infection and cerebral palsy [editorial]. JAMA 1997;278:247–8.

37. Nelson KB, Dambrosia JM, Grether JK, Phillips TM. Neonatal cytokines and coagulation factors in children with cerebral palsy. Ann Neurol 1998;44:666–75.

38. Eklind S, Mallard C, Leverin AL, Gilland E, Blomgren K, Mattsby-Baltzer I, Hagberg H. Bacterial endotoxin sensitizes the immature brain to hypoxic—ischaemic injury. Eur J Neuroscience 2001;13:1101–6.

39. Dammann O and Leviton A. Brain damage in preterm newborns: biological response modification as a strategy to reduce disabilities. J Peds, 2000:136(4):433–8.

CHAPTER 27

Pathogenesis and Pathophysiology of Neonatal Encephalopathy and Cerebral Palsy

GARY D. V. HANKINS AND MICHAEL SPEER

*I*n 1862, the orthopedic surgeon William John Little advanced the hypothesis that the dominant causes of cerebral palsy were prematurity, asphyxia neonatorum, and birth trauma (1). Little was partially correct inasmuch as a cesarean delivery exposed the mother to unacceptable risks, to life or limb and medical decisions weighed heavily in favor of the mother as opposed to the fetus. Accordingly, prolonged labors and difficult vaginal extractions that now have long since been abandoned were at that time routine. Nevertheless, these proposed causes for cerebral palsy by far outlived these practices and in many circles remained unchallenged, whether by ignorance or convenience. However unintended, Little is the father of what has now become a global childbirth litigation industry (2). Payments to children with cerebral palsy are some of the largest and, in some states, are more than $40 million per case. Is it not egregious that legal fees often approach or exceed the actual dollar awards that the injured child receives? Obstetric health care providers, hospitals, and pregnant women are at crisis stage because liability insurance costs have forced many obstetric providers to withdraw these services in the United States (3–5). The crisis also is international: The British National Health Service currently is facing a medical negligence bill of $4.2 billion (6).

How then do we best proceed in the interest of both the women and children we strive to care for and our profession, which we hope to preserve? Although many potential roads may eventually lead to these destinations, the most direct approach would appear to be research and education. Additionally, these are our areas of strength and areas in which the most immediate impact can be made. They are areas in which each of us bears responsibility, especially with regard to the education of ourselves, our patients, the public, and the media.

The research journey, begun years ago, has progressed substantially over the past 25 years. In 1986, Nelson and Ellenberg observed that "despite earlier optimism that cerebral palsy was likely to disappear with the advent of improvements in obstetric and neonatal care,

there has apparently been no consistent decrease in its frequency in the past decade or two" (Fig. 27-1) (7). They concluded that the inclusion of information about the events of birth and the neonatal period accounted for a proportion of cerebral palsy only slightly higher than that accounted for when consideration was limited to characteristics identified before labor began. These observations were further strengthened 12 years later in a Western Australia case–control study (8, 9). An end point for these studies was moderate or severe newborn encephalopathy, as opposed to cerebral palsy, realizing that many such cases of neonatal encephalopathy do not result in cerebral palsy (8, 9). Similarly, it was observed that the causes of newborn encephalopathy are heterogeneous and many causal pathways start either preconceptionally or in the antepartum period (10). Looking specifically at the intrapartum period, the authors observed that there was no evidence of intrapartum hypoxia in more than 70% of cases of newborn encephalopathy and that isolated pure intrapartum hypoxia accounted for only 4% of moderate to severe newborn encephalopathy (Fig. 27-2). Additionally, intrapartum hypoxia may have been superimposed on preconception or antepartum risk factors with preexisting insult in 25% of cases. In another study, substantially similar results were reported; intrapartum asphyxia was the possible cause of brain damage in only 8% of all of the children with spastic cerebral palsy (11). In the final analysis, the incidence of neonatal encephalopathy attributed to intrapartum hypoxia, in the absence of any other preconception or antepartum abnormalities, is estimated to be approximately 1.6 per 10,000 infants (8, 9).

These facts then would seem to support the evolving concept that cerebral palsy results from the combination of the genetic makeup of the individual and the subsequent collision of that individual during development with the intrauterine and extrauterine environment to which they are exposed, for the first several days, months, or years of life. As examples, the South Australian Cerebral Palsy Research Group has recently reported that

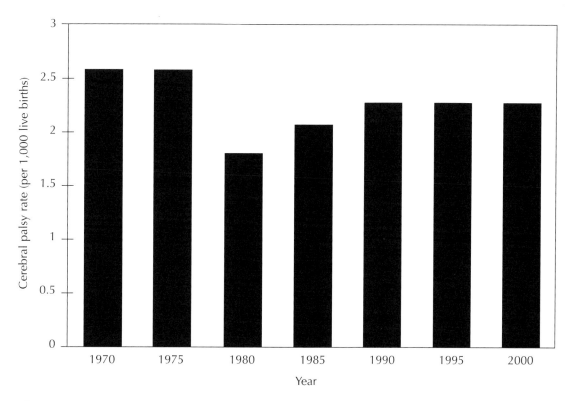

Fig. 27-1. Cerebral palsy rates per 1,000 live births, 1970–2000. (Data from Hankins GDV, Speer M. Defining the pathogenesis and pathophysiology of neonatal encephalopathy and cerebral palsy. Obstet Gynecol 2003;102: 628–36.)

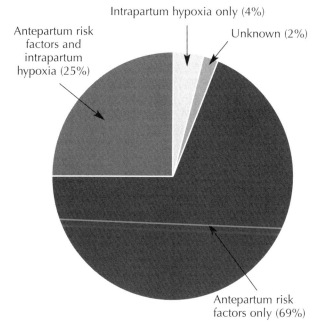

Fig. 27-2. Distribution of risk factors for newborn encephalopathy. (Badawi N, Kurinczuk JJ, Keogh JM, Alessandri LM, O'Sullivan F, Burton PR, et al. Intrapartum risk factors for newborn encephalopathy: the Western Australian case–control study. BMJ 1998;317:1554–8. Copyright © 1998. Reprinted with permission from the BMJ Publishing Group.)

inheritance of the gene mutation MTHFR C677T approximately doubles the risk of cerebral palsy in preterm infants. A combination of homozygous MTHFR C677T and heterozygous prothrombin gene mutation increased the risk of quadriplegia five fold in all gestational ages (12). This clearly is an example of genetic inheritance leading to cerebral palsy. The same report also demonstrated that perinatal exposure to the neurotropic herpes group B viruses nearly doubled the risk of cerebral palsy relative to the control group (13).

It also can be stated with certainty that the pathway from an intrapartum hypoxic–ischemic injury to subsequent cerebral palsy must progress through neonatal encephalopathy and that hypoxic–ischemic encephalopathy is a minor component of the broader diagnostic category of neonatal encephalopathy (8, 9).

Criteria

Criteria to define an acute intrapartum hypoxic event as sufficient to cause cerebral palsy, based on scientific evidence, was first proposed by The American College of Obstetricians and Gynecologists (ACOG) (14). As knowledge was advanced by research, criteria were further refined by the International Cerebral Palsy Task

Force Consensus Statement (15). Most recently, the criteria have been reviewed again and information has been updated by ACOG and the American Academy of Pediatrics Task Force on Neonatal Encephalopathy and Cerebral Palsy (16). Inherent in the review was liberal use of expert consultants and concurrent review, input, and endorsement from many professional societies and organizations, including the Centers for Disease Control and Prevention, U.S. Department of Health and Human Services, Child Neurology Society, March of Dimes Birth Defects Foundation, National Institute of Child Health and Human Development, National Institutes of Health, Royal Australian and New Zealand College of Obstetricians and Gynaecologists, Society for Maternal–Fetal Medicine, and the Society of Obstetricians and Gynaecologists of Canada. Accordingly, the latter publication is the most extensively peer-reviewed document on this subject published to date.

A description of the criteria required to define an acute intrapartum hypoxic event sufficient to cause cerebral palsy follows. This is a modification and update of the International Cerebral Palsy Task Force Consensus Statement (15). The use of these criteria will help to evaluate the probability that the pathology causing cerebral palsy occurred during labor.

Essential Criteria to Define an Acute Intrapartum Event Sufficient to Cause Cerebral Palsy (Must Meet All Four)

1. Evidence of a metabolic acidosis in fetal umbilical cord arterial blood obtained at delivery (pH level less than 7 and base deficit of at least 12 mmol/L). It has been demonstrated that a realistic pH level threshold for significant pathologic fetal acidemia (ie, a pH level associated with adverse neonatal sequelae) is less than 7 (17–20). The metabolic component (ie, base deficit and bicarbonate) is the most important variable associated with subsequent neonatal morbidity in newborns with an umbilical artery pH level less than 7 (21). A base deficit of 12 mmol/L or greater is a reasonable cutoff criterion (22).

2. Early onset of severe or moderate neonatal encephalopathy in infants born at 34 or more weeks of gestation (15, 23). Neonatal encephalopathy is a clinically defined syndrome of disturbed neurologic function in the earliest days of life in the near-term and term infant. If an intrapartum insult is severe enough to result in ischemic cerebral injury, abnormalities will be noted in the neurologic examination within 24 hours after birth. The examination is characterized by abnormalities in 1) cortical function (lethargy, stupor, coma with or without seizures), 2) brainstem function (ie, pupillary and cranial nerve abnormalities), 3) tone (hypotonia), and 4) reflexes (absent, hyporeflexia) (24, 25). Outcome is related to the maximum grade of severity (24). Thus, for infants with mild encephalopathy (stage I), outcome is invariably favorable. Moderate encephalopathy (stage II) is associated with an abnormal outcome in approximately 20–25% of cases, and severe encephalopathy (stage III) is associated with a poor outcome in all cases (25).

Many cases of severe neonatal encephalopathy are not associated with intrapartum hypoxia, and the list grows continually (8, 9, 26, 27). The associations with neonatal encephalopathy are diverse, with a representative listing in Figure 27-3.

3. Cerebral palsy of the spastic quadriplegic or dyskinetic type. Spastic quadriplegia and, less commonly, dyskinetic cerebral palsy are the only types of cerebral palsy associated with acute hypoxic intrapartum events (23, 28). Although spastic quadriplegia is the most common subtype of cerebral palsy associated with acute hypoxic intrapartum events, it is not specific to intrapartum hypoxia (28). Unilateral brain lesions are not the result of birth asphyxia; studies relating birth complications to neurologic outcome indicate that hemiparetic cerebral palsy is not a result of known intrapartum asphyxial complications (29, 30). Hemiplegic cerebral palsy, spastic diplegia, and ataxia have not been associated with acute intrapartum hypoxia (30). Any progressive neurologic disability is, by definition, not cerebral palsy and is not associated with acute hypoxic intrapartum events.

Information is increasing concerning another set of risk factors, predisposing to fetal and neonatal strokes and thereby to hemiparetic cerebral palsy or, if bilateral, to spastic quadriparetic cerebral palsy (31–33). Such perinatal strokes commonly involve the middle cerebral artery, and many are related to inherited thrombophilias (of which the most common is the factor V Leiden mutation), acquired disorders including antiphospholipid antibodies, combinations of these factors, and environmental triggers (34–36).

Thromboembolic disease of the mother can be associated with obstetric complications and may be accompanied by placental thrombosis (37). Embolization from the placenta into the fetal circulation is a probable intermediary event (38).

4. Exclusion of other identifiable etiologies, such as trauma, coagulation disorders, infectious condi-

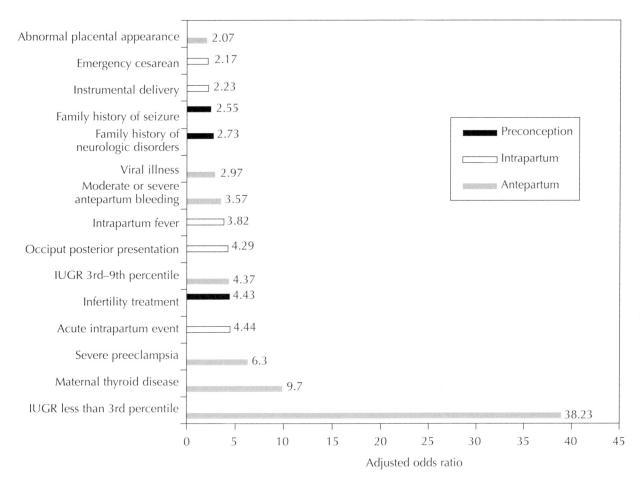

Fig. 27-3. Risk factors for newborn encephalopathy. Abbreviation: IUGR, intrauterine growth restriction. (Data from Hankins GVD, Speer M. Defining the pathogensis and pathophysiology of neonatal encephalopathy and cerebral palsy. Obstet Gynecol 2003;102:628–36.)

tions, or genetic disorders. A large proportion of cerebral palsy cases are associated with maternal and antenatal factors, such as preterm birth, fetal growth restriction, intrauterine infection, maternal or fetal coagulation disorders, multiple pregnancy, antepartum hemorrhage, breech presentation, and chromosomal or congenital abnormalities (7, 11, 30, 39, 40). These causes must be considered and excluded before concluding that intrapartum hypoxia is the cause of cerebral palsy.

Inflammations and infections as well as thromboses and coagulopathies are recognized as being associated with white matter damage and cerebral palsy. Correlates of fetal infection include elevated fetal cytokine levels in both amniotic fluid and fetal blood. Research in animals and humans has shown an association between inflammatory markers and periventricular leukomalacia and neonatal encephalopathy (41–45).

Coagulation disorders such as antithrombin III deficiency, abnormalities of protein C or protein S, pro-

thrombin genetic deficiencies, and the factor V Leiden mutation can lead to stroke (37, 46–48). Also, occlusion of either arterial supply or venous return can cause permanent focal damage. Such damage may rarely be secondary to trauma in pregnancy, especially if it occurs in conjunction with an existing coagulation disorder. Early imaging studies may be very useful in identifying and evaluating a specific cause (49–55).

Numerous genetic and metabolic disorders can present clinically as neonatal encephalopathy; however, although there are many possible genetic causes, the condition in most infants with neonatal encephalopathy does not result from an identifiable genetic cause, and diagnosis during the perinatal period is unlikely unless there is a heightened clinical suspicion based on specific findings or family history. The health care practitioner should attempt to identify such disorders by taking a family history, performing a thorough examination of the infant for dysmorphic features consistent with a genetic etiology, and ordering appropriate laboratory tests if warranted.

Criteria That Collectively Suggest an Intrapartum Timing (Within Close Proximity to Labor and Delivery) but Are Nonspecific for an Asphyxial Insult

1. A sentinel (signal) hypoxic event occurring immediately before or during labor. A serious pathologic event has to occur for a neurologically intact fetus to sustain a neurologically damaging acute insult. Examples of such sentinel events include a ruptured uterus, placental abruption, umbilical cord prolapse, amniotic fluid embolus, maternal cardiopulmonary arrest, and fetal exsanguination from either vasoprevia or massive fetomaternal hemorrhage.

2. A sudden and sustained fetal bradycardia or the absence of fetal heart rate variability in the presence of persistent, late, or variable decelerations, usually after a hypoxic sentinel event when the pattern was previously normal. The most frequently observed fetal heart rate patterns associated with cerebral palsy are those with multiple late decelerations and decreased beat-to-beat variability. However, these patterns cannot be used to predict cerebral palsy because they have a false-positive rate of 99% (56). The high frequency (up to 79%) of nonreassuring patterns found during electronic monitoring of normal pregnancies with normal fetal outcomes makes both the decision on the optimal management of the labor and the prediction of current or future neurologic status very difficult (57).

The International Cerebral Palsy Task Force endorsed the statement by the National Institute of Child Health and Human Development's Research Planning Workshop on electronic fetal heart rate monitoring, which presented recommendations for standardized definitions of fetal heart rate tracings (58).

3. Apgar scores of 0–3 beyond 5 minutes. It is well established that the 1- or 5-minute Apgar score is a poor predictor of long-term neurologic outcome in the individual patient (59). For example, 75% of children with cerebral palsy have normal Apgar scores (59).

There is good correlation between an extremely low Apgar score at 15 and 20 minutes and subsequent neurologic dysfunction. The enhanced correlation most likely reflects that those infants who are most injured and most depressed are resistant to resuscitation efforts. Additionally, in such cases in which chest compressions, mechanical ventilation, or chemical resuscitation are either required or prolonged after

birth, asphyxia may certainly superimpose additional injury. A score of less than 3 at 15 minutes was associated with a 53% mortality rate and a 36% cerebral palsy rate. When a low score persisted at 20 minutes, the mortality rate was almost 60% and more than half (57%) of survivors had cerebral palsy (59).

4. Onset of multisystem involvement within 72 hours of birth. Acute hypoxia sufficient to result in neonatal encephalopathy almost always involves multiple organs and not just the brain (60, 61). Multisystem involvement may include acute bowel injury, renal failure, hepatic injury, cardiac damage, respiratory complications, and hematologic abnormalities (61–63). Evidence of such injury should be sought in every case if an intrapartum cause is in the differential diagnosis.

With initial arterial hypoxemia, fetal cerebral vascular resistance can decrease by at least 50% to maintain cerebral blood flow with minimal impact on oxygen delivery (64, 65). The clinical manifestations of the redistribution of cardiac output during severe asphyxia reflect the involvement of multiple organs (eg, necrotizing enterocolitis, persistent pulmonary hypertension, hypoglycemia, disseminated intravascular coagulopathy, release of nucleated red blood cells, oliguria or anuria, hyponatremia, fluid retention) (60, 63, 66–71).

The timing of laboratory evaluations to help assess organ injury depends on the test. Samples for determination of brain- and myocardial-specific creatine phosphokinase levels should be obtained as soon as possible after delivery because the half-life of these products is measured in hours. However, cardiac troponin I may be detected up to 4 days after myocardial injury (72). Serum aminotransferase levels increase within 12 hours of ischemic injury and peak approximately 24 hours after the acute injury (73). Elevated conjugated bilirubin levels occur later and may not resolve for several weeks after hepatic injury (74). Acute elevations of serum ammonia are associated with severe hepatic injury (75). Although an increase in β2-microglobulin is a sensitive marker of proximal tubular injury, elevated levels may not be associated with clinical renal impairment (67). Marked renal ischemia will result in acute tubular necrosis with oliguria and azotemia with progressive elevation of serum creatinine and blood urea nitrogen over several days after the acute ischemic insult (63, 76). Elevated levels of plasma concentrations of arginine vasopressin after perinatal asphyxia also are found up to 48 hours after delivery (77).

Lymphocyte and nucleated red blood cell counts are elevated among neonates with fetal asphyxial injury. Both counts appear to be more elevated and to remain elevated longer in newborns with antepartum injury than in infants with intrapartum injury. However, the rapid normalization of lymphocyte counts in the neonate limits the clinical usefulness of these counts to the first several hours after birth (69, 70).

5. Early imaging study showing evidence of acute nonfocal cerebral abnormality. Several patterns of brain injury may result from a hypoxic–ischemic episode in the fetus and depend on the severity of cerebral hypotension, the maturity of the brain at the time of injury, and the duration of the event (51).

   Early brain edema suggests recent insult. In the term infant, evaluation with magnetic resonance imaging (MRI) and diffusion imaging show reduced motion of water within hours of the injury (54, 55). Between 24 hours and 7 days, other findings include elevated lactate levels and hyperintensity of gray matter. Later findings reveal cortical thinning and a decrease in the underlying white matter. In mild to moderate injury, the affected areas of the brain lie close to the inner table of the skull near the midline. In contrast, when the injury is more severe, the deeper brain substance is involved (77). Magnetic resonance imaging is the optimal mode of evaluation of early injury (49).

Subsequent to the publication of the International Cerebral Palsy Task Force findings, three important papers on neuroimaging have been published. The first of these publications dealt with an earlier gestation than covered by the International Cerebral Palsy Task Force, which was restricted to term and near-term infants (78). In contrast, this study was of preterm infants of 23–34 weeks of gestation. The significant findings included the fact that in this specific population, intrapartum hypoxia–ischemia as manifested by metabolic acidosis was rarely associated with white matter injury and was not different from that seen in premature neonates without injury.

Another study divided the population into two groups (79). The first group was defined as those with neonatal encephalopathy, with or without seizures, and evidence of perinatal asphyxia. This group consisted of infants with neonatal encephalopathy, defined by abnormal tone pattern, feeding difficulties, altered alertness, and at least three of the following criteria:

1. Late decelerations on fetal monitoring or meconium staining
2. Delayed onset of respiration
3. Arterial cord blood pH level less than 7.14
4. Apgar score less than 7 at 5 minutes
5. Multiorgan failure

The second group consisted of infants who had seizures within 72 hours of birth but who did not meet the criteria for neonatal encephalopathy. In the first group, brain imaging showed evidence of an acute insult without established prior injury or atrophy in 80% of infants. Magnetic resonance imaging showed evidence of established injury in only two infants (less than 1%), although tiny foci of established white matter gliosis, in addition to acute injury, were seen in 3 of 21 infants on postmortem examination. In the second group, acute focal damage was noted in 62 (69%) infants. Two (3%) infants also had evidence of antenatal injury. The authors concluded that although their results cannot exclude the possibility that antenatal or genetic factors might predispose some infants to perinatal brain injury, their data strongly suggest that events in the immediate perinatal period are most important in neonatal brain injury. A valid criticism of this study is the criteria selected for inclusion in the first group. Either late decelerations on fetal monitoring or meconium staining are notoriously poor predictors of intrapartum asphyxia. There are numerous causes of delayed onset of respirations, and many babies will be born with blood pH levels less than 7.1 and almost all will be neurologically intact. What the results of this study failed to reveal is how many of the total population would have met at least 3 of the 5 criteria that were listed for inclusion in the acute injury group.

Another study reported that the watershed pattern of injury was seen in 78 newborns (45%), the basal ganglia–thalamus pattern was seen in 44 newborns (25%), and normal MRI results were seen in 51 newborns (30%) (80). Antenatal conditions such as maternal substance use, gestational diabetes, premature ruptured membranes, preeclampsia, and intrauterine growth restriction did not differ among the injury patterns. The basal ganglia–thalamus pattern was associated with more severe neonatal signs, including more intensive resuscitation at birth, more severe encephalopathy, and more severe seizures. The basal ganglia–thalamus pattern was most closely associated with impaired motor and cognitive outcome at 30 months of age. These authors concluded that the patterns of brain injury in infants with term neonatal encephalopathy are associated with different clinical presentation and different neurodevelopmental outcomes. Further, and contrary to prior epidemiologic studies, they noted that measured prenatal factors did not predict the pattern of brain injury. As with the previously described study, the authors noted that the MRI findings in their cohort were consistent with the recent, rather than chronic brain injury in most patients and the antenatal conditions measured were remarkably similar between newborns with normal and abnormal MRI results. These observations highlighted the potential of interventions to ameliorate brain injury in the newborn. The authors felt that the dissociation of antenatal risk factors from the severity of the clinical presentations supports the hypothesis that the cause of brain injury in neonatal encephalopathy is distinct from these antenatal risk factors. They further noted that the watershed pattern had predominantly cognitive impairments at 30 months of age that were not detected at 12 months of age. The cognitive deficits in this group often occurred without functional motor deficits. They hypothesized that abnormal outcome after neonatal encephalopathy may not be limited to cerebral palsy and often requires follow-up beyond 12 months of age to be detected.

Summary

How are we to resolve the epidemiologic studies with the more recent conclusion from imaging studies? Because newborns with severe encephalopathy are more likely to be identified for research studies in the intensive care nursery and these newborns are more likely to have the basal ganglia–thalamus injury pattern, it is possible the prospective MRI studies of neonatal encephalopathy will overrepresent perinatally acquired injury as compared with population-based epidemiologic surveys. Because population-based retrospective studies identify a preponderance of antenatal risk factors and smaller prospective cohort studies identify the perinatal occurrence of brain injury, there is a pressing need to establish the mechanistic link between prenatal risk factors and the cause of brain injury. This link is critical to the prevention of acquired neonatal brain injury and may be achieved with the development and application of more accurate in utero measures of brain injury, such as fetal MRI.

Both ACOG and the American Academy of Pediatrics acknowledged that their 2003 summary would require updating as the scientific database and knowledge on the topic expanded. They also stated that only with more complete understanding of the precise origins of the pathophysiology of neonatal encephalopathy and cerebral palsy could logical hypotheses be designed and tested to reduce this occurrence. Additionally, they recommended numerous important areas of research. We would again emphasize the need for funding and studies to address this very important issue in neurodevelopment, neuroimaging, and potential improvements in outcomes for individuals worldwide.

References

1. Little WJ. On the influence of abnormal parturition, difficult labours, premature births, and asphyxia neonatorum, on the mental and physical condition of the child, especially in relation to deformities. Trans Obstet Soc Lond 1862;3:293–344.
2. Blumenthal I. Cerebral palsy—medicolegal aspects. Journal of the Royal Society of Medicine 2001;94:624–7.
3. Dyer C. NHS faces rise in negligence payments. BMJ 2001;323:11.
4. Birchard K. No-fault awards for babies with cerebral palsy in Ireland? Lancet 2000;356:664.
5. American College of Obstetricians and Gynecologists. Red Alert: Women's health care at risk: the professional liability crisis Washington, DC: ACOG; 2002.
6. Ferryman A. NHS faces medical negligence bill of £2.6bn. BMJ 2001;322:108.
7. Nelson KB, Ellenberg JH. Antecedents of cerebral palsy: multivariate analysis of risk. N Engl J Med 1986;315:81–6.
8. Badawi N, Kurinczuk JJ, Keogh JM, Alessandri LM, O'Sullivan F, Burton PR, et al. Intrapartum risk factors for newborn encephalopathy: the Western Australian case-control study. BMJ 1998;317:1554–8.
9. Badawi N, Kurinczuk JJ, Keogh JM, Alessandri LM, O'Sullivan F, Burton PR, et al. Antepartum risk factors for newborn encephalopathy: the Western Australian case-control study. BMJ 1998;317:1549–53.
10. Freeman JM. Introduction: Prenatal and perinatal factors associated with brain disorder. In: Freeman JM, editors. Prenatal and Perinatal Factors Associated With Brain Disorder. Bethesda (MD): National Institutes of Health; 1985.
11. Blair E, Stanley FJ. Intrapartum asphyxia: a rare cause of cerebral palsy. J Pediatr 1988;112:515–19.
12. Gibson CS, MacLennan AH, Hague WM, Haan EA, Priest K, Chan A, et al. Associations between inherited thrombophilias, gestational age, and cerebral palsy. Am J Obstet Gynecol 2005;193:1437.
13. Gibson CS, MacLennan AH, Goldwater PN, Haan EA, Priest K, Dekker GA, et al. Neurotropic viruses and cerebral palsy: population based case-control study. BMJ 2006;332:76–80.
14. American College of Obstetricians and Gynecologists. Fetal and Neonatal Neurologic Injury. Washington, DC: ACOG; 1992.
15. MacLennan A. A template for defining a causal relation between acute intrapartum events and cerebral palsy: international consensus statement. BMJ 1999;319:1054–9.
16. American College of Obstetricians and Gynecologists' Task Force on Neonatal Encephalopathy and Cerebral Palsy, American College of Obstetricians and Gynecologists, American Academy of Pediatrics. Neonatal Encephalopathy and Cerebral Palsy: Defining the Pathogenesis and Pathophysiology. Washington, DC: ACOG; 2003.
17. Goldaber KG, Gilstrap LC, III, Leveno KJ, Dax JS, McIntire DD. Pathologic fetal acidemia. Obstet Gynecol 1991;78:1103–7.
18. Winkler CL, Hauth JC, Tucker JM, Owen J, Bromfield CG. Neonatal complications at term as related to the degree of umbilical artery acidemia. Am J Obstet Gynecol 1991;164:637–41.
19. Gilstrap LC, III, Leveno KJ, Burris J, Williams ML, Little BB. Diagnosis of birth asphyxia on the basis of fetal pH, Apgar score, and newborn cerebral dysfunction. Am J Obstet Gynecol 1989;161:825–30.

20. Sehdev HM, Stamilio DM, Macones GA, Graham E, Morgan MA. Predictive factors for neonatal morbidity in neonates with an umbilical arterial cord pH less than 7.00. Am J Obstet Gynecol 1997;177:1030–4.

21. Andres RL, Saade G, Gilstrap LC, Wilkins I, Witlin A, Zlatnik F, et al. Association between umbilical blood gas parameters and neonatal morbidity and death in neonates with pathologic fetal acidemia. Am J Obstet Gynecol 1999; 181:867–71.

22. Low JA, Lindsay BG, Derrick EJ. Threshold of metabolic acidosis associated with newborn complications. Am J Obstet Gynecol 1997;177:1391–4.

23. Rosenbloom L. Dyskinetic cerebral palsy and birth asphyxia. Dev Med Child Neurol 1994;36:285–9.

24. Sarnat BH, Sarnat MS. Neonatal encephalopathy following fetal distress. A clinical and electroencephalographic study. Arch Neurol 1976;33:696–705.

25. Volpe JJ. Neurology of the Newborn, 4th ed. Philadelphia (PA): WB Saunders; 2001.

26. Nelson KB, Leviton A. How much of neonatal encephalopathy is due to birth asphyxia? Am J Dis Child 1991;145: 1325–31.

27. Adamson SJ, Alessandri LM, Badawi N, Burton PR, Pemberton PJ, Stanley FJ. Predictors of neonatal encephalo-pathy in full-term infants. BMJ 1995;311:598–602.

28. Stanley FJ, Blair E, Hockey A, Petterson B, Watson L. Spastic quadriplegia in Western Australia: a genetic epidemiological study. I: Case population and perinatal risk factors. Dev Med Child Neurol 1993;35:191–201.

29. Michaelis R, Rooschuz B, Dopfer R. Prenatal origin of congenital spastic hemiparesis. Early Hum Dev 1980;4: 243–55.

30. Nelson KB, Grether JK. Potentially asphyxiating conditions and spastic cerebral palsy in infants of normal birth weight. Am J Obstet Gynecol 1998;179:507–13.

31. Govaert P, Matthys E, Zecic A, Roelens F, Oostra A, Vanzielegem B. Perinatal cortical infarction within middle cerebral artery trunks. Arch Dis Child Fetal Neonatal Ed 2000;82:F59–F63.

32. Miller V. Neonatal cerebral infarction. Semin Pediatr Neurol 2000;7:278–88.

33. Sreenan C, Bhargava R, Robertson CM. Cerebral infarction in the term newborn: clinical presentation and long-term outcome. J Pediatr. 2000;137:351–5.

34. Harum KH, Hoon AH, Jr., Casella JF. Factor V Leiden: a risk factor for cerebral palsy. Dev Med Child Neurol 1999;41:781–5.

35. Chow G, Mellor D. Neonatal cerebral ischaemia with elevated maternal and infant anticardiolipin antibodies. Dev Med Child Neurol 2000;42:412–3.

36. Gunther G, Junker R, Strater R, Schobess R, Kurnik K, Heller C, et al. Symptomatic ischemic stroke in full-term neonates: role of acquired and genetic prothrombotic risk factors. Stroke 2000;31:2437–41.

37. Kraus FT, Acheen VI. Fetal thrombotic vasculopathy in the placenta: cerebral thrombi and infarcts, coagulopathies, and cerebral palsy. Hum Pathol 1999;30:759–69.

38. Thorarensen O, Ryan S, Hunter J, Younkin DP. Factor V Leiden mutation: an unrecognized cause of hemiplegic cerebral palsy, neonatal stroke, and placental thrombosis. Ann Neurol 1997;42:372–5.

39. Blair E, Stanley FJ. When can cerebral palsy be prevented? The generation of causal hypotheses by multivariate analysis of a case-control study. Paediatr Perinat Epidemiol 1993;7:272–301.

40. Grether JK, Nelson KB. Maternal infection and cerebral palsy in infants of normal birth weight. JAMA 1997;278: 207–11.

41. Kadhim H, Tabarki B, Verellen G, De Prez C, Rona AM, Sebire G. Inflammatory cytokines in the pathogenesis of periventricular leukomalacia. Neurology 2001;56:1278–84.

42. Martinez E, Figueroa R, Garry D, Visintainer P, Patel K, Verma U, et al. Elevated amniotic fluid interleukin-6 as a predictor of neonatal periventricular leukomalacia and intraventricular hemorrhage. J Matern Fetal Investig 1998;8:101–7.

43. Yoon BH, Romero R, Yang SH, Jun JK, Kim IO, Choi JH, et al. Interleukin-6 concentrations in umbilical cord plasma are elevated in neonates with white matter lesions associated with periventricular leukomalacia. Am J Obstet Gynecol 1996;174:1433–40.

44. Yoon BH, Jun JK, Romero R, Park KH, Gomez R, Choi JH, et al. Amniotic fluid inflammatory cytokines (interleukin-6, interleukin-1 beta, and tumor necrosis factor-alpha), neonatal brain white matter lesions and cerebral palsy. Am J Obstet Gynecol 1997;177:19–26.

45. Yoon BH, Romero R, Kim CJ, Koo JN, Choe G, Syn HC, et al. High expression of tumor necrosis factor-a and interleukin-6 in periventricular leukomalacia. Am J Obstet Gynecol 1997;177:406–11.

46. Kraus FT. Cerebral palsy and thrombi in placental vessels of the fetus: insights from litigation. Hum Pathol 1997;28: 246–8.

47. Nelson KB, Dambrosia JM, Grether JK, Phillips TM. Neonatal cytokines and coagulation factors in children with cerebral palsy. Ann Neurol 1998;44:665–75.

48. de Veber G, Andrew M. Cerebral sinovenous thrombosis in children. N Engl J Med 2001;345:417–23.

49. Barkovich AJ. MR and CT evaluation of profound neonatal and infantile asphyxia. AJNR Am J Neuroradiol 1992; 13:959–72.

50. Barkovich AJ, Westmark K, Partridge C, Sola A, Ferriero DM. Perinatal asphyxia: MR findings in the first 10 days. AJNR Am J Neuroradiol 1995;16:427–38.

51. Barkovich AJ. The encephalopathic neonate: choosing the proper imaging technique. AJNR Am J Neuroradiol 1997; 18:1816–20.

52. Amess PN, Penrice J, Wylezinska M, Lorek A, Twonsend J, Wyatt JS, et al. Early brain proton magnetic resonance spectroscopy and neonatal neurology related to neurodevelopmental outcome at 1 year in term infants after presumed hypoxic-ischaemic brain injury. Dev Med Child Neurol 1999;41:436–45.

53. Hanrahan JD, Cox IJ, Azzopardi D, Cowan FM, Sargentoni J, Bell JD, et al. Relation between proton magnetic resonance spectroscopy within 18 hours of birth asphyxia and neurodevelopment at 1 year of age. Dev Med Child Neurol 1999;41:76–82.

54. Cowan FM, Pennock JM, Hanrahan JD, Manji KP, Edwards AD. Early detection of cerebral infarction and

hypoxic ischemic encephalopathy in neonates using diffusion-weighted magnetic resonance imaging. Neuropediatrics 1994;25:172–5.

55. Robertson RL, Ben-Sira L, Barnes PD, Mulkern RV, Robson CD, Maier SE, et al. MR line-scan diffusion-weighted imaging of term neonates with perinatal brain ischemia. AJNR Am J Neuroradiol 1999;20:1658–70.

56. Nelson KB, Dambrosia JM, Ting TY, Grether JK. Uncertain value of electronic fetal monitoring in predicting cerebral palsy. N Engl J Med 1996;334:613–8.

57. Umstand MP, Permezel M, Pepperell RJ. Intrapartum cardiotography and the expert witness. Aust N Z J Obstet Gynaecol 1994;34:20–3.

58. National Institute of Child Health and Human Development Research Planning Workshop. Electronic fetal heart rate monitoring: Research guidelines for interpretation. Am J Obstet Gynecol 1997;177:1385–90.

59. Nelson KB, Ellenberg JH. Apgar scores as predictors of chronic neurologic disability. Pediatrics 1981;68:36–44.

60. Perlman JM, Tack ED, Martin T, Shackelford G, Amon E. Acute systemic organ injury in term infants after asphyxia. Am J Dis Child 1989;143:617–20.

61. Hankins GDV, Koen S, Gei AF, Lopez SM, Van Hook JW, Anderson GD. Neonatal organ system injury in acute birth asphyxia sufficient to result in neonatal encephalopathy. Obstet Gynecol 2002;99:688–91.

62. Willis F, Summers J, Minutillo C, Hewitt I. Indices of renal tubular function in perinatal asphyxia. Arch Dis Child Fetal Neonatal Ed 1997;77:F57–F60.

63. Martin-Ancel A, Garcia-Alix A, Gaya F, Cabanas F, Burgueros M, Quero J. Multiple organ involvement in perinatal asphyxia. J Pediatr 1995;127:786–93.

64. Ashwal S, Dale PS, Long LD. Regional cerebral blood flow: studies in the fetal lamb during hypoxia, hypercapnia, acidosis, and hypotension. Pediatr Res 1984;18:1309–16.

65. Koehler RC, Jones MD, Jr., Traystman RJ. Cerebral circulatory response to carbon monoxide and hypoxic hypoxia in the lamb. Am J Physiol 1982;243:H27–H32.

66. Beguin F, Dunnihoo DB, Quilligan EJ. Effect of carbon dioxide elevation on renal blood lflow in the fetal lamb in utero. Am J Obstet Gynecol 1974;119:630–7.

67. Cole JW, Portman RJ, Lim Y, Perlman JM, Robson AM. Urinary beta 2 microglobulin in full term newborns: evidence for proximal tubular dysfunction in term infants with meconium-stained amniotic fluid. Pediatrics 1985;76:958–64.

68. Dauber IM, Krauss AN, Symchych PS, Auld PA. Renal failure following perinatal anoxia. J Pediatr 1976;88:851–5.

69. Korst LM, Phelan JP, Ahn MO, Martin GI. Nucleated red blood cells: an update on the marker for fetal asphyxia. Am J Obstet Gynecol 1996;175:843–6.

70. Phelan JP, Ahn MO, Korst LM, Martin GI, Wang YM. Intrapartum fetal asphyxial brain injury with absent multiorgan system dysfunction. J Matern Fetal Med 1998;7:19–22.

71. Stark H, Geiger R. Renal tubular dysfunction following vascular accidents of the kidneys in the newborn period. J Pediatr 1973;83:933–40.

72. Jaffe AS, Landt Y, Parvin CA, Abendschein DR, Geltman EM, Ladenson JH. Comparative sensitivity of cardiac troponin I and lactate dehydrogenase isoenzymes for diagnosing acute myocardial infarction. Clin Chem 1996;42:1770–6.

73. Seeto RK, Fenn B, Rockey DC. Ischemic hepatitis: clinical presentation and pathogenesis. Am J Med 2000;109:109–13.

74. Hawker F. Liver dysfunction in critical illness. Anaesth Intens Care 1991;19:165–81.

75. Goldberg RN, Cabal LA, Sinatra FR, Plajstek CE, Hodgman JE. Hyperammonemia associated with perinatal asphyxia. Pediatrics 1979;64:336–41.

76. Perlman JM, Tack ED. Renal injury in the asphyxiated newborn infant: relationship to neurological outcome. J Pediatr 1988;113:875–9.

77. Speer ME, Gorman WA, Kaplan SL, Rudolph AJ. Elevation of plasma concentrations of arginine vasopressin following perinatal asphyxia. Acta Paediatr Scand 1984;73:610–4.

78. Graham E, Holcroft CJ, Rai KK, Donohue PK, Allen MC. Neonatal cerebral white matter injury in preterm infants is associated with culture positive infections and only rarely with metabolic acidosis. Am J Obstet Gynecol 2004;191:1305–10.

79. Cowan FM, Rutherford M, Groenendaal F, et al. Origin and timing of brain lesions in term infants with neonatal encephalopathy. Lancet. 2003;361:736–742.

80. Miller SP, Ramaswamy V, Michelson D, Barkovich AJ, Holshouser B, Wycliffe N, et al. Patterns of brain injury in term neonatal encephalopathy. J Pediatr 2005;146:453–60.

CHAPTER 28

Umbilical Cord Stem Cells

KENNETH J. MOISE JR

$\mathcal{T}$he concept of using umbilical cord blood as a source of stem cells for hematopoietic transplantation was first proposed by Edward Boyse in 1983 (1). Subsequent experiments in irradiated mice revealed that murine blood from near-term and neonatal mice contains adequate numbers of hematopoietic progenitor cells to effect bone marrow recovery (2). The first effort at establishing an umbilical cord blood bank was undertaken at Indiana University to harvest cells from the siblings of children needing transplants. Using one of the cord blood units from this first bank, Gluckman et al (3) performed the first related transplant with umbilical cord blood in a 6-year-old boy with Fanconi anemia in 1988 in Paris, France. This was followed 1 year later by the first related umbilical cord blood transplant in the United States (4). Kurtzberg et al (5) are credited with performing the first successful unrelated umbilical cord blood transplant in the United States in 1994.

In 1991, the New York Blood Center established the first public bank for umbilical cord blood through funding provided by the National Heart, Lung, and Blood Institute of the National Institutes of Health (NIH) (6). In 1996, the NIH awarded a multicenter grant to umbilical cord blood banks and transplant centers to study the safety and efficacy of umbilical cord blood transplants. Today, more than 6,000 hematopoietic transplants have been undertaken worldwide using umbilical cord blood for a growing list of indications (Box 28-1).

Almost 15 years after the first successful umbilical cord blood transplant, House Bill 2852 (HR 2852: Cord Blood Stem Cell Act of 2003) was passed in the United States Congress to appropriate 15 million dollars in fiscal year 2004 for the establishment of a national cord blood bank program. Although a similar bill was not passed by the Senate, the omnibus appropriations bill 2673 (HR 2673: Consolidated Appropriations) included 10 million dollars in funding in fiscal year 2004 to establish a national cord blood bank and charged the U.S. Department of Health and Human Services to contract with the Institute of Medicine (IOM) to make recommendations

on the logistics of establishing such a national program. The IOM issued its final report on April 14, 2005 (7).

Primer on Human Leukocyte Antigen Typing

A basic understanding of the human leukocyte antigen (HLA) system is paramount to an appreciation of umbilical cord blood as a source for hematopoietic transplant. The HLA antigens were first discovered in 1958. There are two classes of antigens. Class I antigens are expressed on the surface of almost all nucleated cells in the human body. They have been subclassified as HLA-A, HLA-B, and HLA-C. Class II antigens are expressed on the surface of immune cells and can be induced in some other cell types. These have been subclassified as HLA-DR, HLA-DQ, and HLA-DP. Human leukocyte antigens play a major role in the immune recognition of foreign proteins by binding short peptides and presenting them to T lymphocytes.

The six major genes encoding the HLA antigens are located in the major histocompatibility complex on chromosome 6. Alleles of these genes vary in their nucleotide sequence, resulting in different protein transcription products and subsequently the expression of different HLA antigens. Because an individual receives one chromosome from each of his or her parents, there is a one in four chance of two siblings in a particular family sharing the same HLA type. If two siblings share one common chromosome (50% chance), they are said to be haploidentical.

The HLA genes are the most polymorphic of any found in the human genome, with hundreds of alleles being identified to date at each locus (Table 28-1) (8). New alleles are being continuously discovered. Identified alleles for HLA-A, -B, and -DRB1 alone would allow for over 45 billion combinations, nine times the world's current population. There are two explanations for this. Many of these represent a null allele—a unique HLA antigen is not encoded by this nucleotide change. In addition,

---

BOX 28-1

INDICATIONS FOR CORD BLOOD TRANSPLANT*

Thalassemias
- Thalassemia intermedia (hemoglobin H disease)
- Thalassemia major (hydrops fetalis)
- Thalassemia major (Cooley's anemia)
- Thalassemia intermedia
- E-thalassemia
- E-B thalassemia

Sickle cell disorders
- Sickle cell anemia (hemoglobin SS)
- HbSC disease
- Sickle thalassemia
- Sickle B-thalassemia

Oncologic disorders
- Acute lymphoblastic leukemia
- Acute myeloid leukemia
- Chronic myeloid leukemia
- Autoimmune lymphoproliferative syndrome
- Burkitt's lymphoma
- Cytopenia related to monosomy 7
- Familial histocytosis
- Juvenile myelomonocytic leukemia
- Hemophagocytic lymphohistiocytosis
- Hodgkin's disease
- Non-Hodgkin's lymphoma
- Langerhans cell histiocytosis
- Lymphomatoid granulomatosis
- Myelodysplasia syndrome

Hematologic disorders
- Amegarakarocytic thrombocytopenia
- Autoimmune neutropenia (severe)
- Congenital dyserythropoietic anemia
- Cyclic neutropenia
- Diamond–Blackfan anemia
- Evans syndrome
- Fanconi's anemia
- Glanzmann disease
- Hypoproliferative anemia
- Juvenile dermatomyositis
- Juvenile xanthogranulomas
- Kostmann's syndrome
- Pancytopenia

- Red cell aplasia
- Refractory anemia
- Shwachman syndrome
- Severe aplastic anemia
- Systemic mastocytosis
- Severe neonatal thrombocytopenia
- Congenital sideroblastic anemia
- Thrombocytopenia–absent radius syndrome

Immune deficiencies
- Ataxia telangiectasia
- Cartilage-hair hypoplasia
- Chronic granulomatous disease
- DiGeorge syndrome
- Hypogammaglobulinemia
- IKK γ deficiency
- Immune dysregulation polyendocrinopathy
- Mucolipidosis, Type II
- Myelokathexis
- X-linked immunodeficiency
- Severe combined immunodeficiency
- Adenosine desaminase deficiency
- Wiskott–Aldrich syndrome
- X-linked agammaglobulinemia
- X-linked lymphoproliferative syndrome

Metabolic disorders
- Adrenoleukodystrophy
- Gaucher's disease (infantile)
- Metachromatic leukodystrophy
- Globoid cell leukodystrophy (Krabbe's disease)
- Günther disease
- Hermansky–Pudlak syndrome
- Hurler' syndrome
- Hurler–Scheie syndrome
- Hunter's Syndrome
- Sanfilippo's syndrome
- Maroteaux–Lamy Syndrome
- Mucolipidosis Types II, III
- Alpha mannosidosis
- Niemann–Pick disease, types A and B
- Sandhoff's disease
- Tay–Sachs disease

---

specific combinations of alleles occur together in a phenomenon known as linkage disequilibrium. This limits the number of HLA types that occur in the general population. However, HLA types vary considerably based on race and ethnicity.

Human leukocyte antigen typing can be performed through serologic methods using antisera from multiparous women (low-resolution typing). Newer DNA-based techniques have resulted in an abandoning of serology for typing. Intermediate-resolution typing will define a group of possible alleles that encode for a specific antigen; high-resolution typing uses DNA sequencing to determine the specific allele.

There is no accepted definition of a match for hematopoietic transplantation. In general, a "6-of-6" antigen match refers to compatibility at the HLA-A, -B, and -DRB1

Table 28-1. Known Human Leukocyte Antigen Alleles

Gene	Allele Number	Gene	Allele Number	Gene	Allele Number
A	451	DRB1	438	DQA1	34
B	782	DRB3	43	DQB1	71
C	238	DRB4	10	DPA1	23
DRA	3	DRB5	16	DPB1	124

Data from European Bioinformatics Institute. IMGT/HLA sequence database. Available at: http://www.ebi.ac.uk/imgt/hla/stats.html. Retrieved May 16, 2006.

loci (identical genes would be present on both chromosomes). Typically, matches at the HLA-A and -B loci are performed through intermediate DNA resolution techniques, whereas the HLA-DRB1 match is performed using high-resolution molecular methods. Although there are 12 HLA loci that could potentially affect a hematopoietic transplant, many transplant centers additionally match for the HLA-C and -DQB1 loci (potential "10-of-10" antigen match) (9).

At of the end of 2004, the National Marrow Donor Program included more than 5.6 million adult donors (10). The chance of finding an unrelated adult donor match through the National Marrow Donor Program using low-resolution typing is estimated to be 88% for whites, 80% for Hispanics, and 78% for Asians. Matches for African Americans continue to be problematic, with only 59% being available by 2003. This is secondary to this ethnic community's lack of interest in serving as donors. For a marrow or peripheral blood stem cell collection transplant using an adult donor, the median time from initiation of the formal search to transplant was between 4.2 months and 6.6 months (10). Although the median time frames can be significantly shortened in urgent situations, given the aggressive nature of the hematopoietic disorders that are treated with transplant, many patients who initiate a formal search never actually proceed to transplant. The National Marrow Donor Program also is affiliated with 17 umbilical cord blood banks and now contains an inventory in excess of 40,000 cord blood units.

Primer on Hematopoietic Stem Cell Transplantation

Since the first successful bone marrow transplant in 1968, hematopoietic progenitor cells have been used to treat a variety of leukemic disorders, hemoglobinopathies, and inborn errors of metabolism. Recipients must undergo ablative chemotherapy and sometimes total-body irradiation before transplant to destroy disease and prevent the rejection of the donor cells. Factors that play a role in the success of the transplant include the ages of the patient and the donor, the disorder being

treated, the premorbid condition of the patient, the degree of HLA mismatch, and the total number of stem cells and progenitor cells transplanted (11). Initially, stem cell activity was measured by plating the hematopoietic progenitor cells product on methyl cellulose cultures to measure the colony-forming units after 10–16 days. Because of variability in the assays between laboratories, flow cytometry is now widely used to assess markers on the surface of the hematopoietic stem cell. The CD34 antigen is typically used as a specific marker for stem cells in both bone marrow and cord blood (CD34+ cells). The assay to quantitate the number of CD34+ cells in umbilical cord blood has not been standardized. For this reason, cord blood units are primarily selected based on the measurement of the total nucleated cell count after processing. Engraftment after hematopoietic progenitor cell transplant is measured by the recovery of circulating neutrophils. Neutrophil recovery is usually defined as the time interval from the day of transplant to the first of 3 consecutive days with a circulating level of 500 neutrophils/mm^3. Platelet recovery is usually defined as a count of 20,000 platelets/mm^3 or more unsupported by transfusions for at least 7 days (12). Donor T-lymphocytes in the hematopoietic progenitor cells product can attack the tissues of the recipient in a process known as graft-versus-host disease (GVH). Acute GVH occurs within the first 100 days posttransplant and is graded from I (mild) to IV (severe). Chronic GVH is graded as limited or extensive. Grades III and IV acute GVH occur in 18–50% of HLA-matched marrow recipients from unrelated donors; chronic GVH occurs in 55–75% of these patients (13). Residual T-lymphocytes in the hematopoietic progenitor cell product also may play a beneficial role in the patient with a hematopoietic malignancy; this is known as the graft-versus-leukemic effect.

Advantages and Disadvantages of Cord Hematopoietic Progenitor Cells

The use of stem cells from cord blood has several clear advantages over bone marrow donation or collection of peripheral stem cells from a donor (Box 28-2). The establishment of a national cord blood stem cell program would allow easy access to many donors of a diverse racial and ethnic population. Cord blood units could be located on short notice through a computerized search. Because the cord blood unit is already tested and banked, it would be available in a short time interval. Recent data from the National Marrow Donor Program would indicate that the average time from initiation of a donor search to the request for the cord blood unit for transplant is less than 2 weeks. In contrast, adult donors who can be found through a computerized registry at the National Marrow Donor Program may be difficult to locate because of a change in their geographic location or because they may decline to participate. In addition, the acquisition of bone marrow from an adult donor requires hospitalization and anesthesia and may be accompanied by postoperative pain (the bone marrow is usually aspirated from the pelvic crest under epidural anesthesia). Peripheral blood stem cell units are collected by outpatient apheresis procedures, but most donors must first receive 4–5 injections of a mobilizing agent, most often filgrastim.

Studies of in vitro cultures of CD34$^+$ cells from umbilical cord blood have yielded a higher rate of proliferation than similar cells from marrow (14). In addition, these cells have a greater capacity for self-renewal and long-term growth in culture (15). The greatest limitation to the use of cord blood appears to be the total cell dose

---

Box 28-2

ADVANTAGES AND DISADVANTAGES OF CORD BLOOD

Advantages
- Limitless supply
- Available on short notice for transplant
- No donor attrition compared with bone marrow registry
- Ethnic diversity easier to achieve
- Painless collection of stem cells
- Higher proliferative capacity
- Lower rate of acute graft-versus-host disease

Disadvantages
- Unable to obtain additional "donor" cells for leukocyte infusion or second transplant
- Fewer total hematopoietic progenitor cells because of small volumes
- Slower engraftment (return of circulating neutrophil and platelet numbers)
- Large inventory product (high up-front costs; units may become "outdated" because of changes in banking standards)

(measured as either the total number of nucleated cells or the CD34$^+$ count). This is predominantly related to the volume of blood that can be obtained from a placental collection. The result is that the transplanted cell dose is approximately 10% of a marrow transplant (16). The dose of cells needed to ensure engraftment is subject to ongoing debate. The IOM report suggests that an "effective" cord blood unit is one with at least 2.5×10^7 nucleated cells per kilogram of recipient body weight (7). The lower cell dose in umbilical cord blood units was the determining factor for attempting transplants initially in children using this source of hematopoietic progenitor cells. As interest in using umbilical cord blood in adults has grown, experimental procedures, including ex vivo expansion of the cells and the use of multiple umbilical cord blood units in the same recipient, have been used. The issue of lower CD34$^+$ cell numbers in umbilical cord blood units is thought to be responsible for the longer reported interval for both neutrophil recovery and platelet recovery (signs of engraftment) that occurs after umbilical cord blood transplants compared with marrow transplants. In one recently published study in adults, neutrophil recovery occurred a median of 7 days later in umbilical cord blood transplants compared with unrelated bone marrow transplants; platelet recovery was 60 days compared with 29 days, respectively (12). However, similar rates of treatment-related mortality, treatment failure, and overall mortality were reported. Adjusted 3-year survival rates were 20% for unmatched bone marrow, compared with 26% for unmatched umbilical cord blood (12).

A clear advantage of umbilical cord blood as a source of hematopoietic progenitor cell transplant is that a partial HLA match is better tolerated by the recipient than bone marrow transplant. Several biologic differences may explain this advantage. CD8$^+$ lymphocytes, thought to be the predominant mediators of GVH, are reduced in numbers in umbilical cord blood (17). In addition, cord blood lymphocytes appear to express a more immature phenotype with a decreased ability to produce certain cytokines and an inability to generate cytotoxic effector cells (18). A recent report of outcome with hematopoietic transplantation using different donor sources included 367 recipients of HLA-matched bone marrow, 83 recipients of partially matched bone marrow, and 150 recipients of partially matched umbilical cord blood (12). Acute GVH was similar between partially matched umbilical cord blood and matched bone marrow but was less likely to occur (relative risk 0.66) when umbilical cord blood was used. Compared with partially matched marrow, umbilical cord blood did not seem to demonstrate any advantage in the rate of chronic GVH (12, 16). Because of this tolerance of HLA incompatibility, the current recommendations for a "matched" umbilical cord blood unit include two or fewer HLA disparities at the HLA-A, -B, and -DRB1 loci (a minimum of a "four-of-six" match). Thus, nearly all patients will find a four-of-six match with the current inventory, while the majority will have a five-of-six match (10).

The issue of greater tolerability of HLA-mismatch with umbilical cord blood transplants led to a theoretical concern for a reduced graft-versus-leukemic effect. However, subsequent studies have not substantiated this concern, with no detectable differences in rates of leukemia relapse when bone marrow transplants are compared with transplants using umbilical cord blood (12, 16).

Future Uses of Cord Blood

Perhaps the greatest future for cord blood lies in the possibility for its use for the regenerative treatment of disease. Although cord blood has proved to contain a high concentration of cells that can restore the hematopoietic system, the recent isolation of mesenchymal cells from cord blood has created new possibilities for tissue transplant (19). These cells have been described as fetal stem cells because they can be induced in culture to form a variety of tissues, including bone, cartilage, myocardial muscle, and neural tissue. More importantly, their acquisition from a readily available source does not involve the same controversies as embryonic stem cells from human conceptuses.

Most of the investigations to date using umbilical cord blood for regenerative therapy have been in experimental models for neurologic diseases. Neural and glial phenotype markers can be detected on donor cells that have engrafted in the brain in some studies (20). Other studies have suggested that neurotropic factors found in cord blood may play a role in the improved function that is noted in the experimental models (21). In one animal study, human umbilical cord blood was injected into mice with iatrogenically induced intracranial hemorrhage. Control animals also underwent induction of intracranial hemorrhage but were treated with saline. By day 14, limb placement testing in umbilical cord blood-treated animals resembled controls (21). Intravenous injection of human umbilical cord blood has also proved to delay the onset of neurologic symptoms and improve life expectancy in a mouse model for amyotrophic lateral sclerosis (22). Other potential neurologic diseases under investigation include spinal cord injury, Alzheimer's disease, Parkinson's disease, multiple sclerosis, and acute hypoxic brain injury. Inborn errors of metabolism that result in progressive neurologic deterioration, such as inherited leukodystrophies, Hunter's syndrome, and Hurler's syndrome have been treated successfully with umbilical cord blood transplant after myeloablative chemotherapy. In one study, 20 children with Hurler's syndrome were treated, and it was noted that neurocognitive function stabilized or improved in all 15 of the 17 surviving children who were monitored serially. In another study, the results of umbilical cord blood transplantation in 15 newborns with Krabbe's disease demonstrated normal myelination and neurological development after transplant (24).

Other injured tissues may eventually be targeted with cells generated from umbilical cord blood. These include cardiac muscle (myocardial infarction), gastrointestinal epithelium (inflammatory bowel disease), and hepatocytes (toxic liver damage). In addition, umbilical cord blood may be used as a conduit for cell-based gene therapy.

Acquisition of Cord Blood Units

The Consent Process

The report of the IOM addressed several issues related to patient consent (7). It recommended that cord blood centers establish clear policies as to who must provide consent for donation. A plan to address paternal objection to the donation of cord blood should be developed. One of their additional recommendations was that balanced information for both autologous and allogeneic donation (donation to other individuals) should be provided to the pregnant patient in the antenatal period. In one study, almost one third of participants did not realize that they had the option to discard their cord blood at delivery whereas only 50% were aware that they could place their blood in a private bank (25). Patients also should be informed that they relinquish property rights to a cord blood unit that is donated to a public bank. Sugarman et al (25) noted that half of respondents stated that the reason that they were donating to a public bank was to protect their child's future health. The IOM report also suggested that for public cord banking, the consent process should not include a promise that the cells may be available at a later date for use by the family (7).

An additional recommendation of the IOM was that the consent for the cord blood collection process should optimally be obtained before labor, preferably in the late third trimester. Although transplants using umbilical cord blood are clearly no longer investigative, at present, public banks continue to use consents that are approved through local institutional review boards (IRB). Women may present in early labor without having previously completed the consent procedure but still wanting to make a cord blood donation. In these cases, based on local IRB approval, a "miniconsent" can be signed during labor that allows a cord blood bank to collect a unit of cord blood and obtain maternal blood samples for later testing. A full consent should then be obtained in the first 24 hours after delivery. This is especially important given the infectious disease screening that will be performed. The consent process should include disclosure for units of cord blood that do not meet quality standards. Many of these cord blood units are used for quality control or may be sold or provided by cord blood banks for research purposes. The IOM also stated that patients should be assured that a secure link will be maintained between the cord blood unit and demographic data. This link is maintained for two reasons: 1) new genetic testing may become available, and 2) a cord blood unit that is later being requested for transplant may test positive for a "new disease." In these situations, the IOM suggested that banks should make a reasonable effort to locate and notify the donor or parents (7). In addition, many banks contact patients before issuing a unit of cord blood for transplant to assure the continued good health of the donor (the infant).

Cord Blood Collection

Several perinatal factors have been associated with increased nucleated cell counts in cord blood units. Higher numbers are associated with first-born infants, increased birth weight, prolonged labor, increased gestational age, and white compared with African-American race (26, 27). Smoking is associated with a decrease in nucleated cell counts, presumably through its association with lower birth weight (28). A shortened interval to cord clamping and placing the infant on the maternal abdomen are associated with enhanced cell numbers (26, 29). However, the IOM report strongly discourages any changes in routine obstetric practice to enhance the quality of a cord blood unit (7). In some reports, the mode of delivery, vaginal versus cesarean, does not seem to influence the CD34+ count, whereas other studies indicate higher counts after cesarean delivery (30, 31).

Cord blood is collected at the time of delivery by one of two techniques: either in vivo (while the placenta still remains in utero) (Fig. 28-1) or in vitro in a specialized apparatus (Fig. 28-2). For in vivo collection, the cord is wiped clean and held slightly away from the perineum to avoid contamination with maternal blood. It is then prepped with povidone iodine and alcohol, and a large bore needle is inserted into the umbilical vein. This is connected to a closed collection bag that contains an anticoagulant (usually citrate-phosphate-dextrose). Obstetric health care providers new to cord collection should undergo standardized training on proper techniques. Ongoing quality assurance should be undertaken by the umbilical cord blood bank to ensure that the profiles of collectors do not point to consistent problems such as bacterial contamination or low volume cord blood units.

In vitro collection is usually undertaken by trained collectors outside of the delivery room at a specified location, usually in the labor and delivery suite. The distal end of the umbilical cord is clamped by the obstetric health care provider and the placenta delivered intact. Traction should be avoided to prevent tearing of umbilical vessels at the cord insertion because a break in these vessels results in the need to discard the cord blood unit because of the possibility of bacterial contamination. The placenta is then inserted into a holding device and the cord cleansed and punctured in much the same fashion as during in vivo collection.

A comparison of the two techniques has indicated larger cord blood unit volumes and higher total nucleated cell counts with in vivo collection (30). This may be the result of placental collapse secondary to acute uterine involution after the delivery of the fetus. Alternatively, macroscopic clot formation may occur with the prolonged handling times necessary for in vitro collection (32). A higher incidence of cord blood units exhibiting bacterial contamination also has been reported with in vitro collection (30). From a practical sense, in vivo collection adds minimal time to the delivery process after vaginal delivery. In vivo collection at cesarean delivery increases operative time and can make placental removal more difficult once the uterus has involuted.

Screening of Donors

In the case of donation for public use, donors must undergo extensive screening for both genetic disorders and infectious diseases. This usually includes a review of the obstetric events that might affect the quality of the cord blood unit. The following criteria, established by the National Marrow Donor Program, applies to events at the time of delivery:

- Cord blood is usually not collected from pregnancies of less than 34 weeks of gestation because of the lower total nucleated cell counts associated with the smaller placental and infant size associated with earlier gestational ages.
- A positive carrier state for group B streptococcus, the presence of meconium, and prolonged rupture of membranes (in the absence of suspected maternal infection) are not considered exclusion criteria.
- Multiple gestations are usually excluded because of the possibility of cross contamination and issues with proper labeling of cord blood units at the time of delivery.
- Other exclusion criteria include suspected chorioamnionitis, a malodorous placenta, suspi-

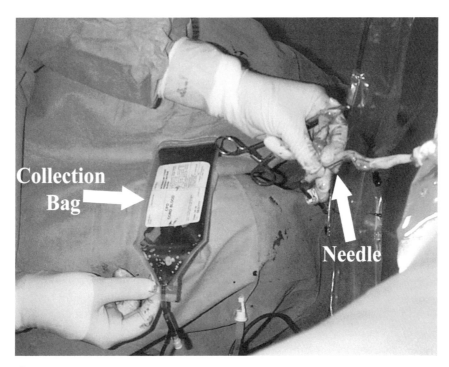

Fig. 28-1. In vivo collection of cord blood. (Moise KJ. Umbilical cord stem cells. Obstet Gynecol 2005;106:1393–407.)

cion of or active genital herpes, extensive vaginal or perineal condylomata, or a tear of the placental plate vessels because of excessive traction. These factors may increase the likelihood for infection in the cord blood unit.

• Any chromosomal or major phenotypic structural abnormality of the neonate excludes an umbilical cord blood unit. All neonates should undergo a physical examination to detect more subtle anomalies that have been associated with congenital hematologic disorders.

Follow-up of the infant (the donor in umbilical cord blood collection) should be undertaken in the first few years of life. Some umbilical cord blood banks contact the parents by telephone or mail a questionnaire at a prescribed interval after birth. In one survey of umbilical cord blood donors, only one fourth of respondents stated that they knew how to contact the bank if their infant became seriously ill (25). Serious illnesses that occurred in mother–infant pairs were only reported to the bank in 2 of 7 cases in this study. Many banks routinely contact parents at the time a cord blood unit is being issued for transplant to assure that the donor child has not developed a disease such as leukemia or a metabolic storage disease that could be transmitted through cord stem cells.

At the time of umbilical cord blood donation, a thorough family history is reviewed for hematologic and

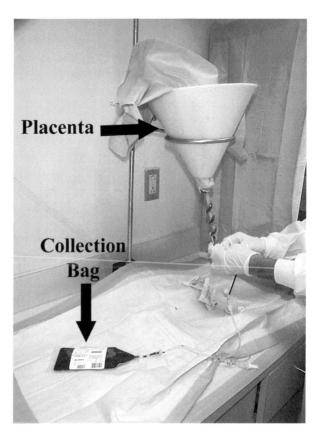

Fig. 28-2. In vitro collection of cord blood. (Moise KJ. Umbilical cord stem cells. Obstet Gynecol 2005;106:1393–407.)

immune abnormalities as well as various malignancies. Testing of the infant donor or the cord blood to exclude the presence of a homozygous hemoglobinopathy is required. Infectious disease screening is undertaken on the infant's mother. A thorough history is reviewed to exclude overseas travel to specific countries, exposure to live viral vaccines, use of illicit drugs, or high-risk sexual behavior. Infectious serologies for viral and bacterial disease, as required by the U.S. Food and Drug Administration (FDA) for any cord blood donation, are drawn at the time of admission to the labor and delivery suite or in the immediate postpartum period. These include testing for hepatitis B and hepatitis C, human immunodeficiency virus (HIV) 1 and 2, human T-lymphotropic virus 1 and 2, West Nile virus, and syphilis.

Processing of Blood

Cord blood can be stored at room temperature for up to 48 hours with minimal effects on cell viability (33). Samples from the cord blood unit are sent for bacterial culture, red blood cell type testing, preliminary HLA testing, and cell counts. The cord blood unit is processed by first adding a hetastarch solution to facilitate separation of the red cells from the mononuclear white cells at the time of centrifugation. The plasma is extracted to result in a final volume of approximately 20 mL. Generally the cord blood unit is mixed with a final concentration of 10% dimethyl sulfoxide, cryopreserved by controlled-rate freezing, and then stored in liquid nitrogen at −196°C. Approximately 20% of the hematopoietic progenitor cells are lost through the thawing process (11). Multiple segments are attached to the specialized storage bag to allow for confirmatory HLA testing without subjecting the cord blood unit to prolonged periods of thawing in case it might later be requested by a transplant center.

Regulations

The cord blood banking industry has been surprisingly unregulated since its inception. In January of 2005, Bone Marrow Donors Worldwide reported the U.S. inventory of public cord blood banks from unrelated donors to be in excess of 87,000 cord blood units. However, almost half of these cord blood units probably do not meet criteria for a usable cord blood unit based on cell count and other collection issues (7). The quality of 268 umbilical cord blood units received at a transplant center between the years 1994 and 2004 from cord blood banks in the United States and Europe was reviewed (34). Fifty-four percent of the cord blood units were determined to have quality control issues, including 21 cord blood units with incomplete or positive test results for transmissible

infectious diseases and four cord blood units with bacterial contamination. Ten percent of the quality control issues were felt likely to affect the overall quality of the cord blood unit. An additional 40% of the cord blood units had problems with documentation of medical history (4% thought to affect cord blood unit quality), and 6% of cord blood units had problems with labeling and documentation (4% thought to affect cord blood unit quality).

Although active in the regulation of donated adult blood products in the United States, the FDA has only recently become involved in the regulation of cord blood banking. The reasons for this are unclear. Many banks have undergone voluntary accreditation through the American Association of Blood Banks or the NetCord-Foundation for the Accreditation of Cellular Therapy. Both organizations have developed specific guidelines for cord blood banking, and both conduct site inspections of the collection facilities. The National Marrow Donor Program has also established standards for cord blood bank participation in its network, providing annual assessments and biannual audits of member banks. In 1997, the FDA proposed regulations for cellular and tissue-based products that included the cord blood banking industry. In January 2004, all facilities collecting cells for hematopoietic transplant were required to register with the FDA. This regulation included private banks. Finally, on May 25, 2005, FDA regulations (21 CFR 1271) for cord blood banking were passed. Although routine inspections are not planned at this time because of a lack of resources, under these new regulations, cord blood banks must notify the FDA of specific adverse reactions in the stem cells they process and allow for FDA inspections. Private banks that involve the collection of autologous cord blood units or cord blood units to be used by a primary family member are currently exempt from the new FDA regulations. The IOM report contained several definitive proposals regarding quality assurance and accreditation of cord blood banks that would participate in a national cord blood program (7). Specifically, the Health Resources and Services Administration should identify and contract with one of the existing organizations that accredit banks to establish uniform standards for collection and quality assurance. Such standards would apply to both public and private banks that participate in the program. It also recommended that the FDA establish a system of licensure of cord blood units intended for clinical transplantation.

Types of Cord Blood Banks

There are three types of cord blood banks: public banks, private banks, and directed-donation banks. Public banks involve allogeneic donation. At the time this chapter was written, there were a total of 30 public cord blood banks operating in the United States (Table 28-2) (Table 28-3) (35, 36). In these situations, blood is collected from the general public in a manner analogous to whole blood donation. The stem cells are then stored in a central facility for public use. These cord blood units must meet rigorous standards for infectious disease testing identical to the blood donor pool for adult blood. Initial HLA testing, red cell blood type, and cell counts are performed. Cord blood units that do not meet certain criteria for cell count or volume are not included in the active inventory. Funding for the establishment of a public cord blood bank is problematic. Initial processing costs typically exceed $1,000 per cord blood unit stored. Most current public banks were initiated with research funding from the NIH or funding from local foundations. Recently, the National Marrow Donor Program has subsidized cord blood banks in its member network. Public banks are allowed to recover some of their costs by charging insur-

ance carriers for cord blood units used for transplant. Fees usually are between $15,000 and $35,000 per cord blood unit (average $25,000). An economic model for the initiation of a public cord blood bank has been developed (37). The establishment of an inventory of 10,000 cord blood units was proposed during the first 3 years. In years 4–7, only 3% of the inventory would be released for transplant, necessitating a charge per cord blood unit of approximately $12,000 to make the venture cost neutral.

Private banks were initially conceived for autologous use by a child who develops a disease later in its life. More recently, private banks have promoted their use for allogeneic donation for siblings or parents. Some private banks offer directed donation at no charge to the patient if there is a sibling or parent with a known disease that can be treated with umbilical cord blood (38). Today, there are more than 24 private banks established in the United States (Table 28-4) (39). In general, cord blood units for private banks are collected on site by an obstetric health care provider and shipped to a central process-

Table 28-2. U.S. Public Cord Banks (National Bone Marrow Donor Program)*

Bank	Location	Web Site
Ashley Ross Cord Blood Bank Program of San Diego Blood Bank	San Diego, California	http://www.sandiegobloodbank.org
Bonfils Cord Blood Services Belle Bonfils Memorial Blood Center	Denver, Colorado	http://www.bonfils.org
COBLT Cord Blood Units Carolinas Cord Blood Bank	Durham, North Carolina	http://cancer.duke.edu/pmbt/ccbb
Carolinas Cord Blood Bank	Durham, North Carolina	http://cancer.duke.edu/pmbt/ccbb
Children's Hospital of Orange County Cord Blood Bank	Orange, California	http://www.choc.org/clincs/blooddonorsvs.cfm
Cryobanks International, Inc.	Altamonte Springs, Florida	http://cryo-intl.com
ItxM Cord Blood Services	Glenview, Illinois	http://www.givcord.org
J.P. McCarthy Cord Stem Cell Bank	Detroit, Michigan	http://www.karmanos.org/cordblood/
LifeCord	Gainesville, Florida	http://www.lifesouth.org/lifecord.html
M.D. Anderson Cord Blood Bank	Houston, Texas	http://www2.mdanderson.org/app/cbb/
New Jersey Cord Blood Bank at the Coriell Institute for Medical Research	Camden, New Jersey	http://www.coriell.org/njcbb
Pudget Sound Blood Center	Seattle, Washington	http://www.psbc.org/cordblood/
Sheba Cord Blood Bank	Tel-Hashomer, Israel	http://eng.sheba.co.il/cbb
St. Louis Cord Blood Bank	St. Louis, Missouri	http://www.slcbb.org
StemCyte International Cord Blood Center	Arcadia, California	http://www.stemcyte.com/
StemCyte Taiwan National Cord Blood Center	LinKou, Taiwan	http://www.stemcyte.com
The Ellie Katz Umbilical Cord Blood Program	Paramus, New Jersey	http://www/communitybloodservices.org

*All National Marrow Donor Program banks collect at specific hospitals in their state/region.
Data from the National Bone Marrow Donor Program. Network Cord Blood Banks. Available at: http://www.marrow.org/cgi-bin/NETWORK/nmdp_cord_blood_banks.pl. Retrieved May 18, 2006.

Table 28-3. Other U.S. Public Cord Blood Banks

Bank	Location	Web Site	Collection Strategy
CORDUS	Lake Mary Florida,	www.cordus.com	Collects only in medical centers where they have trained the staff
CureSource	Charleston, South Carolina	www.curesource.net	Collects only at the University of SC Medical Center (research only)
Family Cord Blood Services*	Los Angeles, California	www.familycordbloodservices.com	Collects from anywhere; additional charge for donation
Gift of Life	Amherst, New York	www.giftoflife.org	Collects from select hospitals in Brooklyn, New York
Ireland Cancer Center at Case Western Reserve University and University Hospitals of Cleveland Umbilical Cord Blood Program	Cleveland, Ohio	http://www.irelandcancercenter.org	Collections only accepted from University Hospitals of Cleveland
Kehila Cord	Brooklyn, New York	No web site available	Collects for the Chasidic Jewish community of Brooklyn, New York
LifeBank USA*	Cedar Knolls, New Jersey	www.lifesouth.org/lifecord/lifecord.htm	Accepts donations from anywhere
Michigan Community Blood Centers Cord Blood Bank	Grand Rapids, Michigan	www.miblood.org/giving_blood/cordblood.html	Collections only at 15 specific hospitals in the state of Michigan
The New York Blood Center National Cord Blood Program	New York, New York	www.nationalcordbloodprogram.org/	Collection sites at five hospitals in New York, Virginia and Ohio
SaneronCCEL	Tampa, Florida	www.saneron-ccel.com	Collects for research only
South Texas Blood and Tissue Center	San Antonio, Texas	http://www.bloodntissue.org/texascordbloodbank.asp	Collections only accepted from San Antonio hospitals
University of Colorado Cord Blood Bank	Aurora, Colorado	www.coloradocord.org	Collects only at Pouder Valley Hospital in Fort Collins
University of Iowa	Iowa City, Iowa	www.uihealthcare.com/depts/cordblood/update.html	Collects only from University of Iowa Hospitals for research purposes only

*Non-National Bone Marrow Donor Program cord banks that accept donations from anywhere.

Data from Parent's Guide to Cord Blood Banks. Available at http://www.parentsguidecordblood.com/content/usa/banklists/listusa.shtml?navid=11. Retrieved on May 17, 2006.

ing laboratory. Because these cord blood units are being collected primarily for autologous use, most banks limit their testing for maternal infectious diseases. Initial HLA typing is not undertaken. Families are charged an initial fee ($1,100–$1,750) followed by a yearly fee for continued storage ($115–$125) (40). If a cord blood unit should later be needed, processing and shipment fees are billed to the health care insurance carrier.

A directed-donation public bank is one in which cord blood is collected at no charge to the patient in situations where a sibling is affected with a disorder in which a cord blood transplant may prove beneficial (Box 28-1). The Children's Hospital Oakland Research Institute is currently the only federally funded bank of this type.

The Public Versus Private Bank Controversy

The banking of umbilical cord blood for private use or public use is mired in emotion with very few facts. Private companies, particularly in the United States, have used direct patient advertising for recruitment, often using a promise of "biologic insurance" for the newborn. One company even offers a college savings plan as part of their package for storing cord stem cells (41). Important issues of future use, quality control, long-term availability, availability to those in need, and costs argue for public banking as a more practical approach to the use of umbilical cord blood.

In a committee opinion on this issue, the American College of Obstetricians and Gynecologists (ACOG) states

Table 28-4. Private Cord Blood Banks

Bank	Location	Web Site
Alpha Cord, Inc.	Atlanta, Georgia	www.alphacord.com
CellMed Biotech	Paramus, New Jersey	www.cellmedbiotech.com
CorCell*	Philadelphia, Pennsylvania	www.corcell.com
Cord Blood Registry*	San Bruno, California	www.cordblood.com
Cord Blood Solutions	Alpharetta, Georgia	www.cordbloodsolutions.com
Cord Partners, a Cord Blood America Company	Los Angeles, California	www.cordpartners.com
Cryobanks International*	Altamonte Springs, Florida	www.cryo-intl.com
Cryo-Cell International	Olsmar, Florida	www.cryo-cell.com
CureSource	Charleston, South Carolina	www.curesource.net
Family Cord Blood Services	Santa Monica, California	www.familycordbloodservices.com
Family Link	Louisville, Kentucky	www.nortonhealthcare.com/specialties/women/obstetrics/cordblood/index.aspx
Genesis Bank	Indianapolis, Indiana	www.thegenesisbank.com
LifeBankUSA*	Cedar Knolls, New Jersey	www.lifebankusa.com
LifeLine Cryogenics	Stamford, Connecticut	www.lifelinecryogenics.com
MAZE Laboratories	Stamford, Connecticut	www.MAZElabs.com/cordblood.htm
MiraCell	Less's Summit, Missouri	www.mira-cell.com
National Children's Leukemia Foundation	New York, New York	www.leukemiafoundation.org/stemc/stemc.htm
Newborn Blood Banking, Inc.	Tampa, Florida	www.newbornblood.com
New England Cord Blood Bank	Boston, Massachusetts	www.cordbloodbank.com
Regenrative Medicine Institute	California	www.rmilabs.com
Securacell, Inc.	Canton, Ohio	www.securacell.com
Stembanc	Cleveland, Ohio	www.stembanc.com
Stemcyte Family*	Arcadia, California	www.StemCyteFamily.com
Viacord	Boston, Massachusetts	www.viacord.com

*Offer charity program to provide free banking to siblings of children with transplantable disease. Data from Parent's Guide to Cord Blood Banks. Available at http://www.parentsguidecord blood.com/content/usa/banklists/listusa.shtml?navid=11. Retrieved on May 17, 2006.

"Parents should not be sold this service without a realistic assessment of their likelihood of return on their investment" (42). Some private banks quote unrealistic odds for the future use of an umbilical cord blood unit stored in a private bank. One private bank cites a frequency of 1:27, with the future possibility of 50% of cord blood units ultimately being used (43). Autologous umbilical cord blood cannot be used to treat inborn errors of metabolism because the genetic mutation is already present in the stem cells. In addition, some subtypes of leukemia are associated with chromosomal translocations that have been found in fetal blood (44). For this reason, many pediatric hematologists will not use autologous stem cells to treat leukemia. In addition, the use of such cells would negate the beneficial graft-versus-leukemic effect that occurs with allogeneic stem cell transplants. This led Johnson (45) to suggest that the chance of an individual using an autologous unit of cord blood is approximately 1:2,700 (Fig. 28-3).

The definition of a "quality" umbilical cord blood unit is still being refined. Initial procedures developed in the NIH Cord Blood Transplantation study called for a minimum cord blood unit volume at the time of the collection of 60 mL or a total nucleated cell count of 6×10^8 or greater if the volume was between 40 mL and 60 mL; cord blood units with volumes of less than 40 mL were discarded (46). Public banks also have numerous other exclusion criteria that are meant to assure quality. Many banks now use a minimum of 1×10^9 total nucleated cell count to define an adequate cord blood unit; this results in as many as 65–70% of cord blood units being discarded after initial collection. The collection of cord blood units for private banking is subject to the pressure of "our only chance to collect cells." Therefore, subopti-

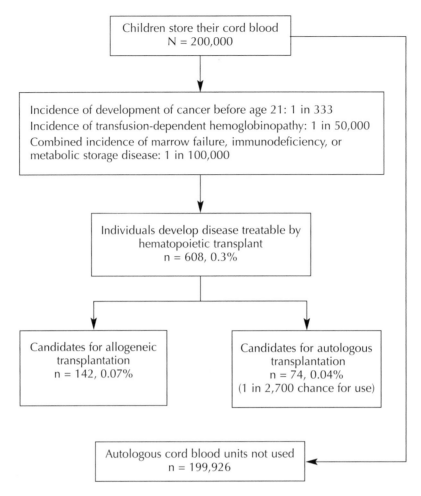

Fig. 28-3. Flow diagram for potential future autologous use of stored umbilical cord blood. (Moise KJ. Umbilical cord stem cells. Obstet Gynecol 2005;106:1393–407.)

mal cord blood units are often sent to the collection facility. At the time of the processing, the private bank will usually contact the parents to have them decide whether to store or discard the cord blood unit. Many likely decide to proceed with storage, with very little knowledge that the cord blood unit could not be realistically used at a later date.

Because umbilical cord blood banking is in its infancy, issues with long-term availability have not arisen. Studies have shown long-term survival of stem cells in cord blood units for up to 15 years after initial freezing (47). Viability of cells after this time has not been substantiated. This, therefore, calls into question the use of autologous stem cells harvested at birth for regenerative medicine many decades later. In addition, private banks must continue to recruit new donors to remain financially viable. What is to happen to privately donated cord blood units if a company becomes insolvent?

The final argument for public banking involves the use of a human resource for the greater good of mankind.

Public banks collect cord blood units from patients with a wide ethnic diversity. Many actually seek out certain ethnic groups that are underrepresented in the national bone marrow registry. Private banking allows those of means to collect stem cells while the less fortunate have no access to this valuable resource. Because of the economics of maintaining a public bank based on current use, many public banks have found it necessary to curtail or even eliminate collection activity (this includes an initial effort by the Red Cross to establish a cord blood bank). The IOM report recommended federal funding for the acquisition of 100,000 new high quality cord blood units (7). On December 20, 2005, President George W. Bush signed into law the Stem Cell Therapeutic and Research Act of 2005 (Public Law 109-129) (48). The law established the C.W. Bill Young Cell Transplantation Program, a network of cord blood banks to facilitate the use of cord blood for transplantation. The bill appropriates $79 million between the years of 2006 and 2010 to establish a national inventory of

150,000 cord blood units. The bill also calls for the FDA to develop licensing requirements for cord blood banks that will contribute cord blood units to the inventory.

All of these reasons have led many organizations and countries to take a stand against private banking. The American Academy of Pediatrics has suggested "...private storage of cord blood for biologic insurance is unwise" (49). In Europe, the practice of private cord blood banking has been banned by law in Italy since 2002. The Royal College of Obstetricians and Gynaecologists states their position as "Routine directed commercial cord blood collection and stem cell storage cannot be recommended at the present time, because of the insufficient scientific base to support such practices..." (50). The French National Consultative Ethics Committee's ...recommendation to decision makers is that they should "encourage a considerable extension of cord public banks for essentially allogeneic purposes, rather than subscribing to the creation of private banks for strictly autologous purposes, the potential therapeutic usefulness of which is, as yet, in no way corroborated" (51). In March of 2004, the European Group on Ethics in Science and New Technologies stated their position as follows: "The legitimacy of commercial cord blood banks for autologous use should be questioned as they sell a service which has presently no real use regarding therapeutic options. Thus, they promise more than they can deliver. The activities of such banks raise serious ethical criticisms" (52). The Maternal/Fetal Medicine Committee of the Society of Obstetricians and Gynaecologists of Canada recommended that "altruistic donation of cord blood for public banking and subsequent allogeneic transplantation should be encouraged when umbilical cord blood banking is being considered by childbearing women…" The committee also stated that the "collection and long-term storage of umbilical cord blood for autologous donation is not recommended because of the limited indications and lack of scientific evidence to support the practice" (53).

Legal Concerns

Before the realization of the value of cord blood, obstetric health care providers routinely allowed the placenta to drain into the kick bucket at the foot of the delivery bed. The discovery of the value of this resource has created the possibility of new legal dilemmas, many of which have gone unrealized.

Parents of the newborn have limited rights to control their child's umbilical cord blood. However, the newborn has not legally abandoned its property rights to his or her own cord blood (54). Because cord banking is still in its infancy, no newborn has reached the age to legally request ownership of his or her stem cells that may be stored in a public bank. The possibility that such a situation may occur in the future is not unrealistic.

Most private banks indemnify the collecting obstetric health care provider from any errors that may occur in the collection procedure at the time of delivery. One may conjecture a situation in which a poor quality cord blood unit (low cell count or bacterial contamination) results from a collection. In a future life-threatening situation for the family, would the obstetric health care provider be held partially liable for suboptimal collection?

Patent issues have become part of the debate in the cord blood industry. An initial patent (U.S. patent 5,004,681) was filed in November 1987 by the Biocyte Corporation regarding the cryopreservation of neonatal and fetal blood and their therapeutic use for hematopoietic reconstitution after thawing. Subsequent patents were filed in November 1988 (U.S. patent 5,192,553), May 1990 (U.S. patent 6,461,645), May 1995 (U.S. patent 6,569,427), and August 2003 (U.S. patent 6,605,275). The latter three patents were filed under the new entity of PharmaStem Therapeutics Inc, which also acquired the rights to the first two patents. PharmaStem filed similar patent claims in Europe and Japan but these claims were ultimately denied on the basis that previously published scientific work had already established the principles that were cited in support of these claims. In the United States, PharmaStem licensed 14 private banks under agreements for undisclosed royalties at the time each cord blood unit was collected (55). The company filed a lawsuit in federal court in Delaware against five other private companies that did not agree to royalty payments. In October 2003, a jury upheld the argument that PharmaStem's patents were enforceable and were willingly infringed by four of the five private cord blood banks, one having settled with PharmaStem before the jury award. The judge initially set aside the verdict pending a request for a post-judgement review. In June 2004, the company sent a warning letter to obstetricians indicating that they were infringing on the patents if they collected cord blood for any of the four remaining companies: Viacord, Cord Blood Registry, CRYO-CELL International, and Corcell. Three months later, in response to the motion for post-judgement review, the court affirmed the jury verdict as to patentability but threw out claims for damages against banks for other reasons. Both PharmaStem and the cord blood banks appealed and, in April 2006, the U.S. Court of Appeals for the Federal Circuit heard oral arguments in the appeal. A second case involving the same parties as well as others on substantially the same issues has been stayed pending decisions from the Federal Circuit on the appeal and the patent reexaminations by the U.S. Patent and Trademark Office (PTO).

The patents themselves, with the exception of patent #6,605,275, have been the subject of various petitions for reexamination brought before the PTO beginning in June 2004. As a result of these petitions, the PTO had ordered a reexamination of each of the patents and in March of 2006 issued orders that rejected all claims contained in patents 6,461,645 and patent 5,004,681 related to certain aspects of the collection, cryopreservation and storage of hematopoietic stem cells from umbilical cord blood. The PTO ruled that these claims were not patentable because of prior publication and knowledge.

Although private banks have been the target of these patent infringement cases, at least two public banks have entered into license agreements with PharmaStem. This latest event may open the door to additional costs for the public banks as this new technology comes into widespread use. Because public banks do not collect fees at the time of collection of the cord blood units, it is likely that royalties will be paid at the time cord blood units are shipped or thawed for transplant.

Summary

Umbilical cord blood represents an exciting new source of hematopoietic stem cells. The obstetrician represents the first line of information and counseling for the pregnant woman regarding the pros and cons of public versus private banking. Several keys points should be considered:

- Pregnant women should be provided balanced information about both private and public cord blood banking during their prenatal course.
- The currently estimated chance of a child requiring a transplant with its own cord blood is 1:2,700. Promising research in regenerative medicine may allow for more applications of autologous cord blood in the future. Many of these applications are, to date, unproved in clinical trials. The long-term viability of stored cord stem cells over many decades for such purposes is untested.
- Private banks for autologous storage are under less stringent FDA regulations for quality control than public banks.
- Legal issues related to patent infringement continue to cloud the collection of cord blood units for private banks.
- Public banks allow for greater access to cord blood by the general population, are more cost effective, and allow for the establishment of ethnic diversity of the cord blood inventory. In situations in which a hospital is not a collection site for a public bank, several cord blood banks will accept patient donations that can be shipped to their storage facility (Table 28-3).
- Directed donation of cord blood should be considered when there is a specific diagnosis of a disease within a family that is known to be amenable to stem cell transplantation. This can be arranged through many public banks, such as the Children's Hospital Oakland Research Institute.

References

1. Wagner JE. Umbilical cord blood stem cell transplantation. Am J Pediatr Hematol Oncol 1993;15:169–74.
2. Broxmeyer HE, Kurtzberg J, Gluckman E, Auerbach AD, Douglas G, Cooper S, et al. Umbilical cord blood hematopoietic stem and repopulating cells in human clinical transplantation. Blood Cells 1991;17:313–29.
3. Gluckman E, Broxmeyer HA, Auerbach AD, Friedman HS, Douglas GW, Devergie A, et al. Hematopoietic reconstitution in a patient with Fanconi's anemia by means of umbilical-cord blood from an HLA-identical sibling. N Engl J Med 1989;321:1174–8.
4. Smith FO, Thomson BG. Umbilical cord blood collection, banking, and transplantation: current status and issues relevant to perinatal caregivers. Birth 2000;27:127–35.
5. Kurtzberg J, Graham M, Casey J, Olson J, Stevens CE, Rubinstein P. The use of umbilical cord blood in mismatched related and unrelated hemopoietic stem cell transplantation. Blood Cells 1994;20:275–83.
6. Rubinstein P, Rosenfield RE, Adamson JW, Stevens CE. Stored placental blood for unrelated bone marrow reconstitution. Blood 1993;81:1679–90.
7. Institute of Medicine. Cord blood: establishing a national hematopoietic stem cell bank program. Available at: http:// www.iom.edu/report.asp?id=26386. Retrieved September 28, 2005.
8. European Bioinformatics Institute. IMGT/HLA sequence database. Available at: http://www.ebi.ac.uk/imgt/hla/stats.html. Retrieved May 16, 2006.
9. Hurley CK, Baxter-Lowe LA, Logan B, Karanes C, Anasetti C, Weisdorf D, et al. National Marrow Donor Program HLAmatching guidelines for unrelated marrow transplants. Biol Blood Marrow Transplant 2003;9:610–5.
10. 2004 Biennal Report of the National Bone Marrow Donor Registry. U.S. Department of Health and Human Services, Health Resources and Services Administration, Healthcare Systems Bureau, Division of Transplantation, U.S. Government Printing Office, 2006.
11. Gluckman E, Koegler G, Rocha V. Human leukocyte antigen matching in cord blood transplantation. Semin Hematol 2005;42:85–90.
12. Laughlin MJ, Eapen M, Rubinstein P, Wagner JE, Zhang MJ, Champlin RE, et al. Outcomes after transplantation of cord blood or bone marrow from unrelated donors in adults with leukemia. N Engl J Med 2004;351:2265–75.
13. Wadlow RC, Porter DL. Umbilical cord blood transplantation: where do we stand? Biol Blood Marrow Transplant 2002;8:637–47.

14. Lansdorp PM, Dragowska W, Mayani H. Ontogeny-related changes in proliferative potential of human hematopoietic cells. J Exp Med 1993;178:787–91.

15. Hao QL, Shah AJ, Thiemann FT, Smogorzewska EM, Crooks GM. A functional comparison of CD34 + CD38- cells in cord blood and bone marrow. Blood 1995;86:3745–53.

16. Rocha V, Labopin M, Sanz G, Arcese W, Schwerdtfeger R, Bosi A, et al. Transplants of umbilical-cord blood or bone marrow from unrelated donors in adults with acute leukemia. N Engl J Med 2004;351:2276–85.

17. Rainaut M, Pagniez M, Hercend T, Daffos F, Forestier F. Characterization of mononuclear cell subpopulations in normal fetal peripheral blood. Hum Immunol 1987;18:331–7.

18. Roncarolo MG, Vaccarino E, Caracco P. Immunologic properties of umbilical cord blood. In: Broxmeyer HA, editor. Cellular characteristics of cord blood and cord blood transplantation. Bethesda (MD): AABB Press; 1998.

19. Bieback K, Kern S, Kluter H, Eichler H. Critical parameters for the isolation of mesenchymal stem cells from umbilical cord blood. Stem Cells 2004;22:625–34.

20. Sanberg PR, Willing AE, Garbuzova-Davis S, Saporta S, Liu G, Sanberg CD, et al. Umbilical cord blood-derived stem cells and brain repair. Ann N Y Acad Sci 2005;1049:67–83.

21. Nan Z, Grande A, Sanberg CD, Sanberg PR, Low WC. Infusion of human umbilical cord blood ameliorates neurologic deficits in rats with hemorrhagic brain injury. Ann N Y Acad Sci 2005;1049:84–96.

22. Ende N, Weinstein F, Chen R, Ende M. Human umbilical cord blood effect on sod mice (amyotrophic lateral sclerosis). Life Sci 2000;67:53–9.

23. Staba SL, Escolar ML, Poe M, Kim Y, Martin PL, Szabolcs P, et al. Cord-blood transplants from unrelated donors in patients with Hurler's syndrome. N Engl J Med 2004;350:1960–9.

24. McGraw P, Liang L, Escolar M, Mukundan S, Kurtzberg J, Provenzale JM. Krabbe disease treated with hematopoietic stem cell transplantation: serial assessment of anisotropy measurements–initial experience. Radiology 2005;236:221–30.

25. Sugarman J, Kurtzberg J, Box TL, Horner RD. Optimization of informed consent for umbilical cord blood banking. Am J Obstet Gynecol 2002;187:1642–6.

26. Donaldson C, Armitage WJ, Laundy V, Barron C, Buchanan R, Webster J, et al. Impact of obstetric factors on cord blood donation for transplantation. Br J Haematol 1999;106:128–32.

27. Askari S, Miller J, Chrysler G, McCullough J. Impact of donorand collection-related variables on product quality in ex utero cord blood banking. Transfusion 2005;45:189–94.

28. Ballen KK, Wilson M, Wuu J, Ceredona AM, Hsieh C, Stewart FM, et al. Bigger is better: maternal and neonatal predictors of hematopoietic potential of umbilical cord blood units. Bone Marrow Transplant 2001;27:7–14.

29. Grisaru D, Deutsch V, Pick M, Fait G, Lessing JB, Dollberg S, et al. Placing the newborn on the maternal abdomen after delivery increases the volume and CD34 cell content in the umbilical cord blood collected: an old maneuver with new applications. Am J Obstet Gynecol 1999;180:1240–3.

30. Solves P, Moraga R, Saucedo E, Perales A, Soler MA, Larrea L, et al. Comparison between two strategies for umbilical cord blood collection. Bone Marrow Transplant 2003;31:269–73.

31. Yamada T, Okamoto Y, Kasamatsu H, Horie Y, Yamashita N, Matsumoto K. Factors affecting the volume of umbilical cord blood collections. Acta Obstet Gynecol Scand 2000;79:830–3.

32. Wong A, Yuen PM, Li K, Yu AL, Tsoi WC. Cord blood collection before and after placental delivery: levels of nucleated cells, haematopoietic progenitor cells, leukocyte subpopulations and macroscopic clots. Bone Marrow Transplant 2001;27:133–8.

33. Hubel A, Carlquist D, Clay M, McCullough J. Liquid storage, shipment, and cryopreservation of cord blood. Transfusion 2004;44:518–25.

34. McCullough J, McKenna D, Kadidlo D, Schierman T, Wagner J. Issues in the quality of umbilical cord blood stem cells for transplantation. Transfusion 2005;45:832–41.

35. National Marrow Donor Program. Network Cord Blood Banks. Available at: http://www.marrow.org/cgi-bin/NET-WOTK/nmdp_cord_blood_banks.pl. Retrieved May 18, 2006.

36. Parent's Guide to Cord Blood Banks. Public Cord Banks in the USA. Available at http://www.parentsguidecord-blood.com/content/usa/banklists/publicbanks/pub-licbanks_new.shtml?na. Retrieved May 18, 2006.

37. Sirchia G, Rebulla P, Tibaldi S, Lecchi L. Cost of umbilical cord blood units released for transplantation. Transfusion 1999;39:645–50.

38. Viacord. Extra measures: Viacord's Case of Need program. Available at: http://www.viacord.com/advantage_extra_measures.htm. Retrieved September 29, 2005.

39. Parent's Guide to Cord Blood Banks. Private cord blood banks in the USA. Available at: http://www.parents-guidecordblood.com/content/usa/banklists/listusa.shtml?navid=11. Retrieved May 18, 2006.

40. CRYO-CELL International, Inc. Competitive matrix: choosing the right cord blood stem cell bank is easier than you think Available at: http://www.cryo-cell.com/service/competitive_ matrix.asp. Retrieved September 29, 2005.

41. CRYO-CELL International, Inc. CRYO-CELL Joins Upromise®. Available at: http://www.cryo-cell.com/serv-ice/ upromise.asp. Retrieved September 29, 2005.

42. American College of Obstetricians and Gynecologists. Routine storage of umbilical cord blood for potential future transplantation. ACOG Committee Opinion 183. Washington, DC: ACOG; 1997.

43. Viacord. What are the odds of a family member being diagnosed with a disease treatable with cord blood? Available at: http://www.viacord.com/what_visitor_quiz.htm. Retrieved September 29, 2005.

44. Greaves MF, Wiemels J. Origins of chromosome translocations in childhood leukaemia. Nat Rev Cancer 2003;3:639–49.

45. Johnson FL. Placental blood transplantation and autologous banking: caveat emptor. J Pediatr Hematol Oncol 1997;19:183–6.

46. Fraser JK, Cairo MS, Wagner EL, McCurdy PR, Baxter-Lowe LA, Carter SL, et al. Cord Blood Transplantation Study (COBLT): cord blood bank standard operating procedures. J Hematother 1998;7:521–61.

47. Kobylka P, Ivanyi P, Breur-Vriesendorp BS. Preservation of immunological and colony-forming capacities of long-term (15 years) cryopreserved cord blood cells. Transplantation 1998;65:1275–8.

48. Office of Legislative Policy and Analysis. Bill Tracking, House Bills – 109th Congress. H.R. 2520 – The Stem Cell Therapeutic and Research Act of 2005. Available at http://olpa.od.nih.gov/tracking/109/house_bills/session1/hr-2520.asp. Retrieved May 15, 2006.

49. Cord blood banking for potential future transplantation: subject review. American Academy of Pediatrics. Work Group on Cord Blood Banking. Pediatrics 1999;104:116–8.

50. Royal College of Obstetricians and Gynaecologists Scientific Advisory Committee. Umbilical cord blood banking. Opinion paper 2. Available at: http://www.rcog.org.uk/index.asp? PageID=545. Retrieved September 29, 2005.

51. French National Consultative Ethics Committee for Health and Life Sciences. Umbilical cord blood banks for autologous use and or for research. Opinion #74. Available at: http://www.ccneethique. fr/english/avis/a_074p3.htm. Retrieved September 29, 2005.

52. European Group on Ethics in Science and New Technologies. Ethical aspects of umbilical cord blood banking. Available at: http://europa.eu.int/comm/european_group_ethics/docs/ avis19_en.pdf. Retrieved September 29, 2005.

53. Armson BA, Maternal/Fetal Medicine Committee, Society of Obstetricians and Gynaecologists of Canada. Umbilical cord blood banking: implications for perinatal care providers. J Obstet Gynaecol Can 2005;27:263–90.

54. Munzer SR, Smith FO. Limited property rights in umbilical cord blood for transplantation and research. J Pediatr Hematol Oncol 2001;23:203–7.

55. PharmaStem Therapeutics, Inc. Licensed Cord Blood Banks. Available at: http://www.pharmastem.com/newsroom.htm. Retrieved May 15, 2006.

Test Your Skills

Complete the answer sheet at the back of this book and return it to ACOG to receive Continuing Medical Education credits. The answers appear on page 396.

Directions: Select the one best answer or completion.

1. Ultrasound measurement of fetal nuchal translucency should optimally be measured at
   A. 4–6 weeks of gestation
   B. 8–12 weeks of gestation
   C. 10–14 weeks of gestation
   D. 16–18 weeks of gestation
   E. 20–24 weeks of gestation

2. Increased nuchal translucency is a specific marker for
   A. Down syndrome
   B. fetal loss before 10 weeks of gestation
   C. nonspecific aneuploidy
   D. glycogen storage abnormalities
   E. fetal normality

3. Universal screening for subclinical hypothyroidism is
   A. mandated by the American Medical Association
   B. strongly supported by the American College of Obstetricians and Gynecologists
   C. mandated by some states
   D. to be implemented on a practice-by-practice basis
   E. not currently recommended

4. The most common cause of hypothyroidism in pregnancy is
   A. Sheehan's syndrome
   B. chronic autoimmune thyroiditis (Hashimoto's thyroiditis)
   C. iodine deficiency
   D. prior radioiodine therapy
   E. prior thyroidectomy

5. The mainstay of the diagnosis of thyroid disease is the measurement of
   A. thyroid-binding globulin
   B. TSH
   C. total T_4
   D. free T_4
   E. free T_4/total T_4 ratio

6. Breastfeeding by women taking levothyroxine is not contraindicated because
   A. levothyroxine is not excreted in breast milk
   B. secreted levels are too low to alter thyroid function
   C. levothyroxine is not absorbed by the newborn
   D. the newborn thyroid is not responsive to levothyroxine
   E. the newborn pituitary is not responsive to levothyroxine

7. Which of the following complications of pregnancy is most common among women with pregnancies complicated by moderate-to-severe chronic renal insufficiency?
   A. Prematurity
   B. Preeclampsia
   C. Anemia
   D. Chronic hypertension
   E. Macrosomia

8. In a study of women with mild renal disease associated with a renal allograft, the likelihood of a successful pregnancy outcome was approximately
   A. 75%
   B. 80%
   C. 85%
   D. 90%
   E. less than 95%

9. In a study by Cunningham and associates, the most common complication of pregnancy seen in women with severe renal disease was
   A. prematurity
   B. preeclampsia
   C. anemia
   D. chronic hypertension
   E. macrosomia

10. When proteinuria (greater than 500 mg/d) is detected in an asymptomatic pregnant woman, end-stage renal disease will occur within the subsequent 5 years in approximately what percent of cases?
    A. 5%
    B. 10%
    C. 15%
    D. 20%
    E. 25%

11. The preferred method of managing all levels of persistent asthma during pregnancy is
    A. antihistamine therapy
    B. inhaled corticosteroids
    C. systemic corticosteroids
    D. allergen desensitization
    E. antiprostaglandin therapy

12. The single best measurement of pulmonary function is
    A. functional residual capacity
    B. forced vital capacity
    C. PEFR
    D. FEV_1
    E. diffusion capacity

13. The best measure of pulmonary function for patient self-monitoring is
    A. functional residual capacity
    B. forced vital capacity
    C. PEFR
    D. FEV_1
    E. diffusion capacity

14. Which of the following answers would suggest the greatest risk of preeclampsia for a patient with chronic hypertension?

    A. A history of hypertension for more than 4 years
    B. Increased maternal age
    C. A history of preeclampsia in a prior pregnancy
    D. Proteinuria early in pregnancy
    E. Diastolic blood pressure greater than 100 mm Hg at baseline

15. When managing a woman with high-risk hypertension during pregnancy, fetal non-stress testing should begin at 28 weeks of gestation and be repeated

    A. twice weekly
    B. weekly
    C. every other week to term
    D. every other week to 36 weeks of gestation, then weekly
    E. monthly to term

16. A 28-year-old G3P0121 patient with antiphospholipid syndrome with prior thrombosis is on chronic warfarin therapy. She is considering pregnancy sometime in the future. She should be advised to switch to anticoagulation therapy with heparin

    A. immediately
    B. as soon as her menstrual period is missed
    C. after the fifth week of gestation
    D. after the eighth week of gestation
    E. after the 12th week of gestation

17. For most patients, fetal surveillance testing for patients with antiphospholipid syndrome should begin no later than

    A. 30 weeks of gestation
    B. 32 weeks of gestation
    C. 34 weeks of gestation
    D. 36 weeks of gestation
    E. 38 weeks of gestation

18. Of the following choices, the most common, clinically significant, inherited thrombophilia is

    A. deficiency of protein C
    B. deficiency of protein S
    C. polymorphisms of the methylenetetrahydrofolate reductase gene
    D. 4G/4G mutation in the type-1 plasminogen activator inhibitor gene
    E. factor V Leiden

19. Thrombophilias have been positively linked to

    A. abortion before 10 weeks of gestation
    B. preeclampsia
    C. placental abruption
    D. intrauterine growth restriction
    E. recurrent abortion

20. When a patient is homozygous for the factor V Leiden mutation, her risk of thromboembolism is increased by a factor of approximately

    A. threefold
    B. fivefold
    C. 15-fold
    D. 30-fold
    E. 100-fold

21. As a part of your initial assessment of a patient who presents for her first prenatal visit, you calculate her baseline BMI to be 31.3. Based on this calculation, she should be classified as
    A. normal weight
    B. overweight
    C. obese, class I
    D. obese, class II
    E. obese, class III

22. A patient seeks care for preconception counseling. You note that she would be classified as obese, class I. The most appropriate recommendation regarding weight management is
    A. a combination of diet and exercise before pregnancy
    B. a low glycemic diet during pregnancy
    C. limiting weight gain during pregnancy to no more than 10 kg (22 lb)
    D. bariatric surgery
    E. no intervention is indicated at this time

23. Obesity has been documented to interfere with the interpretation of which of the following blood or serum tests?
    A. Maternal hematocrit
    B. hCG
    C. AFP
    D. TSH
    E. Three-hour glucose tolerance test

24. When compared with women of normal weight, obese women have an increased risk of diabetes because of an increase in the prevalence of
    A. reduced insulin production
    B. insulin resistance
    C. intraabdominal fat storage
    D. elevated waist/hip ratio
    E. a family history of type 2 diabetes

25. You perform a measurement of plasma glucose one hour after a 50-g oral glucose load, without regard to the time of day or the time of the last meal. The value is reported as 146 mg/dL. The most appropriate next step in the management of this patient should be
    A. a repeat of the test after a 12-hour fast
    B. a repeat of the test after a 3-day glucose load
    C. a repeat of the 50-g test with measurements taken at 30, 60, 120, and 180 minutes.
    D. a full diagnostic 100-g oral glucose tolerance test.
    E. routine prenatal care with no further glucose testing required

26. A primigravid patient with gestational diabetes and normal blood pressure has had good control of her diabetes with diet and exercise alone. She should be advised to begin twice weekly nonstress testing beginning at
    A. 32 weeks of gestation
    B. 36 weeks of gestation
    C. 38 weeks of gestation
    D. 40 weeks of gestation
    E. 41 weeks of gestation

27. The diagnosis of intrauterine growth restriction is established by
    A. physical examination
    B. biophysical profile
    C. ultrasonography
    D. radiographic evaluation
    E. serial maternal weight measurement

28. Which of the following findings would suggest a fetus at greatest risk in a near term pregnancy that has been otherwise uneventful?
    A. Estimated weight less than the 10th percentile
    B. Decreasing growth velocity
    C. Femur length less than anticipated
    D. Abdominal circumference less than predicted by head measures
    E. Fundal height (in centimeters) less than gestational age (in weeks) minus two

29. The WHO defines a stillbirth as one that occurs after
    A. 16 weeks of gestation
    B. 20 weeks of gestation
    C. 24 weeks of gestation
    D. 28 weeks of gestation
    E. 32 weeks of gestation

30. Which of the following is associated with the highest risk of fetal loss after 10 weeks of gestation?
    A. Antiphospholipid syndrome
    B. Fetal thrombophilia
    C. Factor V Leiden
    D. Protein C deficiency
    E. Protein S deficiency

31. The most appropriate technique for the induction of labor in cases of term intrauterine fetal death is
    A. oxytocin
    B. prostaglandin E_2
    C. prostaglandin $F_{2\alpha}$
    D. misoprostol
    E. membrane "stripping"

32. Which of the following findings or conditions would be sufficient to classify a patient's preeclampsia as "severe"?
    A. Proteinuria of 3.9 g in a 24-hour urine collection
    B. Urine dipstick test that shows "4+" protein
    C. Urine output of 750 ml over a 24-hour period
    D. Platelet count of 120,000/mm^3
    E. Abnormal liver enzymes with persistent epigastric pain

33. When compared with normal pregnancies, the perinatal death rate for pregnancies complicated by mild preeclampsia is
    A. 50% lower
    B. 25% lower
    C. unchanged
    D. 25% higher
    E. 50% higher

34. When used to treat severe preeclampsia, the purpose of intravenous magnesium sulfate therapy is to
    A. prevent convulsions
    B. reduce uterine tone
    C. increase placental perfusion
    D. reduce maternal blood pressure
    E. accelerate fetal lung maturity

35. The presence of which of the following findings would be most suggestive of the presence of preterm labor rather than uterine irritability?
    A. Contractions every 8 minutes
    B. Cervical dilation of 2 cm
    C. Cervical effacement of 60%
    D. Intact fetal membranes
    E. Fetal presenting part at zero station

36. A patient presents at 32 weeks of gestation with contractions occurring every 10 minutes. Examination of her cervix finds her to be dilated to 3 centimeters. Based on these findings, the chance that she will deliver within 7–14 days is approximately
    A. 10–20%
    B. 30–40%
    C. 50–60%
    D. 70–80%
    E. greater than 90%

37. In symptomatic women, the optimal threshold to exclude a diagnosis of preterm labor is a cervical length of
    A. 10 millimeters
    B. 15 millimeters
    C. 20 millimeters
    D. 25 millimeters
    E. 30 millimeters

38. When prophylactic cervical cerclage is contemplated, it should optimally be performed
    A. prior to pregnancy
    B. at 5–7 weeks of gestation
    C. at 9–11 weeks of gestation
    D. at 13–16 weeks of gestation
    E. at 18–22 weeks of gestation

39. Which condition would be a contraindication to emergency cervical cerclage?
    A. Cervical effacement of 60%
    B. Cervical dilation of 3 centimeters
    C. Vaginal bleeding
    D. Heavy mucoid vaginal discharge
    E. Bulging membranes prolapsed through the cervical os

40. The most common acute fetal morbidity associated with preterm rupture of the membranes is
    A. umbilical cord prolapse
    B. uteroplacental insufficiency
    C. abruptio placentae
    D. perinatal infection
    E. umbilical cord compression

41. According to the NICHD Maternal–Fetal Medicine Units Network trial, Initial broad-spectrum parenteral therapy for women with preterm PROM at less than 34 weeks of gestation has the greatest impact on
    A. reducing amnionitis
    B. prolonging pregnancy by more than one week
    C. reducing neonatal sepsis
    D. reducing respiratory distress syndrome
    E. reducing the rate of intraventricular hemorrhage

42. When fetal fibronectin is found in cervicovaginal secretions after the 20th week of gestation and before term, the risk of subsequent preterm delivery in the next week or two is approximately
    A. less than 2%
    B. 10–15%
    C. 20–25%
    D. 45–50%
    E. 65–70%

43. Based on literature reviews and meta-analyses of tocolytic therapy, it appears that the role of tocolytic therapy in reducing the morbidity and mortality of preterm birth is to
    A. significantly delay birth for all gestational ages
    B. accelerate fetal lung maturity
    C. reduce preterm births in high-risk groups
    D. reduce the incidence of births before 34 weeks of gestation
    E. allow time for adjunctive therapy

44. To avoid any possible teratogenic effects of 17 α-hydroxyprogesterone caproate, treatment should be withheld until
    A. 8 weeks of gestation
    B. 12 weeks of gestation
    C. 16 weeks of gestation
    D. 20 weeks of gestation
    E. 22 weeks of gestation

45. Based on available evidence, 17 α-hydroxyprogesterone caproate treatment should limited to women with
    A. multiple gestations
    B. a history of prior preterm delivery
    C. shortened cervical length
    D. a history of recurrent abortion
    E. positive fetal fibronectin test results

46. The half-life of Rh Ig is approximately
    A. 72 hours
    B. 7 days
    C. 14 days
    D. 24 days
    E. 34 days

47. An increased rate of false-positive readings of fetal middle cerebral artery peak velocity occur after
    A. 26 weeks of gestation
    B. 29 weeks of gestation
    C. 32 weeks of gestation
    D. 35 weeks of gestation
    E. 38 weeks of gestation

48. A 38-year-old, G5P4014 woman presents for prenatal care at 32 weeks of gestation. A review of her obstetric history reveals that she has had one elective termination of pregnancy and her other pregnancies were delivered by cesarean delivery. She is a 2 pack-per-day smoker. Which aspect of this patient's history suggests the greatest risk for placenta previa?
   A. The patient's age
   B. Increased parity
   C. The number of prior cesarean deliveries
   D. Elective termination of pregnancy
   E. History of smoking

49. The ultrasound finding that carries the highest positive predictive value for diagnosing placenta accreta is
   A. irregularly shaped placental lacunae
   B. thinning of the myometrium overlying the placenta
   C. increased vascularity of the uterine serosa–bladder interface
   D. a retroplacental "clear space"
   E. the presence of lacunae in the placenta

50. Which of the following factors is associated with the highest risk of placental abruption?
   A. Cocaine and drug use
   B. Prior cesarean delivery
   C. Premature rupture of membranes
   D. Multiple gestations
   E. Thrombophilic syndromes

51. The uterine activity most often associated with partial placental abruption is
   A. high-tone, high-frequency, low-amplitude contractions
   B. high-tone, high-frequency, high-amplitude contractions
   C. high-tone, low-frequency, low-amplitude contractions
   D. high-tone, low-frequency, high-amplitude contractions
   E. low-tone, high-frequency, high-amplitude contractions

52. Based on studies of venous thromboembolism prevention in gynecologic surgery, which of the following is the most cost-effective prophylaxis method?
   A. Unfractionated heparin therapy
   B. Low molecular weight heparin therapy
   C. Warfarin anticoagulant therapy
   D. Pneumatic compression devices
   E. Vitamin K supplementation

53. The proposed benefit of low molecular weight heparin therapy compared with unfractionated heparin is
   A. three time per day dosages
   B. fewer bleeding complications
   C. shorter half-life
   D. improved compliance
   E. proved increased efficacy

54. Based on currently available data, patients who have a first episode of a venous thromboembolism should receive anticoagulant therapy for a period of
   A. 2 weeks
   B. 6 weeks
   C. 3 months
   D. 6 months
   E. 12 months

55. The physiologic change associated with pregnancy that is thought to be most responsible for an increased risk of urinary tract infection is
    A. progesterone induced ureteral dilation
    B. ureteral compression at the pelvic brim
    C. vesicoureteral reflux
    D. increased glomerular filtration rate
    E. compression of the bladder by the fetal head

56. The most common bacterial cause of urinary tract infections in women is
    A. *E coli* species
    B. *Enterobacter* species
    C. *Enterococcus* species
    D. *Klebsiella* species
    E. group B streptococcus

57. Based on current national guidelines, culture for group B streptococcus should be carried out at
    A. 28–32 weeks of gestation
    B. 35–37 weeks of gestation
    C. 38–40 weeks of gestation
    D. the time of labor
    E. the time of birth

58. The best strategy to increase the sensitivity of prenatal group B streptococcus screening is to culture
    A. both sexual partners
    B. the rectum and vagina
    C. each trimester
    D. weekly after 32 weeks of gestation
    E. the vagina and pharynx

59. A woman presents at 34 weeks of gestation with premature rupture of the membranes. Regarding prevention of neonatal group B streptococcal sepsis, the most appropriate initial management of this patient is
    A. penicillin prophylaxis
    B. vancomycin prophylaxis
    C. culture of material obtained from the vagina and rectum
    D. Gram stain of cervical mucous
    E. no specific management is indicated

60. Most women who acquired a genital HSV infection will present with
    A. local pain
    B. dysuria
    C. malaise
    D. fever
    E. no symptoms

61. At 12 weeks of gestation, a patient is suspected of having a moderately severe, new-onset genital HSV infection. The most appropriate next step in the management of this patient should be
    A. confirmatory acute and convalescent serologic testing
    B. oral antiviral therapy
    C. intravenous antiviral therapy
    D. CVS for HSV PCR
    E. counseling regarding pregnancy termination

62. Which of the following patients would be at greatest risk of transmitting HSV infection to their neonate?
    A. A patient with three recurrent HSV-2 infections during pregnancy
    B. A patient with new onset genital HSV infection during the third trimester
    C. A patient with oral HSV-1 infection who is breastfeeding
    D. A patient with new onset genital HSV infection before 8 weeks of gestation
    E. A patient with a history of HSV-1 genital infection one year before pregnancy

63. Once HIV antiretroviral therapy is instituted, the success of intervention is monitored by
    A. viral load levels
    B. CD4 counts
    C. resistance testing
    D. phenotypic testing
    E. genotypic testing

64. In HIV cases, phenotypic testing is used to determine the virus'
    A. virulence
    B. genetic subtype
    C. resistance to therapy
    D. global origin
    E. mode of transmission

65. The risk of mother-to-child HIV transmission appears to be most closely linked to
    A. viral load
    B. CD4 count
    C. gestational age
    D. type of antiretroviral therapy
    E. HIV resistance

66. The majority of mother-to-child transmission of HIV occurs at or during
    A. conception
    B. the first trimester
    C. the second trimester
    D. the third trimester
    E. delivery

67. The most frequently observed fetal heart rate pattern associated with cerebral palsy is
    A. prolonged early decelerations
    B. mixed variable and late decelerations
    C. prolonged variable decelerations
    D. multiple late decelerations
    E. sinusoidal fetal heart rate pattern

68. To assess fetal pH above 7.20, fetal scalp sampling for pH fell out of use primarily in favor of the presence of which aspect of fetal heart rate monitoring?
    A. Accelerations
    B. Baseline normality
    C. Long-term variability
    D. Short-term variability
    E. Tachycardia

69. Studies indicate that intrapartum asphyxia is the possible cause of newborn encephalopathy or cerebral palsy in approximately what percent of cases?
    A. 1–2%
    B. 4–8%
    C. 12–15%
    D. 18–22%
    E. 26–32%

70. The optimal mode of evaluating early anoxic brain injury is
    A. magnetic resonance imaging
    B. computed tomography
    C. ultrasonography
    D. electroencephalography
    E. transillumination

71. The greatest advantage of using umbilical cord blood as a source of hematopoietic progenitor cells for transplant is
    A. better tolerance of a partial HLA match
    B. lower cost
    C. improved availability of good HLA matches
    D. increased number of cells available
    E. increased number of CD8⁺ lymphocytes in cord blood

Index

Infection
in cerebral palsy, 339–340
in fetal death, 126–127
Inferior vena cava filter placement, 268
Inflammatory bowel disease, in
intrauterine growth restriction,
115
Inhaled β₂-agonists, in asthma control,
44
Inhaled corticosteroids, in asthma control,
42–43
Insulin action profiles, 104*t*
Insulin pump, 105, 106*f*
Insulin therapy, 103–106
Intrauterine growth restriction
complications of, 118
definitions and standards, 113–114
diagnosis of, 115–116, 118*t*
in fetal death, 127
management of, 116–117, 118*t*
oligohydramnios in, 117
pathophysiology of, 114–115
risk factors for, 116*t*
symmetric versus asymmetric, 116
treatment of, 117–118
Intrauterine transfusion, 234–235
Isolated hypothyroxinemia, 23

K

Karyotype, in case of fetal death, 129
Kleihauer–Betke test
in placenta previa, 240
in placental abruption, 258–259
in Rh alloimmunization, 226
Krabbe's disease, 365

L

Labor. *See* Delivery
Laparoscopic adjustable gastric banding,
89, 90*t*
Leukotriene moderators, in asthma
control, 44
Liley curve, 230
Loop electrosurgical excision procedure,
171–172

M

Magnesium sulfate
contraindications to, 206
dosage and side effects of, 204*t*
in eclamptic convulsion prevention,
151
in preeclamptic convulsion prevention, 142
in preterm delivery prevention,
205–206
Magnetic resonance imaging, in placenta
accreta, 245
Maternal age, as fetal death risk factor,
123

Maternal titer values, 228
Mechanical heart valves, and deep vein
thrombosis therapy, 270
Membrane sweeping, 302
Metabolic syndrome, obesity as risk factor
for, 85–87
Metformin, 103
Methotrexate therapy, in placenta accreta,
246–247
Methyldopa, 57
Misoprostol, 131
Multiple gestations
Down syndrome in, 10
in fetal death, 127–128
fetal heart rate monitoring and, 348*f*
intrauterine growth restriction and,
114*f*, 115
placental abruption in, 255*t*
in preterm delivery, 158, 164, 201
progesterone therapy in, 219, 222

N

Nephropathy, diabetic, 31*t*, 103
Neural tube defect
detection of, in Down syndrome
screening, 11
maternal obesity as risk factor for,
84–85
Nevirapine, 329
Nifedipine, 204*t*, 207–208
Nitric oxide donors, 208–209
Nonalcoholic steatohepatitis, 86–87
Nuchal translucency screening
chorionic villus sampling and, 12
combined testing with first-
and second-trimester serum
markers, 8
combined testing with first-trimester
serum markers, 7
cystic hygroma and, 8–9, 9
description of, 3
interpretation of results in, 11
measurement success rate in, 6
quality control in, 10–11
second-trimester serum screening
and, 11–12
second-trimester ultrasonography
and, 12
studies of, in unselected patient populations, 4–6, 5
test combination choice in, 12–13
ultrasonography criteria in, 4
underascertainment in, 6

O

Obesity. *See also* Weight
bariatric surgery and, 89–90
body mass index and, 83
in children of obese mothers, 93–94
complications of, 94*b*

Obesity *(continued)*
as fetal death risk factor, 123
fetal growth and, 90–92
folic acid deficiencies and, 84–85
gestational diabetes mellitus and,
85–87
intrauterine fetal death and, 87–88
neural tube defects and, 84–85
nonalcoholic steatohepatitis and,
86–87
peripartum risks in, 88–89
pregravid, versus weight gain in pregnancy, 83–84
preterm delivery and, 87
prevalence of, 83
as risk factor in early gestation,
84–85
as risk factor in late gestation, 85–87
sleep apnea and, 87
as ultrasonography impairment, 85
Ohio State University protocol, in
fibronectin screening, 163
Oligohydramnios, 117, 201, 207
Oral corticosteroids, in asthma control,
44–45
Overt hypothyroidism, 20–22
Oxytocin antagonists, 208
Oxytocin initiation, in preterm delivery,
199

P

Parvovirus B19, 126
Penicillin, 294
Periarteritis nodosa, 31*t*
Perinatal autopsy, 129–130
Placenta accreta
balloon catheter occlusion and
embolization in, 246
bladder involvement in, 247
clinical significance of, 243
definition of, 243
diagnostic approach to, 244
hysterectomy in, 245, 246
magnetic resonance imaging in, 245
methotrexate therapy in, 246–247
pathophysiology of, 244
prevalence of, 243
risk factors for, 243–244
therapeutic approach to, 245–246
ultrasonography in, 244–245
Placenta previa
anesthesia in, 243
cerclage in, 242
definition of, 238
delivery in, 242–243
diagnostic approach to, 239–240
management of, 240–242
outpatient versus inpatient management in, 242
pathophysiology of, 239

Answers

1. C, 2. C, 3. E, 4. B, 5. B, 6. B, 7. A, 8. D, 9. C, 10. D, 11.
B, 12. D, 13. C, 14. E, 15. B, 16. C, 17. B, 18. E, 19. C, 20.
E, 21. C, 22. A, 23. C, 24. B, 25. D, 26. D, 27. C, 28. D, 29.
B, 30. C, 31. D, 32. E, 33. C, 34. A, 35. A, 36. C, 37. E, 38.
D, 39. C, 40. E, 41. B, 42. C, 43. E, 44. C, 45. B, 46. D, 47.
D, 48. C, 49. E, 50. A, 51. A, 52. D, 53. B, 54. D, 55. B, 56.
A, 57. B, 58. B, 59. C, 60. E, 61. B, 62. B, 63. A, 64. C, 65.
A, 66. E, 67. D, 68. A, 69. B, 70. A, 71. A